# PRACTICAL ENDOSCOPY
## Tips by Experts

# PRACTICAL ENDOSCOPY
# Tips by Experts

**Second Edition**


*Editor*

**Sunita R Tandulwadkar**

MD FICS Dip Endo (USA and Germany)

Head of Department of Obstetrics and Gynecology, Ruby Hall Clinic

Chief, Ruby Hall IVF and Endoscopy Center

Pune, Maharashtra, India

*Co-editor*

**Nirzari Mangeshikar**

MBBS DNB (OBGY)

III-year PG Student, Ruby Hall Clinic

Pune, Maharashtra, India


*Forewords*

**Togas Tulandi**
**Bomi Bhote**


JAYPEE *The Health Sciences Publisher*

New Delhi | London | Philadelphia | Panama

**Jaypee Brothers Medical Publishers (P) Ltd**

**Headquarters**

Jaypee Brothers Medical Publishers (P) Ltd
4838/24, Ansari Road, Daryaganj
New Delhi 110 002, India
Phone: +91-11-43574357
Fax: +91-11-43574314
Email: jaypee@jaypeebrothers.com

**Overseas Offices**

J.P. Medical Ltd
83, Victoria Street, London
SW1H 0HW (UK)
Phone: +44 20 3170 8910
Fax: ++44 (0)20 3008 6180
Email: info@jpmedpub.com

Jaypee Medical Inc
The Bourse
111 South Independence Mall East
Suite 835, Philadelphia, PA 19106, USA
Phone: +1 267-519-9789
Email: jpmed.us@gmail.com

Jaypee Brothers Medical Publishers (P) Ltd
Bhotahity, Kathmandu, Nepal
Phone: +977-9741283608
Email: kathmandu@jaypeebrothers.com

Jaypee-Highlights Medical Publishers Inc.
City of Knowledge, Bld. 237, Clayton
Panama City, Panama
Phone: +1 507-301-0496
Fax: +1 507-301-0499
Email: cservice@jphmedical.com

Jaypee Brothers Medical Publishers (P) Ltd
17/1-B Babar Road, Block-B, Shaymali
Mohammadpur, Dhaka-1207
Bangladesh
Mobile: +08801912003485
Email: jaypeedhaka@gmail.com

Website: www.jaypeebrothers.com
Website: www.jaypeedigital.com



**Inquiries for bulk sales may be solicited at:** jaypee@jaypeebrothers.com

***Practical Endoscopy: Tips by Experts***

*First Edition*: *2008*

*Second Edition*: **2015**

ISBN 978-93-5152-587-5

*Printed at Ajanta Offset & Packagings Ltd., New Delhi.*

**Dedicated to**

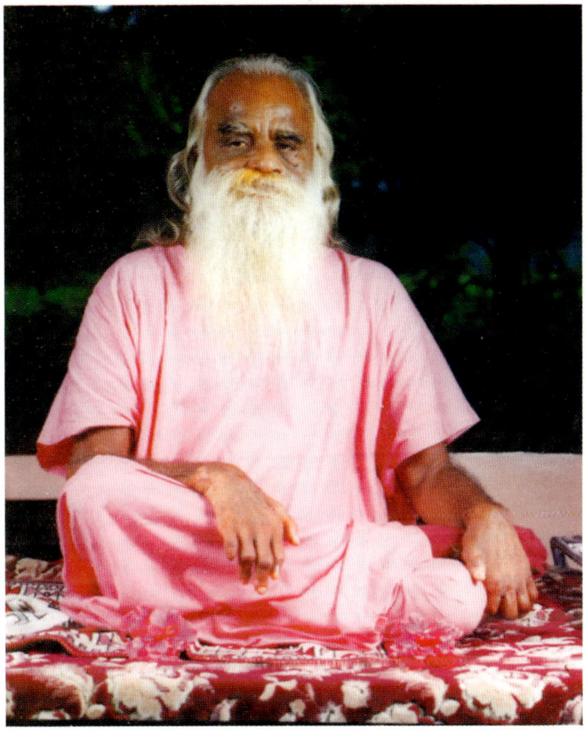

***My Guru***
***Param Pujya Swami Shree Gagangiri Maharaj***

गुरूः ब्रह्मः गुरुः विष्णुः गुरुः देवमहेश्वरः।
गुरुः साक्षात् परं ब्रह्मः तस्मै श्रीगुरुवे नमः।।

Guru Brahma Guru Vishnu Guru Devo Maheshwaraha |
Guru Saakshat Para Brahma Tasmai Sree Gurave Namaha ||

# Contributors

**Ajay Rane, Kannan K, Fiadjoe P**
James Cook University
Townsville, Australia

**Alessandro Loddo, Vito Cofelice, Gian Benedetto Melis**
Clinica Ostetrica e Ginecologica,
Azienda Ospedaliero-Universitaria di Cagliari,
University of Cagliari, Italy

**Andri Nieuwoudt**
Vaginal Reconstructive Surgeon, Gynecologist
The Hague Area, Netherlands

**Bruno J van Herendael, Lisbeth Jochems**
Consultant
ZNA (Zieken Huis Netwerk Antwerpen)
Antwerp, Belgium

**Charles Miller, Kirsten Sasaki**
Advocate Lutheran General Hospital
Illinois, USA

**Devika Chopra**
Ruby Hall Clinic, Pune
Maharashtra, India

**Jorge E Dotto, Paola Da Graca Mila, Miguel A Bigozzi Jr, Jorge E Dotto Jr**
Instituto Argentino de Diagnóstico y Tratamiento, Liga Argentina de Lucha contra el Cáncer
Argentina

**Jacques Hamou**
Universitaire d'Hystéroscopie, Maternité Antoine Béclere,
University of Paris, France

**Liselotte Mettler, Anupama Deenadayal, Ibrahim Alkatout**
University Clinics
Schleswig Holstein
Campus Kiel, Germany

**Nirzari Mangeshikar**
Ruby Hall Clinic, Pune
Maharashtra, India

**Ornella Sizzi, Giuseppe Florio**
Gynecological Endoscopy Department
Nuova Villa Claudia Hospital
Rome, Italy

**Pooja Lodha**
Lead Consultant
Department of Fetal Medicine
Ruby Hall Clinic, Pune
Maharashtra, India

**PG Paul, Renuka Borisa, P Biju**
Paul's Hospital and Gynecological Endoscopy
Training Center, Cochin
Kerela, India

**Prakash Trivedi**
Chief Gynecological Endoscopist and ART Consultant
NILES
Head of Department (OBGYN)
VC Rajawadi Municipal Hospital, Mumbai
Maharashtra, India

**Rafique Parkar**
Director, The International Center for
Minimal Access Surgery
Kenya

**Revaz Botchorishvili, Sara Campos**
Centre International de Chirurgie Endoscopique
France

**Sanjay Gupte**
Gupte Hospital and Center for
Research in Reproduction, Pune
Maharashtra, India

**Sanjay Patel, Yogendra Jhala**
Mayflower Hospital, Ahmedabad
Gujarat, India

**Sevellaraja Supermaniam**
Consultant Obstetrician and Gyñecology
Mahkota Medical Center
Malaysia

**Shailesh Puntambekar**
Galaxy Hospital Institute, Pune
Maharashtra, India

**Sunita R Tandulwadkar**
Head, Department of Obstetrics and Gynecology
Ruby Hall Clinic, Pune
Chief, Ruby Hall IVF and Endoscopy Center, Pune
Maharashtra, India

**Sejal Naik**
Gynec Endoscopist and IVF Consultant
Sunsine Global Multispecialty Hospital
Rahul Hospital and Well Women Clinic, Surat
Gujarat, India

**Wachyu Hadisaputra, Leonita TA Sutrisna**
Departemen Obstetri dan Ginekologi
Fakultas Kedokteran
Universitas Indonesia
Indonesia

# Foreword

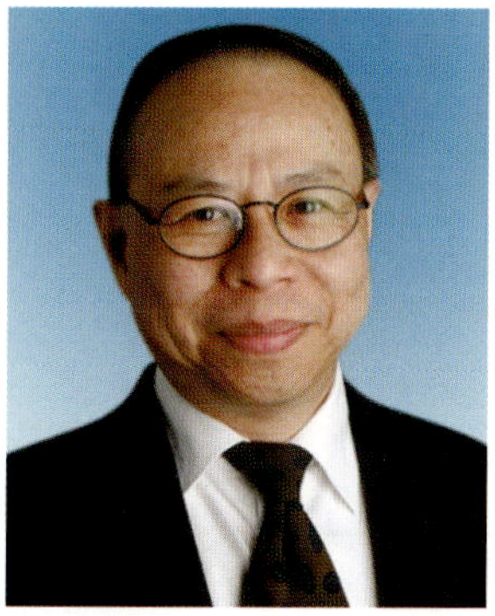

*"There is a single light of science, and to brighten it anywhere is to brighten it everywhere."*
***–Isaac Asimov (1920-1992)***

Many operations that previously required a laparotomy can now be performed with minimally invasive technique. This progress has been adopted everywhere in the world. The clear advantages of laparoscopy and hysteroscopy have achieved a prominent position in the field of gynecology.

The second edition of this book encompasses a variety of minimally invasive gynecology techniques ranging from vaginal surgery, laparoscopy and hysteroscopy. It starts with basic principles of endoscopic surgery, instrumentations and set-up. Among the relatively new developments are the use of laparoscopy with robotic assistance, single incision laparoscopy and transvaginal sling procedures for stress incontinence.

Dr Sunita R Tandulwadkar has dedicated her time and effort to assemble and edit the book. It has beautiful surgical photographs that facilitates understanding of the surgical technique. This edition is a good addition to the medical literature that will be useful for both the trainees and the practicing gynecologists.

**Togas Tulandi** MD MHCM FRCSC FACOG
Professor and Academic Vice Chairman of Obstetrics and Gynecology
Milton Leong Chair in Reproductive Medicine
McGill University, Canada

# Foreword

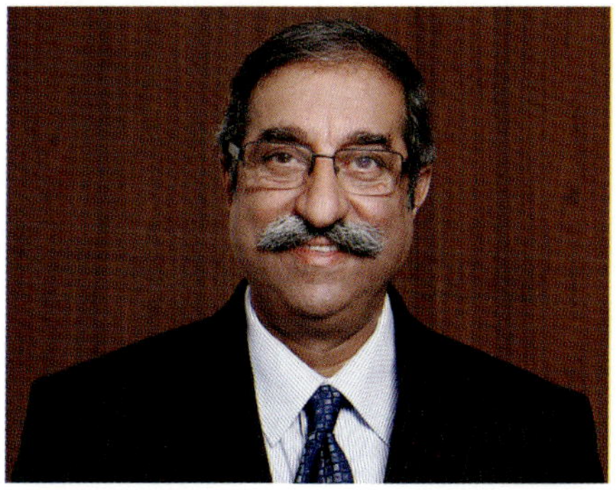

Endoscopic surgery has changed the face of medical surgeries particularly in the spectrum of gynecology. By means of this technology, surgeons are now able to perform the most complex procedures with minimal invasion. With immense pride, I write the foreword of the book *Practical Endoscopy: Tips by Experts* penned by a true master in the realm of gynecological endoscopy. Each chapter describes in-depth the preoperative preparation, steps of surgery, tips and tricks by surgeons along with images of the surgeries.

With each chapter in this book, I am struck by the complexity of work that Dr Sunita R Tandulwadkar has amassed in the last few years since such endoscopic procedures have gained popularity. While I have witnessed Dr Tandulwadkar's natural gift as a gynecologist par excellence, I admire her knowledge and endeavor to pen down her insightful first-hand experiences in the intricate field of endoscopy with which she treats her patients. The well-iterated descriptions and step-by-step pictorial references make this book an interesting read. It has been a pleasure to be associated with such an expert in her field, and I am confident that this book will become an important reference tool guiding surgeons not only now, but also in the times to come.


**Bomi Bhote**
Chief Executive Officer
Ruby Hall Clinic, Pune
Maharashtra, India

# Preface

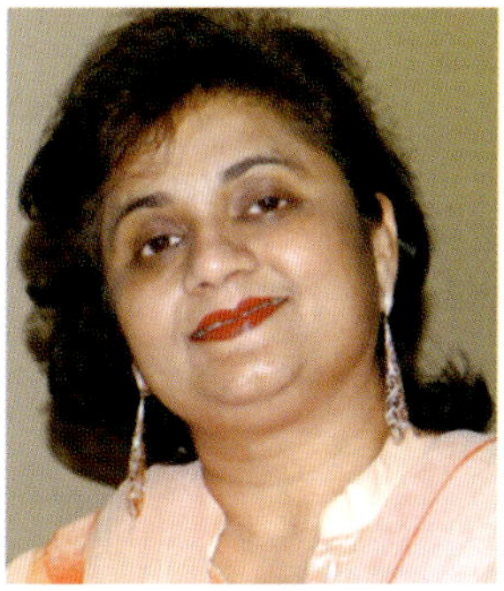

In this 'Information Age', an interested reader can easily locate information on everything from movies to medical care with the click of a finger. When it comes to health and disease, the quality of information is vital.

Many standard books have been published on endoscopy during the last two to three decades to meet the needs of beginners in the field of endoscopy. *Endoscopy Simplified—Practical Tips by Experts* was brought out in 2008, and covered important surgeries related to laparoscopy and hysteroscopy in gynecology. All the practical tips to enhance the surgical performance have been given in an absolutely simplified way, and the book is of great help to beginners as well as practicing endoscopists.

I am extremely pleased and gratified to present the second edition of this book, which I presume will be read by tens of thousands of medical students and medical practitioners. One likes to think that the clinical practice of these practitioners will be influenced by the book and that patient care will be a little more humane, a little more gentle and perhaps a little more effective because some of the practical tips in the book will take root.

In this second edition, we have not only added a few chapters from our side, but we have nearly 12 internationally renowned endoscopy faculty, who have happily contributed. We have tried to cover all aspects of the field, from setting up an endoscopy to guiding regarding energy sources and suturing techniques, and the latest advances like robotic surgery.

A thorough reader of this book will have very little trouble in starting an endoscopy set-up with least complication rates. In order to make the book as useful as possible, other than the practical tips and footnotes at the end of the chapters, the salient feature of the book remains its self-explanatory colorful illustrations.

Although this book will be useful for the medical students as well as the practicing endoscopists, professors in training programs will also find its content germane to their students. We have worked hard to make this book clinically relevant and almost all the chapters include the application of the principles being discussed. Every case draws on the clinical experience and expertise of the authors and illustrates how the principles of the book can be applied in a clinical setting. I am sure you will get an experience as if you are performing surgery while going through the steps of the surgery and the color figures. Also, apart from the practical tips that have been given, each endoscopist can individualize the steps of surgery to enhance the performance.

I wish to thank my colleagues and students in the Department of IVF and Endoscopy, Ruby Hall Clinic, Pune, India, for providing valuable suggestions, which have been indispensible to the accomplishment of my task.

I wish to thank Dr Nirzari Mangeshikar, my third year postgraduate student in OBGY, who has shown tremendous interest in helping me out with each and every section, while compiling this second edition.

Most of all, thanks go to my family, my husband, Dr Rajesh Tandulwadkar, Surgeon Gastroenterologist and GI Endoscopist and my son, Rishi, all took notes for me that found their way into the pages of my book. And, as for my earlier writings, my husband continues to be my first reader and key critic, apart from my great assistance in difficult situations.

**Sunita R Tandulwadkar**

# Contents

## Section 1

## BASIC ENDOSCOPY


**CHAPTER 1. How to Set-up an Ideal Endoscopic Operation Theater** **3**

*PG Paul, Sunita R Tandulwadkar, Renuka Borisa, P Biju, Kannan K, Fiadjoe P*

**CHAPTER 2. Equipment and Instruments in Endoscopic Surgery** **5**

*Sunita R Tandulwadkar*

Anesthesia Work Station *5*

**CHAPTER 3. Energy Sources in Endoscopic Surgery** **11**

*Wachyu Hadisaputra, Leonita TA Sutrisna*

Aim *11*
Fundamentals and Biophysics of Electrosurgery *11*
Types of Energy Source *12*
Use of the Thermal Effect *12*
General Safety Aspects *13*
Prevention of Electrosurgical Injuries *14*
Other Energy Sources *15*

**CHAPTER 4. Medicolegal Issues in Endoscopic Surgeries** **17**

*Sanjay Gupte*

Medicolegal Aspects in Endoscopic Surgeries *17*

**CHAPTER 5. Prevention of Complications in Endoscopic Surgeries** **20**

*PG Paul, Renuka Borisa, P Biju, Kannan K, Fiadjoe P*

Prevention of Preoperative Complication *20*
Prevention of Postoperative Complications *22*
Prevention of Complications During Hysteroscopy *23*

**CHAPTER 6. Port Placement** **24**

*Sunita R Tandulwadkar*

Routine Port Placements *24*
In Difficult Situations, Like *24*

**CHAPTER 7. Laparoscopic Suturing** **27**

*Alessandro Loddo, Vito Cofelice, Gian Benedetto Melis*

Making the Ideal Stitch *28*
Suturing Techniques *28*

## Section 2

# HYSTEROSCOPY

**CHAPTER 8. Diagnostic Hysteroscopy** **37**

*Sunita R Tandulwadkar, Pooja Lodha*

Preoperative Preparation *37*
Anesthesia *37*
Important Equipment *37*
Technique *37*

**CHAPTER 9. Office Hysteroscopy** **42**

*Sunita R Tandulwadkar, Pooja Lodha*

Preoperative Evaluation *42*
Preoperative Preparation *42*
Important Equipment *42*
Technique *42*

**CHAPTER 10. Classification of Microhysteroscopic Images** **44**

*Jorge E Dotto, Paola Da Graca Mila, Miguel A Bigozzi Jr, Jorge E Dotto Jr, Jacques Hamou*

Hysteroscopy Techniques *44*
Classification of Hysteroscopic Images *44*

**CHAPTER 11. Hysteroscopic Myomectomy** **56**

*Sunita R Tandulwadkar, Nirzari Mangeshikar*

Preoperative Evaluation *56*
Preoperative Preparation *56*
Important Equipment *56*
Classification of Submucosal Fibroid *56*
Technique *56*

**CHAPTER 12. Hysteroscopic Management of Intrauterine Adhesions** **62**

*Sunita R Tandulwadkar, Pooja Lodha*

Preoperative Evaluation *62*
Preoperative Preparation *62*
Instrumentation *62*
Technique *62*
Postoperative Care *62*

**CHAPTER 13. Hysteroscopic Cannulation for Proximal Tubal Block** **66**

*Sunita R Tandulwadkar*

Preoperative Evaluation *66*
Preoperative Preparation *66*
Important Equipment *66*
Technique *66*

**CHAPTER 14. Hysteroscopic Resection of Septum** 68

*Sunita R Tandulwadkar, Sejal Naik*

Preoperative Evaluation *68*
Preoperative Preparation *68*
Special Instruments *68*
Technique *68*

## Section 3

# LAPAROSCOPY

**CHAPTER 15. Laparoscopic Hysterectomy** 75

*Sunita R Tandulwadkar*

Preoperative Evaluation *75*
Preoperative Preparation *75*
Important Equipment *75*
Technique *75*
Steps of Laparoscopic Hysterectomy *76*

**CHAPTER 16. Laparoscopic Subtotal and Total Hysterectomy for Multiple Fibroids** 84

*Liselotte Mettler, Anupama Deenadayal, Ibrahim Alkatout*

Microscopic Facts and Fibroid Viability *86*
Costs of Fibroids *86*
Will the Ovaries be Removed or Left in Place? *86*
Laparoscopic Subtotal Hysterectomy *87*
Prerequisites *87*
Steps of Surgery *88*
Laparoscopic Total Hysterectomy (LTH) *91*

**CHAPTER 17. Laparoscopic Hysterectomy in Case of Large Uteri** 111

*Bruno J van Herendael, Lisbeth Jochems*

Preparation of the Surgery *111*
The Ten Step Laparoscopic Hysterectomy *113*

**CHAPTER 18. Laparoscopic Hysterectomy for Previous Cesarean Sections** 118

*Ornella Sizzi, Giuseppe Florio*

Preoperative Evaluation *118*
Preoperative Preparation *118*
Equipment *118*
Technique *118*
Changing of Technique for Previous Cesarean Sections *121*
Steps in Case of Adhesions and Uterus Ventrofixation *121*

**CHAPTER 19. Laparoscopic Hysterectomy in Endometriosis** 126

*Sanjay Patel, Yogendra Jhala*

Hysterectomy in Endometriosis with Frozen Pelvis *126*

**CHAPTER 20. Laparoscopic Radical Hysterectomy** **135**

*Shailesh Puntambekar*

Preoperative Preparation *135*
Instruments and Equipment *135*
Technique *135*
Procedure *135*

**CHAPTER 21. Laparoscopic Myomectomy** **143**

*Sunita R Tandulwadkar, Nirzari Mangeshikar*

Preoperative Evaluation of the Patient *143*
Preoperative Preparations *143*
Instruments and Equipment *143*
Bowel Preparation *143*
Prerequisites *143*
Procedure *143*
Closure of Uterine Flap *144*
Extraction of Myoma *144*
Myomectomy in Difficult Situations *144*

**CHAPTER 22. Laparoscopic Myomectomy for Intramural Fibroids** **153**

*Rafique Parkar*

Indications *153*
Contraindications *153*
Advantages *153*
Principles for a Good Laparoscopic Myomectomy *154*
Preoperative Evaluation/Preparation *154*
Surgical Procedure *154*

**CHAPTER 23. Laparoscopic Management of Benign Ovarian Mass** **160**

*Prakash Trivedi*

Preoperative Evaluation *160*
Preoperative Preparation *160*
Laparoscopic Ovarian Cystectomy *160*
Polycystic Ovarian Drilling *160*
Benign Cystic Teratomas *168*

**CHAPTER 24. Laparoscopic Management of Tubal Ectopic** **171**

*Sunita R Tandulwadkar, Sejal Naik*

Unruptured Ectopic *171*
Salpingostomy *171*
Salpingectomy *172*
Ruptured Ectopic *172*

**CHAPTER 25. Laparoscopic Salpingectomy** **176**

*Sunita R Tandulwadkar*

Preoperative Evaluation *176*
Preoperative Preparation *176*

Criteria for Salpingectomy in an Infertile Patient *176*
Instruments *176*
Procedure *176*

**CHAPTER 26. Conservation Laparoscopic Management of Hydrosalpinx** **180**
*Sunita R Tandulwadkar*
Preoperative Evaluation *180*
Preoperative Preparation *180*
Important Equipment *180*
Surgical Steps *180*

**CHAPTER 27. Laparoscopic Tubotubal Anastomosis** **183**
*Sanjay Patel*
Preoperative Evaluation *183*
Indications *183*
Contraindications *183*
Equipment and Instruments *183*
Sutures, Needles and Energy *183*
Selection of Cases *184*
Intra-operative Evaluation *184*
Surgical Technique *184*
Procedure *187*
Types of Anastomosis 187

**CHAPTER 28. Laparoscopic Management of Endometrioma** **193**
*Sunita R Tandulwadkar*
Preoperative Evaluation *193*
Preoperative Preparation *193*
Important Equipment *193*
Ablation of Cyst Wall *193*
Cystectomy *194*

**CHAPTER 29. Salpingoscopy** **198**
*Sanjay Patel*
Instruments and Procedure of Salpingoscopy *198*

**CHAPTER 30. Laparoscopic Management of Adenomyoma** **205**
*Sanjay Patel, Yogendra Jhala*
Transvaginal Ultrasonography *205*
Adenoma on Laparoscopy *206*
Adenoma on Hysteroscopy *206*
Coexisting Pathologies *208*
Preoperative Adenoma Mapping *208*
AIM of the Adenoma Resection *209*
Technique of Adenomyoma Resection *209*
Technique of Endosuturing: Intra-corporeal Slip Knot Technique *212*
Our Experience *213*

**CHAPTER 31. Anatomy of Pelvic Floor and Laparoscopic Prolapse Repair** **215**

*Revaz Botchorishvili, Sara Campos*

Preoperative Evaluation *215*
Preoperative Preparation *215*
Specific Instruments and Equipment *215*
Prerequisites *216*
Port Placements *216*
Anatomical Landmarks in Port Placement *216*
Key steps of the Procedure *216*

**CHAPTER 32. Laparoscopic Sling Surgery** **224**

*Sunita R Tandulwadkar, Nirzari Mangeshikar*

Laparoscopic Sacro-spinous Fixation for Uterine Prolapse *224*

**CHAPTER 33. Laparoscopic Cervical Cerclage** **228**

*Sunita R Tandulwadkar, Nirzari Mangeshikar*

When to Perform? *228*
Advantages *228*
Disadvantages *228*
Preoperative Evaluation *228*
Preoperative Preparation *228*
Instruments and Materials *228*
Steps of Laparoscopic Cerclage Procedure *228*

**CHAPTER 34. Single Incision Laparoscopic Surgery using Common Laparoscopic Instruments** **231**

*Sevellaraja Supermaniam*

Preoperative Evaluation *231*
Preoperative Preparation *231*
Important Equipment *231*
Technique *231*
Steps for Performing Single Incision Laparoscopic Hysterectomy *234*
Postoperative Management *238*
Other Procedures that can be Performed by this Technique *238*

**CHAPTER 35. Robotic Surgery in Gynecology** **241**

*Charles Miller, Kirsten Sasaki*

Selection of Cases *241*
Preparation for Surgery *241*

## Section 4

# VAGINAL SURGERY

**CHAPTER 36. Vaginal Surgery: Surgical Principles** **249**

*Andri Nieuwoudt*

Anatomical Considerations *251*
Perivaginal Organization *251*
The Role of Surgical Auditing in Defect Specific Surgery *254*

CHAPTER 37. **Nondescent Vaginal Hysterectomy** 258

*Sunita R Tandulwadkar*

Preoperative Evaluation *258*
Preoperative Preparation *258*
Anesthesia *258*
Position *258*
Technique *258*
Modifications *258*
Postoperative *259*

CHAPTER 38. **Newer Concepts of Anterior and Posterior Vaginal Prolapse Repair** 260

*Ajay Rane*

Pelvic Organ Supports *260*
Diagnosis *261*
POP-Q System *261*
Investigations *261*
Urodynamics *261*
Imaging *261*
Ultrasound *261*
Surgical Management *261*
Transobturator Mesh (PERIGEE) *262*
Transobturator Sling (MONARC) *262*

CHAPTER 39. **Apical and Posterior Vaginal Wall Repair** 265

*Andri Nieuwoudt*

Apical and Posterior Vaginal Wall Repair *265*
I. Bilateral Uterosacral Cervicopexy (BUSCer) *268*
II. Bilateral Uterosacral Colpopexy (BUSCol) *273*

CHAPTER 40. **Transvaginal Tape Obturator (TVTO) for Stress Urinary Incontinence** 276

*Prakash Trivedi, Sunita R Tandulwadkar*

Preoperative Evaluation *276*
Preoperative Preparation *276*
Important Equipment *276*
Procedure *276*
Tvt Abbrevo™ *285*

## Section 5

# UNUSUAL CASES

CHAPTER 41. **Uterus Didelphys with Abnormally Placed Ovaries** 289

*Sunita R Tandulwadkar*

**CHAPTER 42. Case of Chronic Twisted Adnexa** **293**

*Sunita R Tandulwadkar*

**CHAPTER 43. 27-year-old Female with Bad Obstetric History with Unicornuate Uterus** **295**

*Sunita R Tandulwadkar, Pooja Lodha*

**CHAPTER 44. Case of Ovarian Fibroma** **297**

*Prakash Trivedi, Sunita R Tandulwadkar*

**CHAPTER 45. Laparoscopy for Benign Uterine, Tubal and Ovarian Pathologies in Adolescent Age Group** **300**

*Sunita R Tandulwadkar, Nirzari Mangeshikar*

Pre-operative Preparations 300
Intra-operative considerations 300
Post-operative considerations 300

**CHAPTER 46. Hysteroscopic Resection of a Large Type 0 Submucous Myoma** **312**

*Sunita R Tandulwadkar, Nirzari Mangeshikar*

**CHAPTER 47. Anti-NMDA Receptor Antibody Encephalitis—A Rare Condition Associated with Ovarian Teratoma** **314**

*Sunita R Tandulwadkar, Devika Chopra*

Investigations *314*
Diagnosis *314*
Histopathology *314*
Patient Recovery *315*

*Index* *317*

# General Guidelines for Beginners

1. Good patient selection.
2. Good preoperative preparation.
3. Plan the surgery ahead.
4. Competent assistance: It is teamwork.
5. Check instrumentation and equipments ahead as it is; technologically-driven surgical modality.
6. Handle all equipment with utmost care.
7. Maintenance of all equipment is the secret of their longevity.
8. All instruments should be cleaned with a brush and water to remove all clots. Ultrasonic cleaners and chemicals are also available to remove all the clots.
9. Instruments should be dried thoroughly before being replaced in their chambers.
10. Sterilization can be achieved as follows:
    i. Metal instruments can be autoclaved.
    ii. Rapid sterilization can be done by placing in Cidex solution for 20 minutes.
    iii. Other instruments (like tubings and cables) can be placed in formalin chambers.
11. Safe port access.
12. Safe use of energy.
13. Gentle dissection, tissue respect.
14. Always remember: Limited view, only two-dimensional visions, no depth perception, therefore, always work under vision.
15. Review your own videos and you will understand your own mistakes which can be subsequently improved.
16. Endoscopic surgery should not be used as a technical gimmick to avoid laparotomy and attract patients. The goal of endoscopic surgery should not be to avoid laparotomy but to achieve highest surgical skills.
17. Quality of surgery inside is much more important than recovery one or two weeks later.
18. Every surgeon should pioneer his own technique in such a way that it gives the best of the results.
19. Every gynecologist should himself or herself decide which surgery he/she can do endoscopically.
20. With experience, the comfort level will definitely expand.
21. The flexible surgeon is familiar with all available techniques so that the best approach is selected for the individual patient.
22. Endoscopic surgery should not be 'in competition' but should be 'complimentary'.
23. Every surgery, open or endoscopic, has its own share of complications. The greatest hazard to the patient is not the surgery but the 'Surgeon'.
24. Every surgery should pick up the right surgical technique for the right patient, understanding his/her limitations and mastery over the technique.
25. Endoscopic surgeries are good for both the patients and the surgeon, it must always be remembered:

***"First do no harm!"***

# DO'S AND DON'TS

## DO's

*Surgeon*

### *"I think It's OK" - Syndrome*

**Be aware of the words "I think it's OK".**

**The surgeon must determine whether the organ in question is or is not injured. If the conclusion is that it is injured, proper steps are taken to deal with it. The matter should not be put aside for period of observation.**

- Be aware of any changes taking place in the operating room during the procedure or between the cases.

1. Personnel.
2. Equipment not working.
3. Running out of critical supplies.
4. In fact, just about any thing that can have an effect on operating surgeon or his/her performance.

*Assistant*

**Assisting is a very special part of any operative procedures.**

**The purpose of the assistance is not only to assist, but to enhance the performance of operating surgeon.**

***A good assistant can make a good case even better***
***A bad assistant can turn a good case into a disaster***

**Make suggestions that might help the procedure.**

**The surgeon and assistant should wok as a team, and each team member has his/her task to do.**

## DONT'S

*Assistant*

**Do not try to do the procedure.**

**In operative laparoscopy, two surgeons can make great team if they work together. Remember the more you work together, the more you will actually.**

***"WORK TOGETHER"***

***A good operative laparoscopy is a four-handed procedure.***

**Do not let your mind wonder back to Mayo's stand or back table. If you are trying to assist someone and you let your attention drawn away from that person, you break line of communication.**

***"Freeze, don't move!"***

**During the actual procedure your best move as an assistant is sometimes.**

***"No move at all!"***

***" The flexible surgeon is familiar with all available techniques so that the best approach is selected for the individual patient"***

Section

1

# Basic Endoscopy

Chapter

1

# How to Set-up an Ideal Endoscopic Operation Theater

*PG Paul, Sunita R Tandulwadkar, Renuka Borisa, P Biju, Kannan K, Fiadjoe P*

## INTRODUCTION

- Well-equipped, well-organized and well-spaced operating room is essential for successful laparohysteroscopic procedures.
- The arrangement of instruments and equipment is important for safety and efficiency.
- Ceiling mounted instrument carts avoid gas tubing and electrical wires on the floor.
- Electrosurgical generator and suction irrigation device are kept on a separate trolley for avoiding spill of irrigation fluid on other equipment.
- Ideally operation theater should be square in shape with minimum measurement of 20 × 20 square foot and should be large enough to accommodate all the equipment (Fig. 1.1).
- The OT table should have capability for Trendelenberg and reverse Trendelenberg positions with right and left tilt. The table should have adjustment to go as below as 2 feet so that one can operate comfortably even with very obese patients. The height of the table should be below the waist of the surgeon for maximum efficacy. For short surgeons, use of stepping platforms is extremely valuable.
- To avoid fatigue and further consequences of the shoulder joint, surgeons should take precautions to see that his/her patient's position is in such a way that he/she does not have to abduct the upper extremity beyond 45° angle unless he/she is using contralateral port.
- A well-equipped Boyle's apparatus for general endotracheal anesthesia is essential to maintain proper oxygenation and relaxation during the procedure along with an ET $CO_2$ and pulse oximeter monitoring.
- The surgeon stands by the patients left side at an angle facing the patient's contralateral foot. Usually, the first assistant stands opposite the surgeon, i.e. on the right side of the patient, while a second assistant sits between the legs of the patient and helps in uterine manipulation. Rarely in cases of advanced surgery, where even first assistant is using two ipsilateral ports, one more assistant is needed to hold the camera, who can stand at the head end, next to the anesthetist.
- The nurse and the instrument table are positioned on the left side of the surgeon for easy accessibility.
- Second trolley is arranged on the foot end of the patient, easily accessible to the left hand of the sister and the right hand of the second assistant.
- Endoscopic equipment cart (Fig. 1.2) should carry:
  - Main video monitor
  - Endovision camera
  - Recording system
  - Light source
  - The $CO_2$ insufflator to allow continuous monitoring of inflation rate and intra-abdominal pressure
  - Electrosurgical generators/harmonic/other energy sources
  - Endomat/hysteromat
  - Morcellator.

  One can also have hanging unit which can carry monitor, camera, recording system, light source and $CO_2$ insufflator.

  If its mobile cart ensure that wheels are good for easy mobility of the unit.
- For laparoscopic surgery this cart with monitor should be placed at the foot end of the table, usually at the patients right foot while for hysteroscopic surgery, the monitor is placed toward the patient's right shoulder.
- Another monitor should be placed at the head end of the patient, which benefits the second assistant and the nurse/technician.
- It is not only the surgeon but assistants, nursing staffs and even ward boys who should be familiar with the functioning of all the equipment for better outcome.
- The place of each and every equipment and instrument should be fixed and everyone should be aware of their placement.

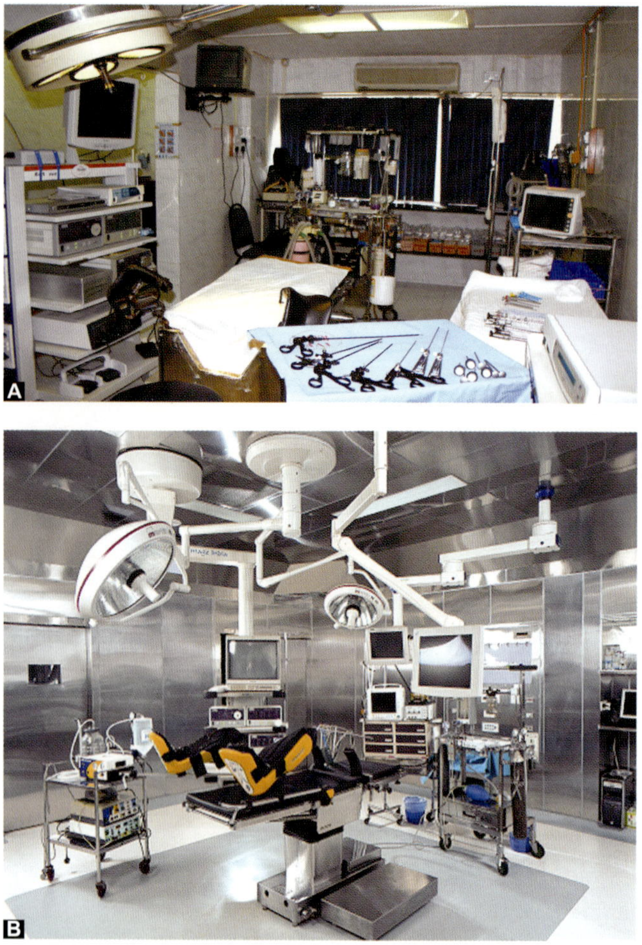

**Figs. 1.1A and B:** OT layout

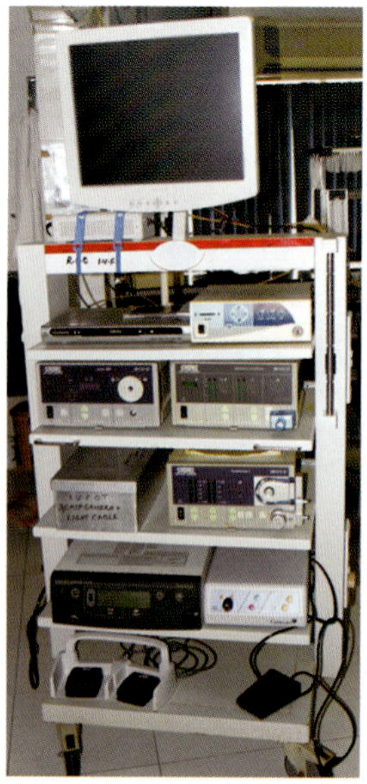

**Fig. 1.2:** Mobile cart

- Sterilization system for the instrument could be either autoclaving, gassing of individual instrument or formalin sterilization by keeping in formalin chambers. It depends on individual's choice as long as it gives 100% assurance of sterility.
- One of the video monitors should have facility to record in multisystem form. One of the most important aspects in endoscopy setup is the facility of proper documentation. The DVD recording is the most easiest and simplest installable modality. Many computer softwares are available to record the live surgery as well as for the data base maintenance, which helps in quick analysis of the total patient information.

**TIPS**

- These are the minimum required gadgets for safe and hastle-free environment in the operation theaters that one needs to have.
- One can keep on enhancing the operation theater with more gadgets (e.g. extra monitors, large monitors, other energy sources, backup equipment, etc.) with time.
- As the surgeon spends more time in the operation theater, other advancements in each gadget happen over the period.

Chapter 2

# Equipment and Instruments in Endoscopic Surgery

*Sunita R Tandulwadkar*

## INTRODUCTION

Gynecologic endoscopic surgery has been evolving continuously and rapidly.

Goal of this chapter is to describe the basic equipment required for endoscopic surgery as well give an overview of the equipment required for advanced laparoscopic surgery.

So acquire the basic equipment and embark on your journey with full enthusiasm after acquiring training in the field of course.

The following equipment are a part of the video tower cart:

## ANESTHESIA WORK STATION

Following are essential for all general anesthesia cases:

- Good quality Boyle's apparatus with fresh soda lime (Fig. 2.1).
- Electrocardiogram tracing.
- Noninvasive arterial pressure monitor.

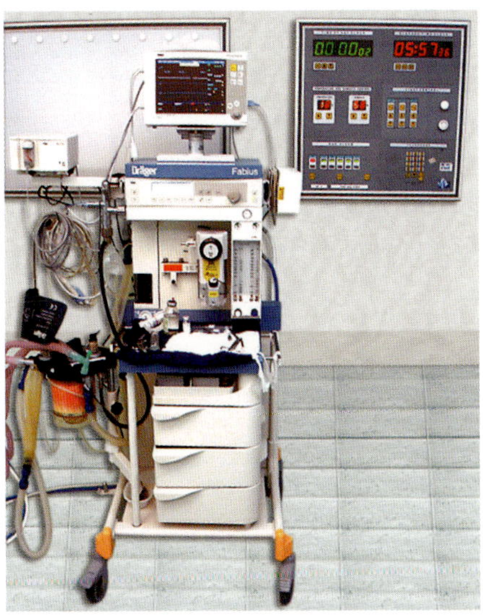

**Fig. 2.1:** Boyle's machine

- Airway pressure.
- Pulse oxymeter.
- End tidal carbon dioxide (ET $CO_2$) which detects drop in the oxygen level.
- Capnograph shows $CO_2$ retention.
- Defibrillators are essential for all general anesthesia cases.

### $CO_2$ Insufflator

$CO_2$ insufflator allows regularized flow and maintenance of optimum intra-abdominal pressure with adjustable pressure and gas flow.

It consists of:

- $CO_2$ insufflators with jumbo $CO_2$ cylinders.
- $CO_2$ filter is essential for generating pure $CO_2$ and thereby reducing postoperative pain.
- Thermoflator—used to decrease peritoneal irritation by providing warm $CO_2$ and prevents continuous fogging of the optics.

### Endoscopic Camera with Camera Control Unit (CCU)

The picture should be at low lux/low intensity.

Glare should be reduced when the light intensity is high.

Available in two types, both are acceptable:

- Single chip.
- Three chip—better picture quality useful in finer work like tuboplasty, severe endometriosis, etc.

### Light Source

- Most commonly used bulbs are xenon bulbs and halogen bulbs. Xenon bulbs generate high intensity of pure white light, which lasts longer and gives best color production but is expensive.
- An ideal endoscopy center should have one good light source with another standby light source.

## Light Cables

- Advanced endoscopic surgeries require fiberoptic cables of at least 4–5 mm diameter.
- Light carrying capacity of the cable depends on the number of fiberoptic bundles.

## Endomat/Hysteromat

- It is useful in centers where operative hysteroscopies are done routinely.
- It has three settings—inflow rate, pressure and suction pressure.
- For hysteroscopic surgeries, normally pressure of 100-150 mm of Hg, with flow rate of 300 mL/min and suction pressure of 50 mm of Hg is optimum. Pressure bags can be used as an alternative.
- They should have a Y tube connection for uninterrupted flow.

## Suction Irrigation System

- It is a must for every endoscopic theater.
- It can also be used for aqua dissection.

## Electrosurgical Generator (Fig. 2.2)

- A separate electrosurgical unit with separate bipolar and monopolar foot switches is essential for endoscopic surgery.
- Placement of cautery foot switch is very important to avoid accidental injuries (Fig. 2.3).

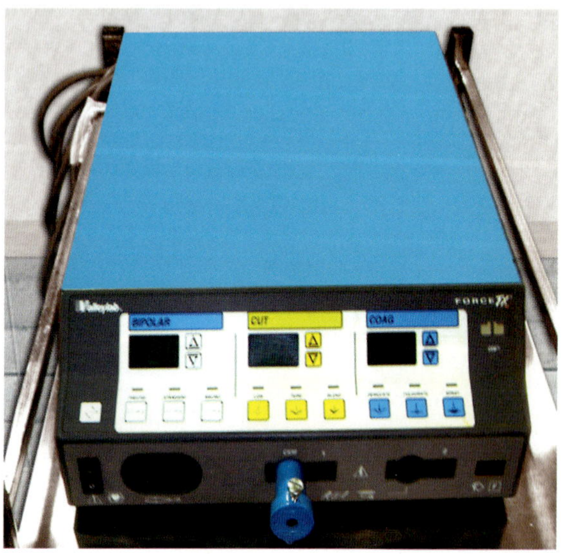


**Fig. 2.2:** Electrosurgical generator

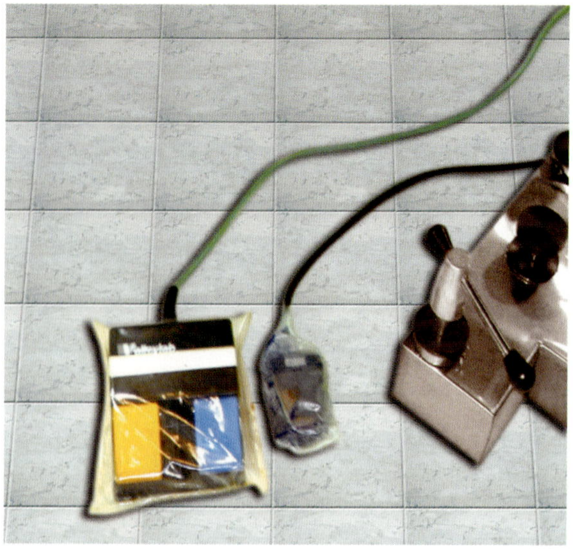

**Fig. 2.3:** Placement of foot switches in relation to operation table

## Leg Stirrups (Fig. 2.4)

- Padded Allen stirrups provide good support and proper position.
- Disadvantage is the cost.
- Ordinary leg stirrups with 45° angle can be used, but care has to be taken when surgery is extended.

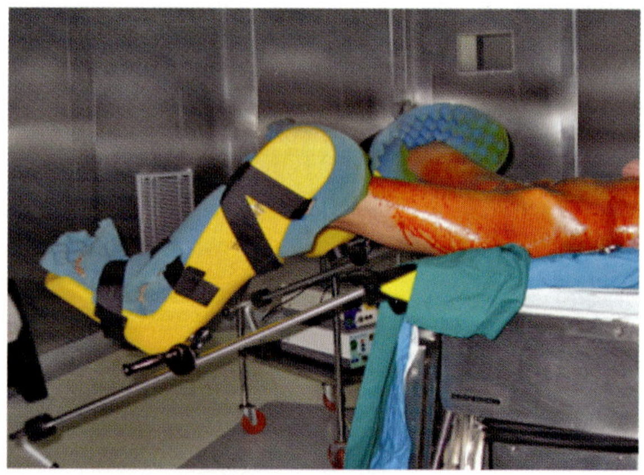

**Fig. 2.4:** Leg stirrups

## Hand Instruments

### *Veress Needle (Fig. 2.5)*

- It is used to create pneumoperitoneum.
- It has a spring mechanism, which protects the viscera from the sharp needle edge.

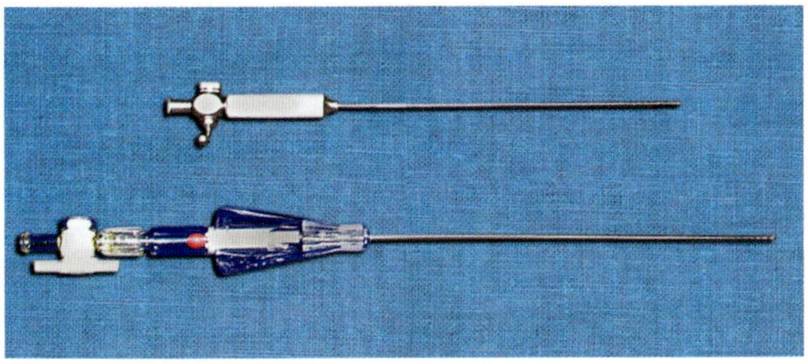

**Fig. 2.5:** Veress needle—disposable and reusable

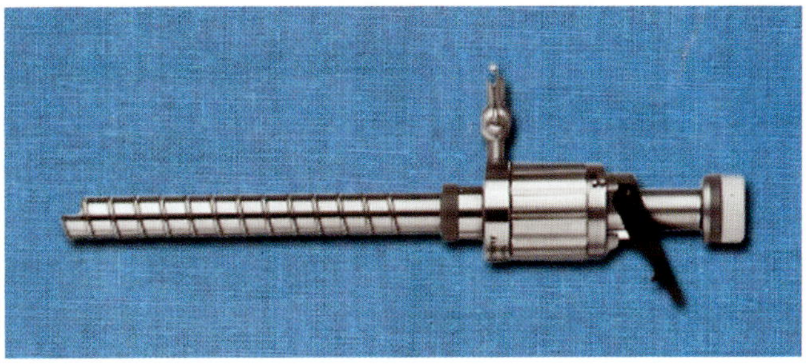

**Fig. 2.6:** Endotip

### *Trocars (Figs 2.6 and 2.7)*

- Various trocars are available in the market.
- Trocars usually have 2 types of valves to prevent the escape of gas. Trumpet valves are airtight but it grips the instruments and prevents smooth movement of telescope as well as operating instruments. So flap valve trocars are preferred.
- Pyramidal shape trocar is easy to insert.
- The conical trocar tip requires a stronger thrust to insert.
- Introduction of auxiliary trocars is always carried out under vision.
- Trocars come in different diameters 3 mm, 5 mm, 10 mm and 12 mm.

### *Endoscopes (Figs 2.8 and 2.9)*

- Most commonly used laparoscopes are 0° and 30°, 5 mm and 10 mm.
- In 0° scope, the direction of view corresponds to natural approach and facilitates orientation.
- Thirty degree laparoscope is advantageous during dissection in the pouch of Douglas and in case of multiple fibroids where one has to see beyond the fibroids.

### *Forceps/Graspers (Figs 2.10 and 2.11)*

- They are available in different sizes and shapes.
- Ideal grasper should be medium sized with a rounded tip and serrated jaws so that it can grasp tissue and act as a blunt probe with jaws closed.
- **Maryland dissector** resembles the curved artery of open surgery.
- **Serrated traumatic tissue graspers** are designed for holding structures such as cyst wall, while **claw forceps** are useful for holding tough tissues like cervix at the time of hysterectomy or small myomas.
- **Tenaculum** are used along with morcellators for holding myoma and are available as 5 mm and 10 mm.
- **Bipolar forceps** are the key to success of endoscopic surgery. Everyone should have a good pair of these forceps. We recommend bipolar forceps with good grip and dissector type, so that it can be used as dissector and grasper which accelerates surgical speed.

### *Scissors (Fig. 2.12)*

- Can be curved, straight or hooked.
- Some have electrical adapters.

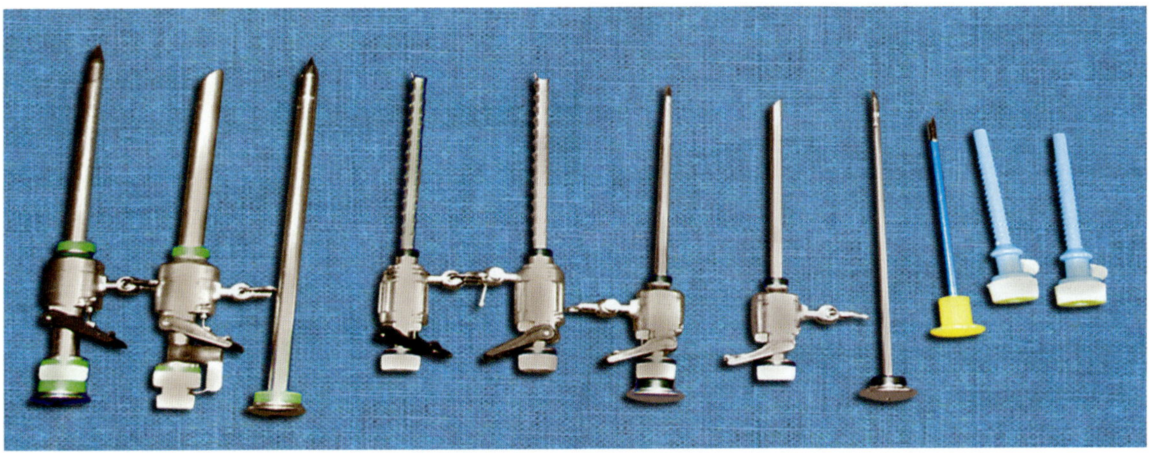

**Fig. 2.7:** Trocars and cannulae

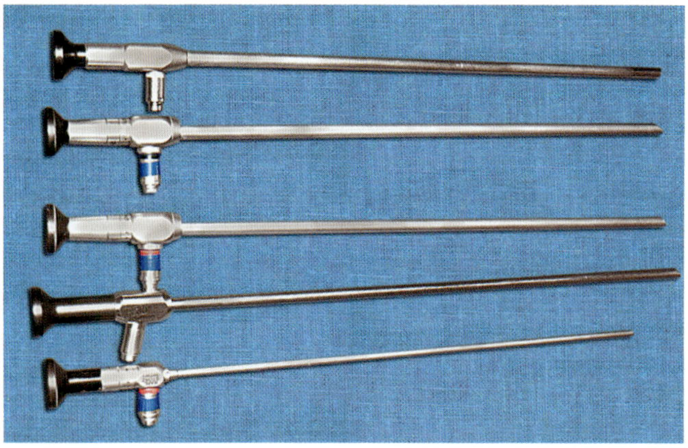

**Fig. 2.8:** Laparoscopes

**Fig. 2.9:** 10 mm laparoscopes 0° and 30°

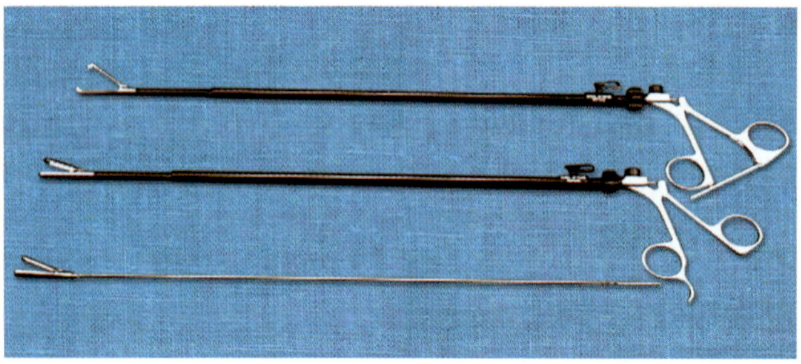

**Fig. 2.10:** 10 mm claw and spoon forceps

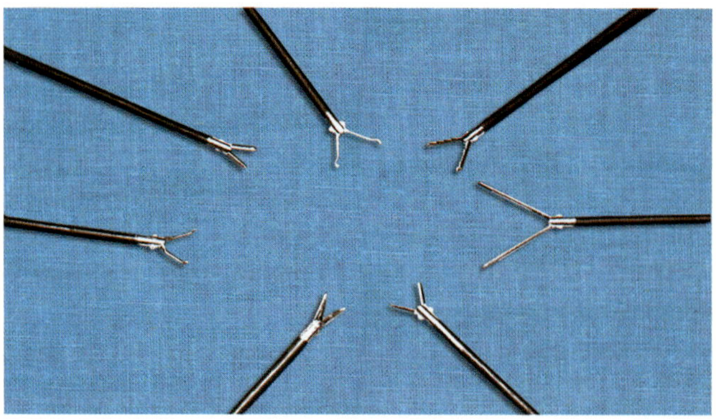

**Fig. 2.11:** Graspers—traumatic and atraumatic

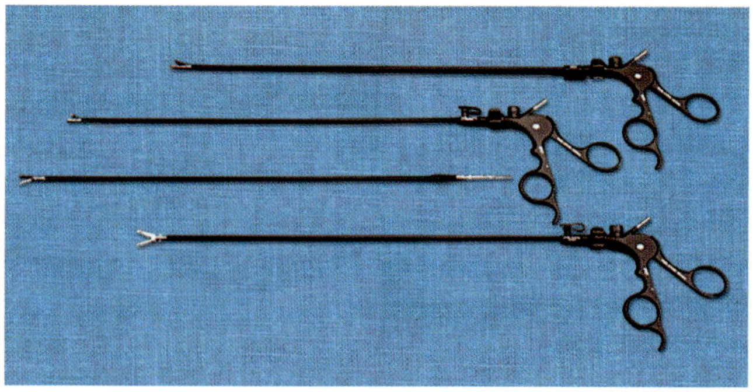

**Fig. 2.12:** Scissors

### *Suction Irrigation Cannula (Fig. 2.13)*

- Available in 5 mm and 10 mm.
- The one end is connected to irrigation whereas other end to the suction tube.
- It can also be used for aqua dissection.
- The suction tip can have single or multiple holes as per the individual's choice.

### *Monopolar Needle (Fig. 2.14)*

- It has a very fine needle with pin control used in cases of PCO drilling, puncturing of cysts and to take a fine incision for salpingostomy in cases of unruptured ectopic pregnancy, tubo-tubal anastamosis, etc.

### *Monopolar Spatula/Hook*

- It can be used to make a precise incision.

### *Needle Holders (Fig. 2.15)*

- One should definitely have a pair of excellent quality needle holders, we recommend left handed curve needle holders so that suture loops can be glided off easily.
- In case of myomectomy and hysterectomy during vault closure, left handed tooth forceps helps to have good grip of uterine flaps.

### *Myoma Screw*

- They are introduced into the myomas, which allow stabilizing the myoma, maneuvering it and applying traction to improve visibility, access and better performance of surgery.
- Some use it in total laparoscopic hysterectomy for uterine manipulation (instead of vaginal manipulator).

### *Clip Applicator*

- They are used for hemostasis of medium sized vessels. One can have 3 mm and 5 mm clip applicators.

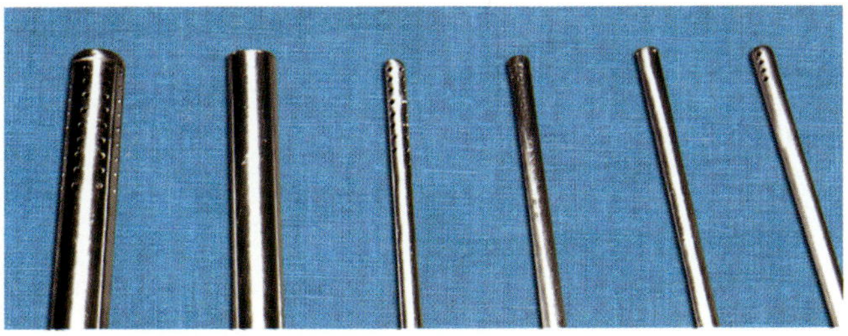

**Fig. 2.13:** Suction irrigation cannulae—5 mm and 10 mm with different tips

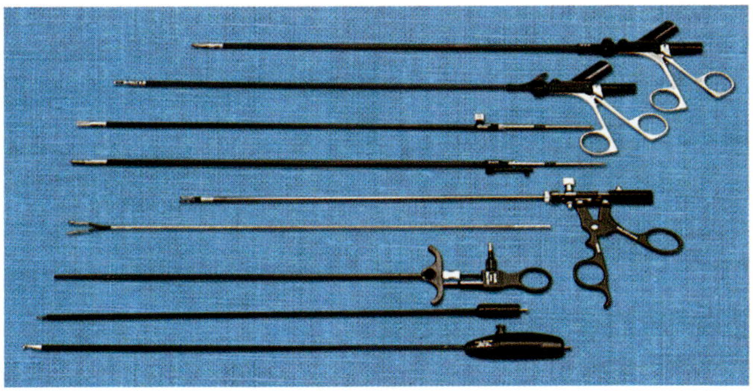

**Fig. 2.14:** Bipolar and unipolar forceps

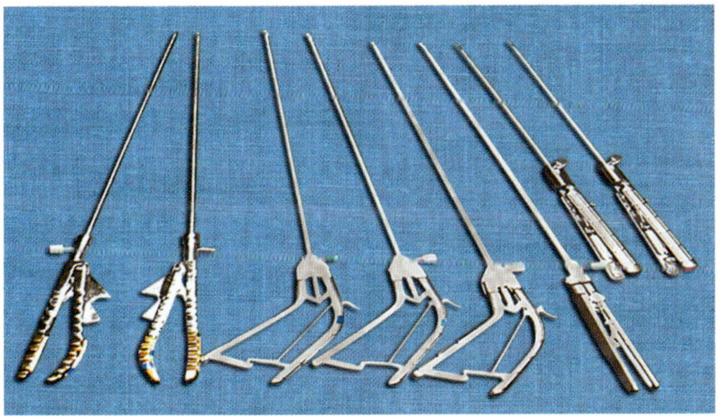

**Fig. 2.15:** Laparoscopic needle holders

### *Uterine Manipulator*

- It is used to mobilize or stabilize the uterus during surgery.

#### Self-designed (Fig. 2.16)

It has a handle with notch for the thumb to know internal curvature of the instrument—

- Notch anterior—curve anterior.
- Notch posterior—curve posterior.
- Handle makes the job of the vaginal assistant easy.

#### Long Sturdy Rod with Angle (Fig. 2.17)

Long sturdy rod with angle helps to manipulate bulky uterus even of 18 weeks easily.

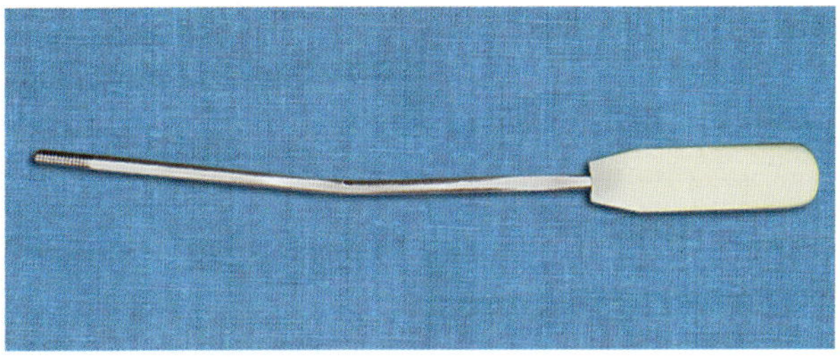

**Fig. 2.16:** Self-designed manipulator

#### Tip

Tip is serrated to avoid perforation of uterus with manipulator.

Same handle if put in the posterior fornix in reverse way can be used for taking posterior colpotomy incisions, as it does not conduct electricity.

#### Electronic Tissue Morcellator (Fig. 2.18)

It is used to morcellate myoma into small bits and remove it piecemeal.

#### Laparoscopy Specimen Retrieval Bag

It facilitates removal of specimen from the abdominal cavity and avoids contamination of the abdomen with its contents.

Most important aspect of endoscopic surgery is to have a proper operation theater setup, instruments and adequate facilities to deal with complications.

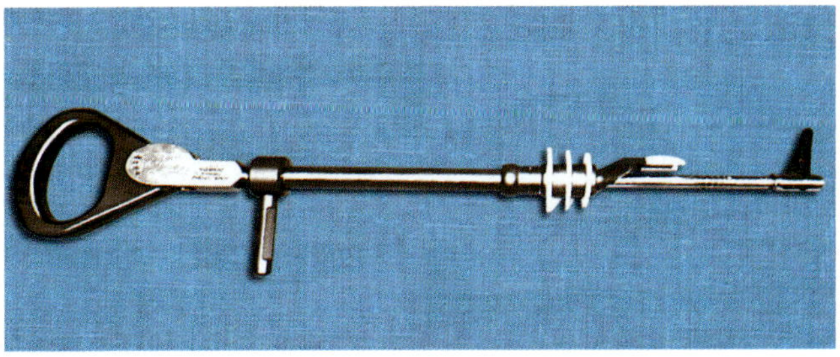

**Fig. 2.17:** Clermont-Ferrand uterine manipulator

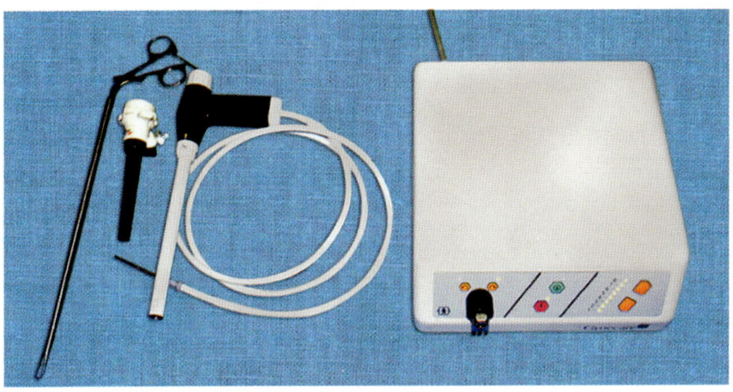

**Fig. 2.18:** Electronic tissue morcellator

***A set of good quality instruments is better than a cupboard full of standard ones.***

## TIPS

- Tip is serrated to avoid perforation of uterus with manipulator.
- Handle all equipments with utmost care.
- Maintenance of all equipments is the secret of their longevity.
- All instruments should be cleaned with a brush and water to remove all clots. Ultrasonic cleaners and enzymes are also available to remove all the clots.
- Instruments should be dried thoroughly before being replaced in their chambers.
- When the xenon light source is kept in contact with the skin/ drape, there is burning of that part suggesting that if this aspect is ignored during surgery, the patient may have electrical burns.
- Light cables are always kept in the larger circular pattern to avoid breakage of the inner fibers.
  In endoscopic surgery, you cannot look at the foot switches every time before cauterizing. Your left foot senses the foot switches. So it is important to have fixed position of monopolar and bipolar foot switches. If you are used to keep the bipolar foot switch medially, always keep it medially only. This will avoid accidental thermal injury especially if accessory instruments carrying both these cautery currents are inside at a time. If one is using the ultrasonic energy source (i.e. harmonic), then hand instrument with hand activation facility should be used.
- Sterilization can be achieved as follows:
  - Metal instruments except the telescopes can be autoclaved.
  - Rapid sterilization can be done by placing in cidex solution for 20 minutes.
  - Other instruments (tubings/cables) can be placed in formalin chambers.

***"It is not the instruments that makes the surgery safe but it is the surgeon who makes the use of instruments safe for the patients"***

# Chapter 3

# Energy Sources in Endoscopic Surgery

*Wachyu Hadisaputra, Leonita TA Sutrisna*

## INTRODUCTION

Learning energy sources is of paramount importance in doing endosurgical procedure.

A clear understanding of its physics and its application to surgical procedure is necessary.

It is equally important to maximize safe delivery of these energy sources.

## AIM

1. To discuss and understand the fundamental therapeutic modalities of the available energy sources.
2. To discuss the inherent risks and advantages of each.

## ELECTROSURGERY

### FUNDAMENTALS AND BIOPHYSICS OF ELECTROSURGERY

Electrosurgery is the surgical use of high-frequency electric current that produced by electron movement. Electrons revolve around the nucleus of an atom and flow from one atom's orbit to the other orbit. When this mechanism happened, it will make a flow of current. The force that provides the electron's ability to travel from one atom to the other atom is the voltage. The electron has encounter resistance, which produce heat, is called impedance. Only a closed electrical circuit allows electron to circulate.

In electrosurgery, there are some common terms include current, voltage and resistance. Current can be described as flow of electrons in a certain period of time. Current measured in amperes. Voltage is the force that drives the current or flow of electrons, measured in volts. In electrosurgery, voltage is provided by the generator, and current is delivered to the tissues through the electrode tip of the instrument. Resistance is obstacle to the flow of current that measured in ohms. Resistance is similar with impedance. In the electrosurgery use in clinical patient, the source of electron flow and voltage came from the electrosurgical generator (ESG). Circuit is an uninterrupted pathway of flowing electrons and Ohm's Law describes the actions of a given circuit :

$$\text{Voltage} = \text{Current} \times \text{Resistance}$$

A current can be driven in a circuit by an electromotive force supplied by a generator just as water can be driven by a pump. Each monopolar circuit consists of the generator, an active electrode, the patient and the patient-return electrode. Some pathways can be used to ground for leakage current, like OR table, stirrups, staff members and equipment. The impedance from the patient's tissues producing heat when the electrons overcome the impedance. The higher inherent resistance needs the greater voltage for the current to pass. Also, as more superficial tissues are cauterized, they become less electrically conductive, increasing their resistance and requiring higher amounts of the voltage for current to penetrate to the tissues.

The transformation of electrical energy into heat can be describe by Joules Law and the following formula :

$$\text{Energy} = (\text{Current}/\text{Cross-sectional area})^2 \times \text{Resistance} \times \text{Time}$$

Heat given off is a function of current density (current per cross-sectional area), time and resistance. The heat produced is proportional to the surface area of electrode. Larger electrodes will require longer periods of current application to achieve the same large heat production.

When an oscillating current is applied to tissue, the rapid movement of electrons through the cytoplasm of cells cause the intracellular temperature rising. In general, thermal damage to tissue is reversible in below 45°C. As tissue temperature exceed 45°C, the proteins in the tissue become denatured and losing their structural integrity. The liquid in the tissue will evaporate when it reach above 90°C. Once the tissue temperatures reach 200°C, the remaining solid components of the tissue are reduced to carbon.

## TYPES OF ENERGY SOURCE

Electrosurgical generators can apply energy in either a monopolar or bipolar fashion. In the monopolar system, the current from the generator pass from the active electrode through the patient and out of the body through a dispersive electrode pad connected to the generator to form a complete circuit. The active electrode is at the surgical site (Fig. 3.1). Bipolar does not require a dispersive return electrode pad because the active electrode and the return electrode are integrated into the energy delivery forceps (Fig. 3.1) with the target tissue to complete the circuit. The damage produced in the tissue is limited and the risk of thermal injury in distant tissues is lower. The advantage of bipolar modality over monopolar modality has been depicted in Table 3.1.

In general, electrosurgical generators provide energy delivery in two types of modes: continuous and interrupted. The continuous mode is referred to the "cut" mode, the interrupted mode is referred to the "coag" or coagulation mode.

There are various forms of electric current :

- Direct current (DC): The electron flow continuously in the same direction. This type of current is used for therapeutic purposes, for example acupuncture and pain electrotherapy.
- Pulsed current: A relatively high amount of energy at short interval. It is used for nerve stimulation.
- Alternating current (AC): The current changes direction periodically between two electrodes (bidirectional). This type of current is used in electrosurgery.

When an electric current flows through biological tissue, we can observe thermal effect, electrolytic effect and faradic effect. The amount of heat in thermal effect depends on the intensity of the electrical current, the resistance of the tissue and the duration of current flows. The electrolytic effect can cause polarization of the electronic compound which can cause potential damage. To avoid this effect, the electrosurgery uses alternating current with constant reversal of polarity. Faradic effect is the reaction in the nerve ending when the electric current passing through the tissue. The reaction includes muscle contraction and pain.

This time, the modern concept of electrosurgery performed safely at frequencies above 100 kHz. This high

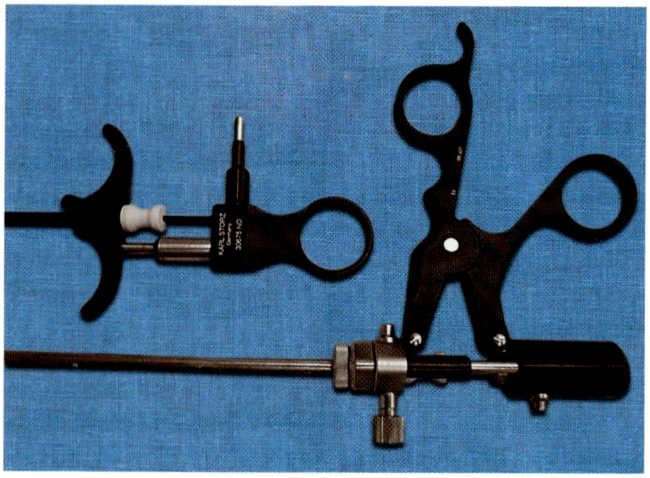

**Fig. 3.1:** Electrosurgery forceps: Monopolar (left) and bipolar (right)

frequency electric current can avoid the negative effect of neuromuscular stimulation that ceases at 10,000 cycles/second (10 kHz). This is important to minimize nerve and muscle stimulation. The possible effects of applying current to the tissue are fulguration, desiccation/coagulation or vaporization/ablation. An electrosurgical generator can produces 60 cycle current and increases the frequency to over 300,000 cycles per second which can pass through the patient with minimal neuromuscular stimulation and no risk of electrocution. Electrosurgical units operating in the frequency range of 300,000 to 600,000 Hz (300 kHz to 600 kHz) typically offer the best balance of safety and performance, instead of low-frequency current, which has a "faradic effect" with possible muscular twitching, pain, even ventricular fibrillation, and cardiac arrest (Fig. 3.2).

## USE OF THE THERMAL EFFECT (FIG. 3.3)

There are two basic methods of thermal tissue destruction, which is used in electrosurgery.

### Cutting

When a high current density is applied to the tissue, the heating of the intracellular fluid is increased so fast from 37°C to 100°C. There is no time for the water to evaporate. The vapor pressure leads to explosion of the cellular membranes (evaporation). The separation of tissues

**Table 3.1:** The bipolar modality has some advantages compared to the monopolar

| *Monopolar Modality* | *Bipolar Modality* |
|---|---|
| The current passes through many tissues outside the surgeon's visual control before it can return to the electrosurgical generator | The current flow through the tissue is restricted to the area between two jaws of the electrode, which is under the direct vision of the surgeon |
| High risk of thermal injuries in distant tissues | The risk of thermal injuries in distant tissues due to direct contact of instrument, faulty insulation or diffusion of the electrical current is reduced |
| This modality interferes with other electronic equipment connected to the patient at the same time | The risk of interference with other electronic equipment (ECG, pacemakers and others) connected to the patient at the same time is lower |

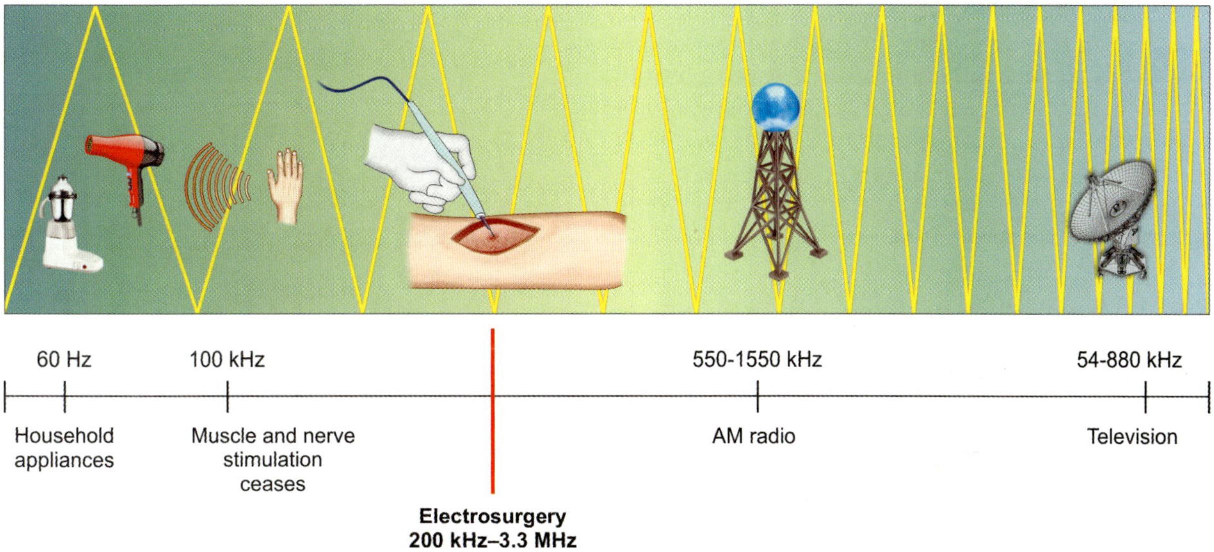


**Fig. 3.2:** Applications of different current frequencies

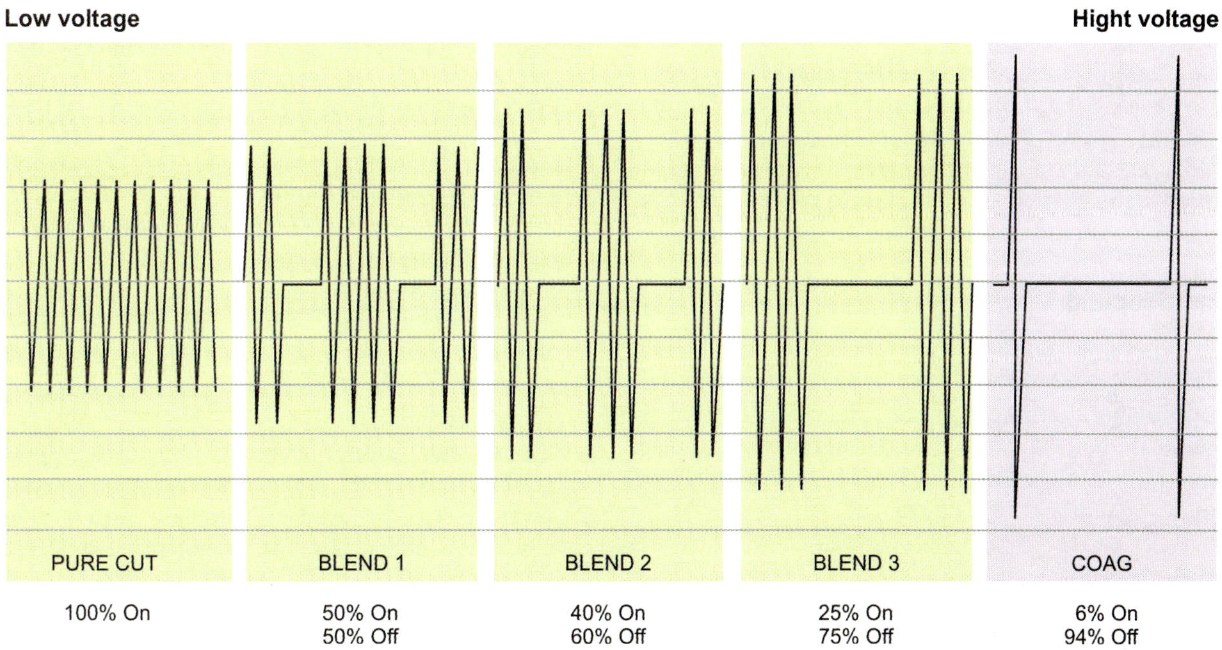


**Fig. 3.3:** Relationship between voltage and thermal effect

can be used to cut. This modality is more powerful and generally less penetrating. It also allows precise cutting with minimal coagulation and also reduce operating time.

With thicker or wider electrodes, the contact area and also the potential for thermal injury are increased. The electrosurgical cutting effect is used on vascular tissue, such as adhesiolysis and also for peritoneal endometriosis resection.

### Coagulation

For coagulation, a low current density is applied so that the tissue temperature increases slowly, giving the water enough time to evaporate. In order to overcom the high impedance of air, the coagulation waveform has significantly higher voltage than the cutting current. Use of a high voltage coagulation current has implications during minimally invasive surgery.

Some surgeons cut with the coagulation current. It may be necessary to adjust power settings and electrode size to achieve the desired surgical effect. The advantage of coagulation with the cutting current is that a much lower voltage is used.

## GENERAL SAFETY ASPECTS

### Grounded Electrosurgery Systems

The electrical current is a continuous flow of electrons. It has an entry and exit site. So the current must return to some place and through the current division phenomenon. The current can split and follow the pathways to ground. The circuit to ground is completed whether it travels the intended electrosurgical circuit to the patient return electrode or to an alternative ground. Patient will have a risk of burns at the alternative grounding site if the resistance of the alternative path is low and the current flowing to ground is concentrated.

### Isolated Electrosurgical Systems

If the circuit to the patient return electrode is interrupted, an isolated generator will deactivate the system because the current cannot return to its source. This type of generator will reduce the risk of burns at the alternative sites but do not protect the burns caused by the return electrode. The quality of the conductivity and contact area at the plate or patient interface must be maintained to prevent burn injury at the return electrode site.

### Patient Return Electrodes

The function of the patient return electrode is to collect and remove current from the patient safely. To eliminate the risk of current density, the plate should present a large contact area to the patient with low impedance, on conductive tissue as close as possible to the operative site. The plate site should be a well vascularized muscle mass.

### Direct Coupling

Direct coupling occurs when the user accidentally activates the generator while the active electrode is near another metal instrument. It can cause a potential risk of significant patient injury. The generator should not be activated while the active electrode is touching or in close proximity to another metal object.

### Insulation Injury

Many surgeons routinely use the coagulation current, which has a relatively high voltage. The concentrate current can caused significant injury. Simply by using the cutting current, the surgeon can obtain the coagulation effect and reduce the insulation failure without high voltage. By lowering current density the rate at which heat is produced is reduced.

### Capacitive Coupling during Laparoscopy

There are three systems of capacitive coupling, including metal trocar system, plastic trocar system, hybrid trocar system. In metal trocar system, the conductive active electrode is surrounded by a conductive metal trocar. A capacitor creates an electrostatic field between the two conductor, a conductor can induce a current in the second conductor. In plastic trocar system, capacitance cannot be entirely eliminated with an all-plastic cannula. Capacitance is reduced, but is not eliminated. In hybrid trocar system, a metal cannula is held in place by a plastic anchor. The capacitive coupled current may exit from adjacent tissue to the patient return electrode that can cause significant injury.

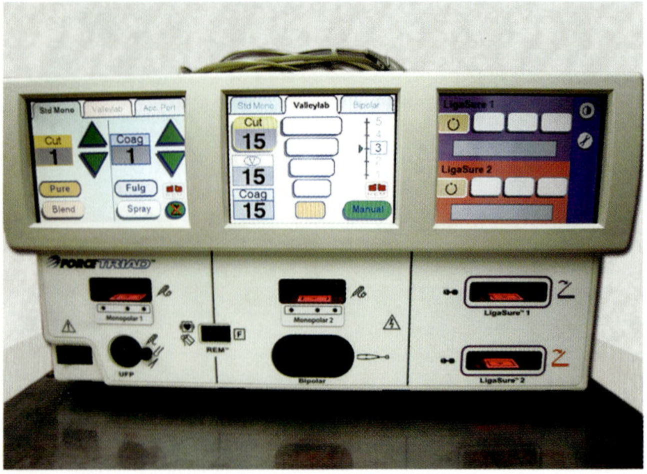


Fig. 3.4: Electrosurgery machine

## PREVENTION OF ELECTROSURGICAL INJURIES

The following steps for preventing electrosurgical injuries:

1. A thorough understanding of the biophysical principles of radiofrequency electrical energy is essential. For example, when the generator output cannot accomplish tissue effect as expected, we should check the ground plate or its connection.
2. Do bowel preparation if it is anticipated that the large bowel is at risk. The use of an orogastric tube is recommended.
3. Choose the proper current waveform mode. In monopolar surgery, either the cutting or coagulation waveform can be used to achieve a cutting effect or fulguration effect. Use the lowest possible generator setting that will achieve the surgical effect and never exceed the power settings recommended by the manufacturers. And also, use a low voltage waveform. Larger diameter scissors will require a higher power setting and will have a bigger footprint on the tissue.
4. Improve dexterity and hand-eye coordination through sequential phases of training, include didactic phase, laboratory experience, observation and/or assistance, and preceptorship. To minimize the chances of direct trauma, activate the electrode only when whole tissue is in the field of vision.
5. Avoid hybrid trocar sleeves. The use of completely metal trocar cannulas can reduce the risk of capacitive coupling. Select an all-metal trocar system as the safest option. It can be avoided by using multiple, short activation times that allows normal tissue to remain cool.
6. Use electrosurgical accessory safety equipment when possible. Do not activate in an open circuit and in close

proximity to or direct contact with another instrument. Use bipolar eletrosurgery where possible.
7. Frequent cleaning of the electrode tip is recommended.
8. Organize a laparoscopic team that includes a biomedical engineer, perioperative nurses, and other operation room personnel.

## OTHER ENERGY SOURCES

### Laser

Many media are used to produce laser light in gynecology including $CO_2$, argon gases, Nd:YAG and KTP crystals for purpose of hemostasis and cutting.

#### *Precautions*

- Operation rooms should be labeled.
- All the staff in the OT should wear protective goggles.
- Laser plume can cause respiratory damage.
- Increased equipment costs.

#### *Advantages*

- Tissue near an incision is protected, since there is little contact with surrounding skin or other tissue.
- The heat produced by lasers sterilizes the surgical site, thus reducing the risk of infection.
- Less operating time may be needed because the precision of the laser allows for a smaller incision.
- Healing time is often shortened, there is less bleeding, swelling, or scarring.

#### *Disadvantage*

- Strict safety precautions must be observed in the operating room.

### Ultrasound Dissector/Ultrasonic Scalpel/ Harmonic Scalpel (Fig. 3.5)

#### *Principle*

- The instrument operates by means of a blade that vibrate longitudinally at a frequency of 55.5 kHz. The end of the device oscillates at about 50,000 cycles/sec, which results in precise cutting.
- The scalpel coagulates and cuts by using lower temperatures than electrosurgery or lasers.
- Ultrasonic scalpel technology controls bleeding by coaptive coagulation at low temperatures (50 to 100°C). Vessels are tamponaded and sealed by a protein coagulum.
- Coagulation occurs by means of a protein denaturation when the blade couples with protein, denaturing it to form a coagulum that seals small coapted vessels, when the effect is prolonged, secondary heat is produced that seals larger vessels.

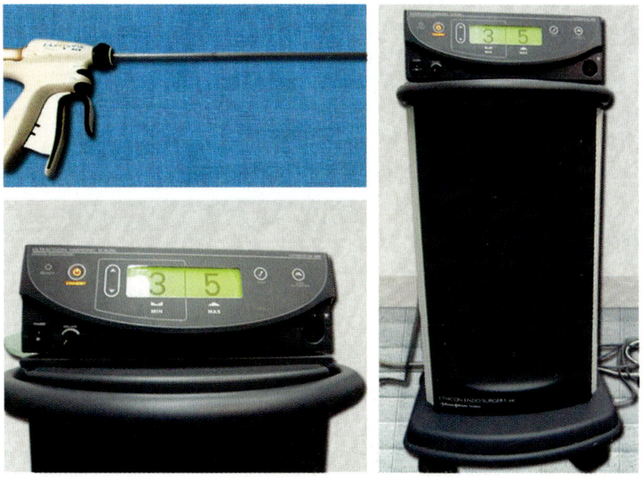

**Fig. 3.5:** Harmonic scalpel machine and forcep

#### *Advantages*

- Minimal lateral thermal tissue damage.
- Minimal charring and desiccation.
- Fewer instrument exchanges simplify procedure steps as it coagulates and cut.
- No electricity to or through the patient.
- Greater precision near vital structures.
- Minimal smoke for improved visibility in the surgical field.
- Lesser wear and tear.

#### *Disadvantages*

- Slower than other energy sources.
- Ultrasonic tip has a limited life span.
- Disposable attachments increase the cost per patient.
- Can not be used as vessel sealing device for vessels with diameter more than 3 mm.

### Argon Beam Coagulator

- Argon beam coagulator used in both open procedures and minimally invasive surgery.
- More effective and cost efficient than conventional electrosurgery.
- Delivers current to the tissue in a directed beam of ionized argon gas.
- Flow of gas blows away blood and debris from the surgical field and produces a coagulated surface that is more uniform and shallower than that produced in standard electrosurgical coagulation.
- Coagulates bleeding tissue faster with reduced blood loss and tissue damage.
- Produce less smoke than conventional electrosurgery.

### Gyrus PK Tissue Management System

The Gyrus PK Tissue Management System instruments provide a unique technology called Vapor pulse coagulation (VPC) and plasma kinetic cutting forceps.

### *Vapor Pulse Coagulation (VPC)*

- Produce faster, more uniform results with pulsed energy instantly delivered in a controlled manner.
- VPC's pulse-off periods allow tissue to cool and moisture to return to the targeted area, greatly reducing hot spots and coagulum formation.
- Results in evenly coagulated target tissue; minimal thermal spread, less sticking, and enhanced hemostasis.
- It does require its own generator, which works in tandem with the instruments manufactured by Gyrus PK.
- This bipolar device is capable of reliably sealing/dividing arteries as large as 6 mm, but it is recommended restricting its use to vessels no larger than 5 mm in diameter to allow a safety margin.
- Thermal spread affects only the area surrounding the divided vessel.

### *Plasma Kinetic Cutting Forceps*

- The second device, the Plasma Kinetic Cutting Forceps, utilizes advanced, solid-state generator software to deliver pulsed energy with continuous feedback control.
- The cycle stops once the device senses that tissue response is complete.
- The cool-down phase ensures that collagen and elastin matrix reforms without tissue fragmentation.

**MESSAGE BOX**

- Electrosurgery is the surgical use of high-frequency electric current that produced by electron movement.
- In electrosurgery, there are some common terms include current, voltage and resistance.
- Electrosurgical generators can apply energy in either a monopolar or bipolar fashion.
- When an electric current flows through biological tissue, we can observe thermal effect, electrolytic effect and faradic effect.
- There are two basic methods of thermal tissue dectruction, which is used in electrosurgery, cutting and coagulation.
- There are many others energy source which is used in surgery, include laser, ultrasound dissector, argon beam coagulator, Gyrus PK tissue management system, and the ligasure system.

## The Ligasure System (Valleylab, Boulder, Colorado)

- Uses a unique combination of pressure and energy to create vessel fusion.
- Melting the collagen and elastin in the vessel walls, and reforming it into a permanent, plastic-like seal accomplish is this fusion.
- A feedback-controlled response system automatically discontinues energy delivery when the seal cycle is complete, eliminating guesswork and minimizing thermal spread to approximately 2 mm for most ligasure instruments.

Chapter

4

# Medicolegal Issues in Endoscopic Surgeries

*Sanjay Gupte*

## MEDICOLEGAL ASPECTS IN ENDOSCOPIC SURGERIES

- Any therapeutic procedure, surgical or medical requires to be offered to the patient within the framework of what is 'ethical.' 'Ethical' implies that the benefits of treatment clearly outweigh the risks of the procedure.
- One has to understand that laparoscopic surgery is a technically driven modality of treatment, which requires training, experience and is typically characterized by a long learning curve till the surgeon establishes skills.
- Evidences in literature have shown that most of the complications occur during the learning curve of the surgeon and therefore, to offer safe technique to patient, it is important to identify your own limitations and capabilities.
- It is imperative that the technique that you use is standardized and the equipment and the instrumentation be of standard quality. This not only offers comfort to the surgeon but also safety and goes a long way in avoiding complications.
- More than 80% of the clinical situations in gynecology today are tackled laparoscopically. The literature unfortunately lacks clear-cut guidelines as to what should and should not be done laparoscopically. These guidelines to be evolved require uniformity of practice, standardization of techniques and modalities. This modality being skill driven also depends upon the competence of the operating surgeon and therefore the need to understand one's own capabilities and limitations. The disease also requires to be properly evaluated and complications, if any, foreseen prior and evaluated.
- It is not only the problem in the court and the public litigation which should be a cause of concern to the surgeon but also the fact that any untoward occurrence or complication receives rejection from the community and therefore one should practice laparoscopy with utmost responsibility and established standards to allow this modality to evolve, progress and receive acceptability.
- One should be utmost careful while selecting the patient, disciplined while performing the surgery and have an open mind toward the need of conversion to the open approach, if the need so arises in the interest of the patient. The need to convert to the open modality should not be considered as a complication of laparoscopic surgery. At any cost, one should not cause any harm to the patient.
- Laparoscopic surgery has distinct advantages and some very important limitations. These require to be understood by the surgeon while offering this mode of treatment to the patient. The patient should be taken into confidence like any other treatment modality that we offer, so that there are no misunderstandings, false assurances and consequently unpleasantness on the part of the patient.
- It is important that a proper preoperative counseling is offered which will go in the long run to avoid any litigations from the patient arising out of this unpleasantness.
- There are no clear cut guidelines for what is right and what is wrong. But the surgeon should, with responsibility be absolutely thorough in documentation and recording of all the events of the surgical session and its aftermath. There are important directives of the Supreme Court with respect to the informed consent in such situations, which were evolved as a result of a case, related to laparoscopic surgery contested in the Supreme Court in the year 1995 under the CPA 1986 Section 21 of Negligence compensation.
- The Supreme Court of India has come out with very important judgment in the case of Sameera Kohli vs Dr Mandhanda, case no. CA 1949 of 1004 decided on 16th January, 2008.

The story goes as such—

The appellant went to the respondent clinic with her mother. On admission, the appellant's signatures were taken on consent form for diagnostic and operative laparoscopy on 10th May 1995—Appellant was put under GA and was subjected to a laparoscopic examination. When the appellant was still unconscious, assistant doctor came out of the operation theater and took the consent for hysterectomy from the appellant's mother, who was waiting outside. Thereafter, the respondent performed an abdominal hysterectomy and bilateral salpingo-oophorectomy and this case went against the respondent resulting in the Supreme Court summarizing the principles relating to consent as follows:

1. A doctor has to seek and secure the consent of the patient before commencing a treatment (the term treatment includes surgery also). The consent so obtained should be real and valid which means that; the patient should have the capacity and the competence to consent; his consent should be voluntary; and his consent should be on the basis of adequate information concerning the nature of the treatment procedure, so that he knows what he is consenting to.
2. The adequate information to be furnished by the doctor (or a member of his team) who treats the patient, should enable the patient to make balanced judgment as to whether he should submit himself to the particular treatment or not. This means that the doctor should disclose:
   i. Nature and procedure of the treatment and its purpose, benefits and effect
   ii. Alternatives, if any, available
   iii. An outline of the substantial risks
   iv. Adverse consequences of refusing treatment.
3. But there is no need to explain remote or theoretical risks involved, which may frighten or confuse the patient and result in refusal of consent for the necessary treatment. Similarly, there is no need to persuade a patient to undergo a fanciful or unnecessary treatment. A balanced should be achieved between the need for disclosing necessary and adequate information and at the same time, avoid the possibility of the patient being deterred from agreeing to a necessary treatment or offering to undergo an unnecessary treatment.
4. Consent given only for a diagnostic procedure, cannot be considered as consent for the therapeutic treatment. Consent given for a specific treatment procedure will not be valid for conducting some other treatment procedure. The fact that the unauthorized additional surgery is beneficial to the patient, or that it would save considerable time and expense to the patient or would relieve the patient from pain and suffering in future, are not grounds of defense in action in tort for negligence or assault and battery. The only exception to the rule is where the additional procedure though unauthorized, is necessary in order to save the life or preserve the health of the patient and it would be unreasonable to delay such unauthorized procedure until patient regains consciousness and takes a decision.
5. There can be common consent for diagnostic and operative procedures where they are contemplated. There can also be a common consent for a particular procedure and an additional or further procedure that may become necessary during the course of surgery.
6. The nature and extent of information to be furnished by the doctor to the patient to secure the consent need not be of the stringent and high degree mentioned in Canterbury, but should be of the extent which is accepted as normal and proper by a body of medical men skilled and experienced in the particular field. It will depend upon the physical and mental condition of the patient, the nature of treatment, the risk and the consequences attached to the treatment.
7. In view of our finding, that there was no consent by the appellant for performing hysterectomy and salpingo-oophorectomy, performance of such a surgery was an unauthorized invasion and interference with appellant's body, which amounted to a tortuous act of assault and battery and therefore a deficiency of service. But as noticed above, there are several mitigating circumstances. The respondent did it in the interest of the appellant. As the appellant was already 44 years old, and was having serious menstrual problems, the respondent thought that by surgical removal of the uterus and ovaries, she was providing permanent relief. It is also possible that the respondent thought that the appellant may approve the additional surgical procedure when she regained consciousness and the consent by appellant's mother gave her the authority to do the same.
8. This is a case of respondent acting in excess of consent but in good faith and for the benefit of the appellant. Though the appellant has alleged that she had to undergo hormone therapy, no other repercussions is made out as a result of the removal. The appellant was already fast approaching the age of menopause, and in all probability required such hormone therapy. Even assuming that AH-BSO surgery was not immediately required, there was a reasonable certainty that she would have ultimately required the said treatment for a complete cure.
9. On the facts and circumstances, we consider that interests of justice would be served if the respondent is denied the entire fee charged for the surgery and in addition, directed to pay Rs. 25,000 as compensation for the unauthorized AH-BSO surgery to the appellant.

10. This particular Supreme Court ruling along with the elaborate case has been on purpose included for each one of us to be able to device a proper consent under the guidelines laid down by the Supreme Court of India.
11. Proper equipment has to be available.
12. Careful case selection is important.
13. Detailed communication complications and develop a standardized system and a habit to remain within the ethical framework.

## TIPS

- The surgeon should be adequately trained as regards the procedure and informed consent is vital.
- Standard techniques should be followed.
- The procedure and especially the precautions taken should be documented.
- Possibility of complications, especially in a high risk patient, should be counseled well in advance.
- Postoperative instructions and follow-up should not be neglected.

Chapter

5

# Prevention of Complications in Endoscopic Surgeries

*PG Paul, Renuka Borisa, P Biju, Kannan K, Fiadjoe P*

## INTRODUCTION

Complications are inherent in any surgical procedure and laparoscopy is no exception. Since complications can occur even with a relatively easy procedure, it is imperative that all surgeons must learn to recognize the complications expeditiously and manage the events.

The risks increase exponentially with the complexity of procedures, the inexperience of the surgeon and with any deviation from the standard techniques.

The learning curve for laparoscopic procedures is lengthy and the risk of complications is greatest in the early period of the surgeon's learning.

**Preoperative complications** can be at different stages, such as given below.

## PREVENTION OF PREOPERATIVE COMPLICATION

### During Anesthesia

- Proper preoperative workup of the patient with cardio-respiratory assessment.
- Sensitivity of the drugs to be checked.
- Monitoring of the patient with pulse oxymetry, cardiogram and ET $CO_2$ to prevent complications.
- Prolonged ventilation with difficult intubation may fill the stomach with air and make it prone for injury with Veress needle or trocar hence Ryle's tube instillation is necessary to decompress the stomach just prior to veress insertion.
- Ryle's tube instillation to prevent Mendelson's syndrome.
- General anesthesia combined with epidural in long cases helps to keep bowel collapsed and decrease oozing.

### During Positioning of Patient

Prevention of nerve injuries especially those involving the brachial plexus, ulnar, femoral and common peroneal nerves.

- Padded Allen stirrups provide good support and allow proper positioning which can be changed in a draped position during surgery.
- In lithotomy position, good cushion support prevents injury to common peroneal nerve (Fig. 5.1).
- Shoulder rest should be placed laterally on acromio-clavicular joint to prevent injury of brachial plexus (Fig. 5.2).
- Placing the left arm extended at the elbow joint, pronated and tucked loosely by the side of the body and the right arm flexed and kept on the chest as if on a sling can prevent both ulnar and brachial plexus injuries (Figs 5.3A and B).

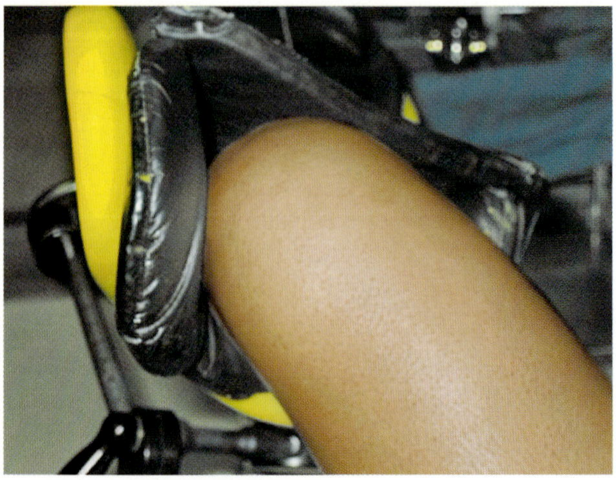

**Fig. 5.1:** Care of popliteal fossa

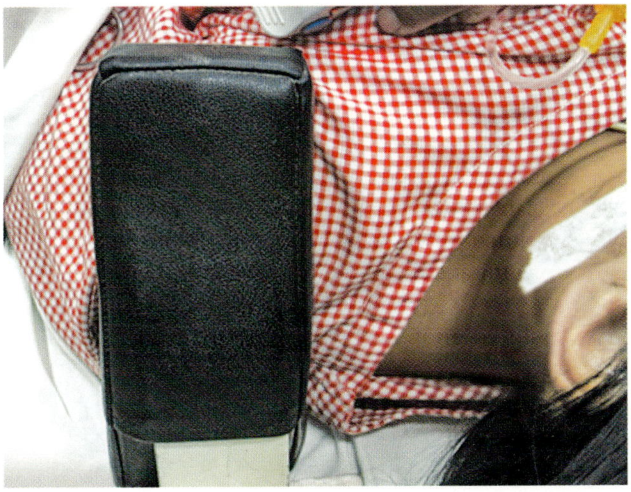

Fig. 5.2: Care of Shoulders

## During the Technique

### *Prevention of Complications due to Pneumoperitoneum*

- Pneumoperitoneum pressure should not exceed more than 15 mm of Hg to avoid cardiorespiratory embarrassment and injuries to major vessels.
- Entry of veress needle or trocar in peritoneal cavity should be confirmed before starting inflow of $CO_2$ to prevent complications due to extra-peritoneal insufflation.
- Embolization can be prevented by use of $CO_2$ for pneumoperitoneum than air.

### *Prevention of Trocar or Veress Needle Injuries*

Most of the vessel injuries are mainly due to technical errors and hence these need to be corrected by —

- Proper stabilization of abdominal wall during trocar insertion.
- Avoid forceful and jerky trocar insertion, guard trocar with index finger tip to prevent sudden and wrong entry of trocar. Screwing motion gives better control than direct thrusting.
- Visualization of inferior epigastric vessels before insertion of ancillary trocars.
- Direction of entry of trocar should be towards the tip of coccyx (Fig. 5.4).
- All accessory trocars should be placed under vision.
- In cases of previous scarred surgery, (laparoscopic/laparotomy) it is preferable to use Palmer's point for primary trocar insertion (Fig. 5.5).
- Do not give head low position unless primary port is taken.

### *Prevention of Bowel Injuries*

- Good bowel preparation is must prior to any laparoscopic surgery.
- Open trocar entry by Hasson's technique or Palmer's point entry in cases of previous scarred surgery.
- Instruments with defective insulation should be discarded and not repaired.
- Avoid dangling of instruments especially monopolar and bipolar forceps at a time inside the peritoneal cavity at the beginning and learning curve.
- Use of plastic abdominal wall grips with metal cannula should be avoided to prevent bowel injury by direct coupling.

### *Prevention of Urinary Tract Injuries*

- Bladder should be emptied adequately before veress or primary trocar insertion.

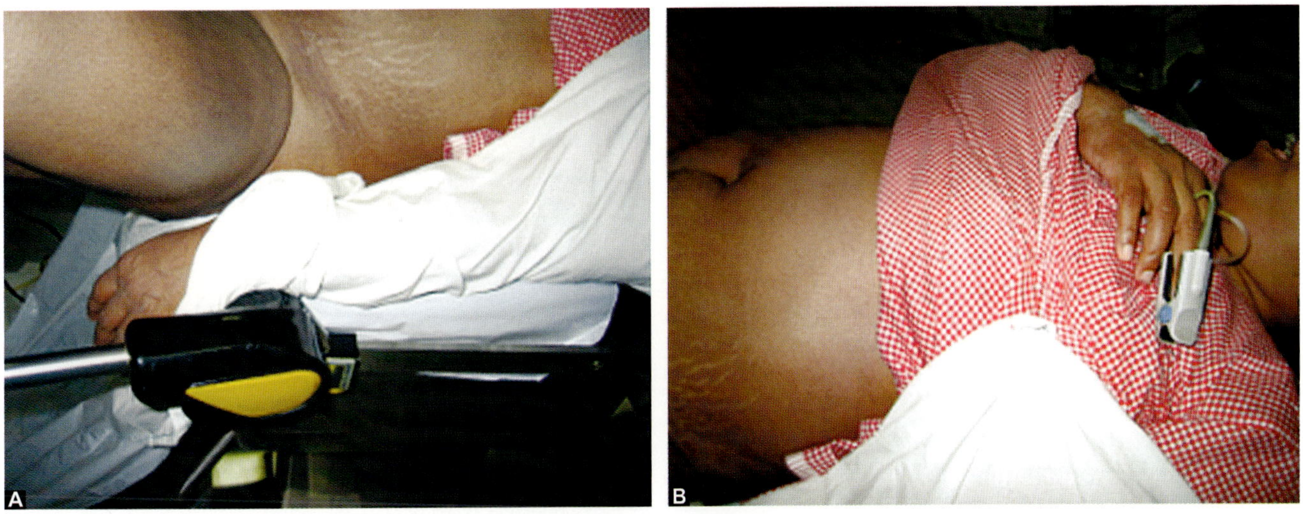

Fig. 5.3A and B: Care of arms

***Every surgery open or endoscopic has its own share of complications. The greatest hazard to the patient is not the surgery but the 'Surgeon'***

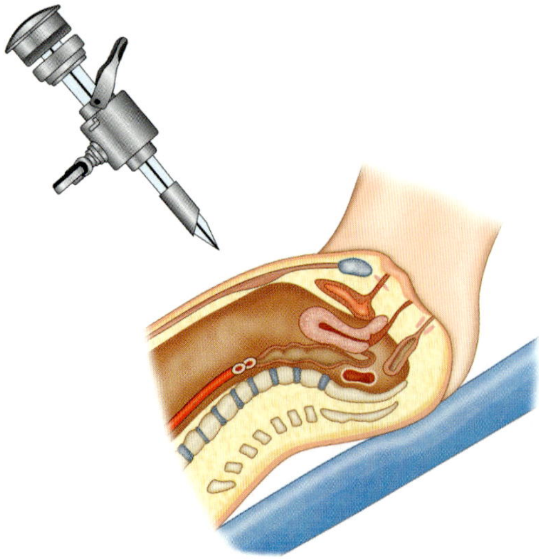

**Fig. 5.4:** Correct direction of entry of trocar

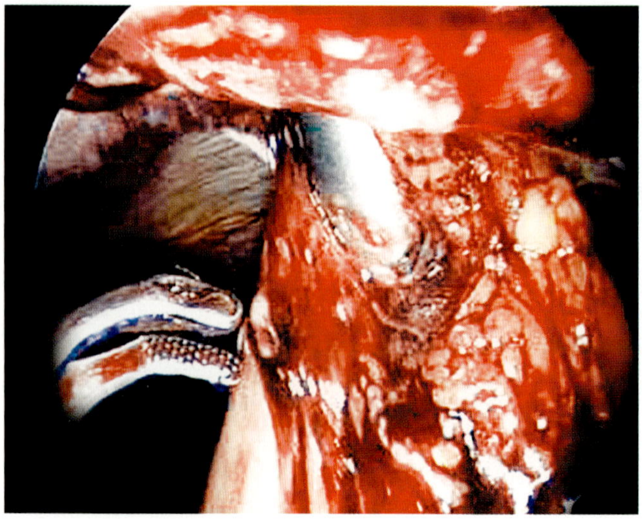

**Fig. 5.5:** Entry of primary trocar directly in bowel

- Good tissue planes and proper dissection of bladder during the procedure prevents bladder injuries.
- While performing hysterectomy—tips to prevent bladder and ureteric injuries (refer to respective chapters).
- Ureteric stenting in case of extensive adhesions, e.g. endometriosis, prevents injury to the ureter.

### *Prevention of Electrosurgical Injuries*

- Periodic check of instruments is must to find out any break or breach in insulation.
- Whole length of the cautery pad should be in contact with the broad skin surface of the buttock or legs to prevent skin burns.
- All instruments carrying monopolar current should be inspected regularly for insulation. Monopolar cautery can not be used under water or free in air as current spreads or jumps to near by organs.

### *Morcellator Related Injuries*

- The rotating blade of the morcellator should be visible throughout the procedure and it should be retracted when not in use.
- The specimen should be completely separated from surrounding structures and vessels before the morcellation.

## PREVENTION OF POSTOPERATIVE COMPLICATIONS

- Early ambulation.
- Coverage of antibiotics—intraoperative and postoperative period.
- Deep breathing exercises.
- Ensure adequate hydration on previous day especially for patients who are on bowel preparation to prevent postoperative electrolyte imbalance in extensive cases.
- Early suspicion in case of abnormal signs and symptoms.

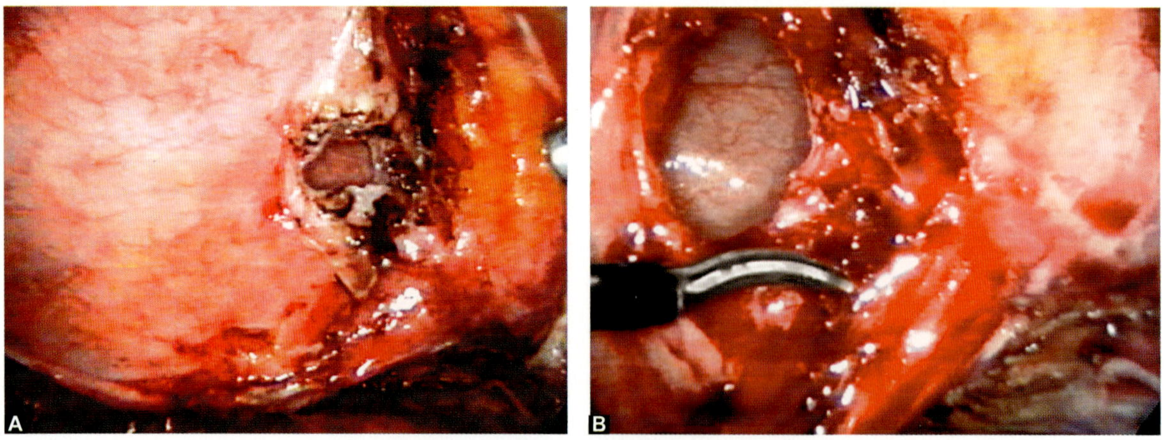

**Figs 5.6A and B:** Inadvertent opening of bladder

***Every surgeon should pick up the right surgical technique for the right patient, understating his/her limitations and mastery over the technique.***

**TIPS**

- Use of stockings and or anticoagulants to prevent deep vein thrombosis.
- Keeping operating time to a minimum by improving surgical skills and standard equipment.
- Suturing rectus sheath whenever incision more than 7 mm is taken and using 'Z' technique for primary trocar insertion can prevent herniation.
- Exposure, identification of anatomic landmarks and careful dissection will reduce the risk of ureteric injury.
- The presence of gas and/or blood in the urinary drainage bag allows early recognition of bladder injury. Cystoscopy is confirmatory.

## PREVENTION OF COMPLICATIONS DURING HYSTEROSCOPY

### Preoperative Prevention

- By using an ideal distending media, in right quantity, water intoxication and hyponatremia can be prevented.
- Uterine perforation is the commonest complication that can be encountered during septum resection, adhesiolysis of Ashermann's syndrome and myomectomy, which can be prevented by—
    - Gentle cervical dilatation.
    - Introduction of hysteroscope under vision.
    - Using energy setting appropriate for the procedure.
    - Making all cutting strokes from fundus toward cervix or lateral alternating technique in case of broader septum.
    - By recognizing thinness of cornual opening and obeying 1st law of holes, i.e. stop digging once inside the holes.
    - By performing simultaneous laparoscopy.
    - During septum resection in its final phase by stopping the resection till small area of bleeding is seen indicating myometrium is reached.
    - Should get reorientation of cavity from time to time by withdrawing telescope till internal os and taking panaromic view.
- Over abduction of the thighs to be avoided.
- Keeping operating time to a minimum.
- Detection of fluid overload by signs and symptoms like transient hypertension followed by hypotension.
- Keep fluid pressures below 80 mm Hg.
- Meticulous accountancy of fluid balance.
- The procedure must be abandoned if the deficit rises to 2 liters or there is evidence of venous congestion.
- In case of suspected electric injury after uterine perforation, laparoscopy may be performed to examine bowel, pelvic blood vessels and aorta.

**TIPS**

- Every surgery open or endoscopic has its own share of complications. The greatest hazard to the patient is not the surgery but the 'Surgeon'.
- Every surgeon should pick up the right surgical technique for the right patient, understating his/her limitations and mastery over the technique."

# Chapter 6

# Port Placement

*Sunita R Tandulwadkar*

Usually in gynecologic endoscopic surgeries, all ports are at and below umbilicus level but position of the ports either in lower or upper abdomen depends upon the size and pathology of uterus and if any previous lower abdominal surgeries done.

## ROUTINE PORT PLACEMENTS

Usually 3 to 4 ports are taken.

### Primary Port

- Taken either infraumbilical or intraumbilical:
  - Veress needle for pneumoperitoneum followed by 10 mm trocar insertion, or
  - Direct 10 mm trocar insertion.

### Ancillary Ports

- Two 5 mm ports on surgeon's side, 10 cm apart
  - Lower port in iliac fossa, approximately 2 fingers medial and 1 finger above anterior superior iliac spine.
  - Upper port 10 cm up and little medial to lower port.
- Third 5 mm port is on the contralateral side usually in line with the primary trocar (A) or can also be taken in similar manner as lower port of ipsilateral side (B) as shown in Figures 6.1.

## IN DIFFICULT SITUATIONS, LIKE

- Previous lower abdominal surgeries
- Large myomas
- Large adenexal masses.

**TIPS**

- Left-sided (surgeon's side) lower 5 mm port should be valveless to carry suture material. Right-sided 5 mm port should have outlet to remove the smoke intermittently.
- Ancillary ports are introduced always under vision.
- Site of ancillary ports is the individual's choice as per the suturing techniques and height of surgeon. For example, one can take one port on each side and third in the suprapubic area.

### Primary Port

- At Palmer's point with 5 mm trocar.
  Under vision, 10 mm trocar is passed at epigastric region (below xiphisternum) or supraumbilical region. 5 mm trocar at Palmer's point is then converted into ancillary port.
- At supraumbilical region 2–3 fingers above umbilicus.

**TIPS**

- While entering Palmer's point, three resistances are encountered:
  - Anterior rectus sheath
  - Posterior rectus sheath
  - Parietal peritoneum.
- Before selection of Palmer's point ensure
  - Deflation of stomach with Ryle's tube
  - Absence of splenomegaly.
- Care has to be taken when primary supraumbilical port is taken, as bifurcation of aorta and inferior vena cava will come directly under the entry of the trocar.

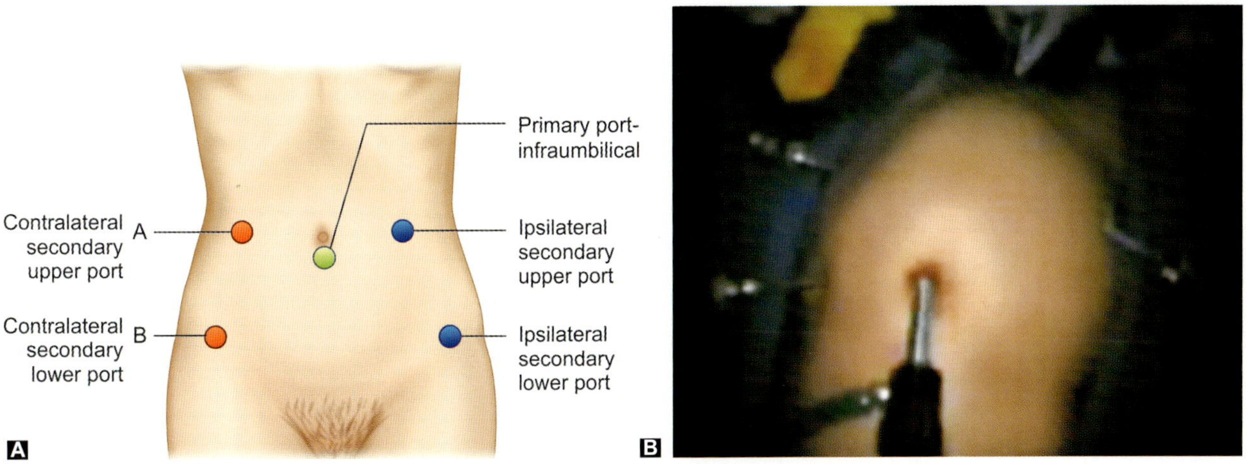


**Figs 6.1A and B:** Routine port placements

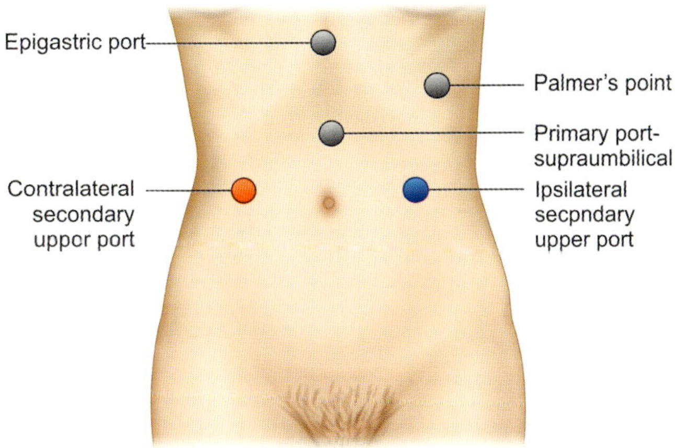


**Fig. 6.2:** Difficult port placements

## Hasson's Technique of Open Trocar Insertion

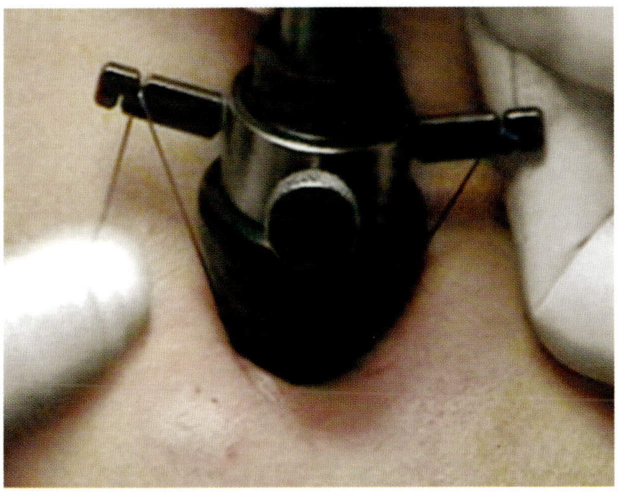

**Fig. 6.3:** Intraumbilical incision

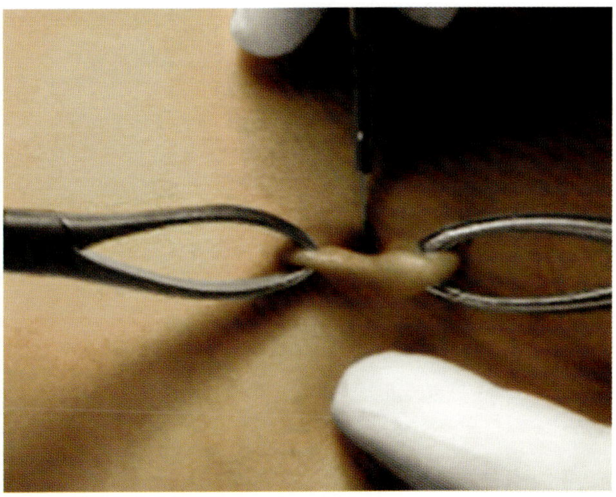

**Fig. 6.4:** Rectus sheath exposed

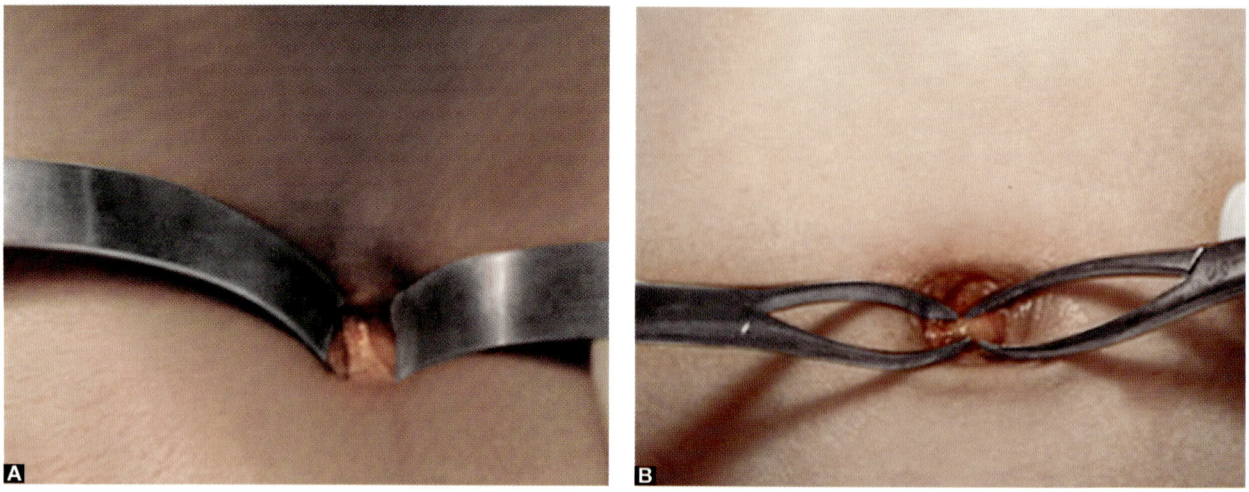

**Figs 6.5A and B:** Rectus sheath hold and cut

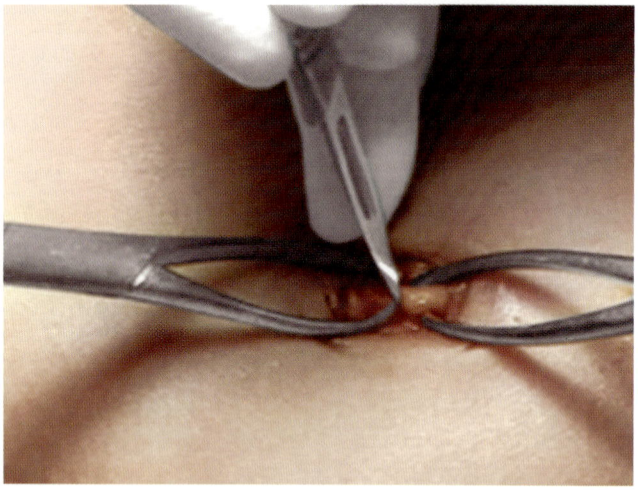

**Fig. 6.6:** Peritoneum dissected

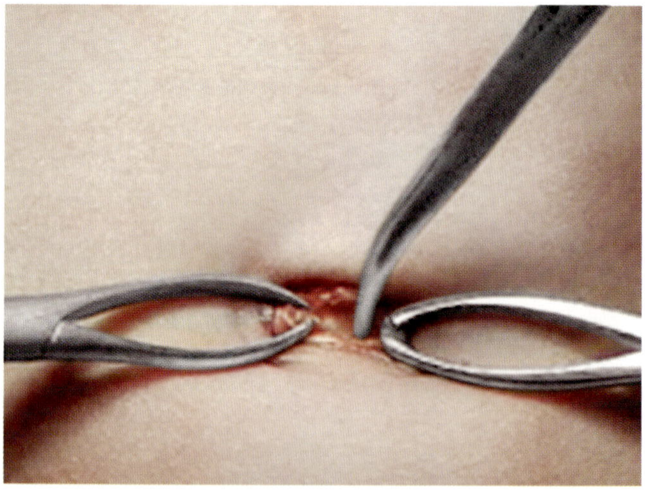

**Fig. 6.7:** Peritoneum opened after taking stitches at rectus, one on each side

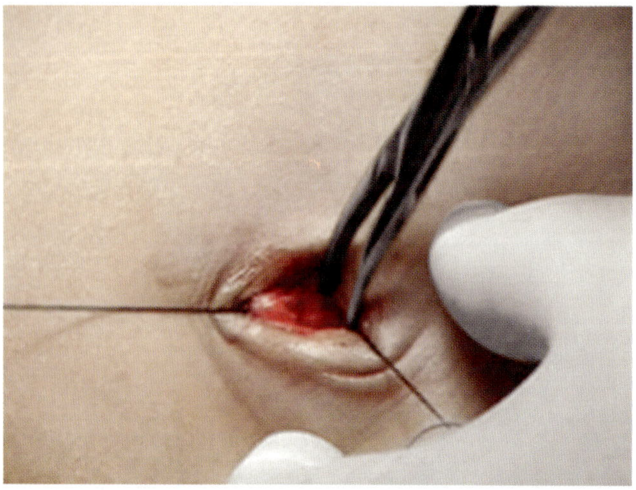

**Fig. 6.8:** Hasson's trocar in place

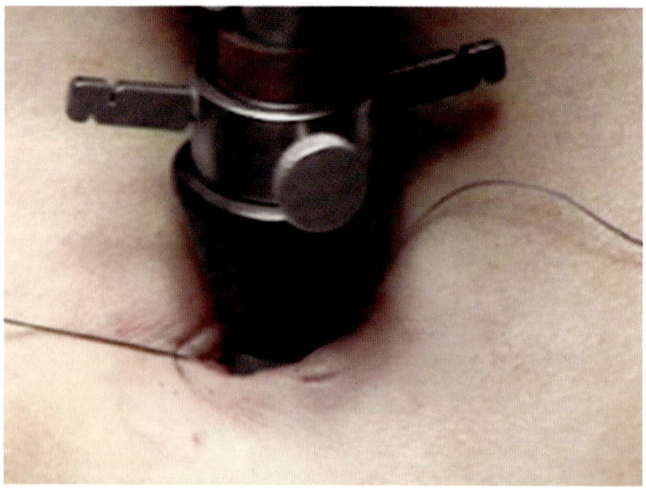

**Fig. 6.9:** Hasson's trocar fixed with stitches taken at rectus

## TIPS

- As the size of the uterus/pelvic pathology increases, the site of port placement shifts higher and higher.
- Port placement should be made in such a way that the tip of the telescope is at least 4 inches above the pelvic pathology which is to be operated so as to get a good field of vision.

Chapter

7

# Laparoscopic Suturing

*Alessandro Loddo, Vito Cofelice, Gian Benedetto Melis*

## INTRODUCTION

The proficiency with laparoscopic suturing is of a crucial importance as it not only allows the performance of a wide range of complex operative scenarios, but also is an essential skill required for dealing with intraoperative complications.

Laparoscopic suturing techniques can be classified as *intracorporeal* and *extracorporeal*.

- In the *intracorporeal technique*, the knot is tied inside the abdominal cavity using two instruments: two needle holder or one needle holder and one assistant forceps.
- In the *extracorporeal technique*, the knot is performed outside the abdominal cavity; afterwards it is pushed inside the abdominal cavity with a knot pusher.

### The Half-knot

This is an incomplete basic knot; it is very easy to untie.

To tie this knot, both the ends of the suture must be pulled in opposite directions with uniform tension. A hypothetical midline divides this knot in two symmetrically identical parts (Fig. 7.1).

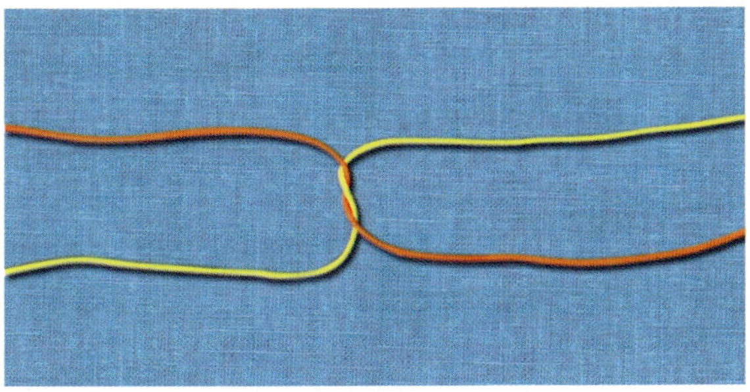

**Fig. 7.1:** Half-knot

### The Slipknot

This is another incomplete basic knot; it is asymmetrical; when tying this knot, each thread has a different role: One remains inactive (passive thread) and the other, called active thread, forms the knot by wrapping around the other one (Fig. 7.2).

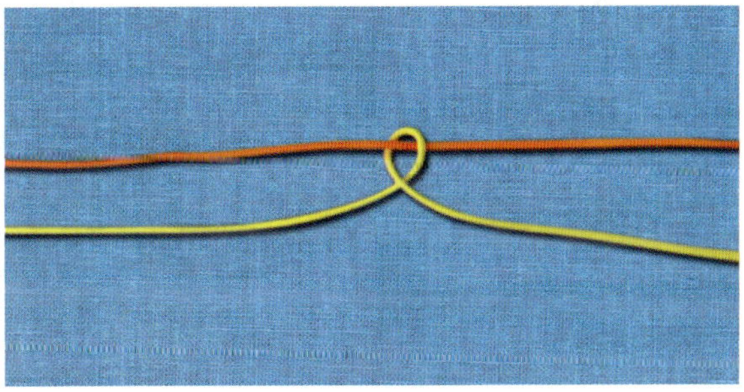

**Fig. 7.2:** Slipknot

The half-knot and the slipknot are the essential bases to build a complete knot, which is composed of a correct sequence of half-knots and/or slipknots.

### The Square Knot

*The square knot* is the sequence of two identical half knots (Figs 7.3 and 7.4).

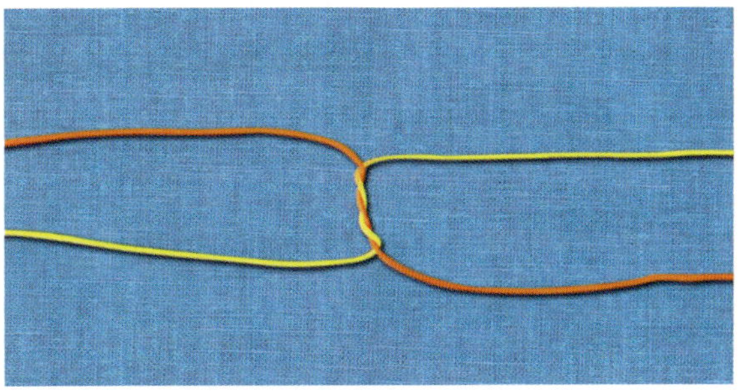

**Fig. 7.3:** Square knot

### The Surgical Knot

*The surgical knot* is a blocking sequence of three half knots or slipknots.

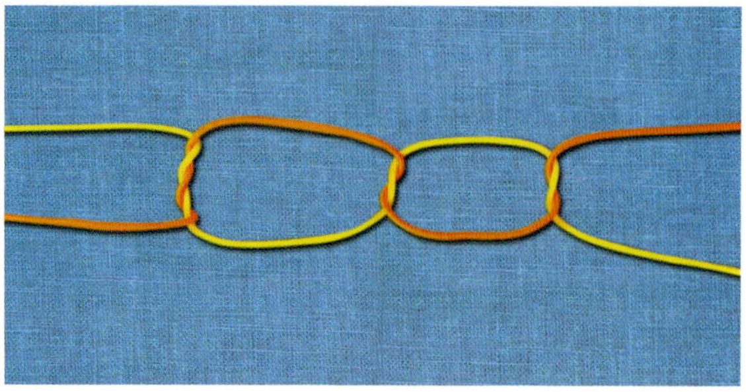

**Fig. 7.4:** Square knot

## The Knot Blocking Sequence

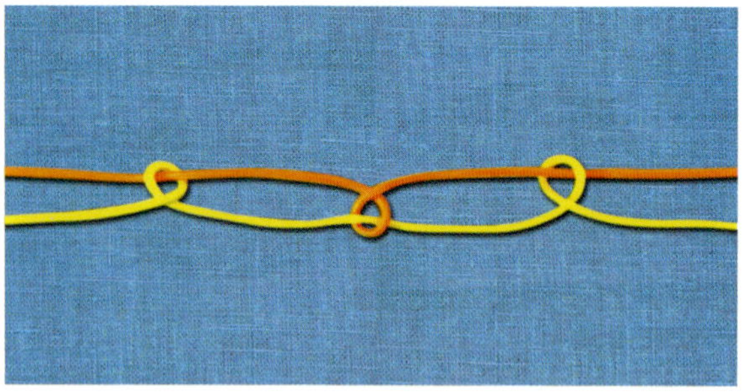

**Fig. 7.5:** Knot blocking sequence

It is a series of half knots and/or slipknots that confers to the knot the maximum strength, which is equal to the maximum tensile strength of the suture that will always break close to the knot (Fig. 7.5).

The block is total and any force applied in an attempt to move the knot in one or the opposite direction will inevitably fail and the result will be the breakage of the suture.

# MAKING THE IDEAL STITCH

In the perfect stitch, the needle penetrates the tissue with an entry angle of 90 degrees in relation to the axis of the wound.

The major axis of the needle holder and the placed needle will form a 90 degrees angle.

So the ideal suturing conditions are achieved if the needle holder is parallel to the suture line and the needle is orthogonal to both suture line and needle holder.

However, in theater, due to fixed trocar sites, the perfect stitch is not always feasible; so all surgical skills of the surgeons should be focused on the idea that you must be able to use both hands to achieve the best position of the needle holder.

At the beginning of a surgical procedure the most ergonomic site for trocar placement should be planned in accordance with the area that needs to be sutured.

Ergonomics in movements and disposing operative trocars is of fundamental importance during the execution of endoscopic suturing because the problems in performing these actions laparoscopically are due to obliged fulcrum point that inhibits a great variety of movements that are easy and feasible when you perform open surgery.

Clearly, the surgeon should be able to perform as close as possible the ideal of a perfect stitch, modifying the access point of needle holders and the angles between needle holder and wound plan and the tissue orientation.

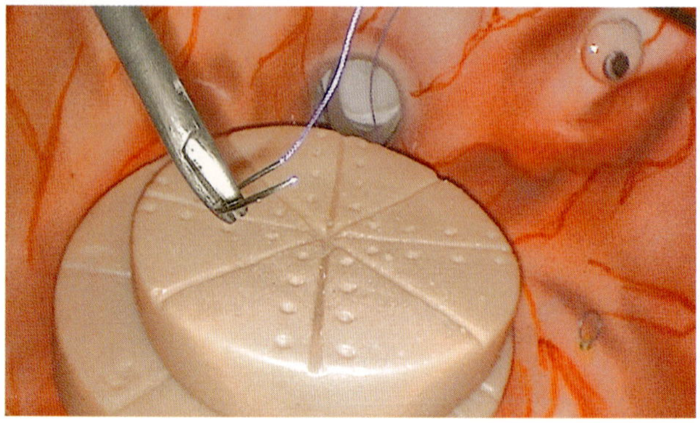

**Fig. 7.6:** Suturing technique

# SUTURING TECHNIQUES

## Intracorporeal Knots

Laparoscopic intracorporeal suturing is one of the most difficult skills in minimally invasive surgery to master.

Intracorporeal knot tying consists of reproduction of the same movements of traditional open surgery with the restriction of degrees of freedom due to fixed trocar sites.

### *Gladiator Rule (Fig. 7.7)*

According to this technique, to tie an intracorporeal knot, it is important to perform the following steps in order:

1. The assistant needle holder picks up the suture 2 cm from the needle.
2. The horizon, defined as the first part of the thread, is created from the assistant needle holder.
3. The needle holder with its open branches acts like the hand of a Roman Imperator, who saved or sentenced to death the gladiator by rotating his thumb (opening the moving branch of the needle holder) up or down, with a 180 degrees rotation around the axis of the needle holder.
4. The needle holder passes behind the thread, called the horizon, with the movable branch open downward. The needle holder then rotates 180 degrees to return to its initial position. The movement is repeated so as to create two turns of thread around the needle holder. This is the basis for a double flat knot. The needle holder grasps the tail of the thread. The two ends are then pulled in opposite directions to create a double flat knot.
5. The " gladiator rule" is repeated a second time to fix the node. In this case, the open branch of the needle holder begins the winding with the movable branch open

upwards, so as to create a reverse knot. The needle holder grasps the tail of the thread. The two ends are then pulled in opposite directions to fix the first knot.

6. The "gladiator rule" is repeated a third time to block the node. In this case, the open branch of the needle holder begins the winding with the movable branch open downwards, so as to create a knot similar to the first one. The needle holder grasps the tail of the thread. The two ends are then pulled in opposite directions to block the first and second knots.

The sequence of knots upon described is a blocking sequence.

In October 2006, the rule was first presented during the 15th ESGE congress in Strasbourg.

In 2013 Mereu et al. published an article about a model course to teach this intracorporeal suturing technique.

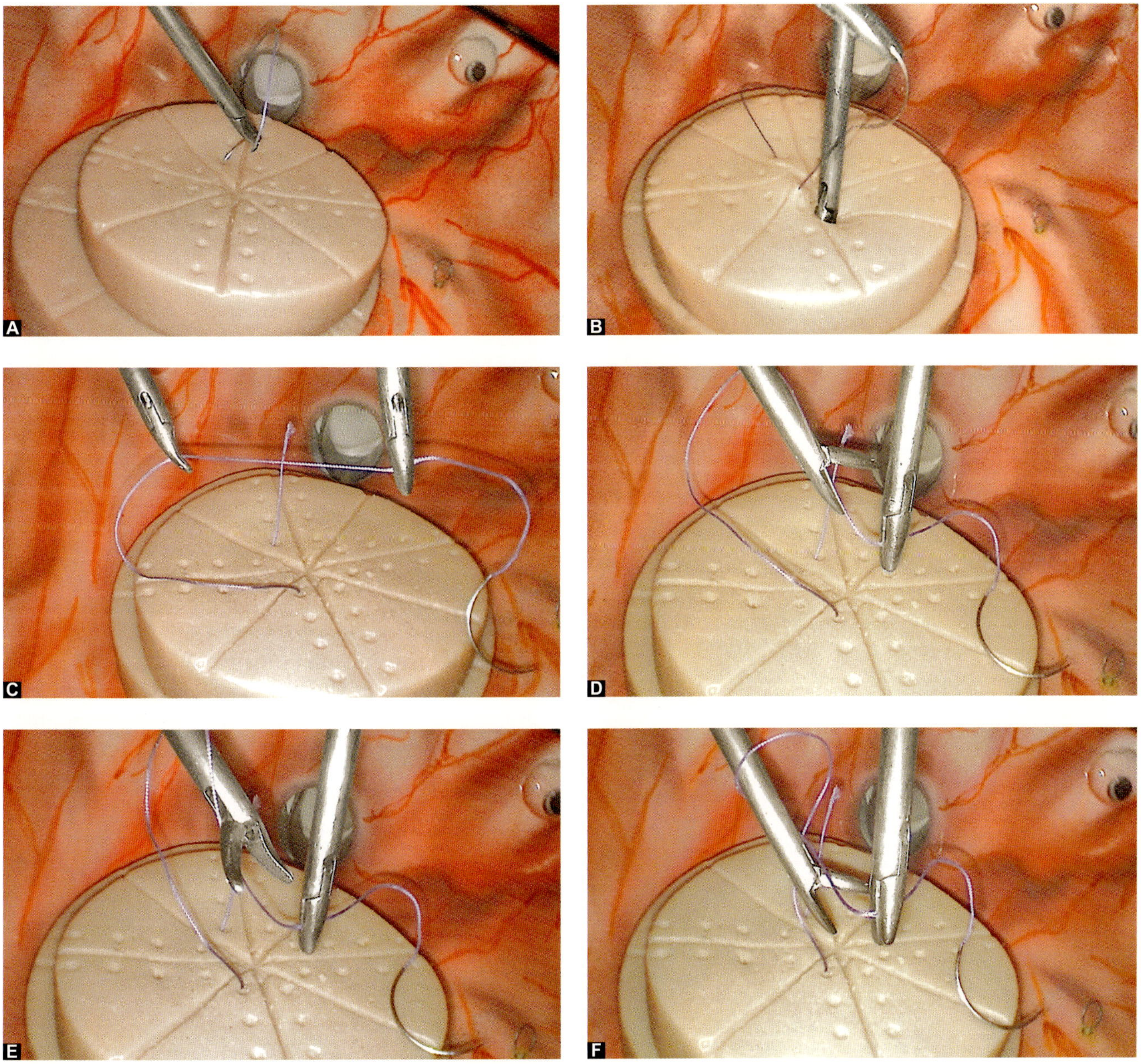


*Contd...*

*Contd...*

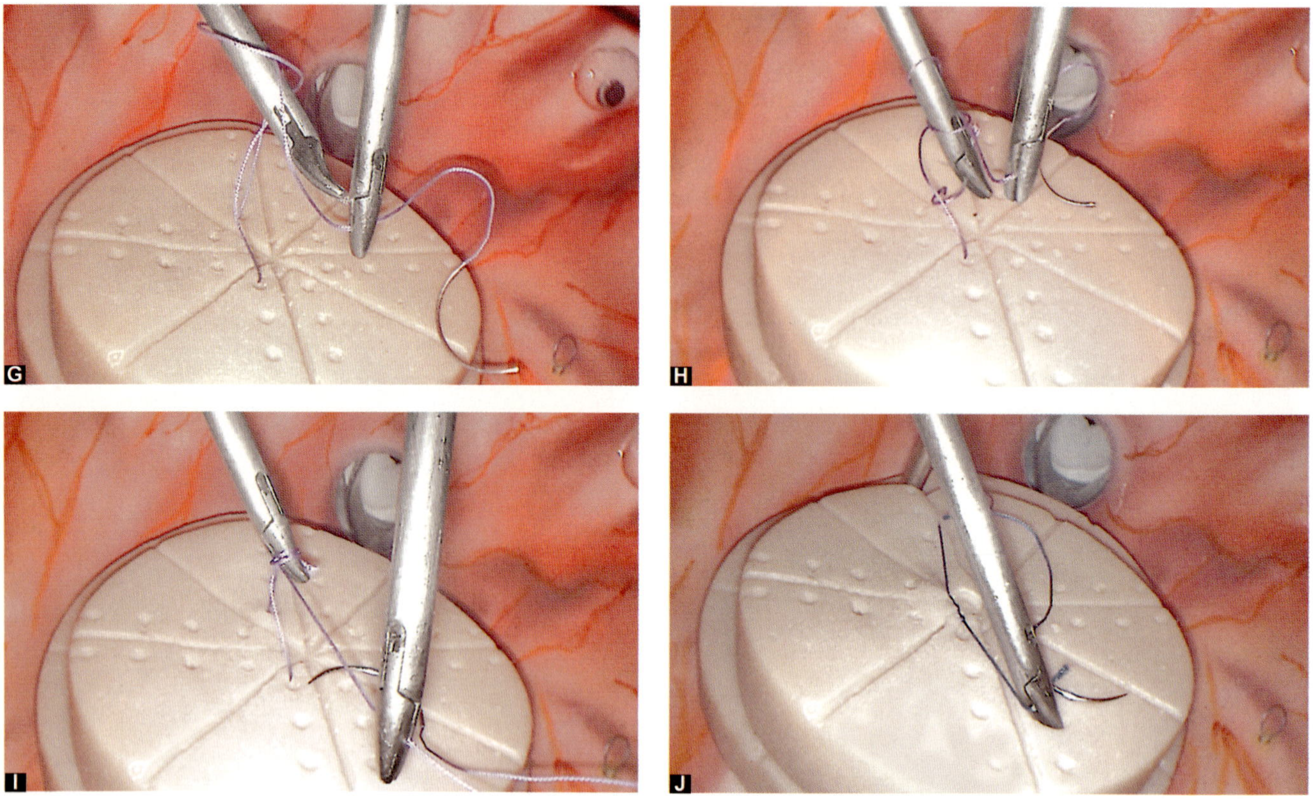

**Figs 7.7A to J:** Gladiator rule

### *C-loop Technique (Fig. 7.8)*

In this alternative suturing technique, you must consider where the tail of the thread exits from the tissue. If the exit is on the right, the right instrument has to form the loop with right concavity (forming a C-loop); the suture has to be wrapped twice around the left -hand needle holder, and the short tail of the thread is pulled through the loops (a square knot is achieved).

Next, the left instrument has to form the loop with left concavity (forming an inverted C–loop); so the thread is wrapped once around the right-hand needle holder, and the short tail is pulled through this loop (an half knot).

Finally, the thread is wrapped around the left-hand needle holder again, and the tail of the thread is pulled through this final loop (surgical knot).

Anyway, the configuration of C-loop or inverted C-loop is a fundamental step for the following wrapping.

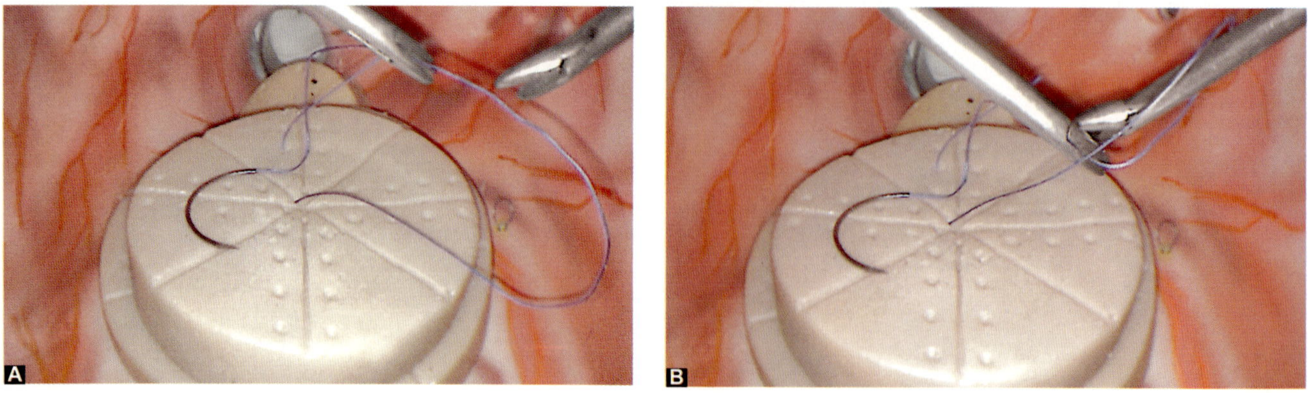

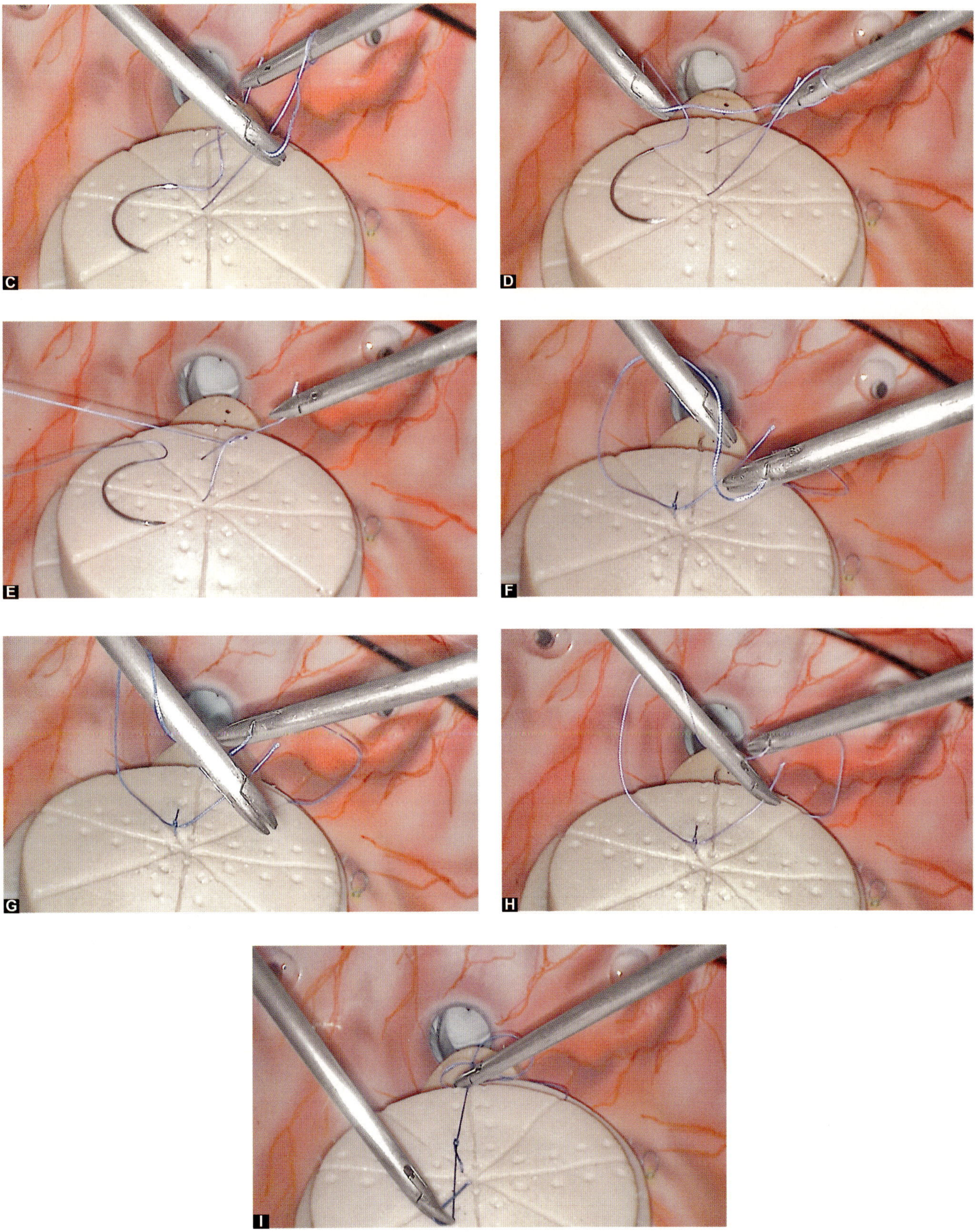


**Figs 7.8A to I:** C-loop technique

## Materials and Methods

We used a multiple-suturing model (EVA II generation ETX A1 LAP; Pro Delphus, Pernambuco, Brazil) as pelvic trainer.

One transumbilical 12 mm-trocar and three 5 mm trocars (two lateral and one soprapubic) were introduced through the ETX 10 abdominal wall (Pro Delphus). A 20 cm 2/0 polyglactin 910 suture (Vicryl®; Ethicon Inc., Johnson and Johnson, Somerville, NJ) on a half-circle cylindrical-section 27 mm needle was used. Laparoscopic instruments included two KOH macroneedle holders (one introduced through the right-side trocar and moved by the right hand of the surgeon and the other introduced through the soprapubic trocar, moved by the left hand of the surgeon, Karl Storz), and one scissors ( Metzenbaum Scissors, Karl Storz) (introduced through the left side trocar and moved by the left hand of the surgeon).

## Extracorporeal Knots (Fig. 7.9)

The knot is totally performed outside the abdominal cavity; after that it is pushed down with a knot pusher in the abdominal cavity.

In an extracorporeal sliding knot can be distinguished a working and a non-working thread.

The non-working thread is the thread that remains passive during knot tying; the working thread has an active rule: it wraps on the passive one during knot preparation.

The suture length should be at least of 100–150 cm in order to permit the execution of the knot outside the abdominal cavity correctly.

Various kinds of extracorporeal knots were proposed: Roeder knot, Duncan loop, Nicky' s knot, Tennessee slider, SMC knot, Weston knot, Meltzer, Tayside knot and others.

All are variants of extracorporeal slip knot.

These knotting techniques are variations in numbers of knots and in wrapping around the axis of passive thread.

Each technique has its supporters and some have been modified to improve; there are some limits with these techniques in terms of size of suture material, the numbers of knots that can be applied at once, and the grade of sliding to perform the knot.

It is important to learn at least one knotting technique and use it when requested.

We have decided to propose and teach the Roeder knot.

*Roeder knot:* It is probably the most efficient among extracorporeal knots; an otolaryngologist first described it to lock the vascular pedicle in tonsillectomy.

It is used to make loops homemade (similar to preformed endo-loops).

The technique is the following: first it is performed a single flat knot (or half knot); then the free tail of the suture wraps three times around the top of a suture loop and locks it with a single throw through the proximal suture leg of the loop. Once the knot is tightened, the free end of the suture is cut to approximately 3 mm.

### *Steps*

1. A single throw is initiated.
2. The free tail of the suture is wrapped around the top of the suture loop.
3. Three additional coils are wrapped around the suture loop.
4. The free tail of the suture is tied around the proximal leg of the loop, from the anterior to posterior, forming a half-hitch.
5. The free tail of the suture is thrown between the second and the last coil.
6. Final configuration of a Roeder knot is achieved.

## Extracorporeal Sliding Knots (Fig. 7.10)

According this technique, extracorporeal half hitches are performed outside the abdominal cavity and then are pushed down in cavity until tightening over the suture line.

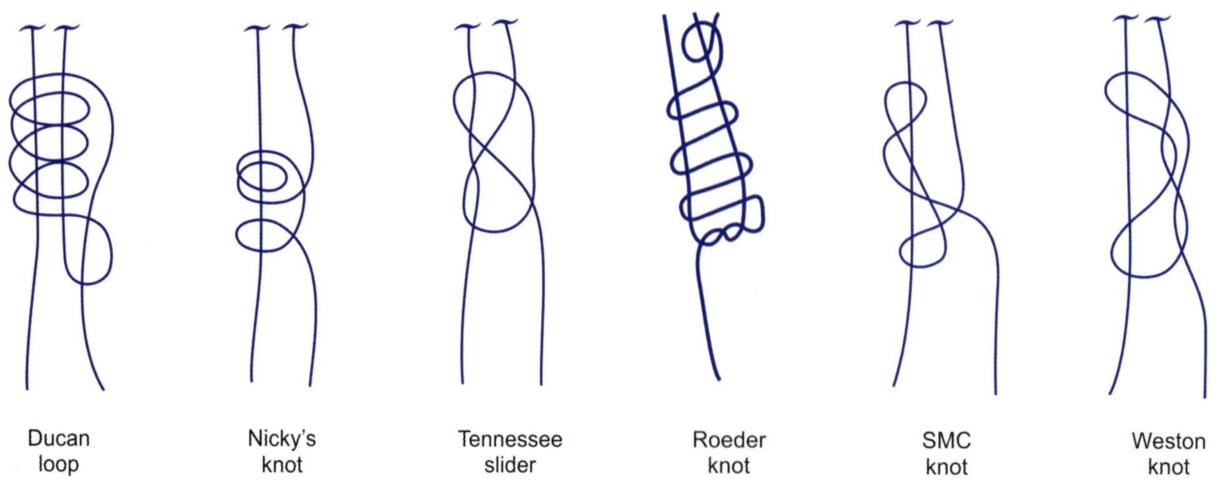


**Fig. 7.9:** Different type of extracorporeal sliding knots

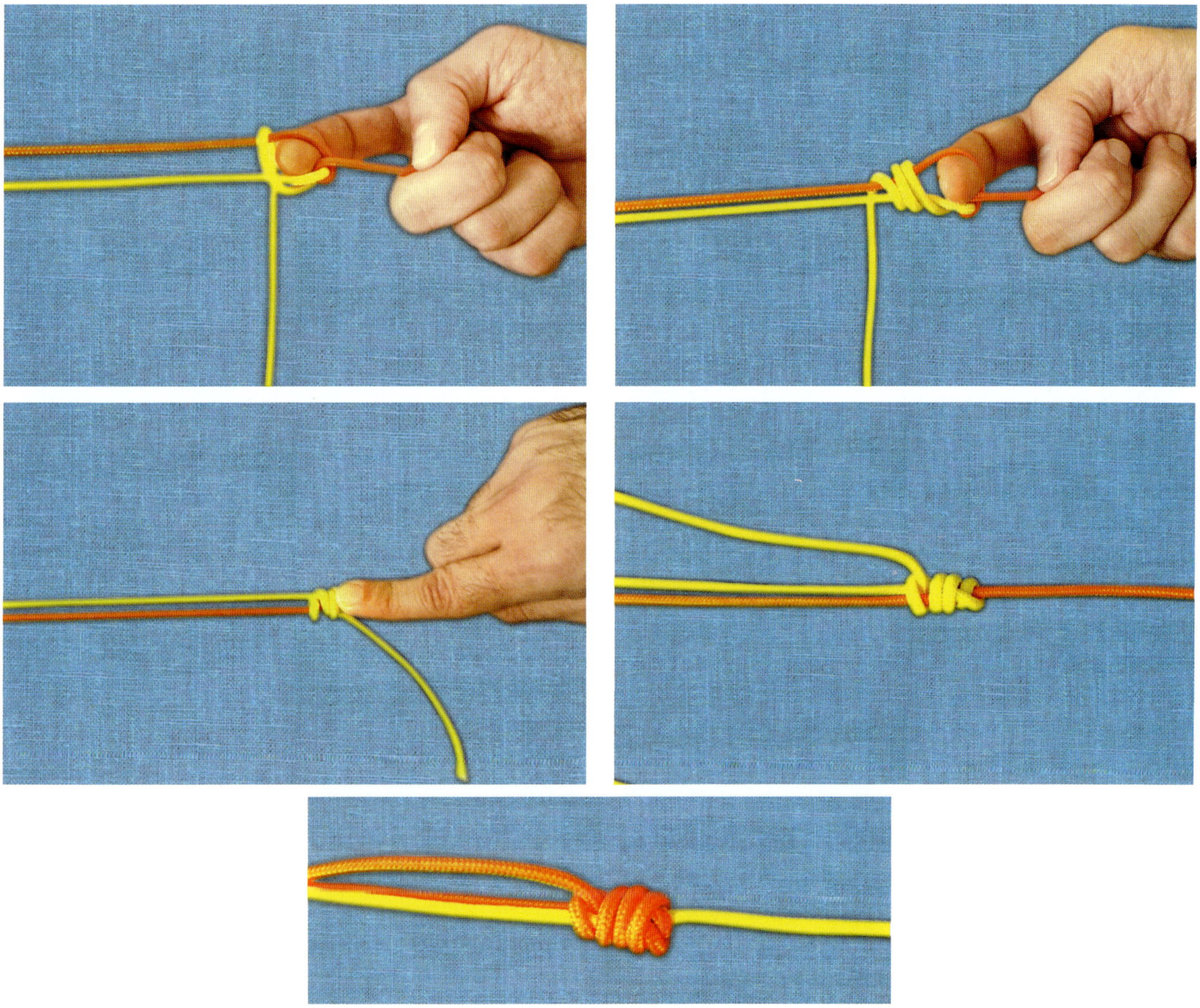

**Fig. 7.10:** Extracorporeal sliding knots

So, a suture is introduced in abdomen, the stitch is passed and the needle with the thread is pulled out the abdomen. While extracting the needle from the abdominal cavity with one instrument, the other one must be positioned on the thread a few centimeters far from the tissue in order to protect and avoid the tearing of the tissue. After that, the knotting procedure can start (according blocking sequence, as performed for intracorporeal technique, like gladiator rule): Each half hitch is pushed in abdomen with a knot pusher; it can be distinguished a non-working thread that remains passive during knot tying and the working one that performs an active role (by wrapping itself on the non-working thread) during knot preparation. During knot tying and pushing, tension must be applied on the non-working thread.

**MESSAGE BOX**

- The proficiency with laparoscopic suturing is of a crucial importance as it not only allows the performance of a wide range of complex operative scenarios, but also is an essential skill required for dealing with intraoperative complications.
- In a perfect stitch, the needle penetrates the tissue with an entry angle of 90 degrees in relation to the axis of the wound.
- However, in theater, due to fixed trocar sites, the perfect stitch is not always feasible; so all surgical skills of the surgeons should be focused on the idea that you must be able to use both hands to achieve the best position of the needle holder.

Section

2

# Hysteroscopy

Chapter

8

# Diagnostic Hysteroscopy

*Sunita R Tandulwadkar, Pooja Lodha*

## PREOPERATIVE PREPARATION

Diagnostic hysteroscopy does not need any other preoperative preparation. It is usually performed in immediate postmenstrual period.

## ANESTHESIA

Under short general anesthesia.

## IMPORTANT EQUIPMENT

Hysteroscope (4 mm) with diagnostic sheath (Fig. 8.1).

## TECHNIQUE

1. 2 Allis forceps are placed on the anterior lip of the cervix to straighten the cervix and the uterus.
2. Cervix is dilated manually with serial dilators to the one size more than the outer diameter of the outer sheath of hysteroscope so as to avoid forceful entry of hysteroscope.
3. Hysteroscope is gently inserted under vision to limit the risk of uterine perforation. The insertion of the scope into uterine cavity is done with inflow on. This inflow of fluid also helps to wash up any blood clots coming in contact with lens tip.
4. The outflow is partially on to make the vision clear. The movement of scope follows the anatomy of cervix.
5. Once inside the cavity, scope is positioned in the center with the distal tip being kept at the distance of 1.5 to 2 mm from the fundus.
6. Fixing the position of the camera in the left hand and holding the light cable in the right hand, scope is rotated by 90° clockwise and 180° anticlockwise, to see right and left cornu respectively. Hysteroscope is withdrawn slowly till internal os. A panoramic view is taken. Hysteroscope is further withdrawn to view and examine the entire cervical canal since better view of cervical canal can be obtained during removal than during insertion (Figs 8.2 to 8.20).

### TIPS

- In case of slight isthmic stenosis, atraumatic dilator, i.e. plastic dilator can be used initially, as it is difficult to create wrong passage with plastic dilator.
- Also, paracervical block can be given with 2% xylocaine.
- Insertion of the scope into uterine cavity is done with inflow on. This inflow of fluid also helps to wash up any blood clots coming in contact with lens tip.

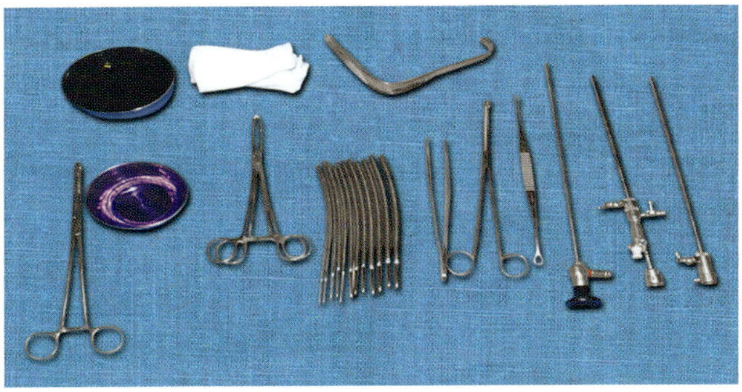

**Fig. 8.1:** Trolley of diagnostic hysteroscopy

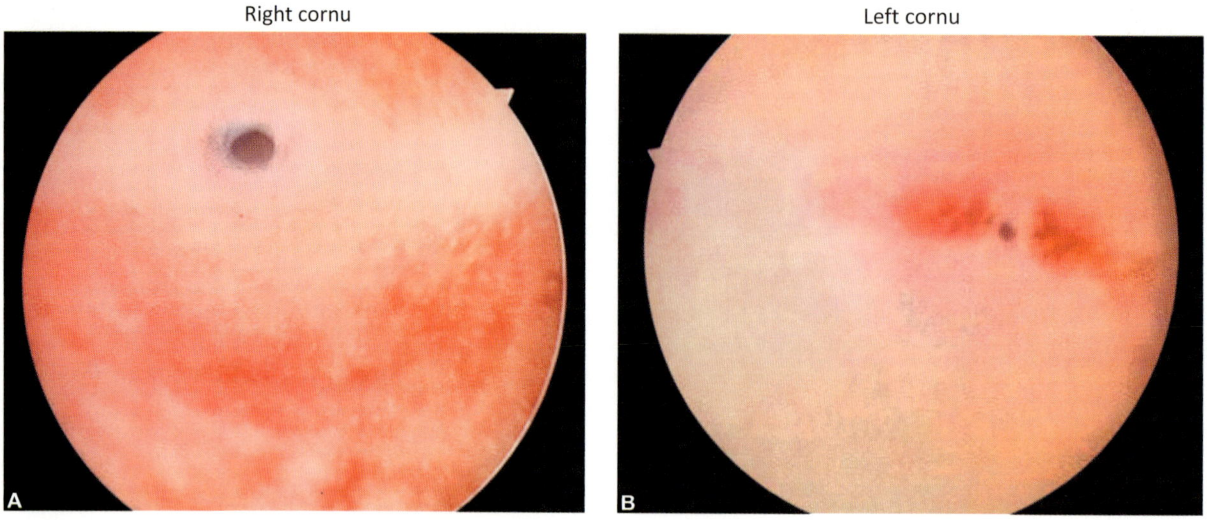


**Figs 8.2A and B:** Rotation of telescope allows visualization of tubal orifice

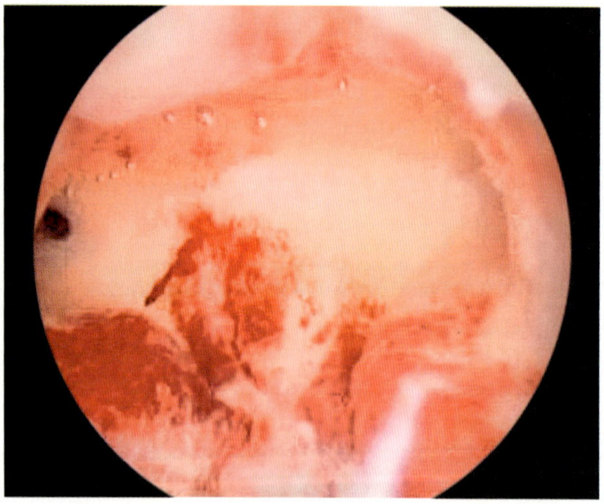

**Fig. 8.3:** Panoramic view from internal Os

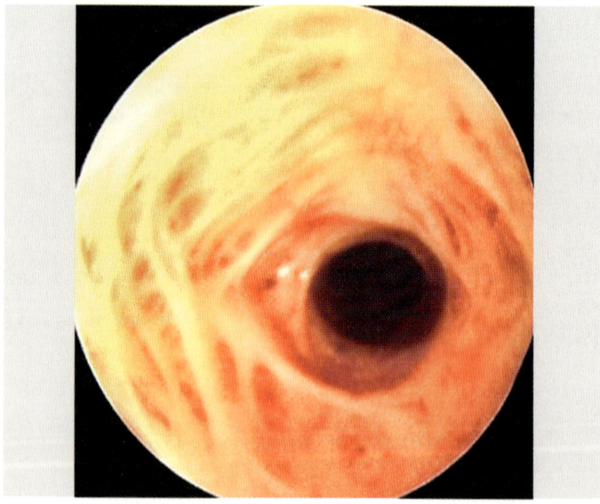

**Fig. 8.4:** Mild stenosis of cervical canal

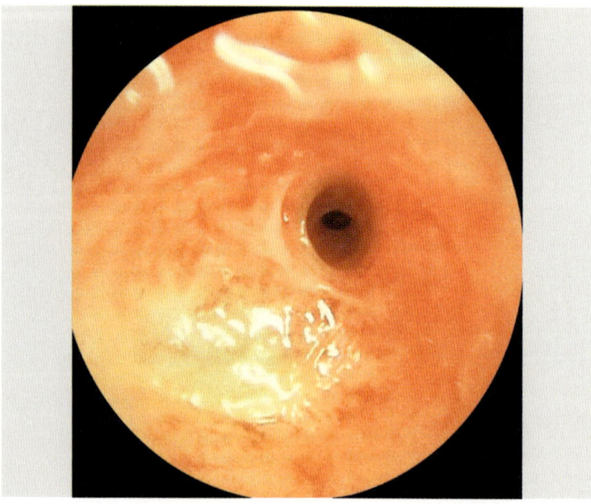

**Fig. 8.5:** Extensive stenosis of cervical canal

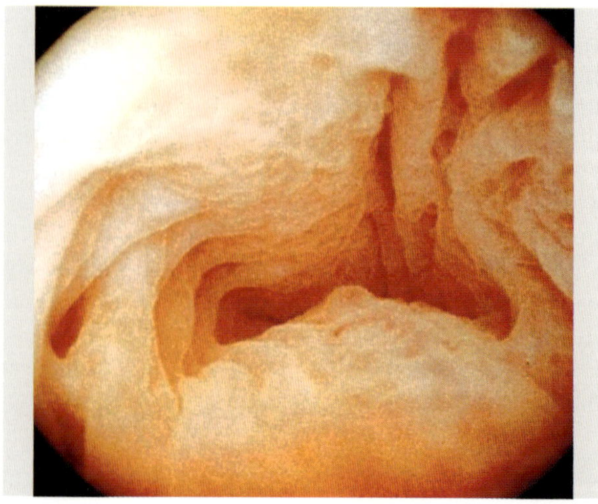

**Fig. 8.6:** Normal cervical canal

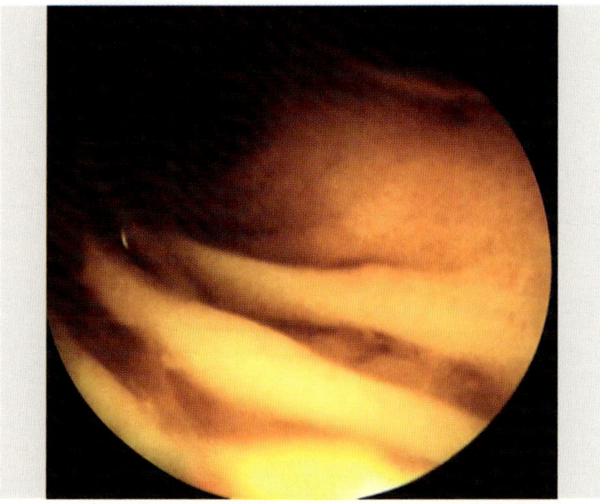

Fig. 8.7: Palmate folds of cervical canal

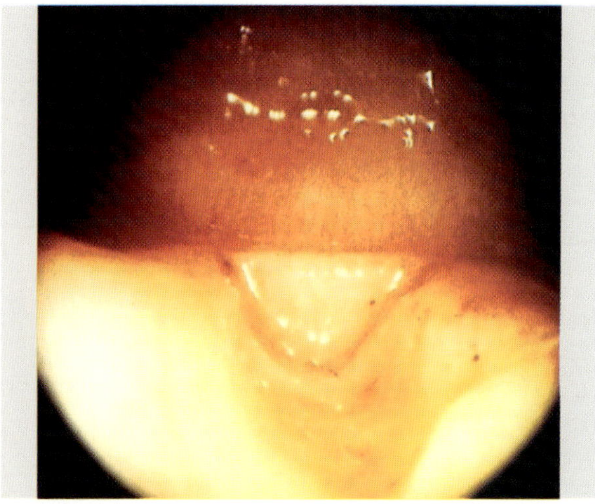

Fig. 8.8: Measurement of endometrial thickness

## Various Pathologies Diagnosed During Hysteroscopy

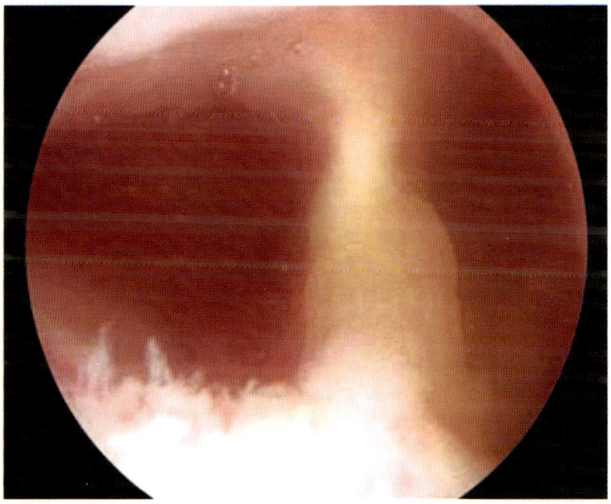

Fig. 8.9: Uterine septum

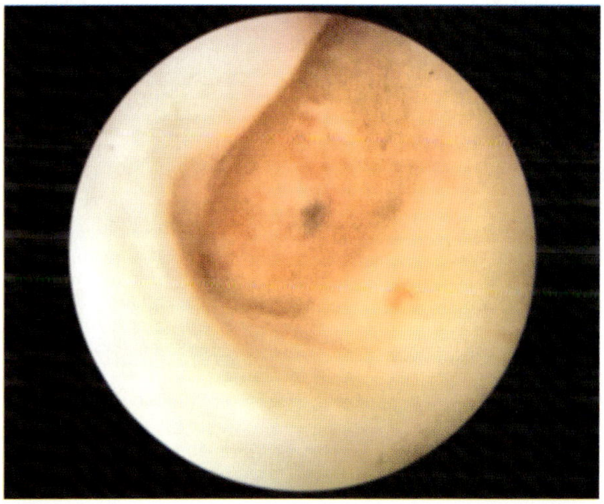

Fig. 8.10: Unicornuate uterus

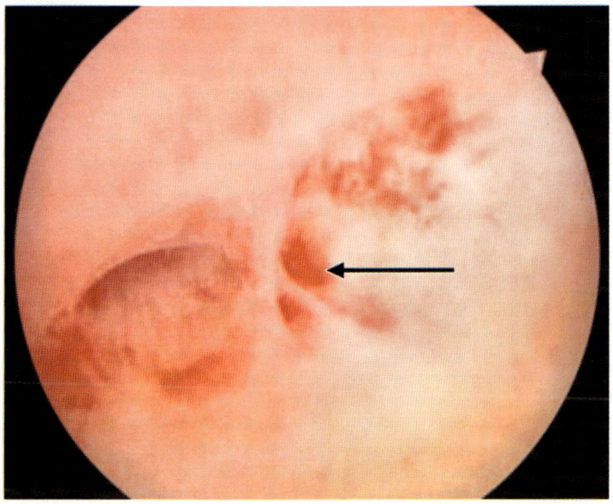

Fig. 8.11: Flimsy adhesions at cornu

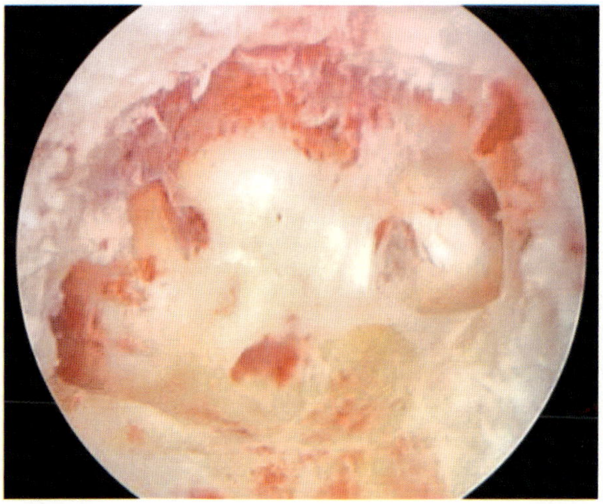

Fig. 8.12: Flimsy adhesions in cavity

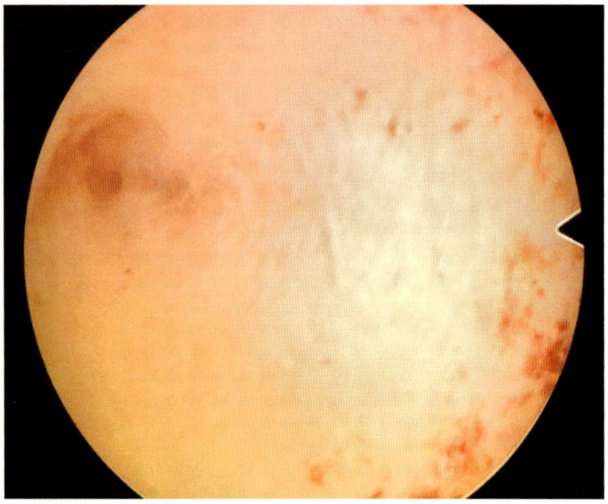

**Fig. 8.13:** Right cornual block

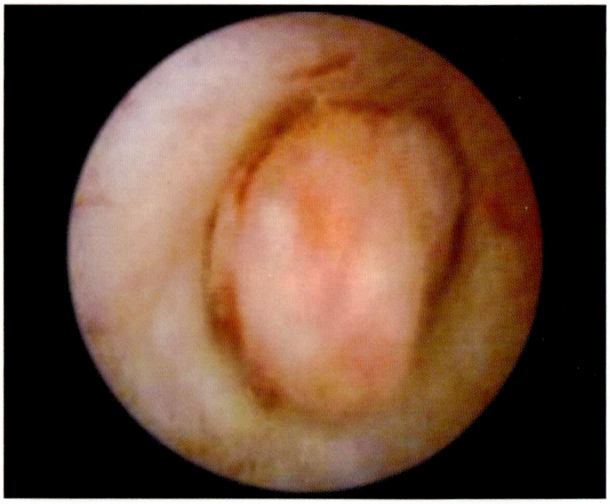

**Fig. 8.14:** Benign endometrial polyp at cornu

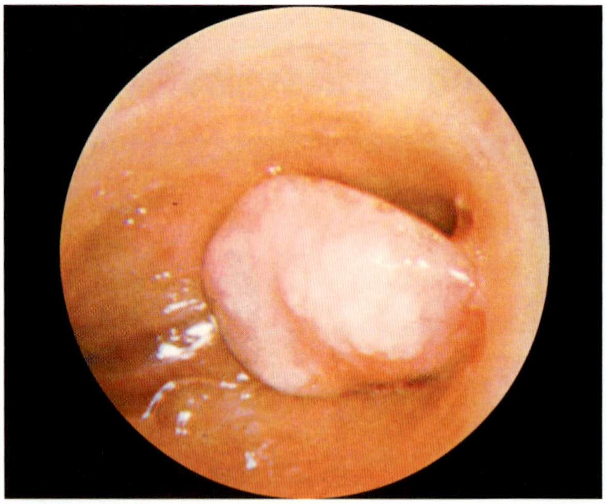

**Fig. 8.15:** Polyp at left lateral wall

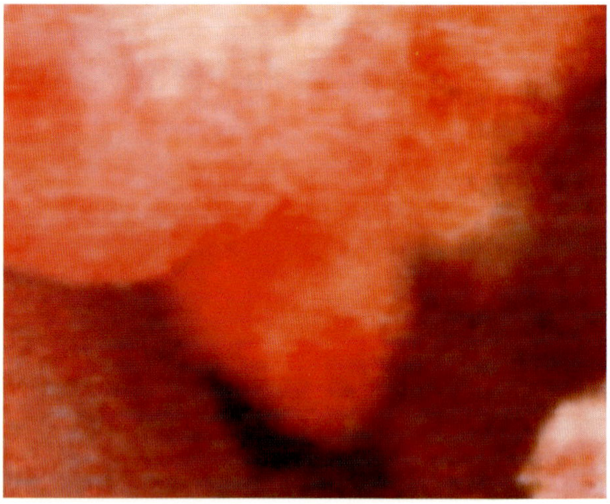

**Fig. 8.16:** Multiple polyps

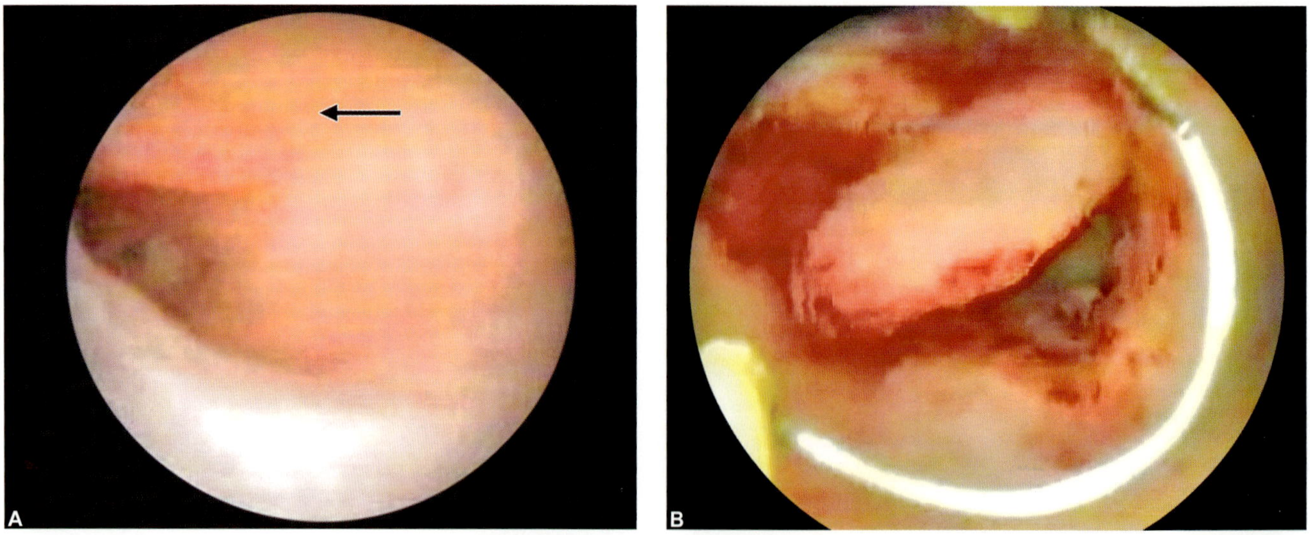

**Figs 8.17A and B:** In benign polyps (single or multiple) we recommend resection with resectoscope without using energy source. This avoids damage to basal endometrium

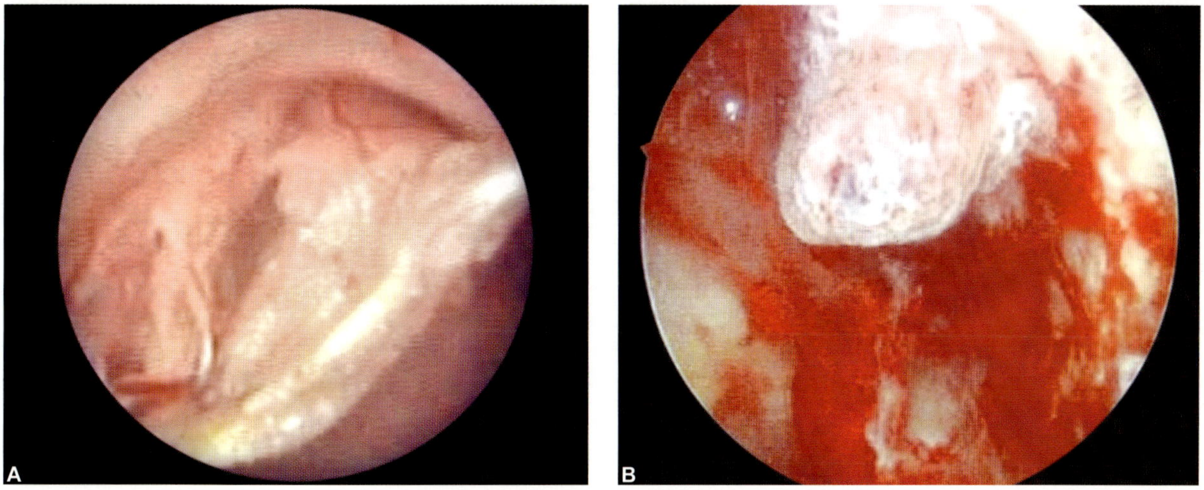


**Figs 8.18A and B:** Malignant endometrial polyps

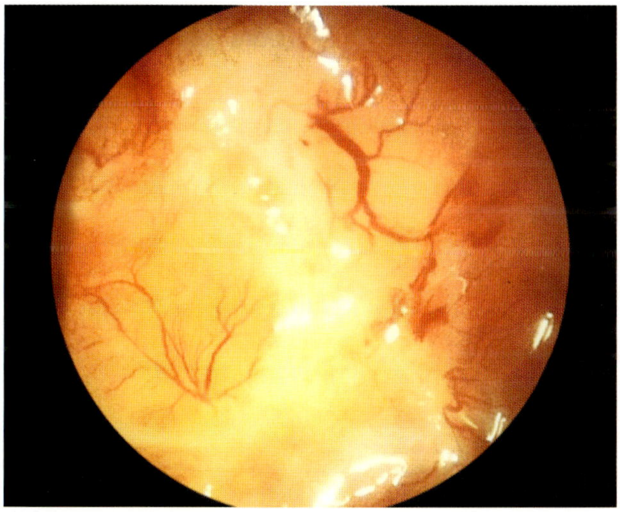

**Fig. 8.19:** Vascular endometrium in endometrial hyperplasia

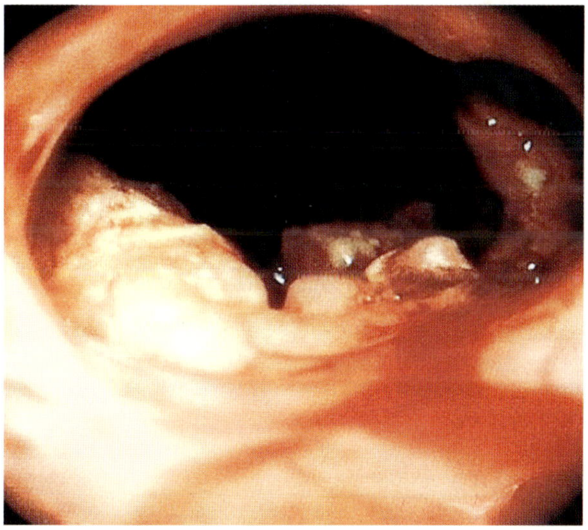

**Fig. 8.20:** Carcinoma endometrium

# Chapter 9

# Office Hysteroscopy

*Sunita R Tandulwadkar, Pooja Lodha*

## PREOPERATIVE EVALUATION

History and general examination of patient.

## PREOPERATIVE PREPARATION

It is done in the immediate postmenstrual period when endometrial thickness is thin.

Office hysteroscopy does not need any other preoperative preparation.

## IMPORTANT EQUIPMENT (FIG. 9.1)

- Versa scope with disposable sheath, (Figs 9.2 to 9.4).
- Betochhi office hysteroscope.

## TECHNIQUE

1. Bimanual examination of uterus to know direction of uterus.
2. Holding of cervix is not required.
3. Hysteroscope with the inflow channel ON is passed through the introitus. Fluid distends the vagina and cervix is identified **(vaginoscopy).**
4. Once the external os is seen, the hysteroscope is negotiated through the external os into the canal, the influx of the fluid keeps on distending the further passage allowing the smooth entry of hysteroscope in uterine cavity under vision (Figs 9.5 to 9.8).
5. Smaller lesions like polyp or a band of intrauterine synechiae can be released with the use of versa point in same sitting.

### TIPS

- In case of patulous introitus, external compression on both sides over labia is given so as to allow sufficient vaginal distension and to minimize fluid wastage.
- In acutely anteverted or retroverted uterus countertraction by applying Allis forceps or vulsellum on the cervix helps to negotiate internal os.

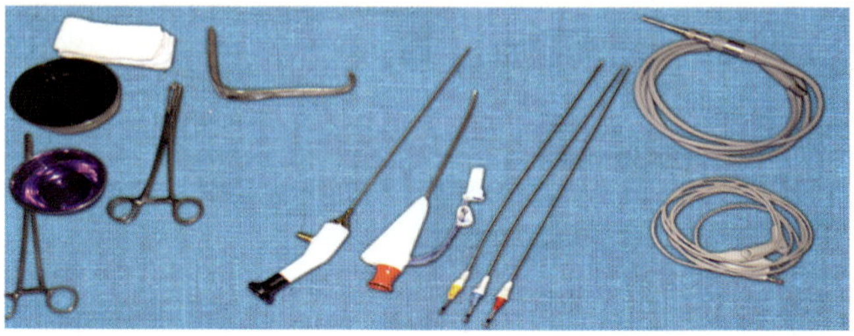

**Fig. 9.1:** Trolley of office hysteroscopy

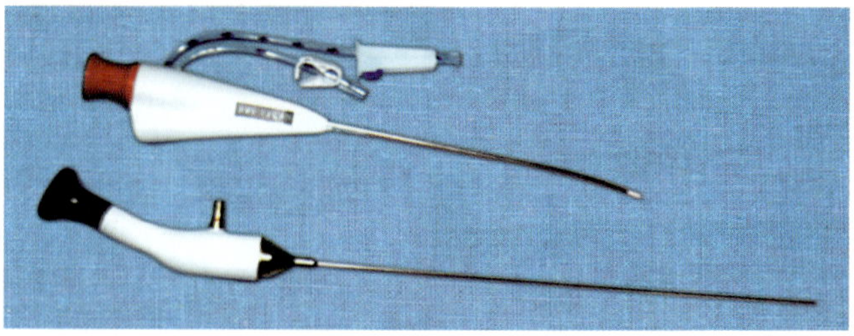

**Fig. 9.2:** Versa scope with operative sheath

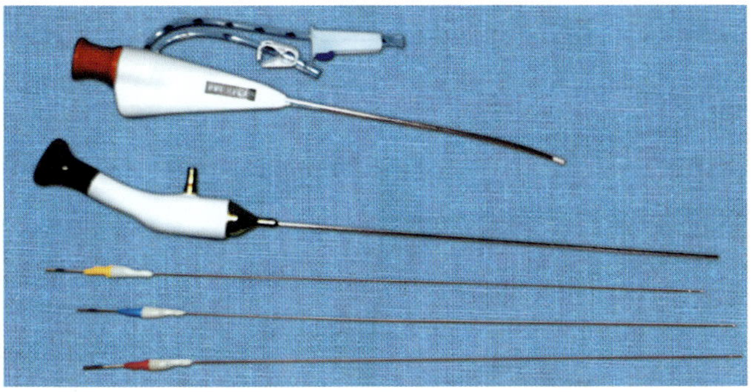

Fig. 9.3: Versa scope with operative sheath with electrodes

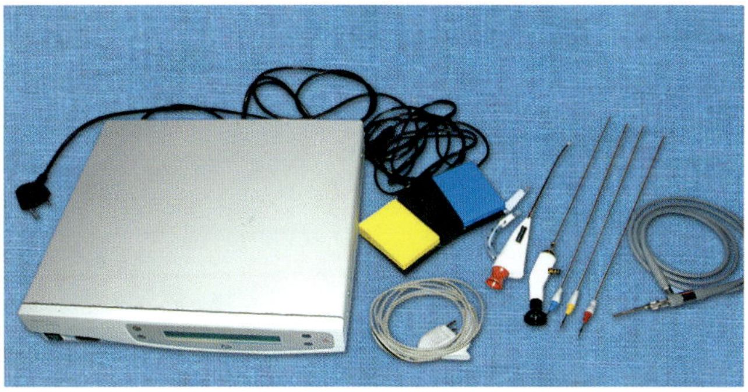

Fig. 9.4: Versa scope with versapoint and operative sheath

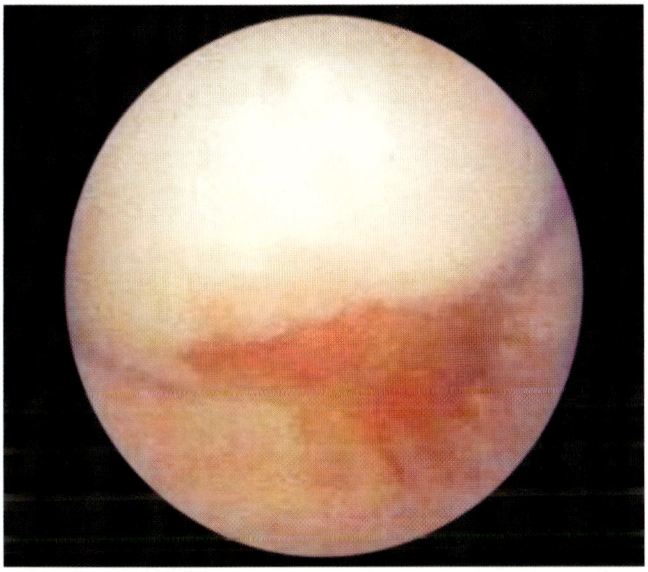

Fig. 9.5: View of external os on vaginoscopy

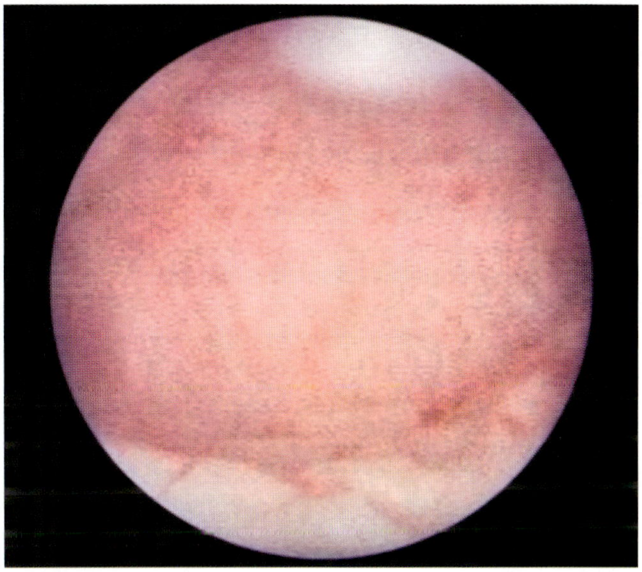

Fig. 9.6: Panoramic view of cavity

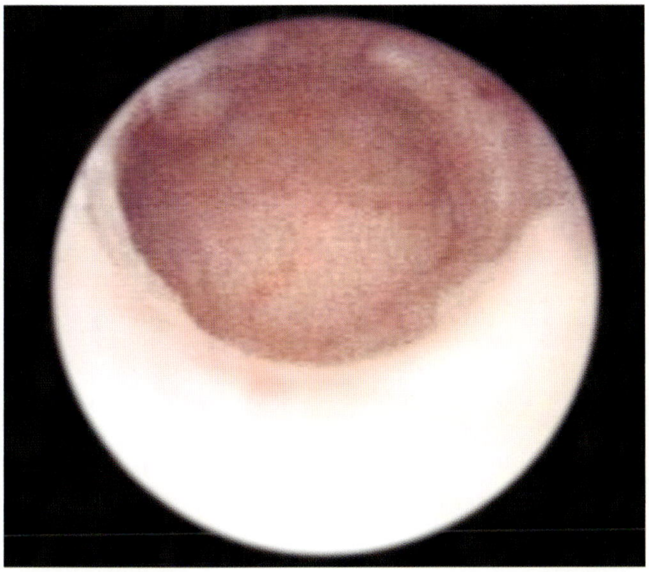

Fig. 9.7: Visualization of cavity while withdrawing the scope

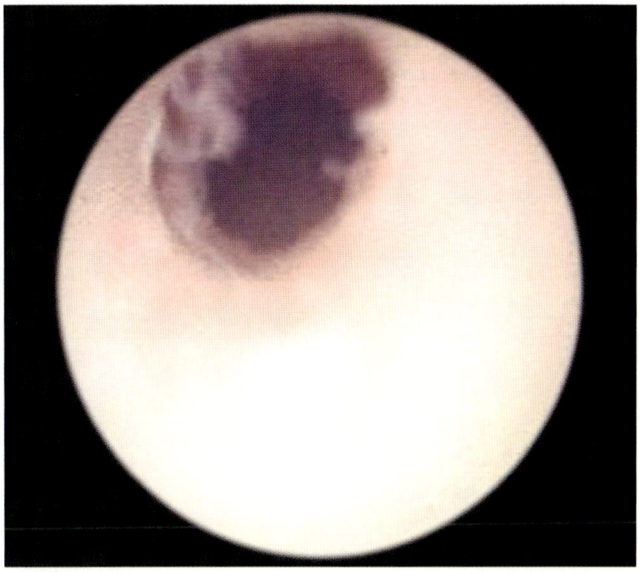

Fig. 9.8: View of internal os while withdrawing the scope

Chapter 10

# Classification of Microhysteroscopic Images

*Jorge E Dotto, Paola Da Graca Mila, Miguel A Bigozzi Jr, Jorge E Dotto Jr, Jacques Hamou*

## INTRODUCTION

Microhysteroscopy is a safe and non-traumatic technique that provides a satisfactory assessment of the uterine cavity, and it is an effective tool for the detection of premalignant lesions and early stages of endometrial cancer. The current state of development of the microhysteroscope provides a high-quality image of the endometrium that allows an approximation to the histological diagnosis of these lesions. In every case, the final diagnosis is histological; however, we consider that a classification of microhysteroscopic images according to the degree of suspicion is both a useful resource for effective communication among the attending gynecologist, the hysteroscopist and the pathologist and a useful guide for selecting the cases and sites for endometrial biopsies.[19]

## HYSTEROSCOPY TECHNIQUES

This study recruited 2342 patients (mean age 50 years, range 35–85 years). 72 of them were excluded from the study due to cervical stenosis or discomfort during the exam, this situation determined that 2270 cavities were examined.

Our patients were divided into two big populations: 834 high-risk patients (high-risk defined by obesity, blood hypertension, diabetes mellitus, history of familial cancer, history of cancer itself: Especially cases of colon and breast cancer) and 1436 low-risk symptomatic patients. They were later divided into 3 groups: Group A: 270 high-risk asymptomatic patients. Group B: 564 high-risk symptomatic patients (spotting, perimenopausal or postmenopausal bleeding) and Group C: 1436 low-risk symptomatic patients.

We usually perform hysteroscopies after menstruation, on day 6 to 14 of the menstrual cycle, in women of reproductive age, and according to indication in postmenopausal women. Neither anesthesia nor preoperative drugs are used. We used the Hamou no. 1, 4 mm, rigid hysteroscope (Karl Storz, Tuttlingen, Germany) with an endoscope, which is 4 mm in diameter, 25 cm long, with 90-degree vision and a fore obliquity of 30 degrees. It has two oculars: One for direct vision, whereas the other is lateral and mobile. The optic system allows up to 1, 20, 60 magnification in panoramic vision and 150 x in contact vision. In our experience 1 x and 20 x are the most useful magnifications for endometrial observation. In cases of cervical stenosis, we use the 2 mm diameter hysteroscope.

A Hamou microhysteroflator ($CO_2$) with an outflow of 40 ml/minute is used for uterine distention. A Sony U 1200 printer is used to print the documentation. Since in our experience, biopsy specimens obtained with the hysteroscope are sometimes inadequate, that is the reason why we prefer to use Kevorkian or Sims curettes. After identifying the biopsy site with the hysteroscope, a biopsy is performed with the microcurette; the hysteroscope is subsequently introduced in order to confirm the adequacy of the biopsy site. Actually we perform the Bettocchi's technique with vaginal approach and saline distension with direct biopsy using the grasper through the 5 French operative channel.

## CLASSIFICATION OF HYSTEROSCOPIC IMAGES

We developed the following classification of hysteroscopic images, based on our experience and on the nomenclature used by Italian authors.

A. Normal hysteroscopy
   1. Reproductive aged women
      - Proliferative phase
      - Luteal phase
   2. Postmenopausal women: Atrophic endometrium.

B. Benign lesions
   1. Endometrial changes due to hormone therapy
   2. Myomas (submucous and intramural)
   3. Adenomas endometrial polyps

4. Endometritis
5. Synechiae
6. Foreign bodies
7. Uterine malformations
8. Placental remnants; placental polyps

C. Low-risk hyperplasia
D. High-risk hyperplasia
E. Carcinoma and other malignant tumors.

## A. Normal Hysteroscopy

- Reproductive-aged women: During the proliferative phase of a normal cycle, the endometrium has a whitish pink appearance; no surface vessels are observed; glandular openings are shallow depressions without evidence of vascularization. The thin mucosa has a compact appearance (Fig. 10.1). During the luteal phase, the surface becomes irregular, and vascular congestion changes the pale mucosal lining to a brighter color. During the luteal phase, less $CO_2$ pressure is required to distend the uterine cavity. The endometrial surface is rough and yellowish red. Because of the presence of stromal edema, it is possible to depress the surface with the distal tip of the hysteroscope (Fig. 10.2).

  At higher magnification, blood vessels can be seen more clearly. Patients must be examined with care since increased mucosal congestion can result in tearing and hemorrhage.
- Postmenopausal women: Atrophic endometrium. The uterine cavity is easily identified; the endometrial surface is whitish, no gland openings are seen and few vessels are recognizable due to atrophy. Telangiectasias and small petechiae can be observed under the surface (Fig. 10.3).

## B. Benign Lesions

- Endometrial changes due to hormone therapy. Several different patterns are observed depending on agents prescribed for dysfunctional metrorrhagia or combined estrogen-progesterone hormone replacement therapy (HRT). Suspicious changes may be evident in a mucosa with cysts, pseudopolyps and angiogenesis, all of which may lead to a wrong presumptive diagnosis of hyperplasia; this pseudohyperplasia pattern is associated with unopposed estrogen therapy (Fig. 10.4).
- Myomas: A submucous myoma is observed as a hemispheric structure with a smooth surface and endometrial lining is solid in appearance under compression with the tip of the hysteroscope, but sometimes pediculated cases can be observed, some submucous myomas are covered with large superficial vessels (Fig. 10.5).

  Intramural myomas can protrude into the cavity and can be identified by diagnostic hysteroscopy.
- Adenomas, endometrial polyps: Because of their typical appearance, endometrial polyps are easy to diagnose; however, when other disorders such as hyperplasia or necrotic myomas are also present, they can be difficult to diagnose and may be considered suspicious.

  Functional adenomas can be multiple and small and have the same progestational transformation as the endometrium.

  They are soft, some are red or reddish, frequently solitary and pediculated (Fig. 10.6).
- Endometritis: The reddish color with "starry sky" white penetration looks similar to colpitis observed with the colposcope (Fig. 10.7), non-specific endometritis can also appear as whitish plaques, friable and easy bleeding (Fig. 10.8). In these cases, it is useful to take biopsies for bacteriological study as well as for histology.
- Synechiae: Hysteroscopy is a useful tool for evaluation of location, extension and constitution of synechiae. Multiple synechiae can make it difficult to observe the uterine cavity leading to an unsatisfactory diagnosis. In some cases, general anesthesia is required for accurate examination.

  Synechiae may be constituted by endometrium, muscle or connective tissue. Endometrial synechiae are fine and friable, they are located in the periphery of the uterine cavity and easily detached (Fig. 10.9). Myofibrous synechiae are thicker and tend to be central or near the tubal ostia (Fig. 10.10). Connective tissue synechiae are large, thick or irregular and may be multiple. The uterine cavity is frequently distorted, and it is therefore difficult to introduce the hysteroscope (Fig. 10.11).
- Foreign bodies: Hysteroscopy makes it possible to assess the uterine device (IUD) in the uterine cavity and its relationship with the uterine wall. Should one of the tips be embedded in the endometrial mucosa, or in the tubal ostium, removal under direct visual control is possible (Fig. 10.12).
- Uterine malformations: Uterus didelphys and uterine septa display characteristic hysteroscopic images (Fig. 10.13).
- Placental remnants, placental polyps: They are dark red and smooth, sometimes with a necrotic white pattern.

The endometrial mucosa is heterogeneous in appearance with projections and marked vascularization.

## C. Low-risk Hyperplasia

The current histological classification groups hyperplasias as simple, including simple hyperplasia and glandular cystic hyperplasia of the old classification system; complex hyperplasia, previously called adenomatous hyperplasia; and atypical hyperplasia.

This classification is concomitant with a range of microhysteroscopic aspects. Endometrial hyperplasia is defined as an exuberant irregular development of endometrial mucosa, which can be either focal or generalized.

The appearance of simple hyperplasia is similar to that of a normal endometrium, with normal glandular

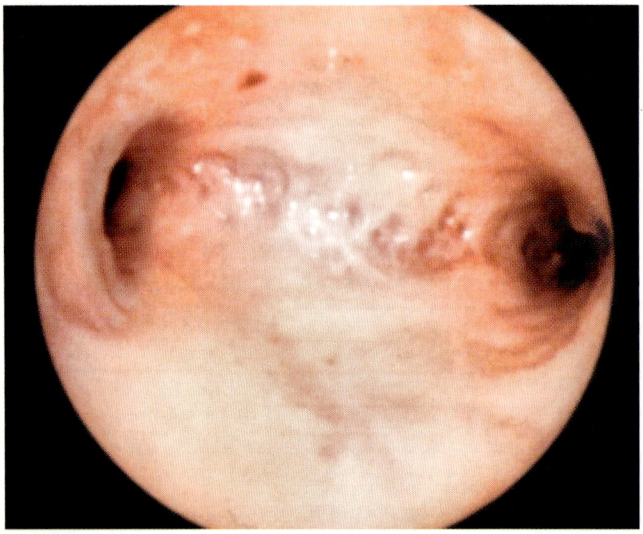

**Fig. 10.1:** Proliferative whitish pink endometrium without surface vessels and compact appearance

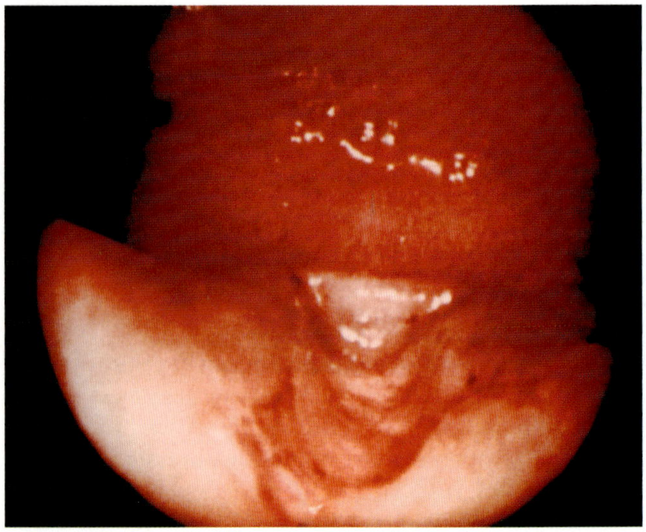

**Fig. 10.2:** Secretory endometrium with an uneven surface and a more intense color. Congestion makes vessels visible. Endoscope produces indentation

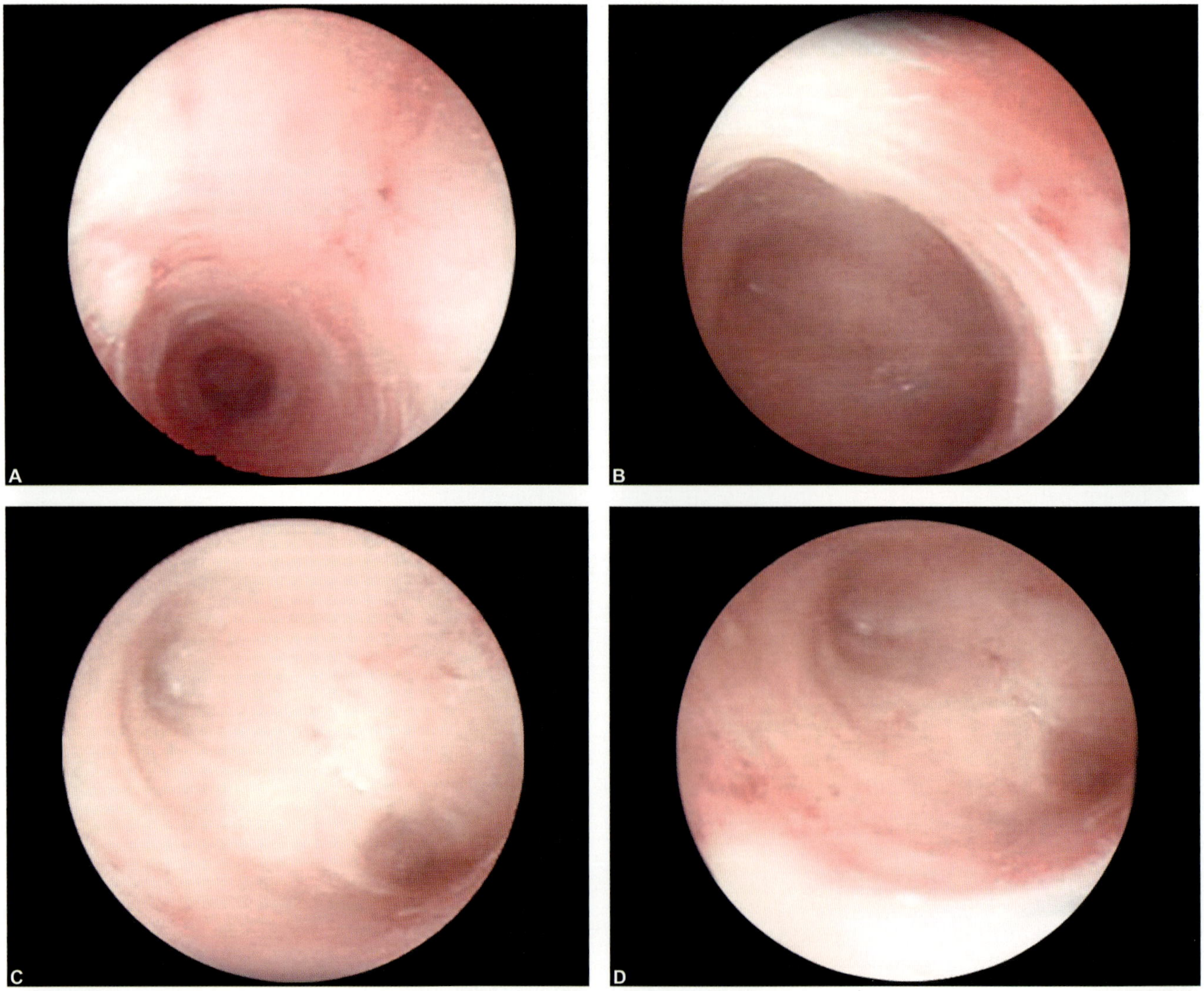

**Figs 10.3A to D:** The cavity is very easily identified. The surface is whitish, no gland openings are seen, very few vessels are present due to atrophy. Petechiae can be seen on the surface due to submucosal bleeding. This shows how thin and friable the epithelium is

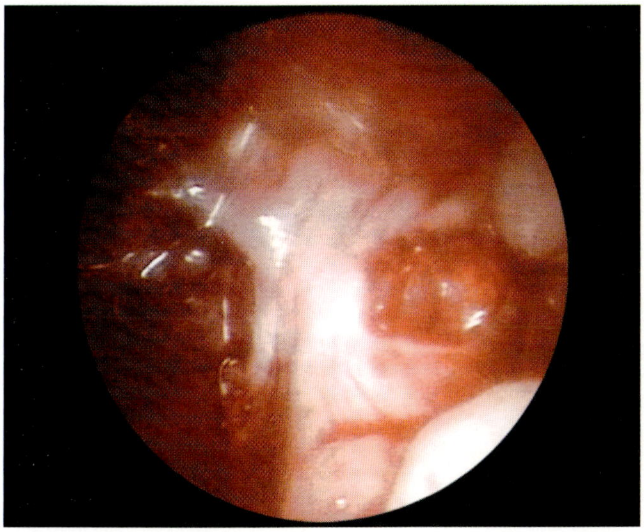

**Fig. 10.4:** HRT modified endometrium, diverse microhysteroscopic appearance. Possible interpretation: hyperplasia, HP correlation: functional basal cell adenoma and endometrium with decidua-like transformation

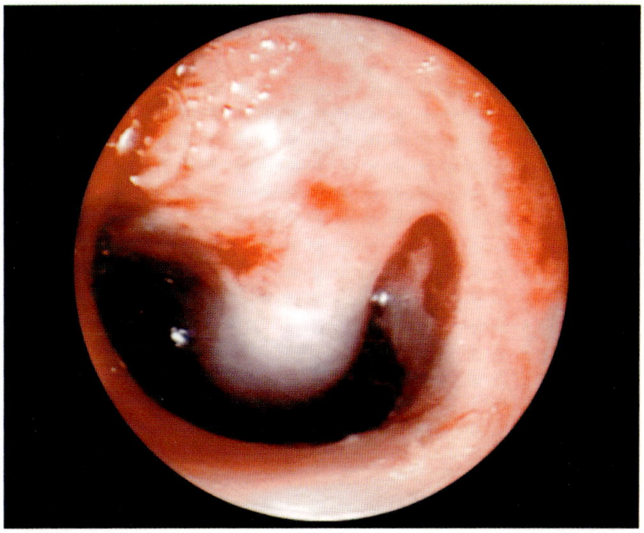

**Fig. 10.5:** Left posterolateral submucosal myoma emerging in the cavity near the left tube orifice. Regular outlines and smooth and whitish surface due to a very thin mucosal lining. Firm consistency.

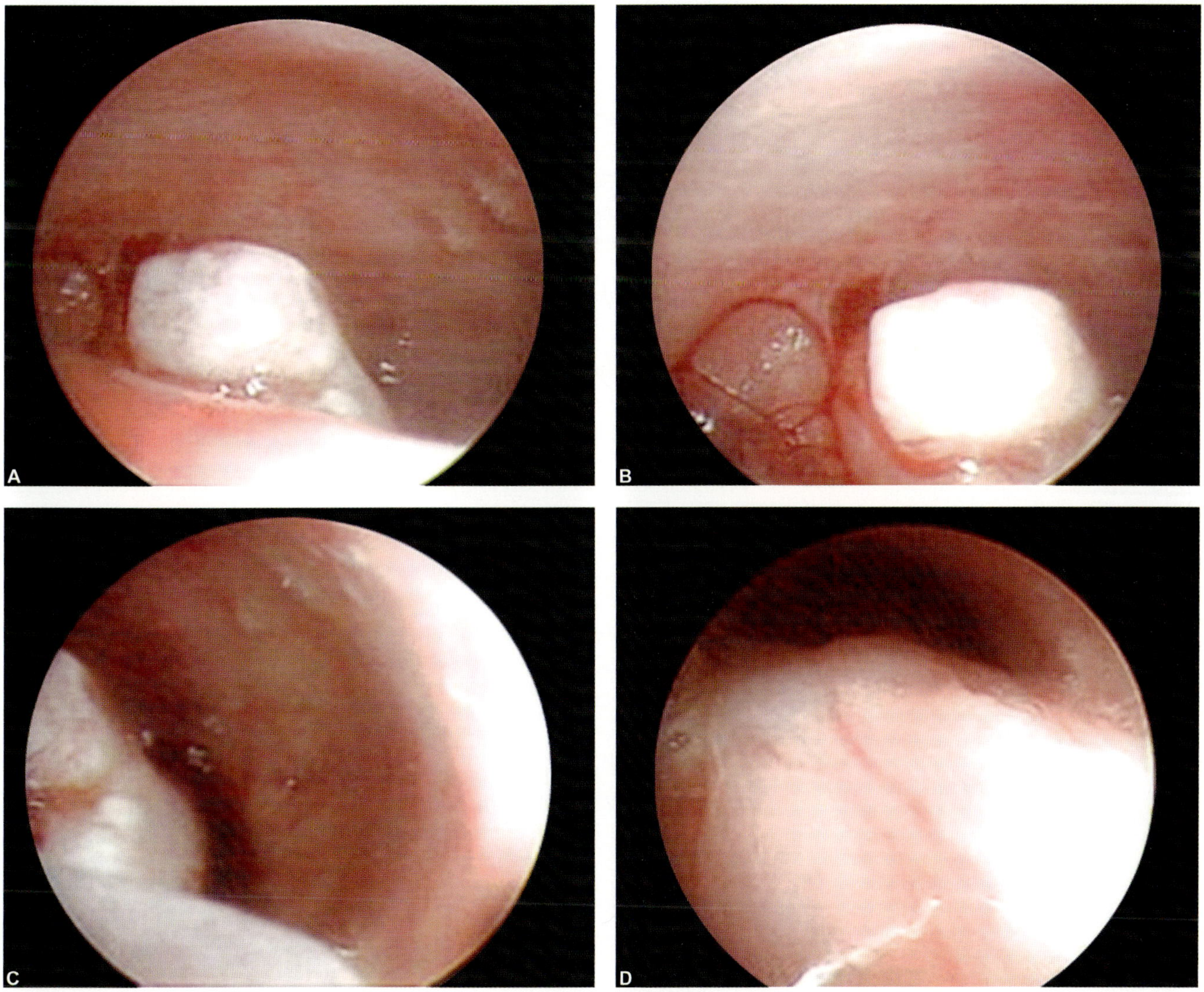

**Figs 10.6A to D:** Whitish endometrial polyp-like growth. On the left, an irregular formation of endometrial mucosa is observed, which reaches into the isthmus. Microhysteroscopic diagnosis: endometrial polyp + low-risk hyperplasia. Histopathologic diagnosis: endometrial polyp + simple hyperplasia

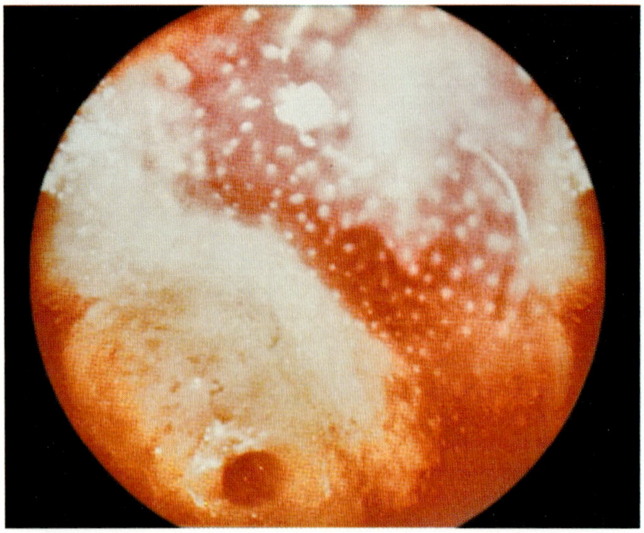

**Fig. 10.7:** Endometritis close to left ostium visualized as a reddish area with abundant punctuation

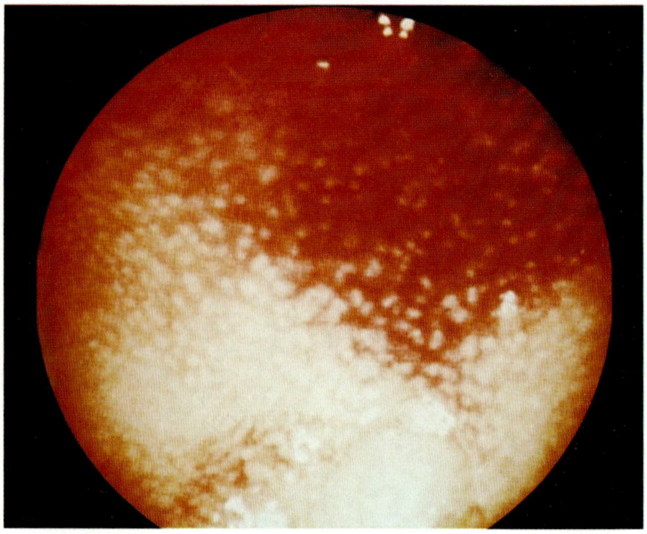

**Fig. 10.8:** Endometritis in the whole cavity, white plaques that can bleed readily

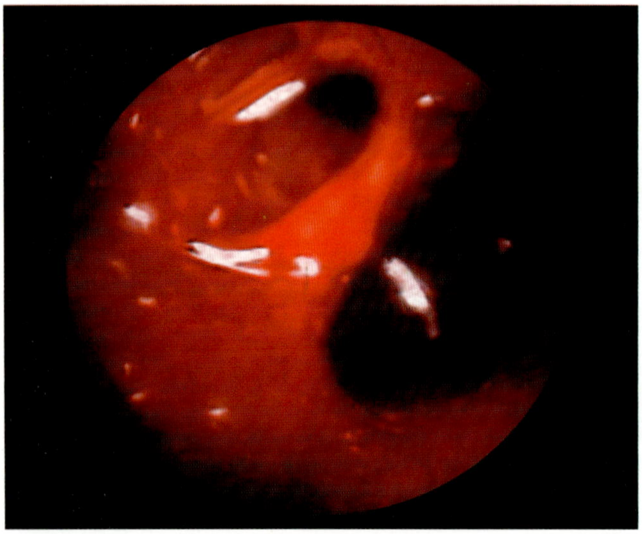

**Fig. 10.9:** Fine and fragile endometrial synechiae, which can be easily ruptured with the tip of the endoscope

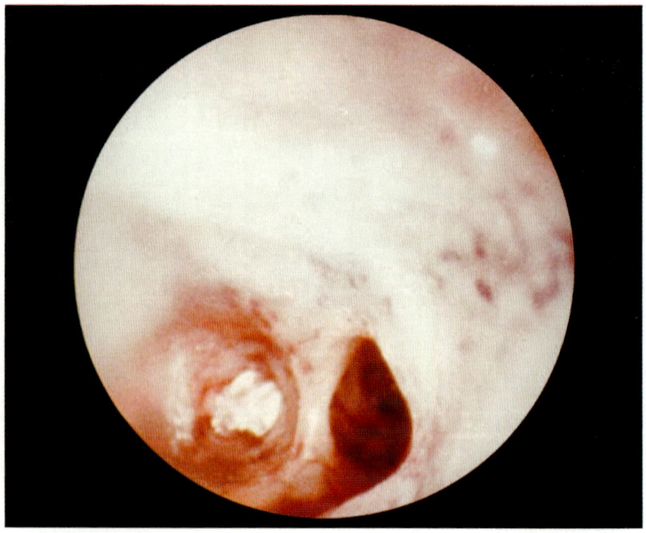

**Fig. 10.10:** Myofibrous synechiae are thicker in this case, located close to the tubal ostium. Remaining endometrium is atrophic

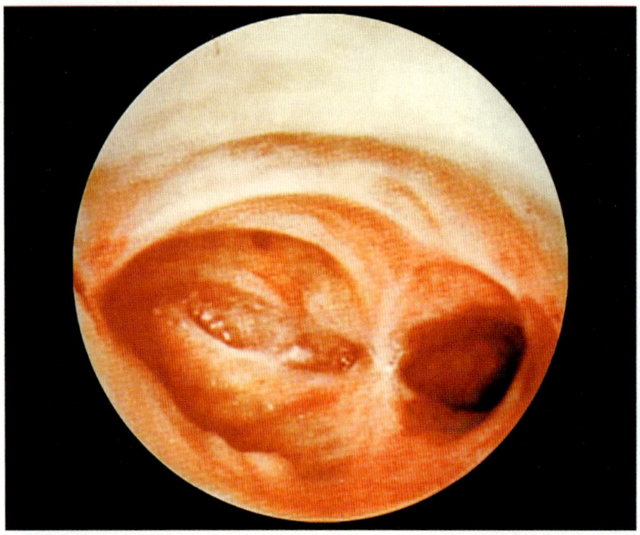

**Fig. 10.11:** Connective tissue synechiae with partial debridement

distribution, but thicker. This can be measured through the depression (>7 mm) produced by the distal tip of the endoscope (Fig. 10.14).

In classic glandular cystic hyperplasia (GCH), the opening of the glands forms a relief including small cysts. This relief is sometimes related to cystic atrophy (apparently due to involution or regression of some CGH features).

This type of hyperplasia produces several different images (Fig. 10.15).

In polypoid hyperplasia, several polyps of different sizes can be observed. They present marked vascularization and interpapillary bridges (Fig. 10.16).

## D. High-risk Hyperplasia

The endometrial surface shows polypoid proliferation as well as interpapillary bridges that can be evident on a hemorrhagic background. Only through histology, can this

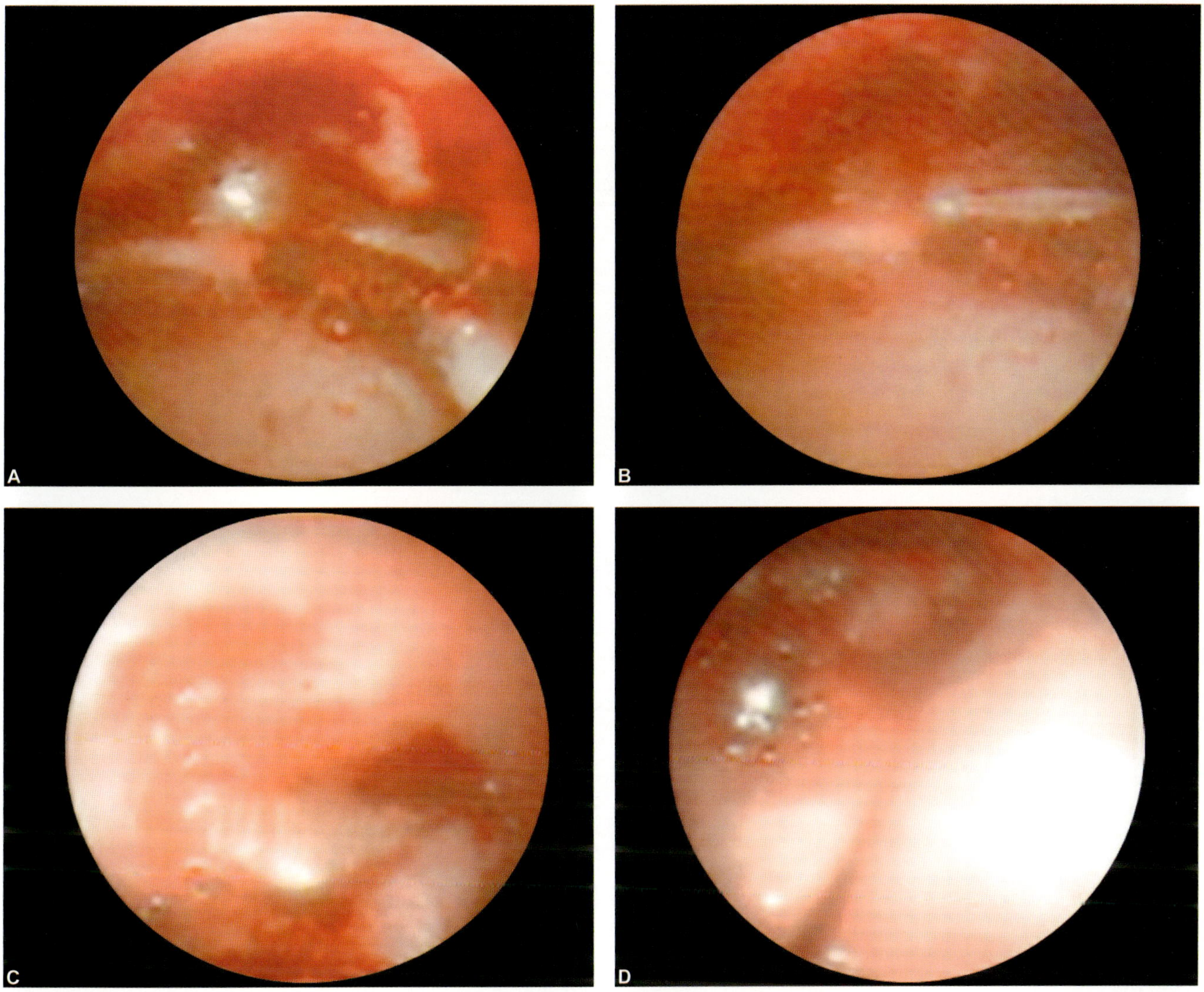


**Figs 10.12A to D:** IUD position in relation to the uterine cavity walls. In lower quadrants, one of the IUD ends is embedded in the left orifice. Device thread visible.

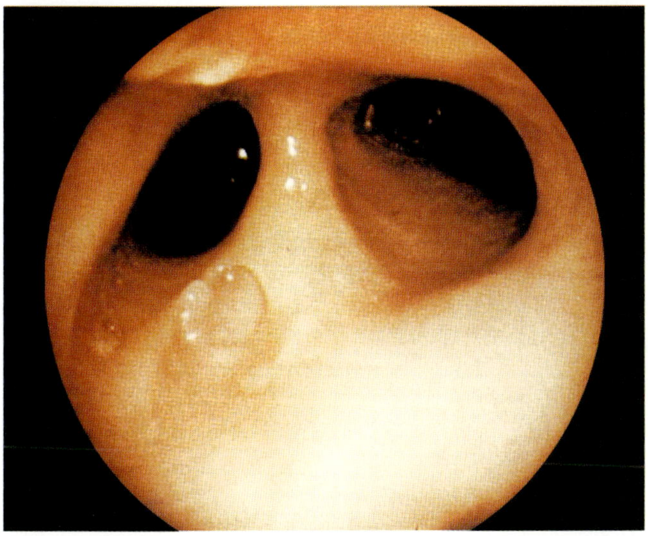

**Fig. 10.13:** Uterine malformation, septum in fundus

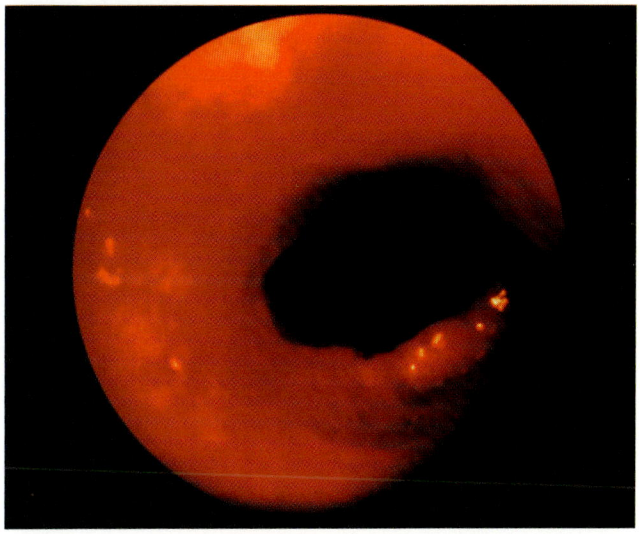

**Fig. 10.14:** Small, whitish, protruding, well-defined area in right horn ostium. Microhysteroscopic diagnosis: Low-risk hyperplasia. Histopathologic diagnosis: Simple hyperplasia

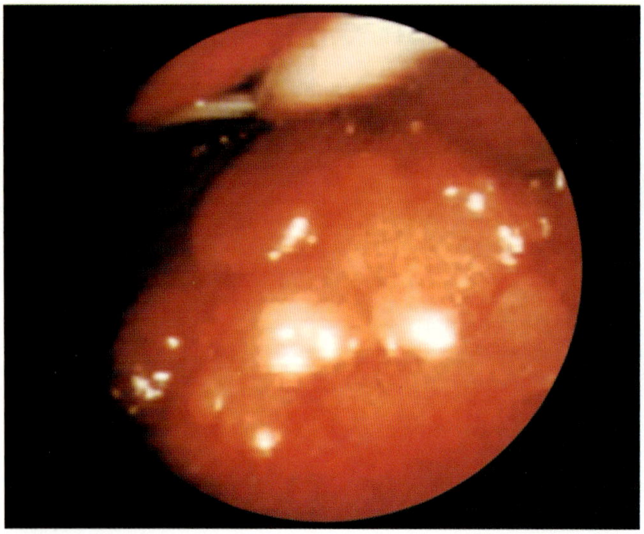

**Fig. 10.15:** Patient with an IUD with exuberant endometrial proliferation and small cysts formation. Microhysteroscopic diagnosis: IUD + low-risk hyperplasia. Histopathologic diagnosis: IUD + simple hyperplasia

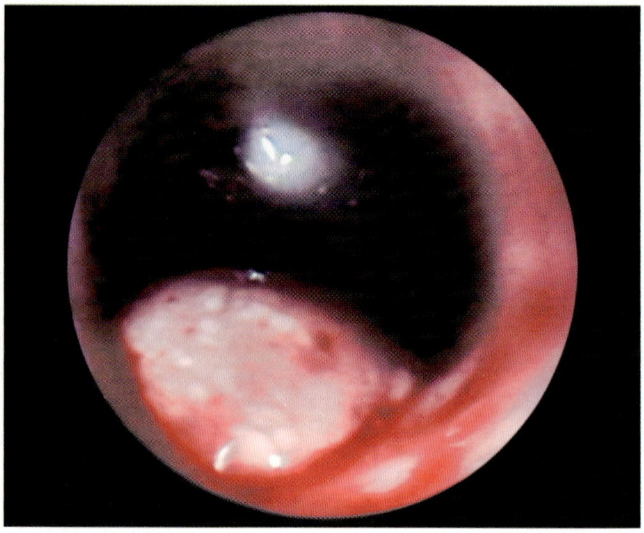

**Fig. 10.16:** Low-risk hyperplasia. Extension toward the endocervical duct can be observed. HP: Simple hyperplasia.

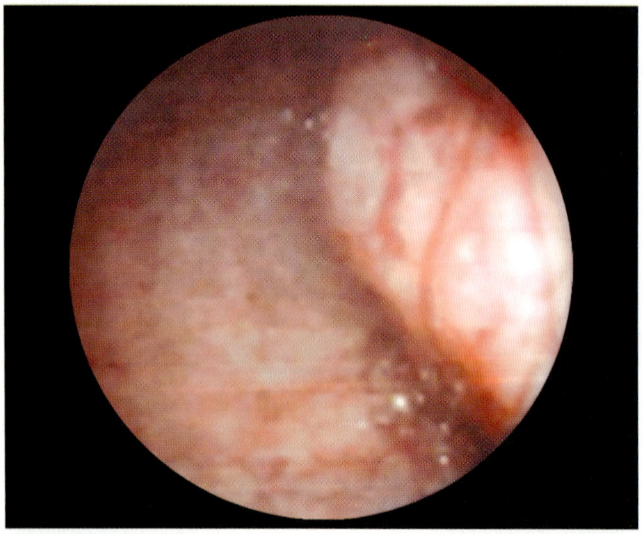

**Fig. 10.17:** Polypoid structure. Background with irregular mammillated surface. Microhysteroscopic diagnosis: High-risk polypoid hyperplasia. HP: complex hyperplasia (adenomatous)

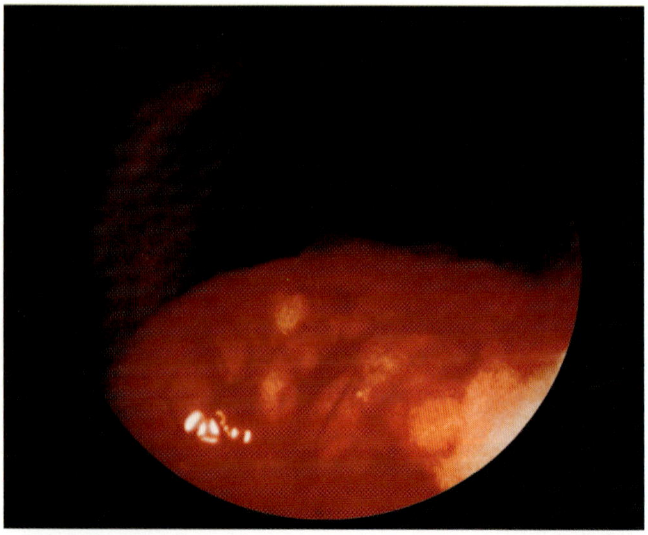

**Fig. 10.18:** Mucosa with exophytic proliferation with areas of congestion hemorrhage and a whitish tone in regions presenting more rapid growth, mammillated surface. Microhysteroscopic diagnosis: high-risk hyperplasia. HP: complex hyperplasia

condition be appreciated. Adenomatous hyperplasia has an irregular mammillated surface, and an imprint is left by the hysteroscope on the surface (Figs 10.17 to 10.19).

## E. Carcinoma

The appearance of carcinoma under microhysteroscopy is multiple and varied, but if visualized the image is characteristic. The lesion may be circumscribed or diffuse. The focal lesion may be described as a whitish exophytic polypoid proliferation with atypical vascularization and hemorrhagic areas (Fig. 10.20), or else papillary with a cerebroid aspect (Fig. 10.21) and including necrotic areas (Fig. 10.22).

An architectural derangement with partial necrotic or hemorrhagic areas is generally observed. Vascularization is completely disorganized. Moreover, it is possible to find endometrial carcinomas in atrophic endometrium. Similar observations have been published in the literature[17,18] (Fig. 10.23).

Carcinoma may also appear as suspicious looking polypoid formation in its implantation base or in combination with other pathologies (Figs 10.24 and 10.25).

In the asymptomatic group we found a lobular breast carcinoma metastasis confirmed with immunohistochemistry (Figs 10.25 and 10.26).

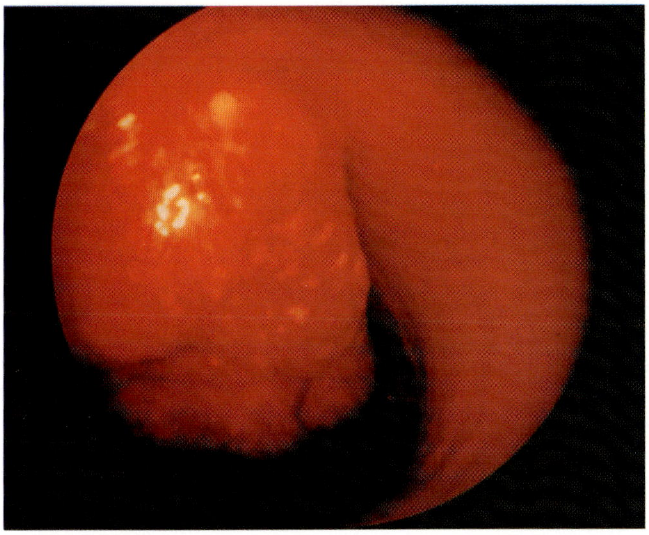

**Fig 10.19:** Hysteroscopic image showing mucosal proliferation with greater vascularity. Hysteroscopic diagnosis: high-risk hyperplasia. Histopathologic diagnosis: atypical hyperplasia

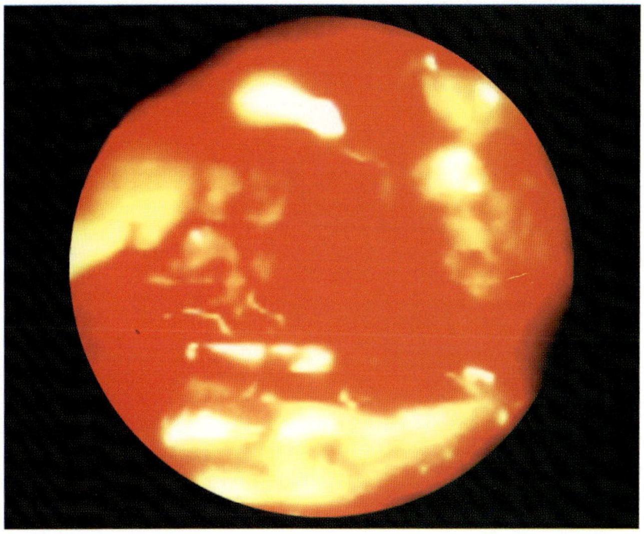

**Fig. 10.20:** Mucosa with exophytic masses with ulcerative zones, necrotic and hemorrhagic foci. The normal structure of the cavity can no longer be distinguished. Tubal orifices cannot be identified. Microhysteroscopic diagnosis: Endometrial adenocarcinoma

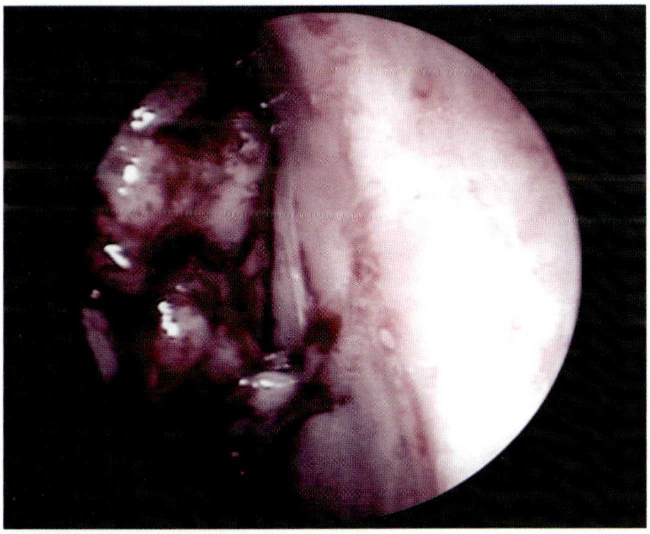

**Fig. 10.21:** Uterine cavity with exophytic hemorraghic proliferation, with necrotic and whitish brain-like areas. Microhysteroscopic diagnosis: endometrial adenocarcinoma. Histopathologic diagnosis: endometrial adenocarcinoma

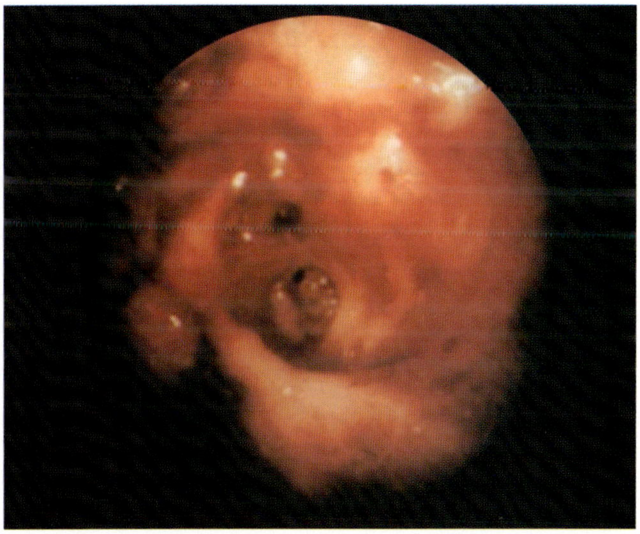

**Fig. 10.22:** Uterine cavity occupied by exophytic hemorrhagic proliferation, necrotic zones and whitish brain-like areas. Microhysteroscopic diagnosis: endometrial adenocarcinoma; HP diagnosis: endometrial adenocarcinoma

It is very important to emphasize that the classification for effective communication among the gynecologist, the hysteroscopist and the pathologist based on suspicion, but the final diagnosis, in every case, must be confirmed by histopathology.

With hysteroscopy, efforts are aimed at identifying pathologic foci for guided biopsies under microhysteroscopic control. Direct macroscopic observation will clearly show the extent of the affected area, the topography, and the distance to the isthmus and endocervix.

Our classification is based on the study of 2342 women (mean aged 50 years, range 35-85 years); of these 72 (4, 8% were withdrawn from the study due to cervical stenosis or discomfort during examination (absolute failures).

- Evaluated population: 2342, mean age 50 years (range 38-85 years).
- 72/2342 3.1%—absolute failures due cervical stenosis or discomfort.
- Studied patients : 2.270.

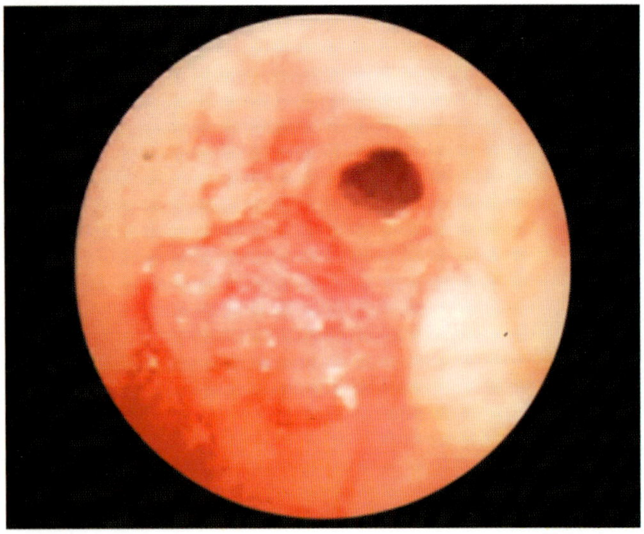

**Fig. 10.23:** Adenocarcinoma near left ostium confirmed by histopathology. The uterine cavity exhibits characteristic whitish atrophic endometrium with a limited number of vessels and petechiae.

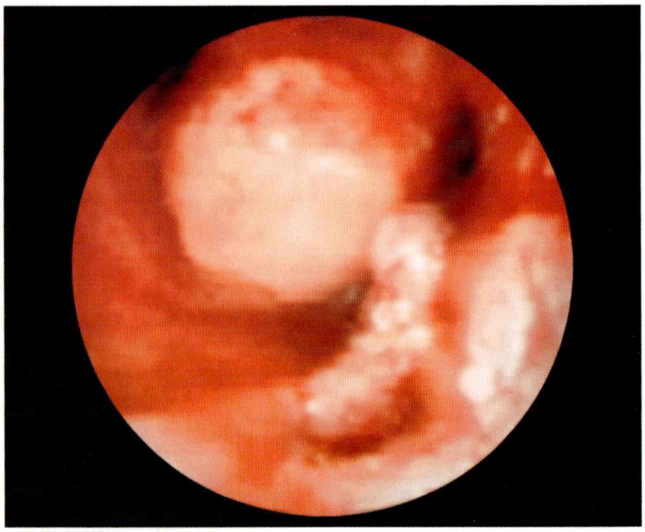

**Fig. 10.24:** Submucosal myoma in the fundus of uterine cavity on left wall in front of left ostium. Microhysteroscopic image of a small carcinoma. Microhysteroscopic diagnosis: small carcinoma. HP diagnosis: endometrial carcinoma

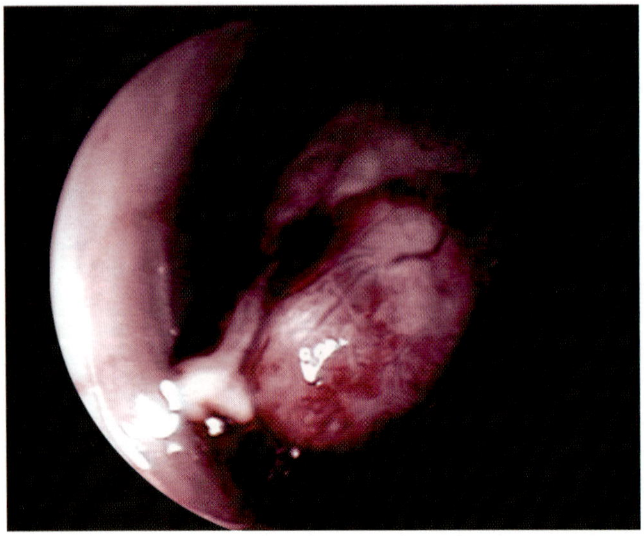

**Fig. 10.25:** Microhysteroscopic image: suspicious looking polypoid structure, grayish color and greater vascularization in its implantation base. HP: well differentiated G1 adenocarcinoma with necrotic (grey) area, probably evolving from pre-existing endometrial adenoma with histology of an endometrium in proliferative phase

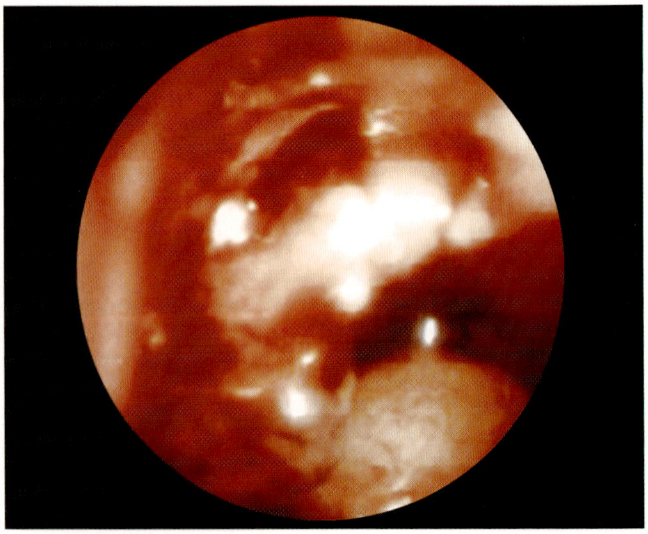

**Fig. 10.26:** Suspicion of malignancy + submucosal myoma HP: Endometrial metastases of lobular breast carcinoma

- High-risk group (HRG): Obesity, hypertension, diabetes mellitus, nulliparity, family cancer, personal cancer (e.g. colon, breast).

In 24 (1.7%) of 1436 patients, the study failed to be completed due to the presence of synechiae that prevented complete cavity visualization (Table 10.1). These cases were classified as relative failures.

In the case of simple hyperplasia, it is sometimes difficult to distinguish dysfunctional forms or HRT-produced endometrial modifications, and the same applies to the differential diagnosis between high-risk hyperplasia and highly differentiated adenocarcinoma.

Table 10.1 correlates microhysteroscopic images and their corresponding histologic confirmation in all 2270 patients. This includes 24 women for whom no presumptive diagnosis of suspicion was made, despite microhysteroscopic studies, due to the presence of synechiae (relative failures). The figures in bold type in the diagonal in this table show the number of cases for which images leading to suspicion and histologic findings

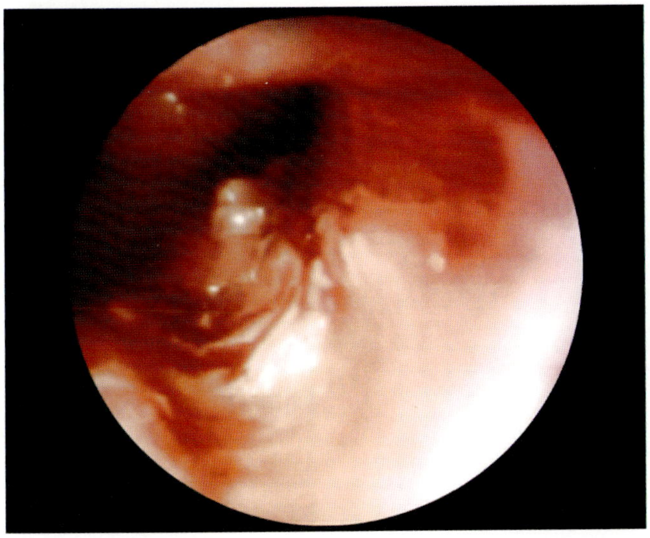

**Fig 10.27:** Suspicion of malignancy + submucosal myoma HP: Endometrial metastases of lobular breast carcinoma

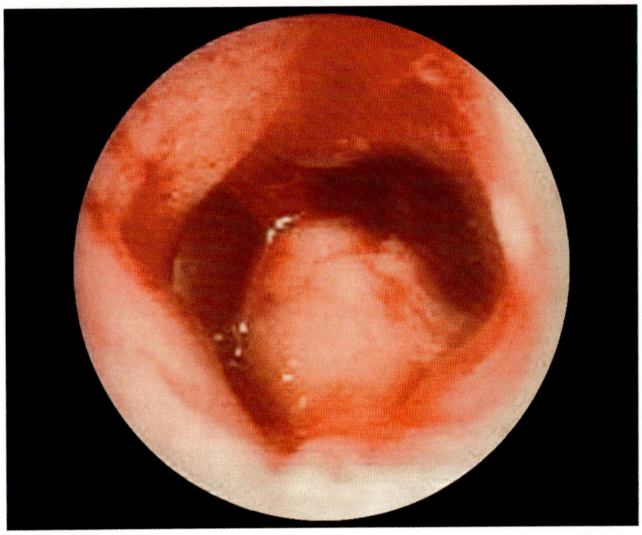

**Fig. 10.28:** Suspected microhysteroscopic diagnosis: high-risk hyperplasia due to associated disorders (overdiagnosis) histopathologic diagnosis: polypoid adenoma, simple hyperplasia (CGH) + necrobiotic myoma

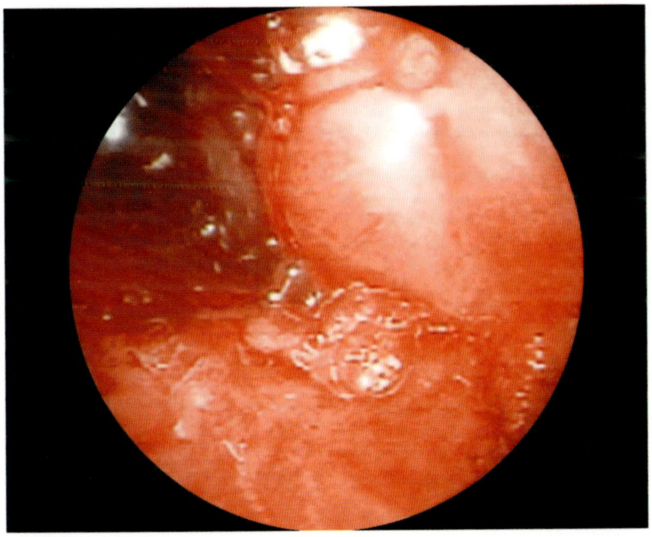

**Fig. 10.29:** Submucosal myoma visualized on the left with focus of high-risk hyperplasia (mixed disorders overdiagnosis) HP: necrobiotic myomas + cystic atrophy

coincided. Cases where disease was overdiagnosed are found under the main diagonal. 18 cases that were diagnosed by microhysteroscopy as low-risk hyperplasia were considered benign according to histologic findings; these patients had been on HRT, and the relevant visual characteristics had been overdiagnosed (Fig. 10.4). 12 cases overdiagnosed as high-risk hyperplasia were in fact cases of simple hyperplasia with associated mixed disorders: 4 simple hyperplasias (GCH) plus necrobiotic myomas and 4 polypoid adenomas (Fig. 10.28), and 4 multiple adenomas with cystic atrophy (Fig. 10.29). When multiple cystic atrophies are associated with other conditions such as necrobiotic myomas, the microhysteroscopic image can be suspicious.

Underdiagnosed cases are found in the upper part of the table, above the diagonal in bold type. Three carcinomas were confirmed on the basis of histologic findings in which the complete cavity could not be visualized due to the presence of multiple synechiae. These cases were included in the benign lesions group.

## Kappa coefficient : 0.966

The Kappa value in this case indicated a very good agreement between suspicion based on images and histologic confirmation

NHI = normal hysteroscopic image; BL = benign lesion

LRH = low-risk hyperplasia; HRH = high-risk hyperplasia; CA = carcinoma; NH = normal histology; BH = benign histology; SH = simple hyperplasia; CH = complex hyperplasia.

| | |
|---|---|
| Sensitivity | 173/176, 98.3% |
| Specificity | 2076/2094, 910.1% |
| Positive predictive value | 173/191, 90.6% |
| Negative predictive value | 2076/2079, 910.9% |

**Absolute failures = 3.1 % (72/2342)**
**Relative failures = 1.1 % (24/2270).**

Inspite of the fact that hysteroscopy has been practiced since the 1980s, it was still necessary to design an image classification such as those available for other endoscopic procedures. Our systematization of hysteroscopic images is based on over 23 years of experience.

**Table 10.1:** Correlation between microhysteroscopic images and histologic confirmation

| | | | | *HISTOLOGY* | | | |
|---|---|---|---|---|---|---|---|
| | | *NH* | *BH* | *SH* | *CH* | *CA.* | *TOTAL IMAGES* |
| | NHI | 1623 | 0 | 0 | 0 | 0 | 1623 |
| | BL | 0 | 453 | 0 | 0 | 3 | 456 |
| HYSTEROSCOPY | LRH | 0 | 18 | 113 | 0 | 0 | 131 |
| | HRH | 0 | 0 | 12 | 21 | 0 | 33 |
| | CA | 0 | 0 | 0 | 0 | 27 | 27 |
| | TOTAL PATHOLOGY | 1623 | 471 | 125 | 21 | 30 | 2270 |

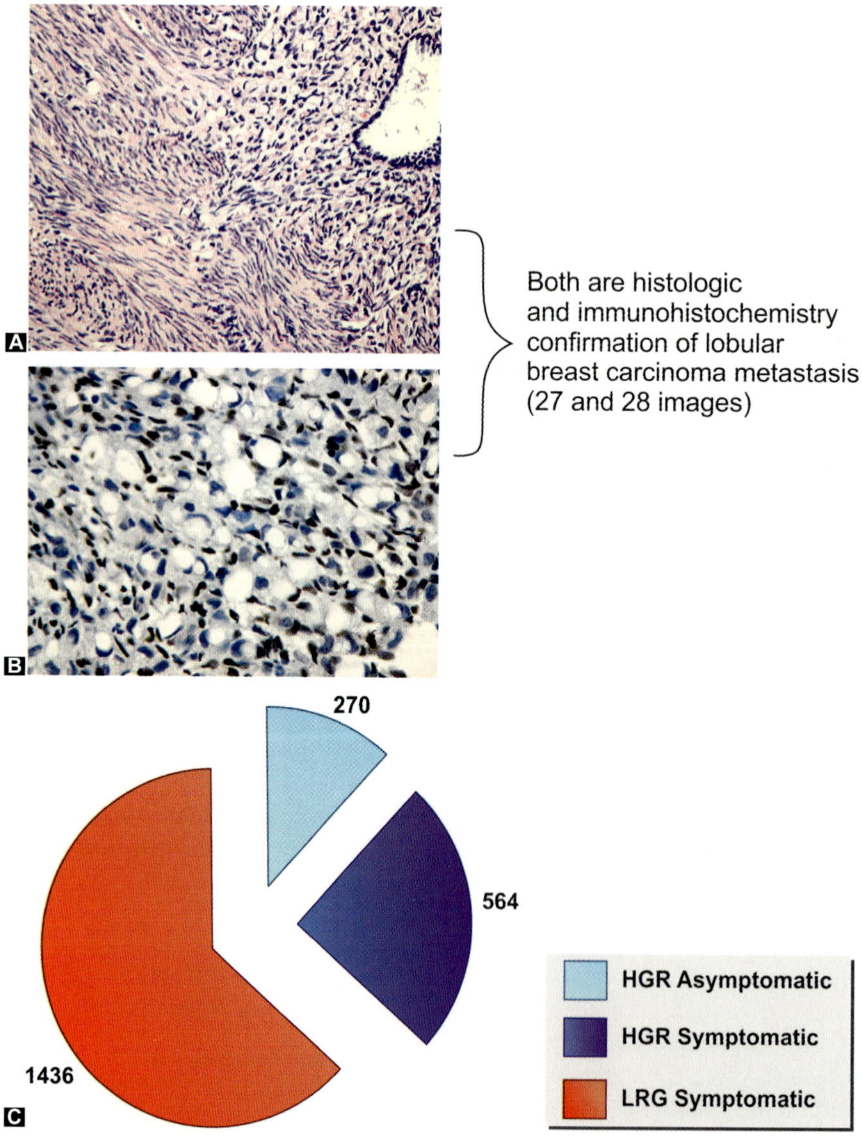


**Figs 10.29A to C:** Microhysteroscopic images and histologic confirmation

Within this framework, it can be stated that this classification is a useful tool for a systematic approach to endoscopic findings. It is also useful for communication between the endoscopist and the attending gynecologist, when the two specialists manage a patient. It is also useful for joint reports drafted by both endoscopists and pathologists. The endoscopist's diagnostic impression can be briefly stated, and a guide in the pathologist's search for malignant or potentially malignant lesions. This diagnostic exploration offers guidance in the case of suspicious lesions or negative biopsies: further investigation of these lesions can help avoid mistaken conclusions. We conclude that the diagnostic method is highly specific and very sensitive in the detection of pathological conditions. Predictive values calculated from specimens indicate that it is also useful to predict endometrial lesions.

Chapter 11

# Hysteroscopic Myomectomy

*Sunita R Tandulwadkar, Nirzari Mangeshikar*

## PREOPERATIVE EVALUATION

- Transvaginal ultrasound (TVS) should be performed to confirm the diagnosis and to assess number, size and location of the myomas.
- It must indicate the extent of myomal intra-mural extension.

## PREOPERATIVE PREPARATION

- It is preferred to do the procedure in immediate post-menstrual period.
- It does not require any particular preparation of the patient.

## IMPORTANT EQUIPMENT

- Biopolar electrode/resectoscope with forward bend loop.
- Hysteromat/pressure bag.
- Normal saline (in case of bipolar energy source) and 1.5% glycine (in case of unipolar energy source).

## CLASSIFICATION OF SUBMUCOSAL FIBROID

It is divided into 3 subtypes:

**Type 0:** Pedunculated fibroid without intramural extension (Fig. 11.1).

**Type I:** Sessile with intramural extension of fibroid of <50% (Fig. 11.2).

**Type II** Sessile with intramural extension of fibroid of >50% (Fig. 11.3).

The degree of intramural extension can be assessed by transvaginal ultrasonography or by hysteroscopy by observing the angle between fibroid and the endometrium at the attachment to the uterine wall.

## TECHNIQUE

1. Diagnostic hysteroscopy is performed to confirm the ultrasonographic findings.
2. Cervix is further dilated to accommodate the bipolar resectoscope. Ensure the free movement of bipolar resectoscope.
3. For leiomyoma resection, a 26 Fr bipolar resectoscope is normally used with 30° telescope. After cervical dilatation, the bipolar resectoscope with the electrosurgical working element (90° cutting loop) is introduced.
4. Distension of the uterine cavity is obtained with normal saline.
5. Irrigation is controlled with an electronic suction and irrigation pump, which automatically controls both intrauterine pressure and flow rate. The system also ensures constant suction and allows us to calculate the precise amount of fluid loss.
6. Intrauterine pressure should be adjusted such that it gives adequate distension and clear vision.
7. Following settings are generally used: Flow rate of approximately 250 mL/minute, pressure of 80–100 mm Hg, monopolar electricity generator at 60–100 watts and suction pressure of 0.25 bar. Fluid balance is recorded by measuring the infused and drained fluid from continuous flow bipolar resectoscope.

8. Resection is performed by placing the electrical loop behind the myoma to be resected and retracting it toward the distal lens of hysteroscope. Myoma is shaved down with slicing technique (Fig. 11.4).
9. Type 0: It is systematically shaved off with the bipolar resectoscope loop until the pedicle is reached. There is no need for hydrostatic massage. In case of large fibroids, too much crowding of pieces can be tackled by removing them with ovum forceps intermittently (Fig. 11.5).
10. Type I and type II: Resection is done by placing the loop behind the myoma and retracting it toward the scope. Myoma is shaved down with slicing technique with cutting loop to the level of myometrium till myoma becomes flat. After having dissected the portion of myoma protruding into the cavity, an attempt is made to remove the part nested deep in the myometrial wall (Fig. 11.6).

    This can be achieved by 2 techniques:
    1. By giving hydromassage by controlled variation of endo-cavitary pressure (opening and closing the endo-uterine aspiration system), myoma will start protruding in the cavity which can be sliced off. Like this we may be able to remove myoma completely in the same sitting. Usually we are able to see pink capsule on myometrium as end result.
    2. Cold knife technique which consists of simple, mechanical passage of the bipolar resectoscope loop along the capsule lining of the myoma, detaching if from the fibrous bridges that anchors it to the uterine wall, without any electrocoagulation.

## TIPS

1. Meticulous attention to intraoperative fluid balance is imperative, if fluid deficit more than 1 to 1.5 liters is detected, serum sodium is measured and hyponatremia, if present, should be treated. For every liter of electrolyte free fluid that is absorbed the sodium will go down approximately 10 mEq /L. This helps surgeon to determine when to stop a case. If deficit is approximately 1500cc it is advisable to put in a Foley's catheter and give diuretic.
2. Absorption of large volumes of electrolyte free, low viscosity fluid especially with large myoma is the trigger of some systemic changes during the operation. Myomectomy of large myomas is liable to hyponatremia, hypo-osmolality, increased CVP, increased PT and aPTT and increased most of the cardio dynamic parameters. These changes deserve performing the procedure by an experienced hysteroscopic surgeon using a quick technique with least possible Normal saline volume and minimal intrauterine pressure to achieve the goal of a safe minimal access surgery.
3. It is advisable not to remove big anterior and posterior fibroids in the same sitting to avoid intraeuterine adhesions/synechiae formations.
4. Type 0 myoma should never be dislodged at the base first, which is the most tempting thing to do. One should avoid this as removal of floating myoma from uterine cavity creates a great problem.
5. While resecting Type I and Type II myoma particular care is taken regarding the intra-uterine pressure. If pressure is very high, fibroids will be pushed deep into the wall making resection difficult and also it may increase the intravasation of fluid. To prevent this, minimal least pressure is kept that gives adequate distension and clear vision.

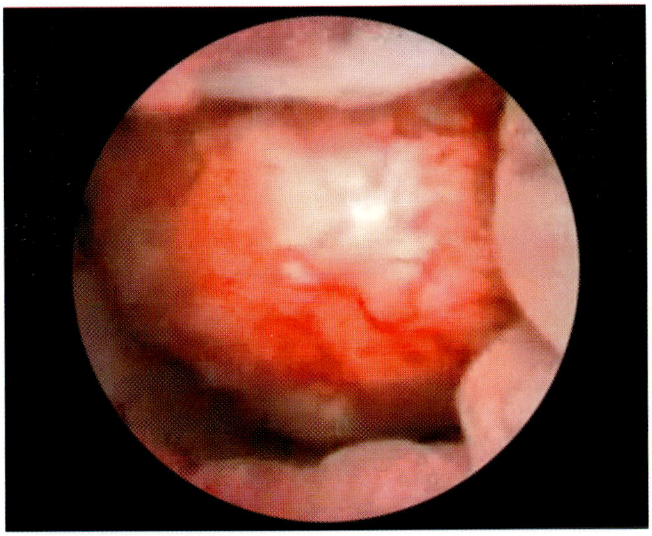

**Fig. 11.1:** Type 0 myoma (intracavitatory-completely in the cavity)

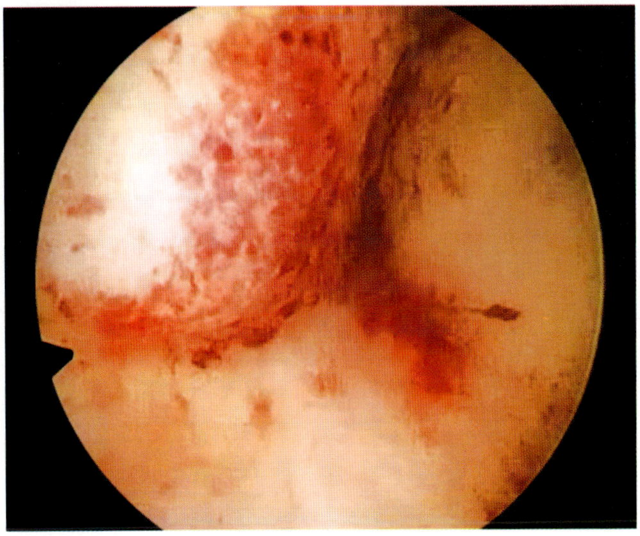

**Fig. 11.2:** Type I myoma (>50% in cavity)

11. The operation can be considered complete when only myometrium can be seen throughout the entire surgical area. Utmost care should be taken to prevent damaging the smooth muscle fiber bundles. If it is impossible to totally remove the intra-mural fibroid in one sitting, in spite of trying the above techniques, because of it is too deep location and/or technical difficulties, the remaining myoma can be coagulated until dry. This effect is achieved by placing the loop in direct contact with remaining wall of the myoma and applying a high coagulation current for approximately 30 seconds. The fibroid can then be treated at a later date (2–3 months later) as over the period intra-mural component of myoma migrates into the uterine cavity.

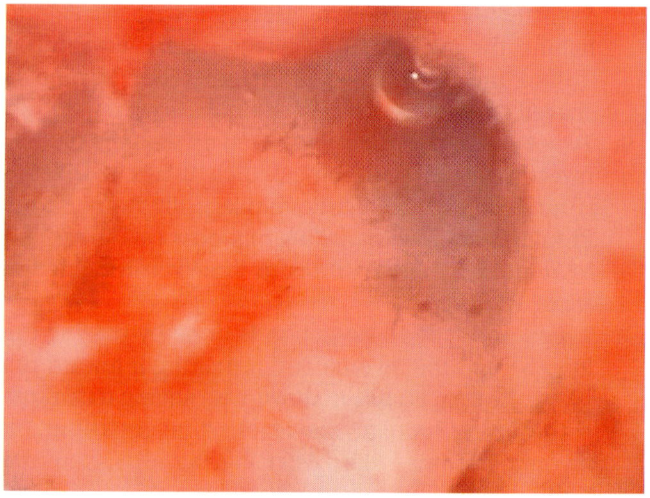

**Fig. 11.3:** Type II myoma (<50% in cavity)

## Resection of Type 0 Myoma

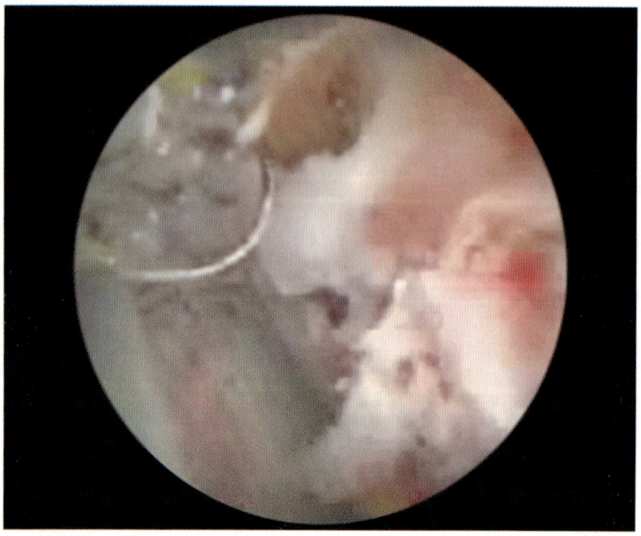

**Fig. 11.4:** Resection of myoma

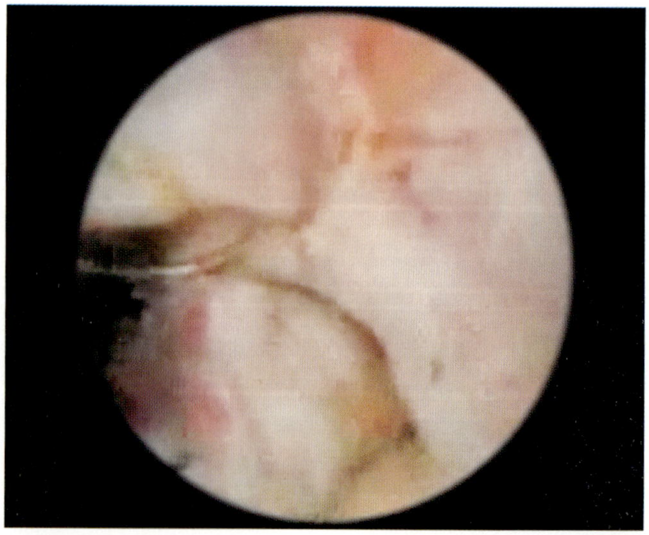

**Fig. 11.5:** Resection till pedicle base

## Hysteroscopic Resection of a Large Type 0 submucous Myoma

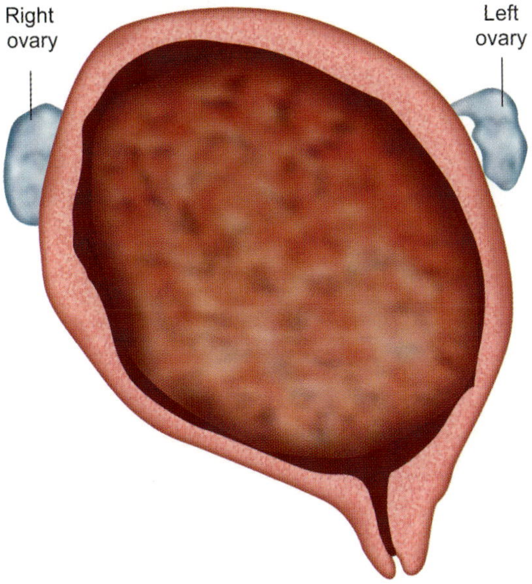


**Fig. 11.6:** Pre-operative sonographic image of the myoma: Type 0 myoma

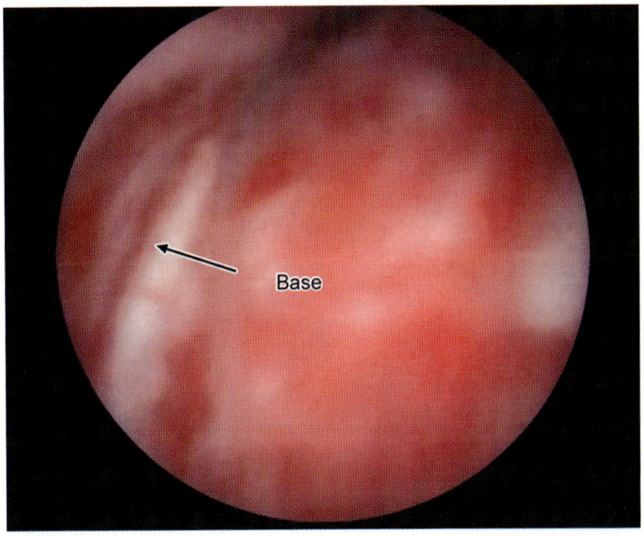


**Fig. 11.7:** Large type 0 submucous myoma with base on the right lateral wall

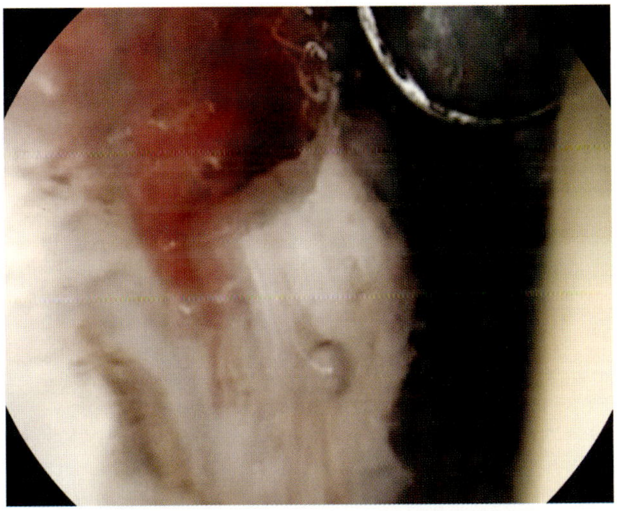

**Fig. 11.8:** Resection of the myoma done using bipolar resectoscope

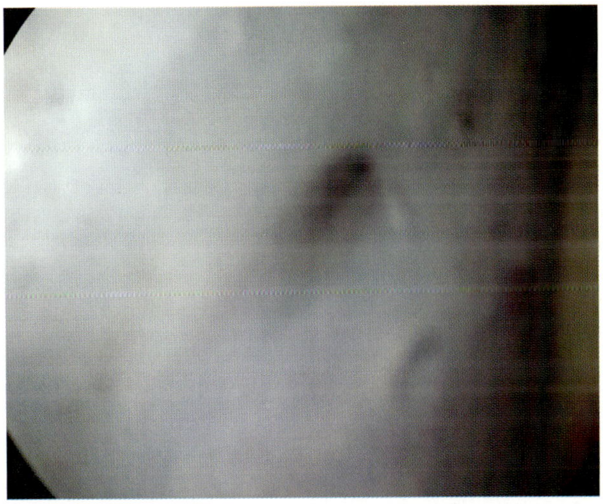

**Fig. 11.9:** Open vessel channels may be encountered

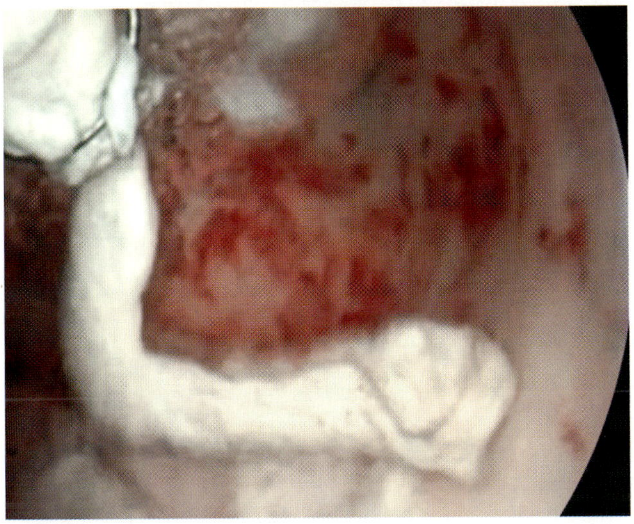

**Fig. 11.10:** End result: Entire myoma removed in one sitting

### TIPS

- In case of large type 0 myomas, one can perform a mini-hysteroscopy initially to discern the extent and identify the base of the myoma.
- Due to large size, there will be overcrowding of the resected pieces; this can be overcome by continuing the resection without wasting time in removal of those pieces. With the flow of fluid, pieces will automatically move laterally maintaining good surgical speed and avoiding blood in the cavity.
- One may encounter large open vessel channels, owing to increased vascularity of the myoma. Again speedy surgery will reduce the risk of complications related to irrigation fluid entering vascular channels, as well as potential hemorrhage.
- One can think of giving pre-operative GnRH analogues, which can shrink the myoma and make it less vascular. This may also allow one to complete the surgery in one go.

## Resection of Type 1 Submucous Myoma by Hydromassage Technique

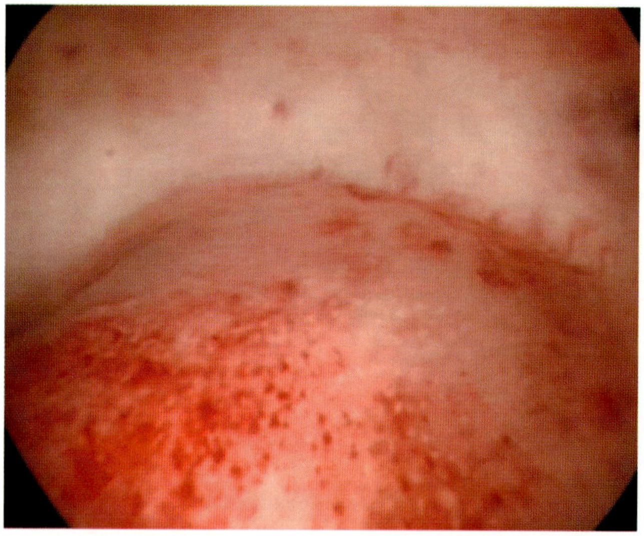

**Fig. 11.11:** Type 1 myoma in posterior wall of uterus

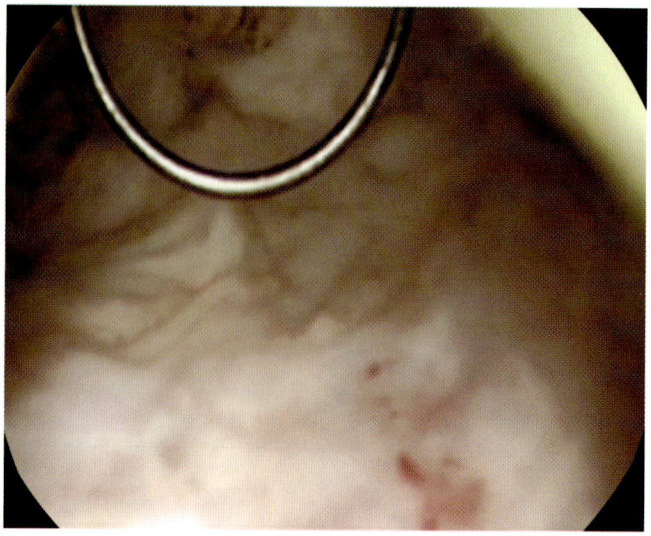

**Fig. 11.12:** Resection with bipolar resectoscope

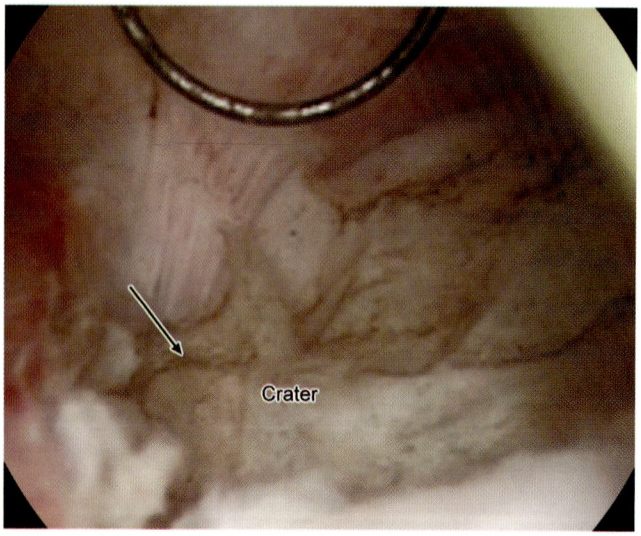


**Fig. 11.13:** Hydromassage to delineate and loosen up the myoma capsule from underlying basal endometrium and myometrium

### TIPS

- In case of a type 1 myoma with a well-defined capsule, one can use 'hydromassage' technique; by opening and closing the outflow channel, in order to loosen up the myoma from its bed.
- This will enable one to remove the myoma from its bed without use of energy source or minimal energy source at the base, thus minimizing the damage to the underlying endometrium and myometrium.

## Resection of Type II Myoma

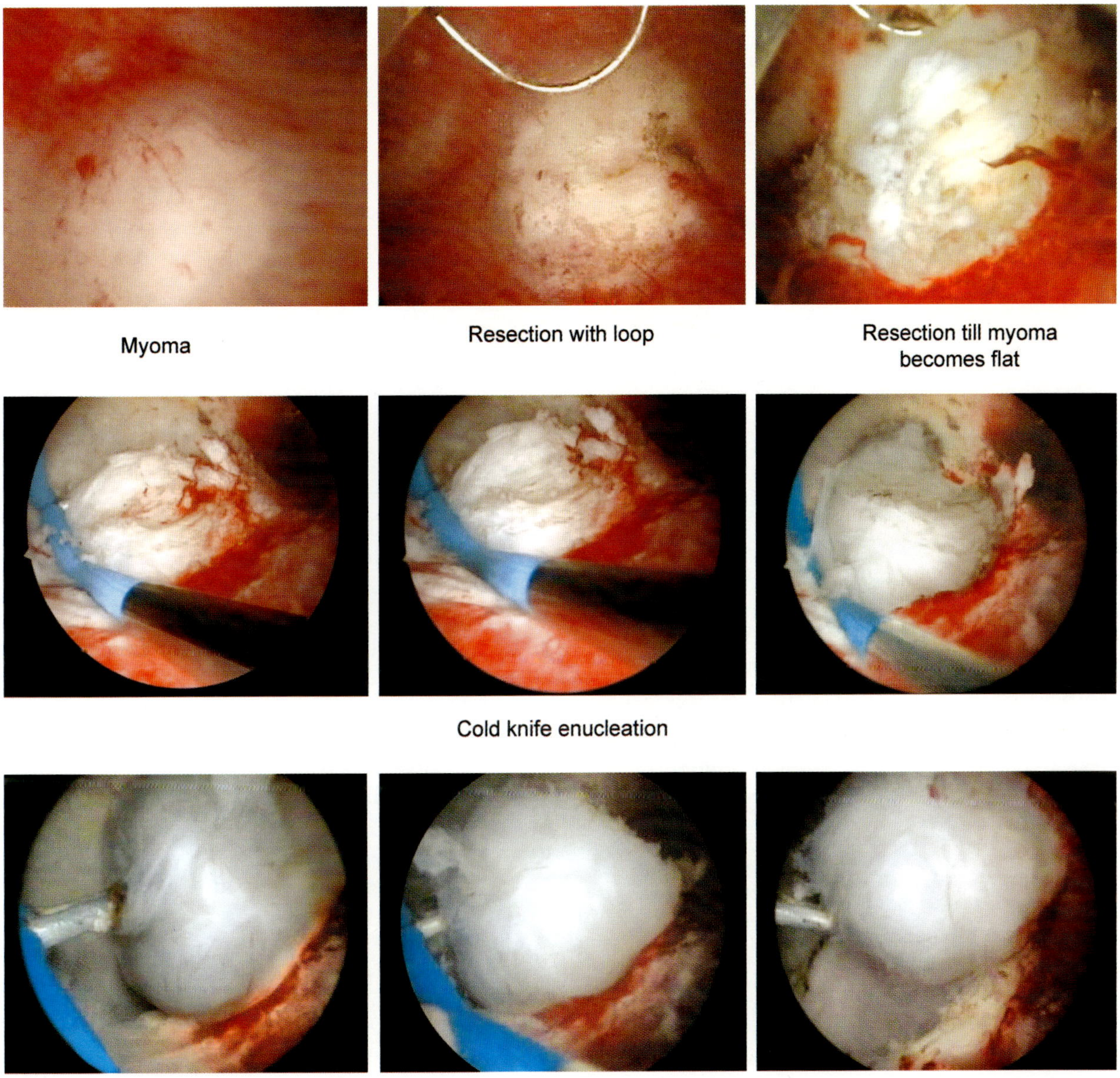

Myoma

Resection with loop

Resection till myoma becomes flat

Cold knife enucleation

Completely enucleated ....encapsule

Completely enucleated with crater in background

**Fig. 11.14**

Chapter

12

# Hysteroscopic Management of Intrauterine Adhesions

*Sunita R Tandulwadkar, Pooja Lodha*

## PREOPERATIVE EVALUATION

- History of oligomenorrhea/amenorrhea following dilatation and curettage or suction and evacuation.
- Hysterosalpingography—may help to outline the extent of uterine cavity occlusion.
- Transvaginal sonography.

## PREOPERATIVE PREPARATION

Usually done immediate postmenstrually, but in patients who have amenorrhea, it can be planned anytime.

## INSTRUMENTATION

- Therapeutic hysteroscope with:
  - Scissors
  - Versa point (bipolar)
  - Monopolar/bipolar needle
  - Resectoscope with Collin's knife.
- Hysteromat/ Pressure bag.
- Glycine 1.5% w/v or normal saline depending on the energy source to be used.

## TECHNIQUE

1. Bimanual palpation should be done to evaluate the position of uterus (Fig. 12.1).
2. Gradual gentle dilatation of the internal os is done.
3. Diagnostic hysteroscopy should be done by using therapeutic sheath to confirm the diagnosis.
4. The set pressure of hysteromat should be between 180–200 mm of Hg with a minimum amount of pure cutting current between 60–80 watts.
5. Either monopolar needle/scissors/versa point is passed through therapeutic sheath to release adhesions (Figs 12.2 and 12.3).
6. If one wishes to use Collin's knife, further dilatation is needed to accommodate resectoscope with the Collin's knife.
7. 1.5% glycine is required whenever cautery current is used (for monopolar/bipolar needle or Collin's knife).
8. One should withdraw the scope till internal os from time to time, to have a panoramic view of cavity for orientation and to avoid going in the wrong plane (Figs 12.4 and 12.5).
9. Adhesiolysis should be stopped once the pink myometrium is reached.

## POSTOPERATIVE CARE

- Estrogen and progesterone treatment—Premarin 0.625 mg, 6 weeks + duphaston 20 mg for latter 4 weeks.
- Second look hysteroscopy if adhesions are moderate to severe and patient is for IVF.

**TIPS**

- Care should be taken not to damage the basal endometrium that may interfere with rapid re-epithelialization of the area.
- In case of severe adhesions, simultaneous laparoscopy is helpful and more than one sitting may be needed.
- Good intra-uterine pressure should be maintained.

***The only criterion for success is a subsequent pregnancy resulting in a viable birth.***

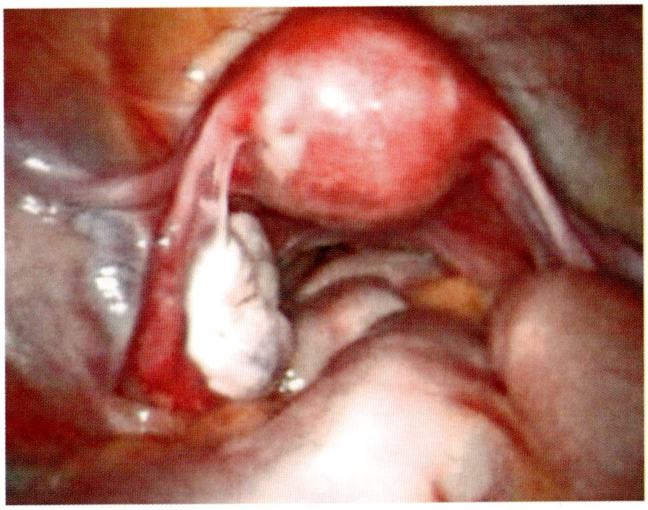

**Fig. 12.1:** Laparoscopy showing normal uterus (hysteroscopy was showing cavity like unicornuate uterus as shown below)

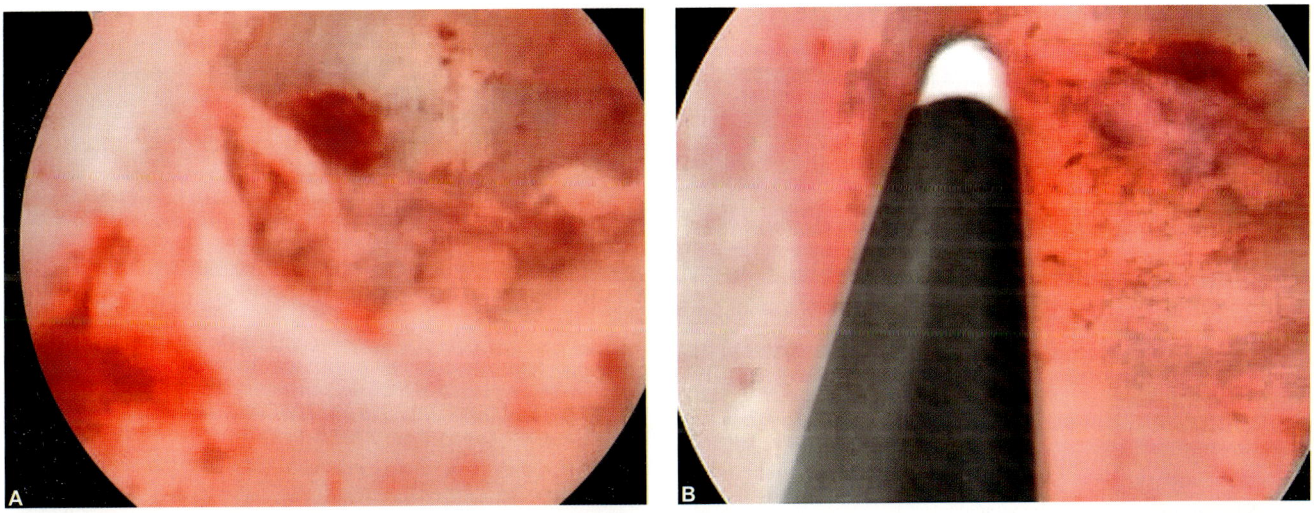

**Figs 12.2A and B:** Hysteroscopy showing intrauterine adhesions on right half of the cavity. With versapoint upper right point is fixed in correspondence with left cornu, no dissection will go in cranial direction from this point, this step avoids fundal perforation

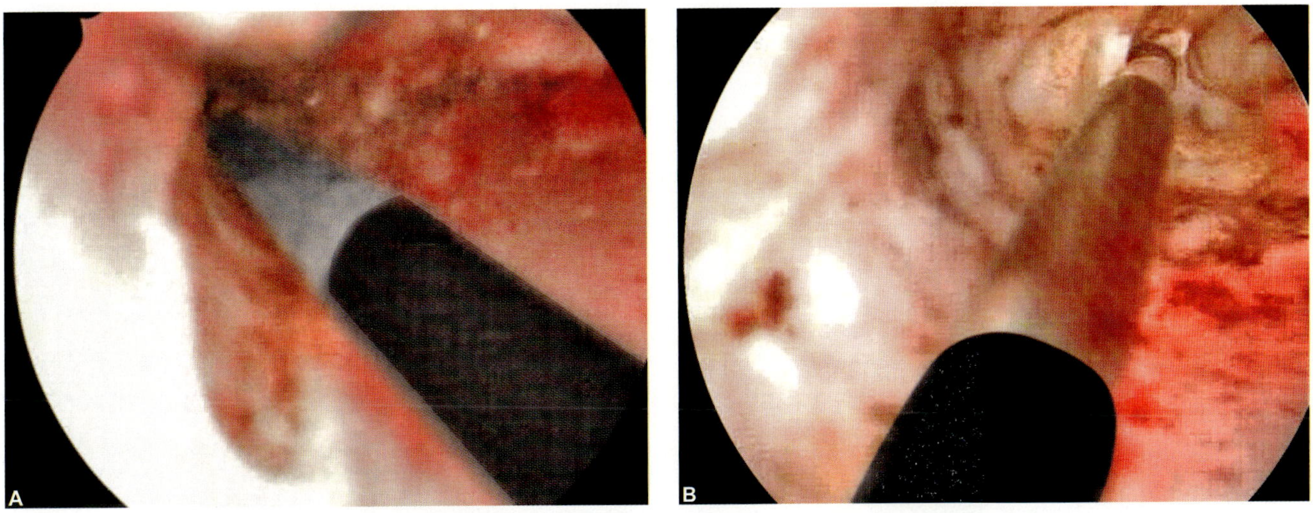

**Figs 12.3A and B:** With versascope lateral and vertical strokes taken so as to release adhesions

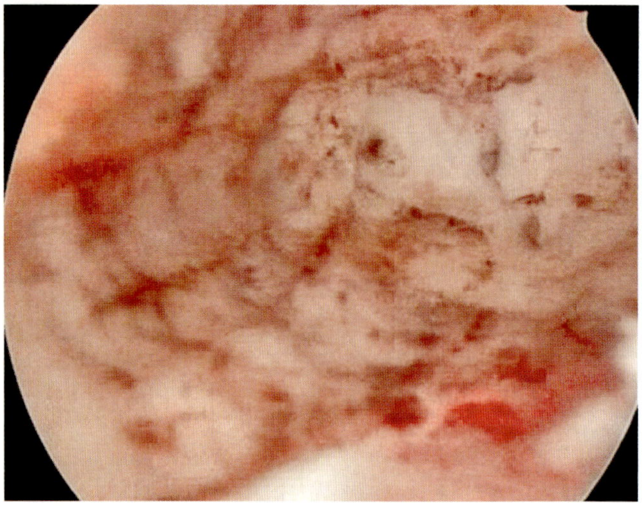

Fig. 12.4: Towards end

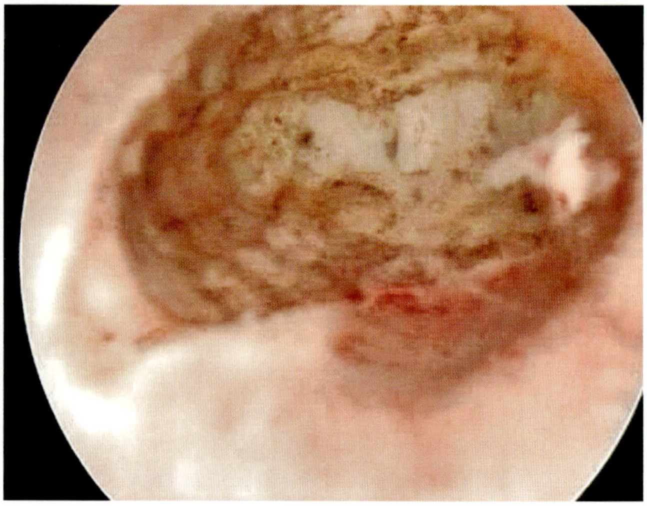

Fig. 12.5: End result (Nearly normal cavity)

## Central Intrauterine Adhesion

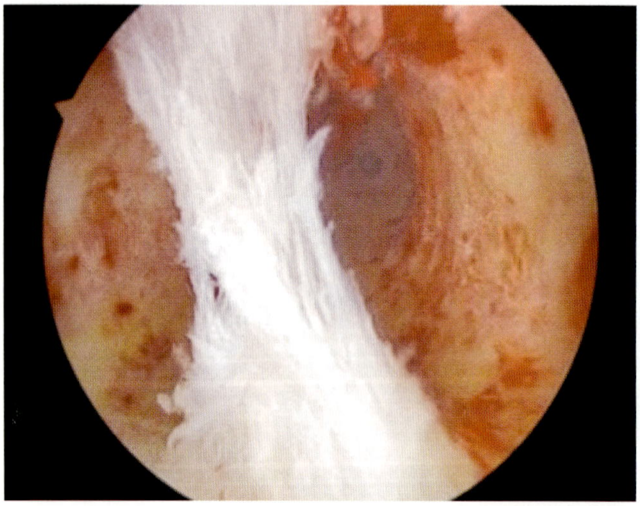

Fig. 12.6A: Band of intrauterine adhesion at isthmus

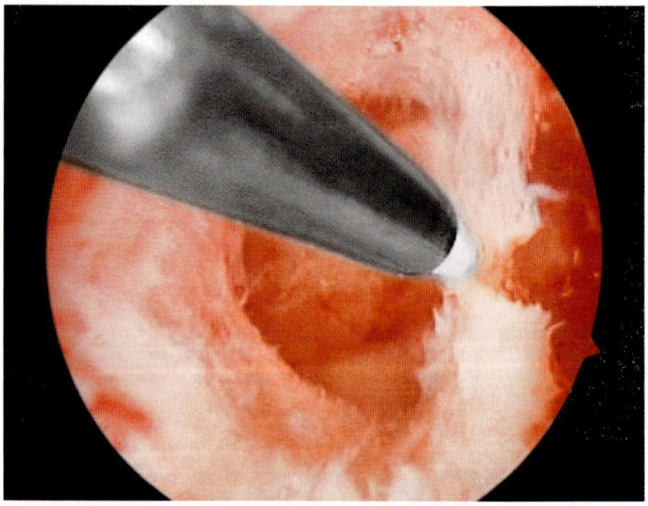

Fig. 12.6B: Adhesion released with versa point

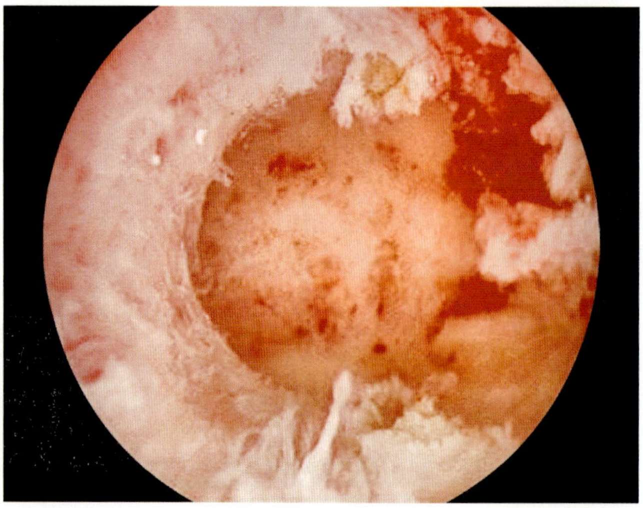

Fig. 12.6C: End result

## Flimsy Adhesion

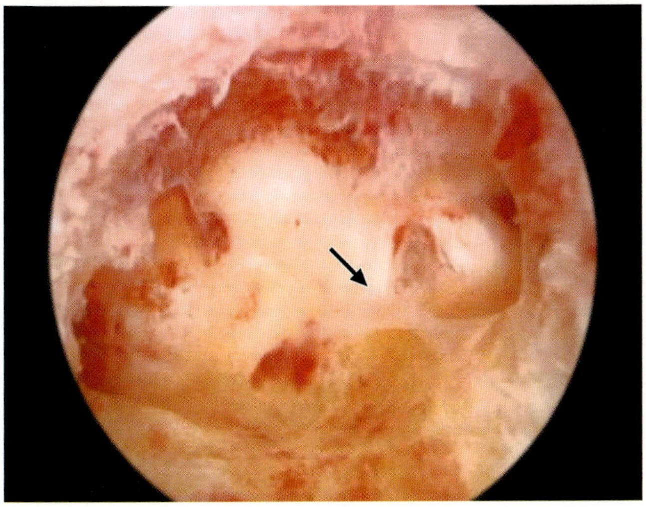

**Fig. 12.7A:** Flimsy adhesions in cavity

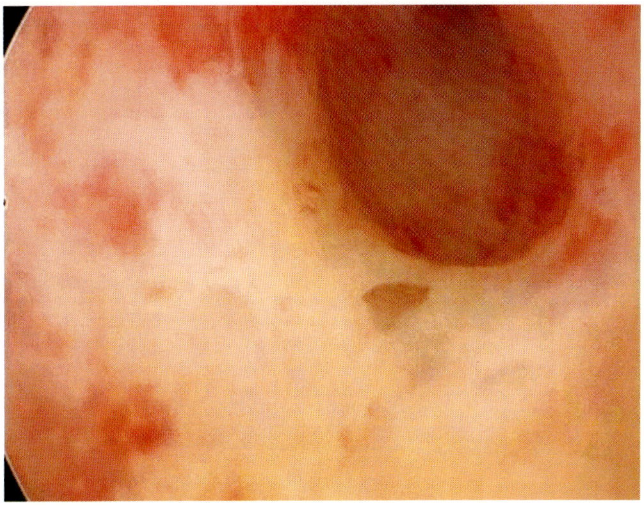

**Fig. 12.7B:** Flimsy adhesions near cornu

Chapter 13

# Hysteroscopic Cannulation for Proximal Tubal Block

*Sunita R Tandulwadkar*

## PREOPERATIVE EVALUATION

- History of infertility
- Hysterosalpingography can give a false positive diagnosis of cornual block.

## PREOPERATIVE PREPARATION

- Cannulation does not need any other preoperative preparation.
- It is performed in the immediate postmenstrual period.

## IMPORTANT EQUIPMENT

- Hysteroscope with therapeutic sheath (single 7 Fr channel is also sufficient).
- Cannulation set with guide wire.

## TECHNIQUE (FIG. 13.1)

1. Bimanual palpation should be done to evaluate the position of uterus.
2. Gradual gentle dilatation of the internal os is done.
3. Hysteroscopy is performed.
4. Approximate site of cornu can be identified.
5. Telescope should be positioned very close to the cornu and the cornu should be positioned at the center of the monitor (so automatically when the guide wire comes out, it will enter the cornu).
6. Once this position is achieved, guide wire and cannula are passed through the operative sheath and is pushed so as to be seen in the field of vision.
7. Guide wire negotiates the cornu and the cannula is guided over it.
8. Cannula is pushed just 2–4 mm beyond the cornu and guide wire is removed.
9. Methylene blue is injected through the distal end of cannula; dye is seen coming out from the fimbrial end of cornu simultaneously by laparoscopy.
10. If cornual block is rigid, cannulation will not be successful.

### TIPS

- Presence of 2 separated monitors, camera and light source for laparoscopy and hysteroscopy each, makes surgery simple and hastle-free.
- The aim of surgery is opening the cornual end of fallopian tube, so never pass guide wire through full length of fallopian tube. It will damage the ciliary and endothelial layer.

## Technique for Hysteroscopic Cannulation

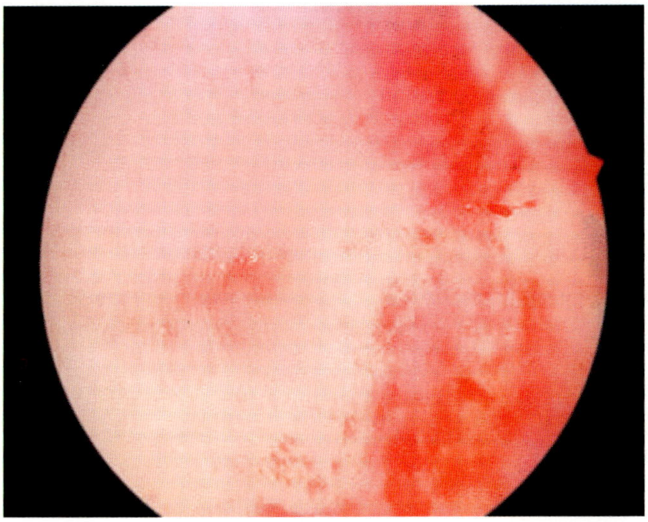

**Fig. 13.1A:** Right cornual block

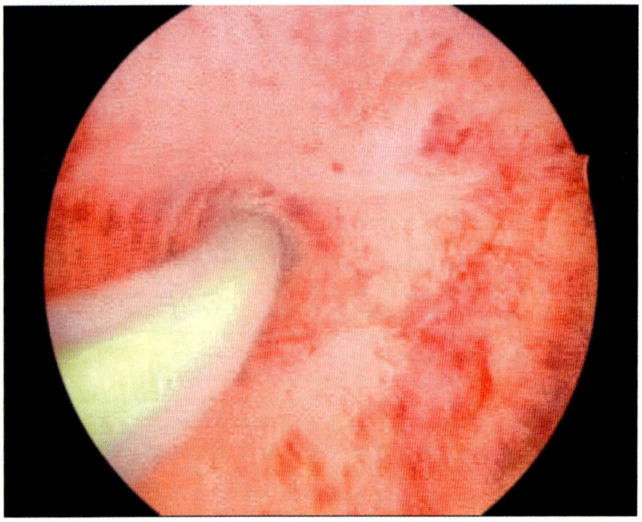

**Fig. 13.1B:** Guide wire passed

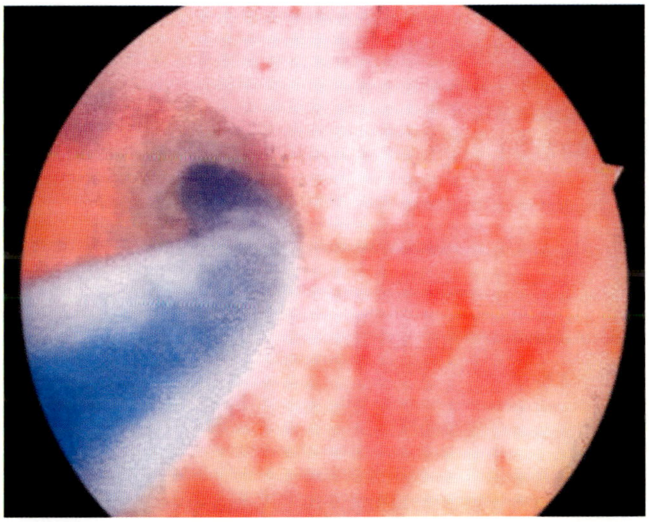

**Fig. 13.1C:** Dye injected

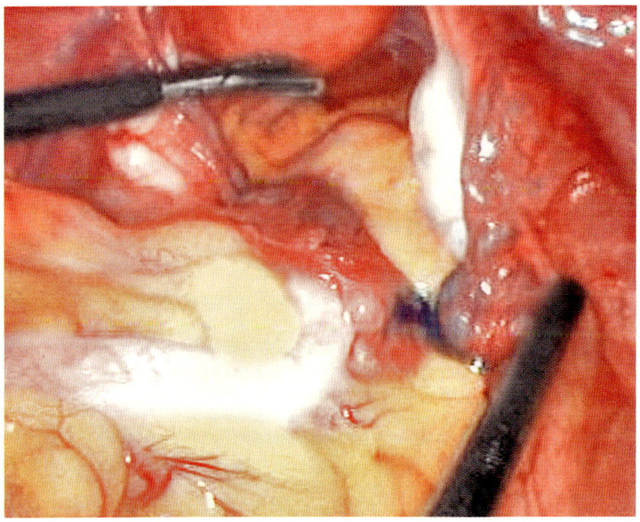

**Fig. 13.1D:** Free spillage seen through laparoscopy

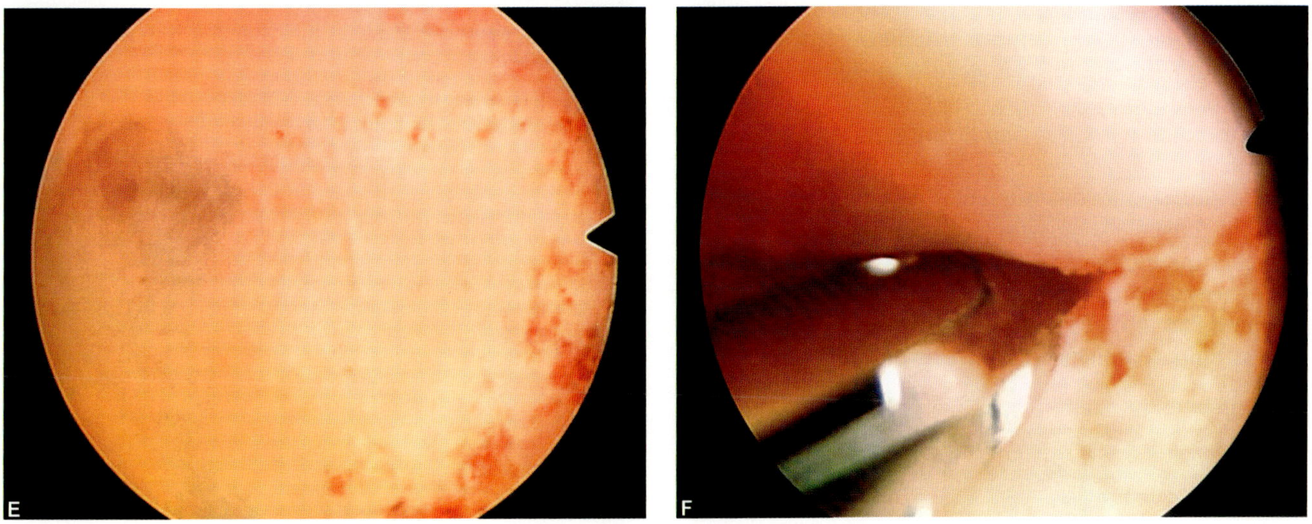


**Figs 13.1E and F:** Occasionally flimsy fibers at cornu can be released with scissors or blunt forceps

Chapter

14

# Hysteroscopic Resection of Septum

*Sunita R Tandulwadkar, Sejal Naik*

## PREOPERATIVE EVALUATION

- Bad obstetric history/infertility.
- 3-D transvaginal sonography.

## PREOPERATIVE PREPARATION

Preferably done in postmenstrual period.

## SPECIAL INSTRUMENTS

- Therapeutic hysteroscope with:
  - Scissors
  - Versa point
  - Monopolar/bipolar needle
  - Resectoscope with Collin's knife
- Hysteromat/ Pressure bag
- Glycine 1.5% w/v or normal saline depending on the energy source to be used.

## TECHNIQUE

First, a diagnostic hysteroscopy is performed to confirm the diagnosis of the septum. (Laparoscopy is needed in case of complete broad septum to differentiate from bicornuate uterus).

1. Bimanual palpation should be done to evaluate the position of uterus.
2. Gradual gentle dilatation of the internal os is done.
3. Diagnostic hysteroscopy should be done by using therapeutic sheath to confirm the diagnosis.
4. The set pressure of hysteromat should be between 180 and 200 mm of Hg with a minimum amount of pure cutting current between 60 and 80 watts.
5. Both the ostia are visualized before the resection of the septum.
6. The septum is visualized.
7. Either monopolar needle/scissors/versa point is passed through therapeutic sheath to release adhesions.
8. Incision is taken from the distal to the cephalic end.
9. When it is thin septum, incise it from distal to cephalic which causes fibroelastic band to retract.
10. In case of broader septum, 1st step is a lateral alternating technique of side-to-side resection up to 0.5 cm from fundus. Then the remainder is removed sweeping from cornu to cornu to avoid damage to this area.
11. Panaromic view is obtained from time-to-time by withdrawing the telescope till the internal os for getting judgement in cases of broad septum.
12. End result is visualizing both ostia in one line.

### TIPS

- Always see both ostia before starting for resection of septum.
- While resection, always stay in the midline of the septum.
- Care should be taken not to damage the basal endometrium that may interfere with rapid re-epithelialization of the area.
- Good intra-uterine pressure should be maintained.
- It is better to have 2–3 cm space remaining than overdoing the resection, as it may cause thinning of fundal myometrium and chances of rupture in subsequent pregnancy.

## Resection of Complete Septum

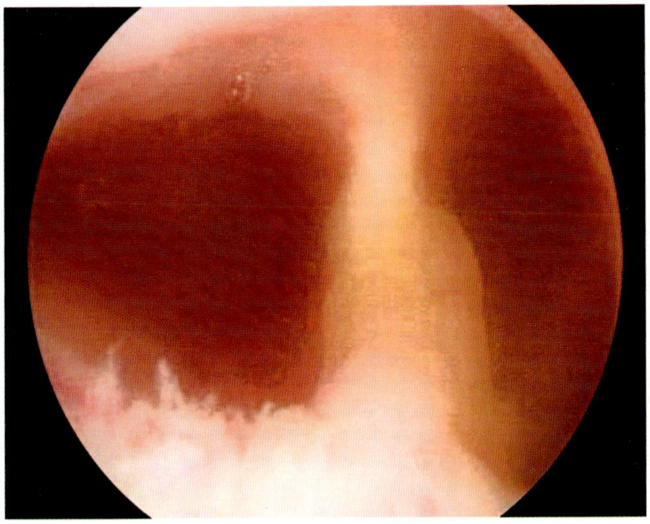

**Fig. 14.1A:** Complete septum upto internal os

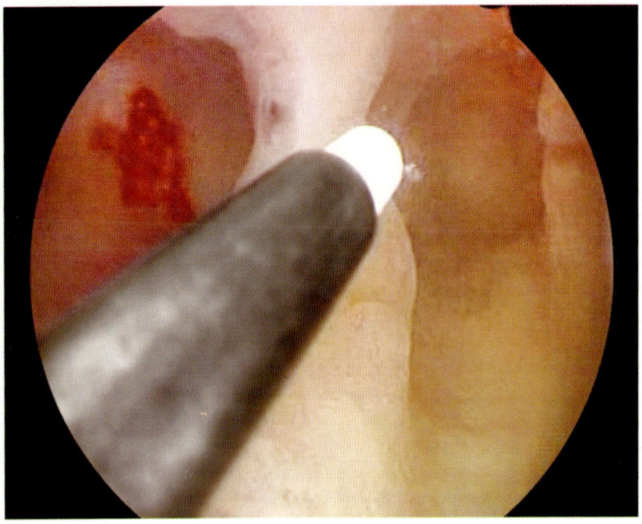

**Fig. 14.1B:** Resection with versapoint

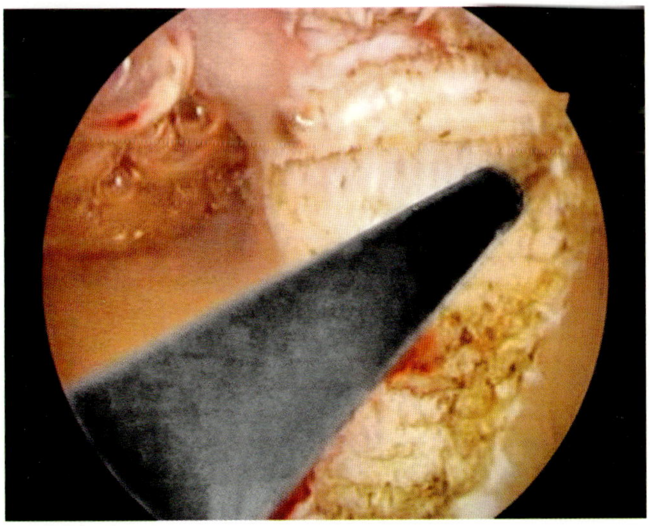

**Fig. 14.1C:** Resection in process

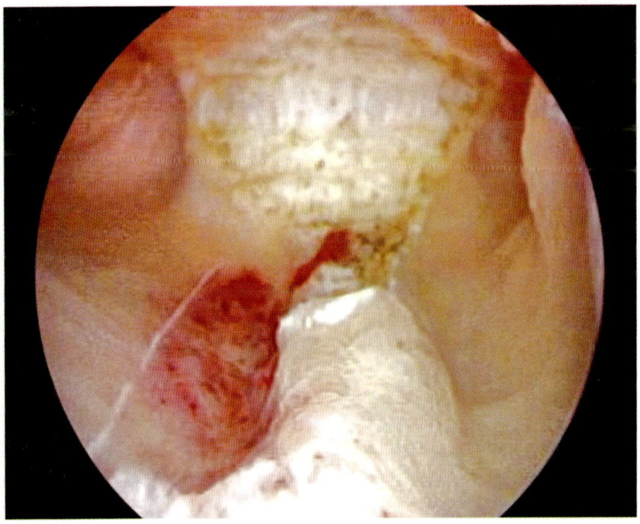

**Fig. 14.1D:** Resection towards end

## Resection of Partial Broad base Septum with Collin's knife

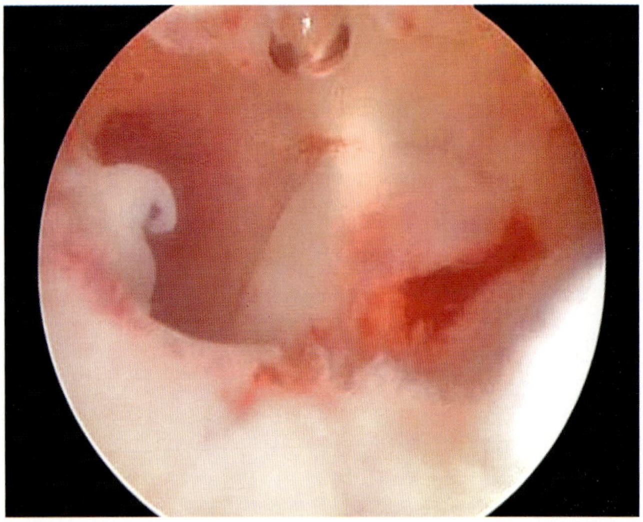

**Fig. 14.2A:** Partial broad septum

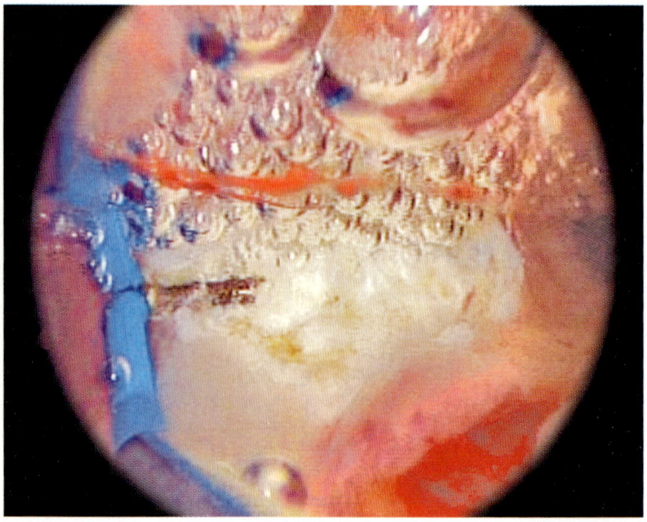

**Fig. 14.2B:** Side-to-side resection in process using Collin's knife

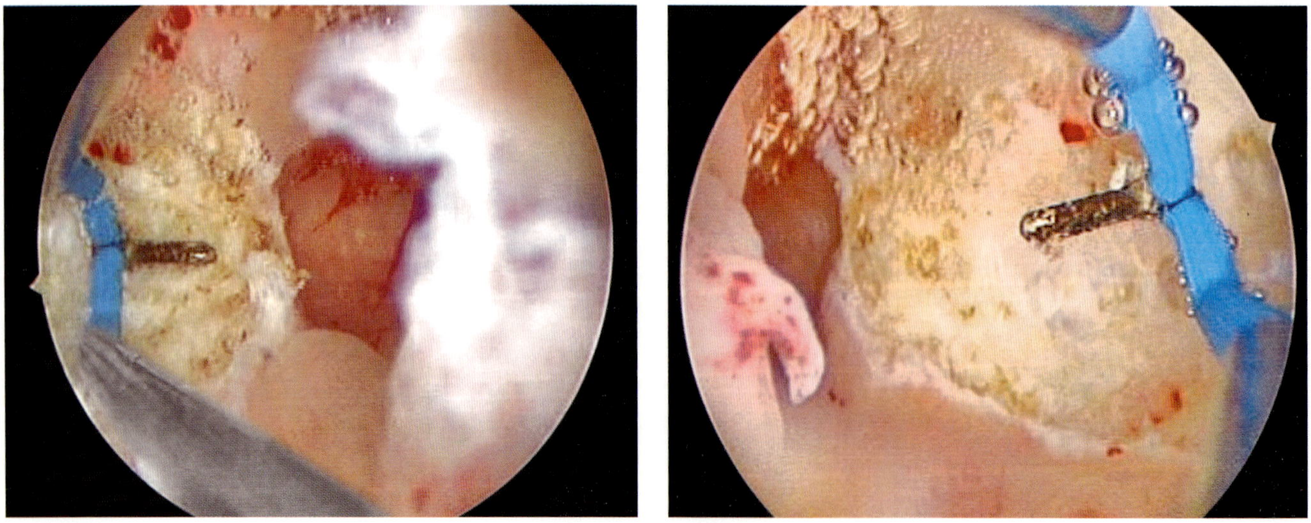

**Fig. 14.2C:** Resection towards end

## Resection of Partial Broad-based Subseptate Uterus with Versapoint

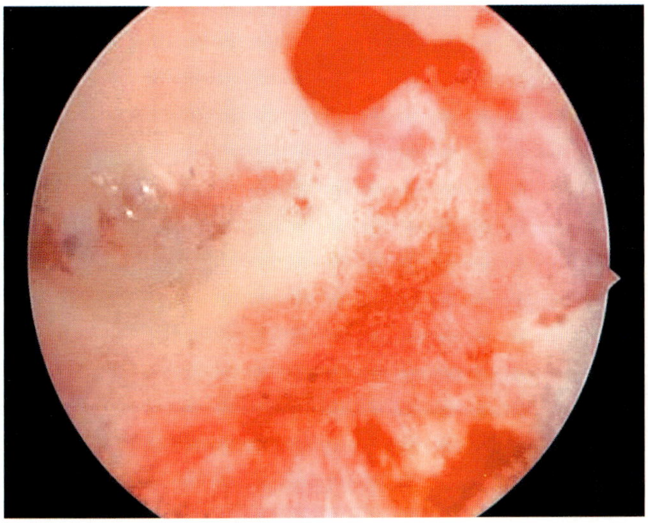

**Fig. 14.3A:** Subseptate uterus

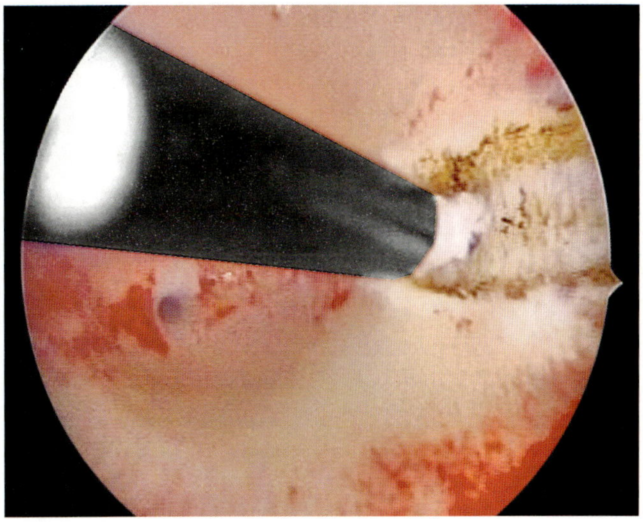

**Fig. 14.3B:** Resection with versapoint

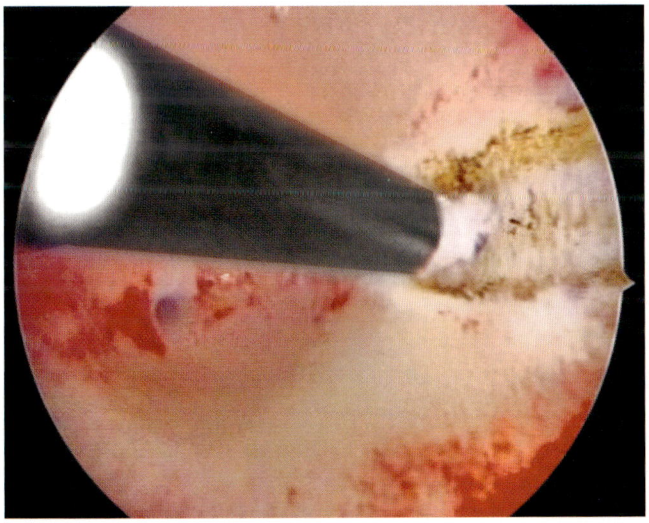

**Fig. 14.3C:** Resection in process

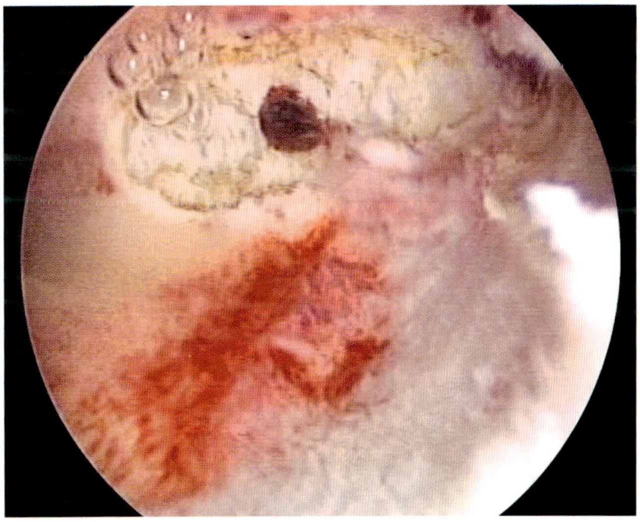

**Fig. 14.3D:** End result

Section

3

# Laparoscopy

Chapter

15

# Laparoscopic Hysterectomy

*Sunita R Tandulwadkar*

## PREOPERATIVE EVALUATION

Proper case selection is necessary (depending on the skills and laparoscopic surgeon).

## PREOPERATIVE PREPARATION

### Bowel Preparation

- *Diet*—one day prior to surgery, soft diet till afternoon followed by clear liquid diet (about 8–10 glasses) and then, nil by mouth for 8 hours prior to surgery.
- *Peglec powder*—dissolve the pack in 2 liters of water to be given over 2–3 hours on previous evening.
  or
- Exelyte solution 90 mL to be added in 300 mL of limca/fruit juice to be given on previous evening.

No need for admission for the above preparation. Patient can be admitted 6 hours prior to surgery (High-risk cases need prior admission, evaluation and fitness).

### Position of Patient

Patient is placed in a low modified lithotomy position (Fig. 15.1) on the Allen stirrups with adjustable and padded leg rest.

If Allen stirrups are not available then standard lithotomy bars with padded rest for the knee joint is suitable, kept at 45° downwards.

## IMPORTANT EQUIPMENT

- One or two 10 mm trocars
- Three or four 5 mm trocars
- 2 nontraumatic graspers
- 1 claw forceps
- 2 scissors (tissue cutting and suture cutting)
- 1 bipolar forceps (and one standby)
- Monopolar spatula or hook

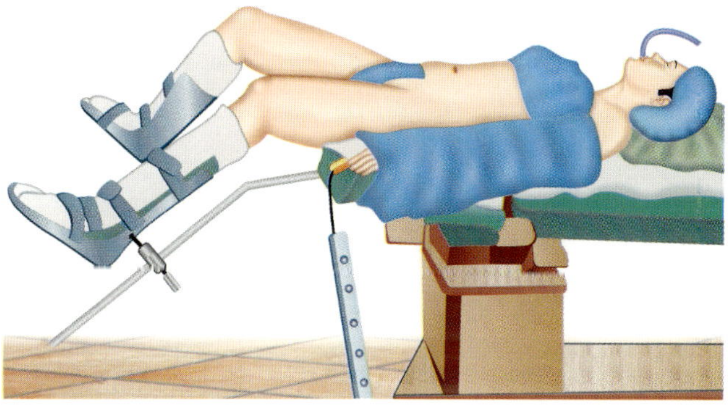

**Fig. 15.1:** Patient's position—modified lithotomy position (extended hips and legs at 135° to the horizontal)

- Uterine manipulator or myoma screw (for manipulation of uterus)
- Pair of needle holders
- Respective grasper if other energy source is to be used.

## TECHNIQUE

### Manipulator

Uterine manipulator [self designed—refer to instrument session (*See* Fig. 2.11)] is inserted to facilitate better mobilization of the uterus.

### Port Placement

1. Position of the ports either in lower abdomen or upper abdomen depends upon the size and pathology of uterus and previous lower abdomen surgeries, if any.
2. Head low only after primary trocar insertion.
3. Secondary trocars can be:
   - Two 5 mm ports on surgeon's side usually 10 cm apart and upper port a little medially. Third 5 mm port is on the contralateral side usually in line with

the primary trocar. Left-sided lower 5 mm port should be valve-less to carry suture material. Right-sided 5 mm port should have outlet to remove the smoke intermittently.

» One on surgeon's side, one in the midline and one on the contralateral side (Individual choice as per the suturing techniques and height of surgeon) (For details, refer to chapter on Port placement).

4. A 10 mm 0° laparoscope or occasionally 30° laparoscope is introduced through primary port. $CO_2$ is used for pneumoperitoneum at a rate of 3–9 liters/minute with a pressure cut off at 15 mm Hg. Then Trendelenburg's position is given.

## STEPS OF LAPAROSCOPIC HYSTERECTOMY

1. Thorough inspection of pelvis (Fig. 15.2) (i.e. examination of uterus, adenexa, anterior and posterior pouch) should be performed first. Correction of anatomy should be done if adhesions are present (Fig. 15.3). Tracing of ureter through its full course from pelvic brim till entry underneath the uterines is must before proceeding for hysterectomy (Figs 15.4 and 15.5).
2. Uterus should be pushed in and to the opposite side when the contralateral ligaments are taken. This causes apparent lengthening of the ligament, which then can be easily cauterized by keeping sufficient length from lateral pelvic wall (Fig. 15.6).
3. Procedure is started with division of infundibulopelvic ligaments (IPL), by using bipolar forceps and dedicated generator. Pull the adnexa on the medial side so that maximum length of IPL can be obtained. Always cauterize its lateral most point first (remember not to cross this point further to avoid injury to ureter). Then cauterization should be done medially. Cautery and cutting should be performed serially so as to involve whole bulk of IPL till one reaches the round ligament (Fig. 15.7).
4. Round ligaments are then coagulated and safely divided by scissors with monopolar cautery or harmonic scalpel (Figs 15.8 and 15.9).
   *Recommend taking IPL first followed by round ligament, (so that both the ligaments can be cauterized and cut in one line) but they can also be taken vice versa.
5. Anterior and posterior lips of broad ligament are separated and cut as much as possible just lateral to uterine wall (Figs 15.10 to 15.12).
6. Maintaining cranial displacement of the uterus with the help of uterine manipulator, uterus is kept in center, midposed and pushed completely in so as to visualize the anterior pouch and bladder margin.
7. Uterovesical fold of peritoneum is then lifted and held in the midline using a Maryland forceps introduced through the right port and cut close to the uterus using a spatula or hook introduced through left upper port (Fig. 15.13). It may be cauterized before cutting to avoid capillary oozing. Usually pneumoperitoneum helps to further create plane. Incision is further extended laterally to the anterior lip of broad ligament to meet the previous cut.
8. Maintaining the position of the uterus, little retroverted, pubocervical ligament can be identified and severed with blunt forceps or cauterized and cut. This allows the bladder to push down easily, exposing 1–2 cm of upper vagina. This step of pushing the bladder completely down and laterally causes lateral displacement of the ureters. We always advocate this step before tackling the uterines (Fig. 15.14).
9. After this uterus is completely anteverted, so as to visualize the posterior lip of broad ligament which is

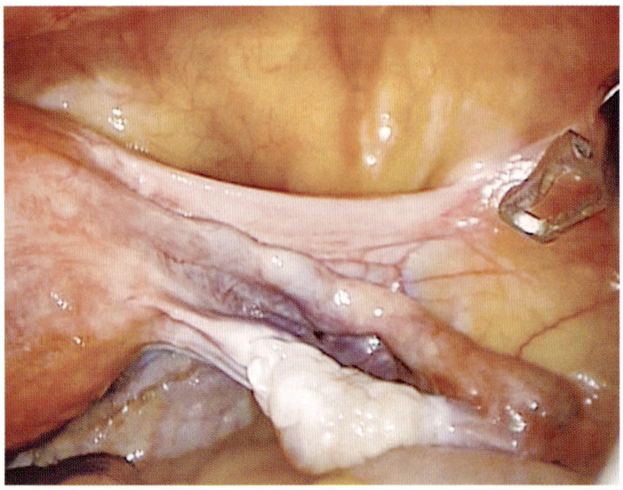

**Fig. 15.2:** Thorough visualization of right adnexa

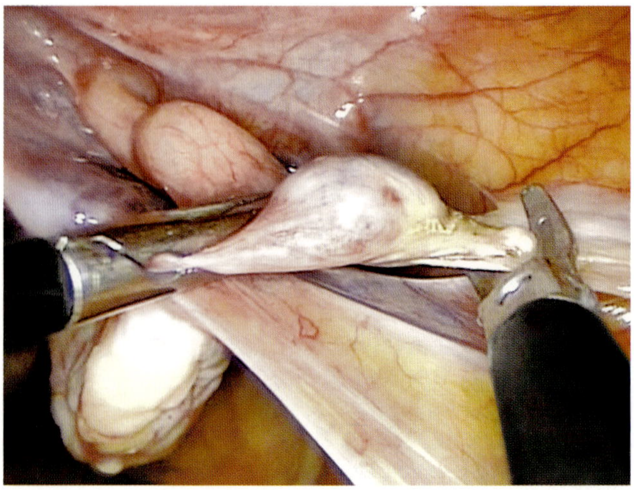

**Fig. 15.3:** Release of adhesions of Fallopian tube from lateral pelvic wall

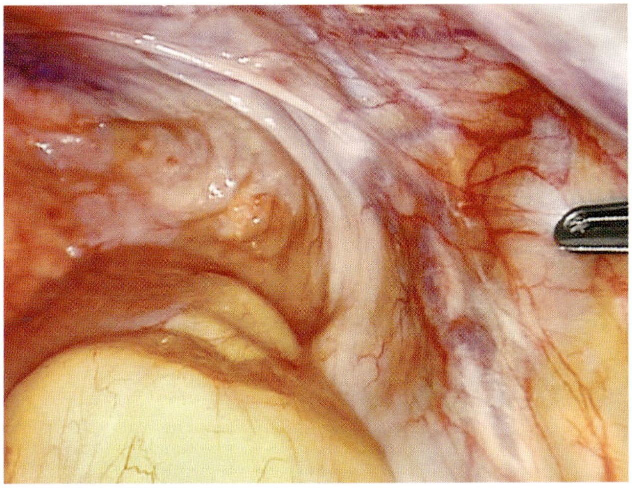

**Fig. 15.4:** Tracing course of right ureter

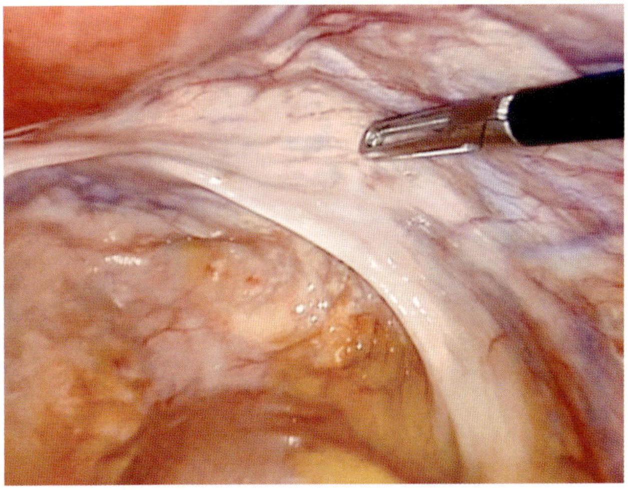

**Fig. 15.5:** Tracing of ureter till its entry beneath uterines

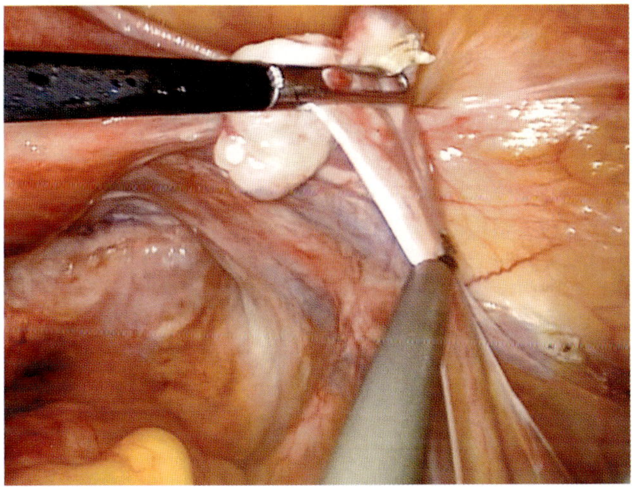

**Fig. 15.6:** Cauterization of infundibulopelvic ligament

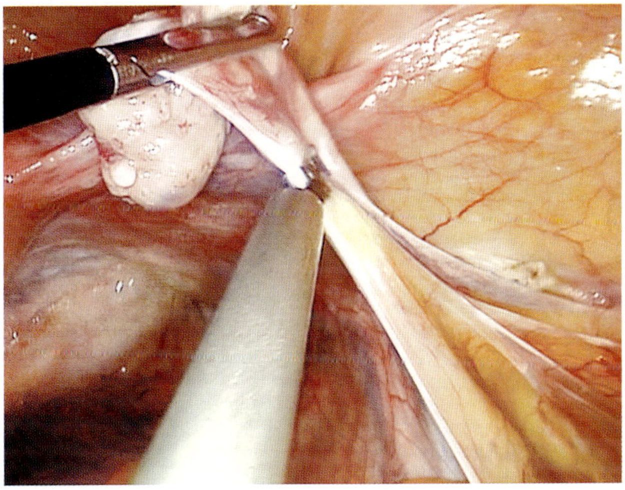

**Fig. 15.7:** Serial cauterization and cutting of infundibulopelvic ligament

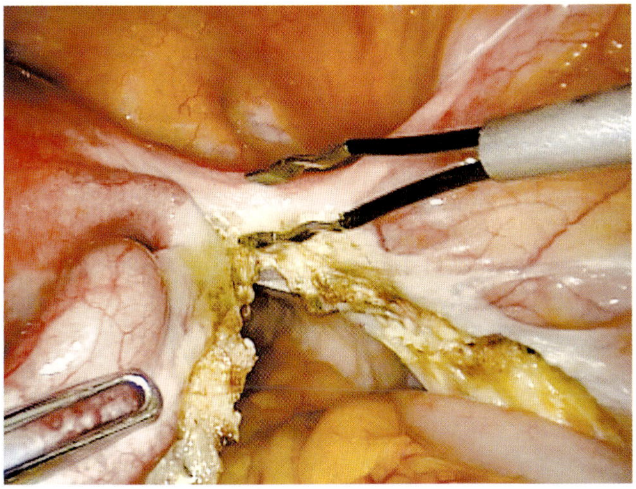

**Fig. 15.8:** Cauterization of round ligament

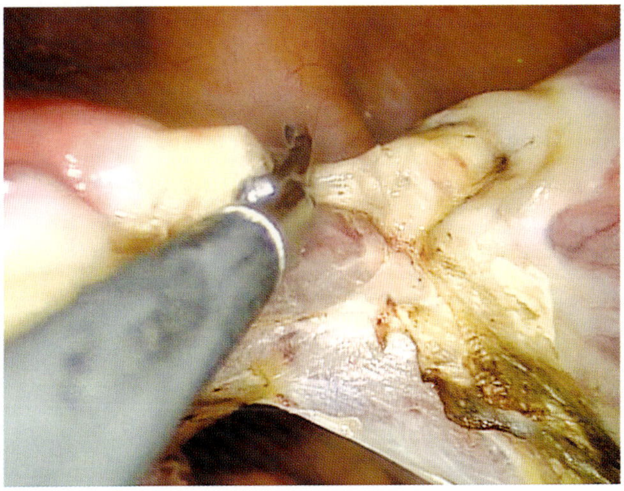

**Fig. 15.9:** Cutting of round ligament

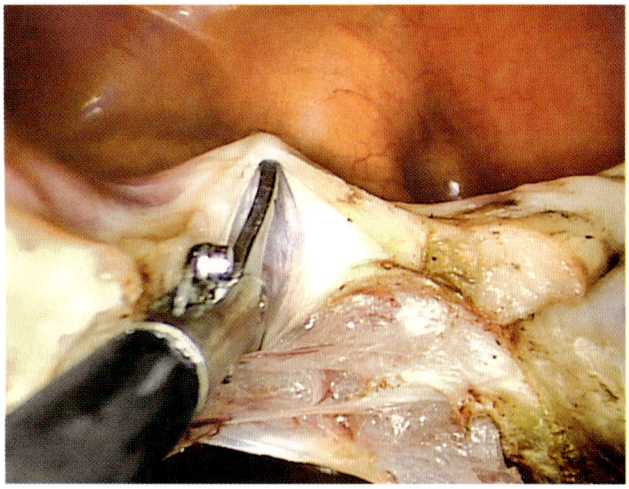

**Fig. 15.10:** Opening of two lips of broad ligament

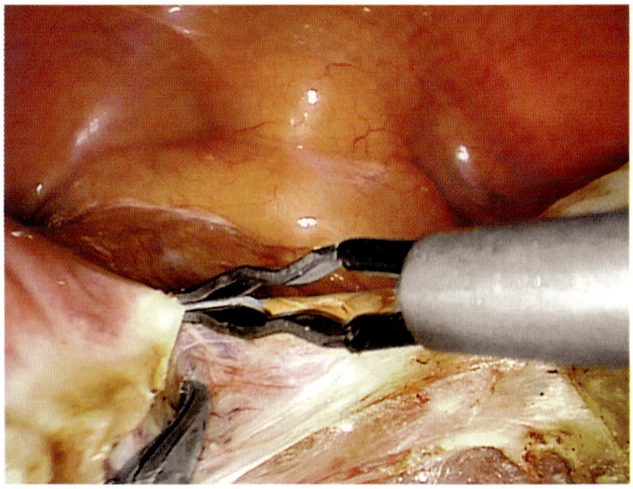

**Fig. 15.11:** Anterior lip of broad ligament being separated

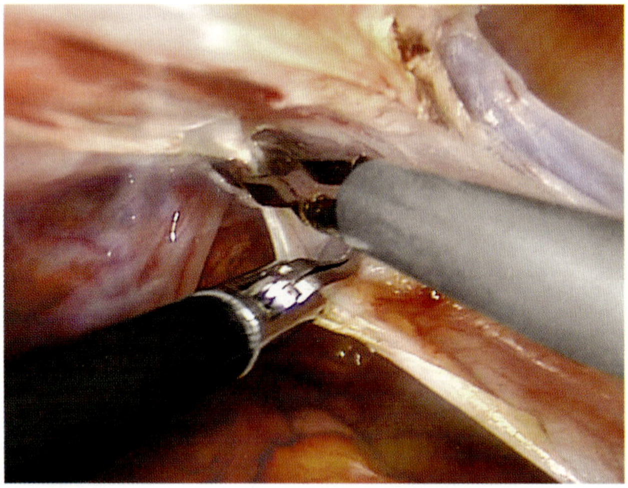

**Fig. 15.12:** Posterior lip of broad ligament being separated and cut lateral to uterine wall

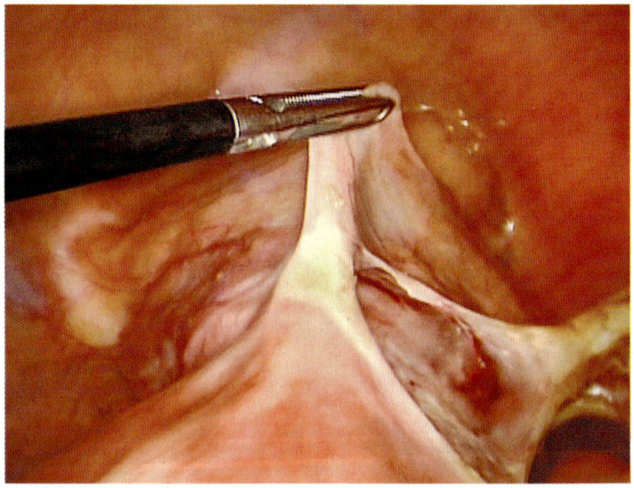

**Fig. 15.13:** Uterovesical fold of peritoneum lifted and cauterized at isthmic level close to uterus

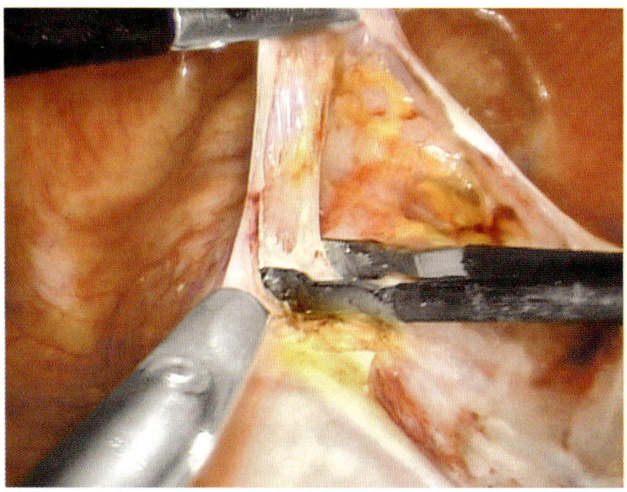

**Fig. 15.14:** Dissection of pubocervical ligament and anterior pouch, pushing bladder down

cut next to uterus up to uterosacral ligament, after blunt separation from the uterine.

10. Once posterior lip of peritoneum is cut, loose areolar tissue is displaced laterally. This step further pushes ureters laterally and since there is breach in continuity of the peritoneum, current will not pass laterally to ureters while cauterizing the uterine artery.
11. Uterine artery is skeletonized for effective dessication. To identify the right uterine artery, the uterus is displaced upwards and to the left side. This will also cause apparent lengthening of the uterines, so that the ureter will be further away from the point of dessication (Figs 15.15 and 15.16).
12. A substantial segment of the skeletonized uterine artery (1-2 cm) is coagulated or sutured (Figs 15.17A to D) and then the pedicle is divided.

    * Vessel sealing device (Gyrus), if available negates the need for suturing the uterine artery.

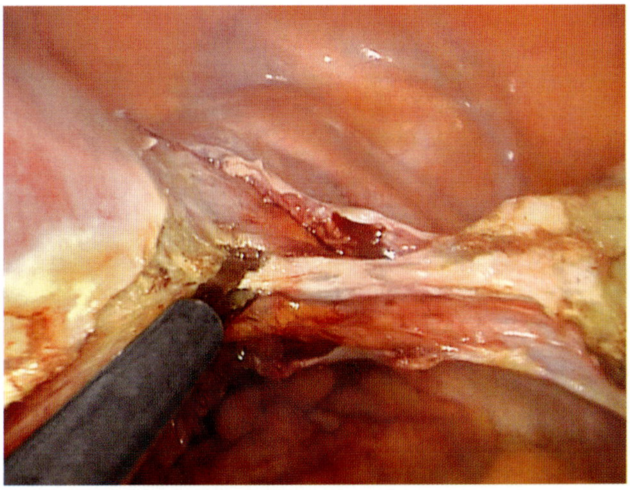

**Fig. 15.15:** Skeletonization of right uterine artery followed by cauterization

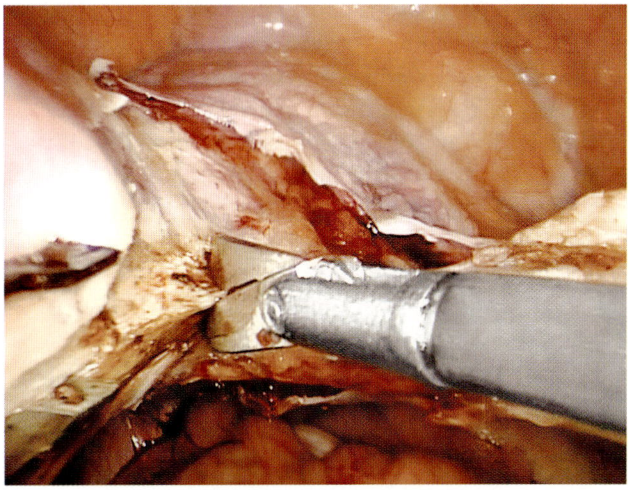

**Fig. 15.16:** Cutting of right uterine artery

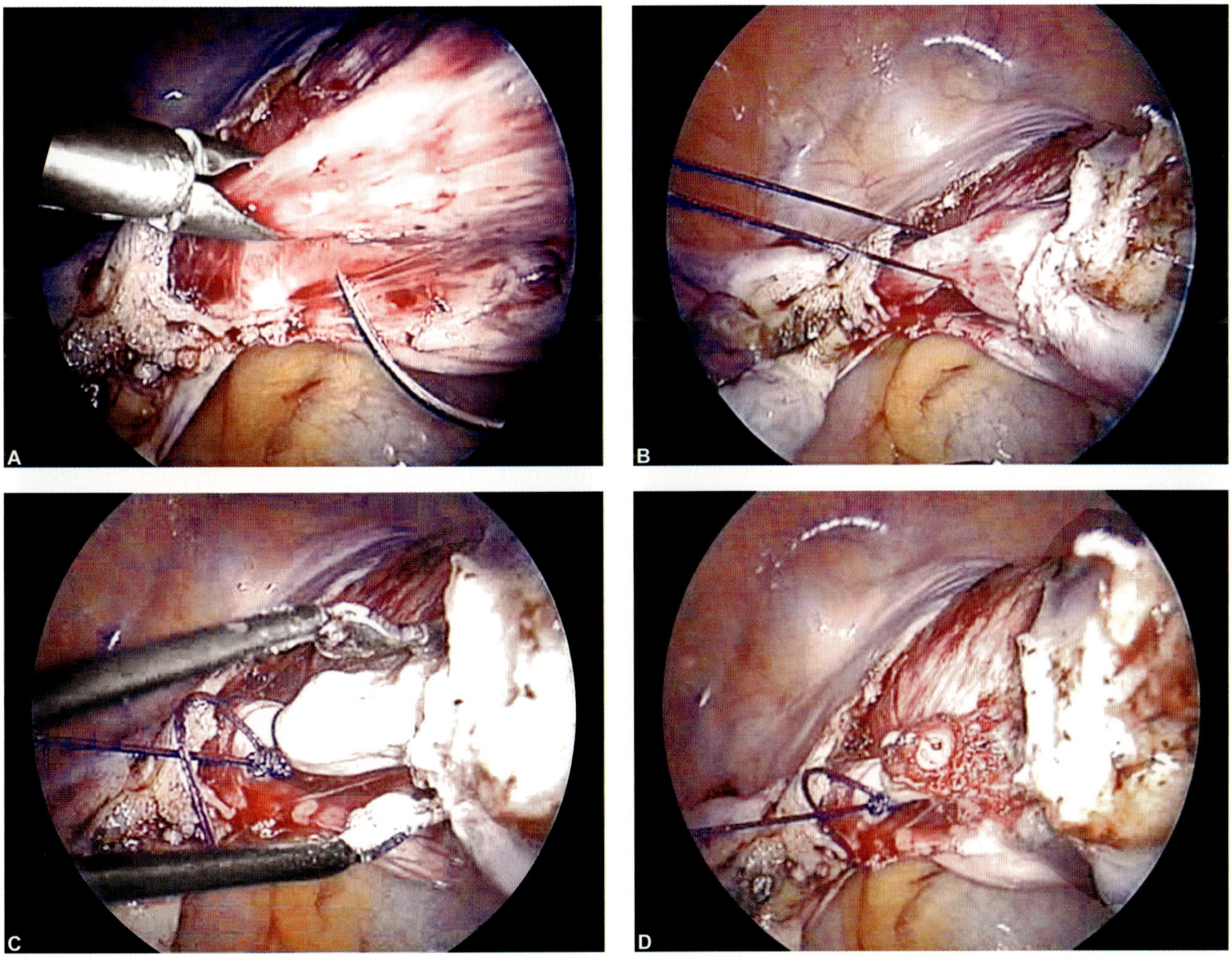

**Figs 15.17A to D:** Left uterine artery ligation

13. Keeping the uterine position same, (completely pushed in and to opposite side) transverse cervical ligament is cauterized and cut medial to the uterine stump till the angle of the vault (Figs 15.18 and 15.19). Before cauterizing it, one should ensure sufficient bladder dissection to avoid thermal spread to the bladder. This anterior displacement and shaving of bladder pillar, transverse cervical ligament and utero-sacral ligament from their attachments maintains the integrity of endopelvic fascia and vascularity.
14. All the steps are done bilaterally.
15. Once you reach the angle of the vault, manipulator is changed to Clermont Ferrand manipulator (Few endosurgeons use this manipulator from the beginning).
16. Maintaining cranial displacement of uterus, blade of the manipulator is thrusted into the anterior fornix in such a way so as to lift the vaginal wall and displace the bladder downwards. Using the monopolar hook, the vault is cut circumferentially over the blade of the vaginal manipulator. The vaginal assistant tactfully rotates the blade so that the surgeon is able to cut the vault over the blade circumferentially. Here, instead of cutting current, if one uses coagulation current, spurters of vault will not bleed. But one should keep sufficient stretch on tissue to be cut, for the coagulation current to work (Figs 15.20 to 15.23).
17. After completing the circumferential incision, the uterus is gently drawn in the vagina and kept in place, which prevents $CO_2$ gas leak.
    - Instead of monopolar spatula, harmonic scalpel with open blade on level 5 setting can be used, without any risks of electrosurgical burns.
18. The angles of vaginal vault along with pubocervical and uterosacral ligaments are closed by endoligature on both sides, re-creating the ring of fascia. One or two more interrupted sutures can be taken over vaginal vault (Figs 15.24 and 15.25). After ensuring hemostasis, a complete peritoneum lavage is done (Figs 15.26 and 15.27).
    - As it is not possible to take uterosacral angle and pubocervical fascia vaginally, (the way it can be taken laparoscopically), vault closure from vagina is never recommended.
    - Continuous locking sutures is not recommended for the vault.
    - In case of laxity of uterosacral ligament, plication stitches are taken on both the uterosacral ligaments, taking care of the ureters.
    - Reconstruction of the vault ring is the most important step to avoid vault prolapse.

In cases where ovarian preservation is done, removal of the Fallopian tubes is done in accordance with GOC (Society of Gynecological Oncology, Canada). Laparoscopic salpingectomy done using bipolar cautery and scissors, while taking precautions not to compromise the ovarian blood supply, especially while cauterizing near the infundibulopelvic ligament.

## Post Hysterectomy Inspection

After closing the vault, saline wash is given and the pedicles are inspected. Bladder, ureters and bowel are also thoroughly inspected.

## Postoperative Management

1. No need to keep Foley's catheter postoperatively, unless excessive bladder handling and dissection is done. Patient is encouraged to walk to the toilet within 2 hours.
2. After 6 hours, clear liquids are given and if tolerated, soft diet can be given in the evening.
3. Patient can be discharged after 24 to 48 hours and can resume her normal activities within a weeks time.

## Problems Anticipated and How to Avoid Them?

### *Opening of the Vaginal Vault*

Division of the lateral part of the cervix is technically difficult as the ascending vaginal vessels may cause troublesome hemorrhage if not coagulated completely. This difficulty can be easily overcome by synchronous movements by the surgeon and the vaginal assistant who pushes the colpotomizer in a proper direction according to the surgeon's choice.

## Removal of Large Masses/Leiomyoma >18 weeks

Preferred methods are:

- All ports in upper abdomen, providing room for vision and surgery.
- Debulking after uterine ligation (Figs 15.28 to 15.33).
- Myomectomy before hysterectomy.
- Securing uterine vessels properly ensuring a bloodless operative field.
- Use of a 30° 10 mm laparoscope aids good anterior and posterior dissection.
- In previous CS cases with large uterus, morcellation reduces lacerations of the vagina during specimen removal.
- Bladder adhesions at isthmus should always be released with sharp dissection by scissors without using energy source or with harmonic scalpel. Throughout the dissection, uterus should be pushed in and is kept midposed, which ensures proper vision and keeps bladder mucosa away from the line of incision.

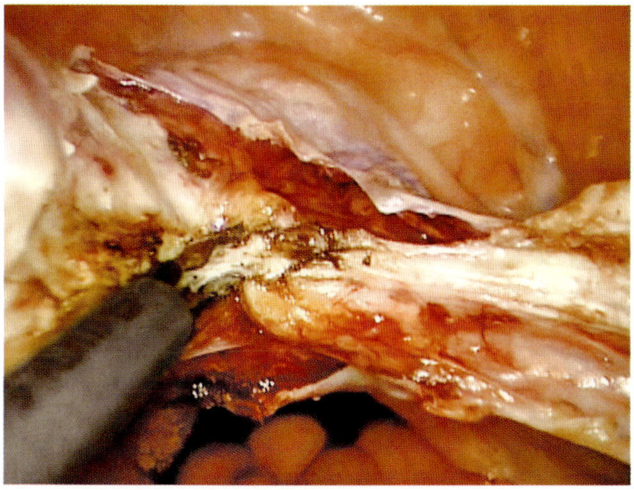

**Fig. 15.18:** Cauterization of Mackenrodt's ligament

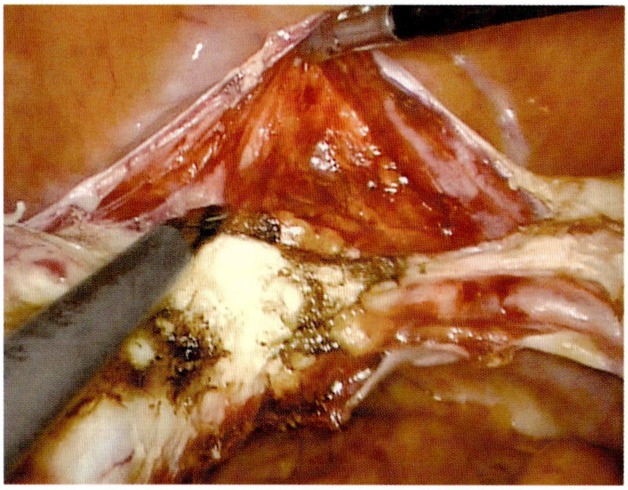

**Fig. 15.19:** Mackenrodt's ligament cut and angle of vault reached on right side

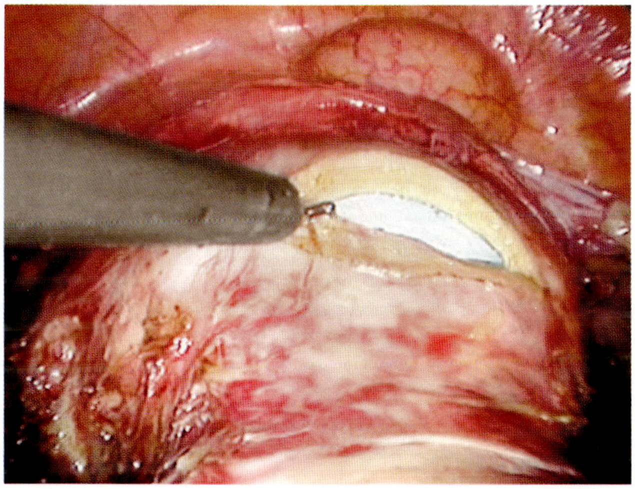

**Fig. 15.20:** Cutting vault with monopolar hook over uterine manipulator

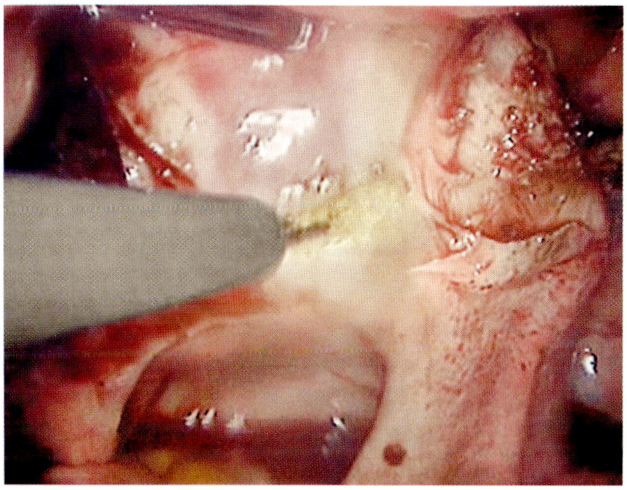

**Fig. 15.21:** Cutting vault in between uterosacrals

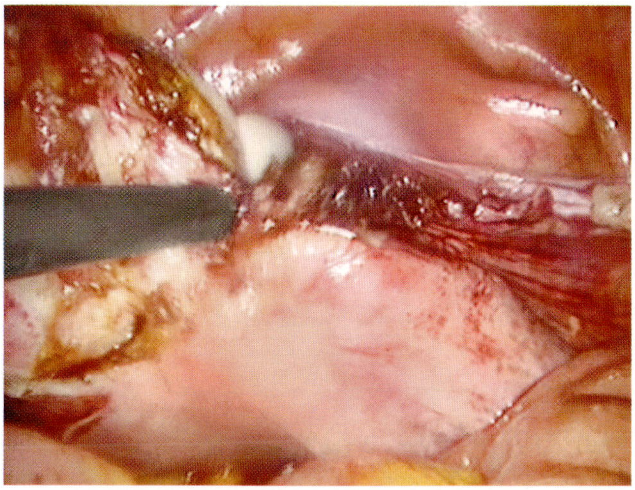

**Fig. 15.22:** Cutting vault circumferentially

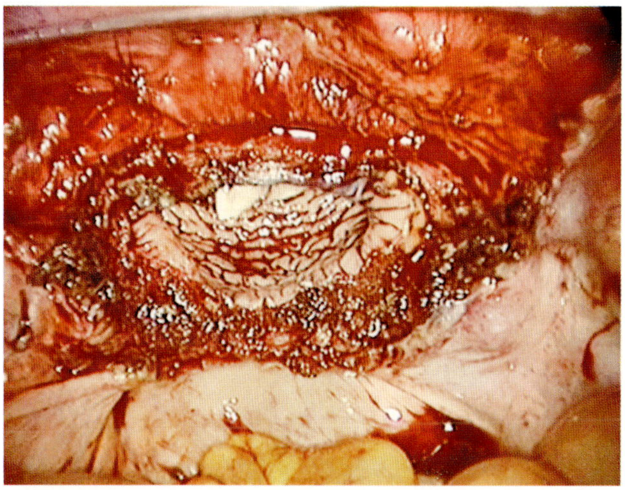

**Fig. 15.23:** Ring of vault after cutting

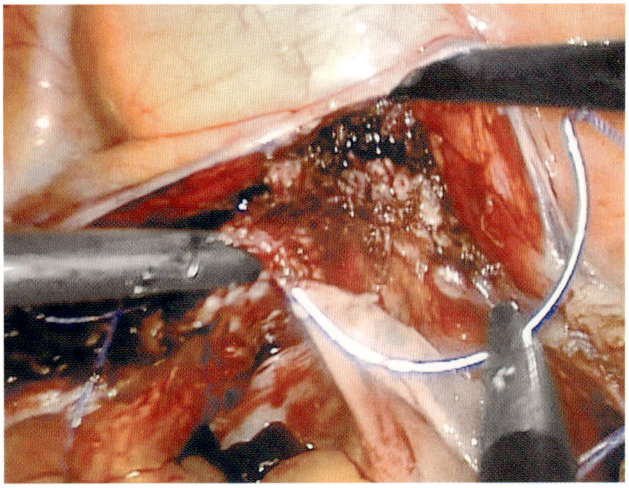

**Fig. 15.24:** Suturing uterosacral ligaments, vaginal angle, and pubocervical fascia separately on both sides

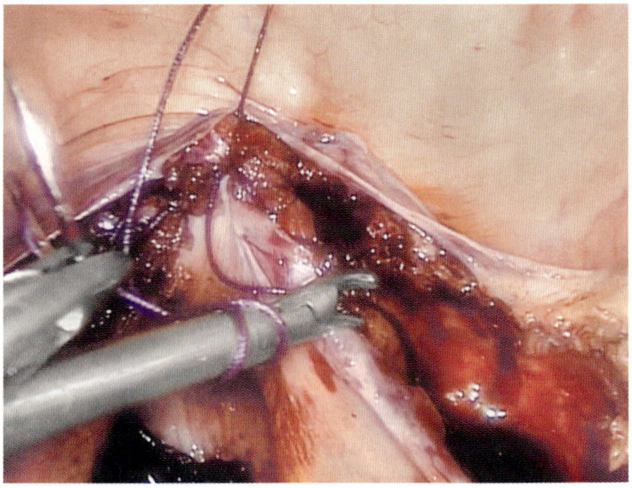

**Fig. 15.25:** Interrupted suture over vaginal vault

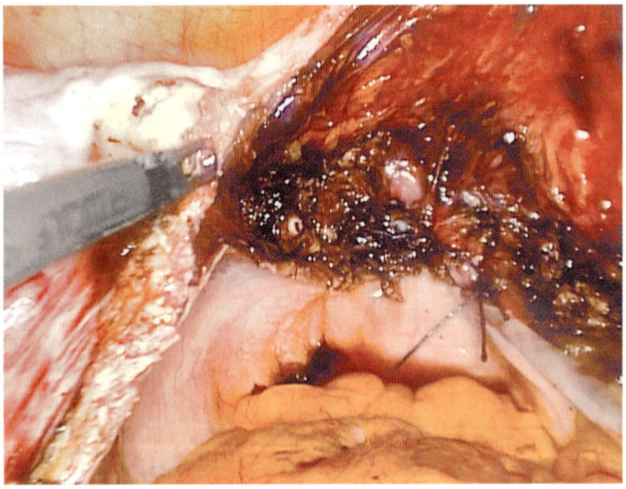

**Fig. 15.26:** Confirming hemostasis of pedicles.

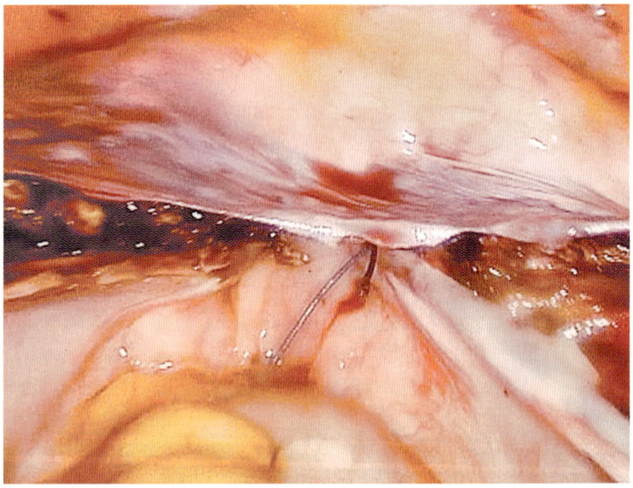

**Fig. 15.27:** End Result: Clean pelvis. Need not suture visceral peritoneum

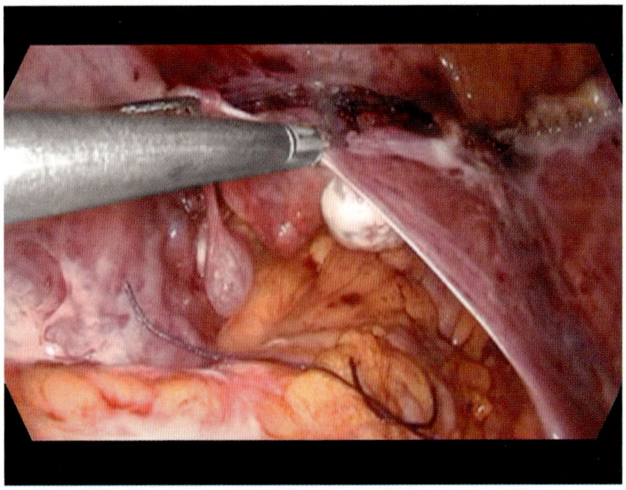

**Fig. 15.28:** Laparoscopic Salpingectomy done using bipolar cautery initially

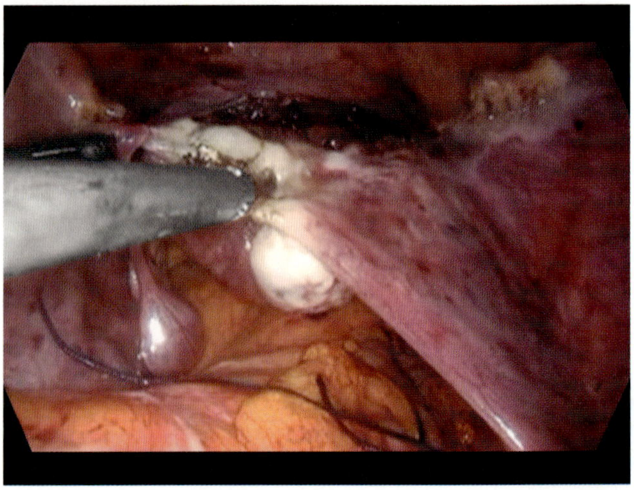

**Fig. 15.29:** After cautery, the tube is cut using either Harmonic scalpel or scissors

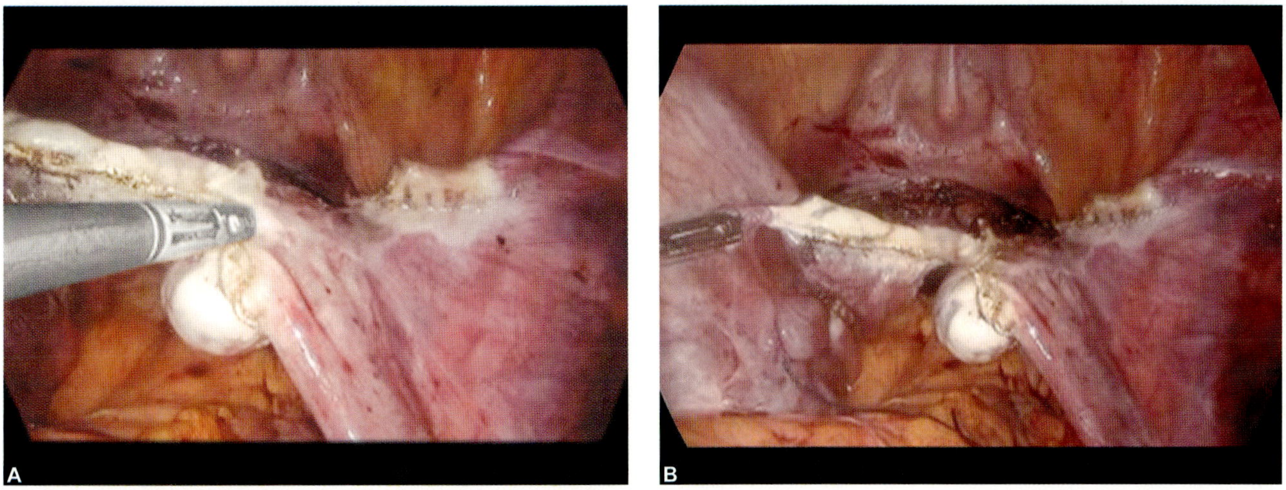

**Figs 15.30A and B:** Precautions taken to avoid any compromise to the ovarian blood supply, during cautery

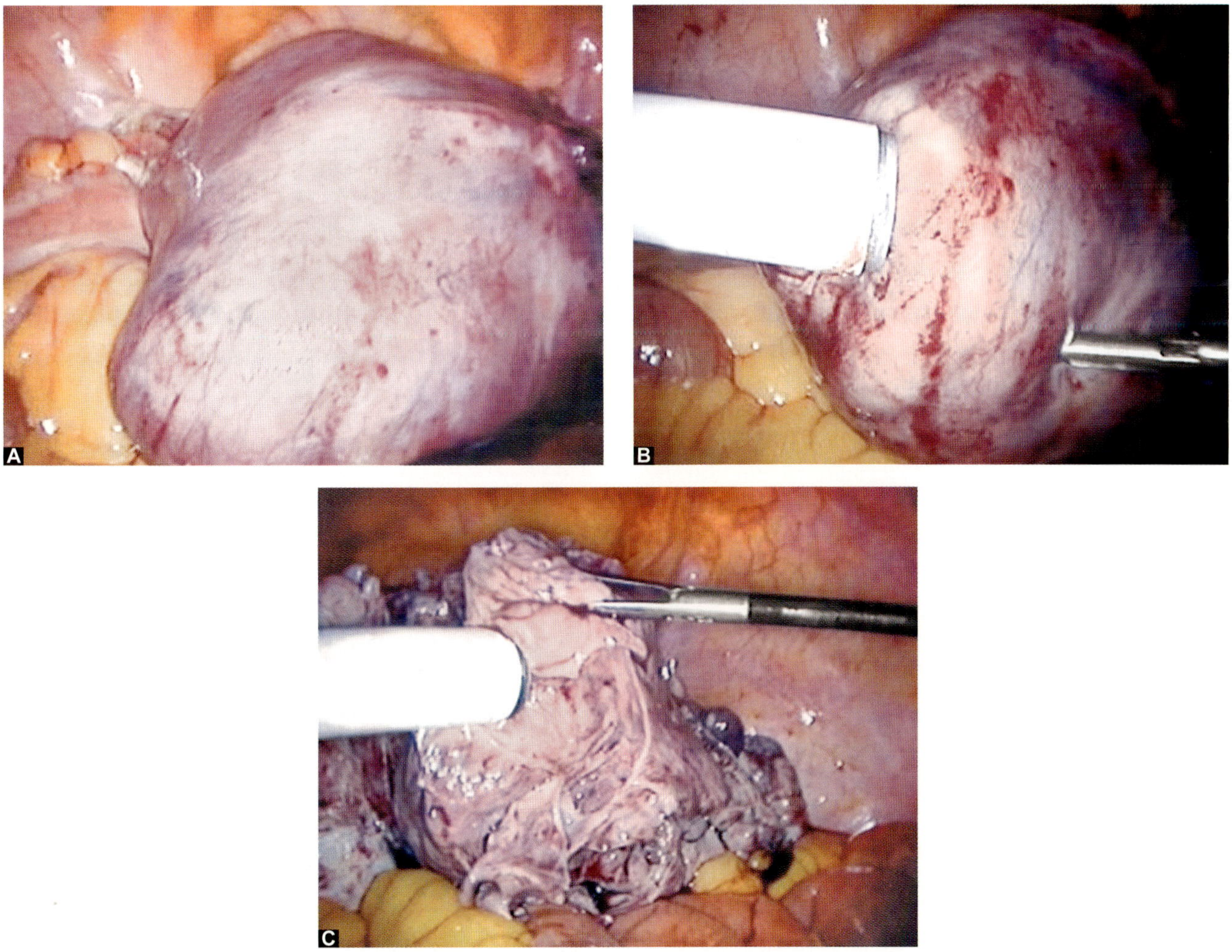

**Figs 15.31A to C:** In situ morcellation of large uterus after uterine ligation

Chapter

16

# Laparoscopic Subtotal and Total Hysterectomy for Multiple Fibroids

*Liselotte Mettler, Anupama Deenadayal, Ibrahim Alkatout*

## INTRODUCTION

### General Introduction

Within today's multiple treatment possibilities for myomas/fibroids as surgical, medical or interventional imaging advances there is still some room left for total hysterectomy (TH) and subtotal hysterectomies (SH) (Figs 16.1A and B). Particularly, the laparoscopic approach for both techniques on the benign side as well as for radical hysterectomies in malignancies of the genital tract becomes more and more accepted and important if family planning is completed. As it is less invasive procedure, indicated patients with myomas can consider a subtotal approach [laparoscopic subtotal hysterectomy (LSH)]. However, only Laparoscopic Total Hysterectomies (LTH) can protect 100% from new fibroid formations, avoid later cervix carcinoma or sarcoma formation, uncontrolled bleedings or any other problems arising from the uterus.

The etiology of fibroid formation remains in spite of numerous theories unclear. While a genetic disposition must be given, as Africans have in a much higher frequency of multiple myomas than Caucasians. Although certain up-regulations and down-regulations in the genes of patients with and without myomas have been described, no clear prevention for fibroids is available. It is known that patients who have close relatives with fibroids are more likely to develop fibroids themselves. This is called family aggregation. In some patients, fibroids are clustered with other disorders. Hereditary leiomyomatosis and renal cell carcinoma syndrome is a rare syndrome involving fibroids. Individuals with the gene that leads to both fibroids and skin leiomyomas are at increased risk for a rare case of kidney cell cancer (papillary renal cell carcinoma).

Understanding which genes are involved in fibroids does not automatically tell us why fibroids develop or how to control them. From our understanding of fibroid behavior, we would guess that genes involved in estrogen or progesterone production, metabolism, or action would be involved. Unfortunately, science is seldom that straightforward. Most guesses regarding these "candidate genes" turn out to be wrong and much study is usually required to find out how these genes lead to disease. There are also small variations called polymorphisms in genes that may play a role in influencing the risk of fibroids. Both polymorphisms and mutations are changes in the sequence of genes, but the difference is in the degree of

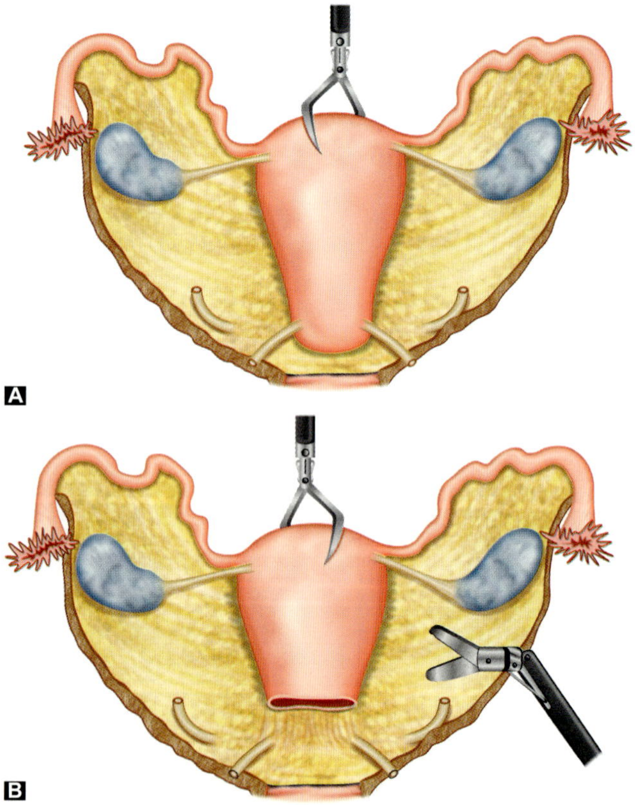

**Figs 16.1A and B:** Overview of subtotal and total hysterectomy in correlation to the surrounding tissue

change. A mutation makes a major change in the gene that leads to a change in the protein the gene is coding for. For example, it can change the amino acid from alanine to glycine or causes the protein to be prematurely cut off.

## The Genetics of Fibroids, Genotype and Phenotype

The discovery of the structure of DNA (deoxyribonucleic acid) by Watson and Crick revolutionized biology and medicine. They discovered that DNA carries the code for life in a ladder like structure and the genes from a single person has been found to take up the space of 400,000 times the distance from the earth to the moon or 1000 times the distance from the earth to the sun = 150 billion kilometers.

Before going further, it is important to define the terms genotype and phenotype. The genotype is the pattern of genes that you inherit. For example, with eye color, brown is a dominant color and is represented by a "B". Blue is a recessive trait and represented by a "b". Therefore, a person can have "BB", "bb", or "Bb" as genotypes for eye color. Each person gets two copies of the gene, one originally from his or her mother and the other from his or her father. The dominant gene will always dominate; it has the power to trump a recessive trait. Phenotype is the physical manifestation, or end result, of the genotype. Although there are three different genotypes (BB, bb, or Bb), there are only two phenotypes: brown eyes and blue eyes. People with the "BB" or the "Bb" genotype have brown eyes because brown is the dominant trait; only the people with the "bb" genotype have blue eyes.

We believe that fibroids are a common phenotype that represents many different underlying genotypes. In other words, in our view, fibroids can arise through multiple different pathways. In this case, "Bb" might represent two different genes that code for the estrogen receptor beta, which influences the action of estrogen on fibroid tissue. A "B" gene may make the fibroid more sensitive to this hormone and therefore more likely to grow. In addition, probably multiple genes influence fibroids, so that in addition to "Bb" we may also have "Pp" for progesterone receptors, "Ff" for fibrotic factors, and so on. This information would be most helpful in advances of treatment, so that the woman who carried a high risk of recurrent fibroids and had completed their family might even choose to have a hysterectomy because their chance of having an additional surgery was so high. We currently have some clinical information (based on physicians' clinical experience with many patients) to predict prognosis for recurrence after abdominal myomectomy, but our clinical information for alternative forms of treatment options is limited.

Finally, understanding the underlying genotype would open up important possibilities for the future. It may, for example, point two ways in which women can modify their risk of disease and lead to prevention of disease. If, for example, a major protein involved in body fat metabolism was found to be abnormally sensitive in women with fibroids, weight loss or preventing weight gain might be an effective strategy for decreasing the risk of fibroids. In this day and age, new therapies can be developed that are targeted to specific abnormalities; this is what happened with chronic myeloid leukemia (CML) and Gleevec, which combats this disease with minimal side effects.

## Evidence for the Role of Genes in the Fibroid Development and Growth

Studies of women with fibroids suggest several reasons to suspect that genes play a role in fibroid formation. The first is that both women in a pair of identical twins are twice as likely to have had a hysterectomy as both women in a pair of fraternal (nonidentical) twins. Identical twins share 100 percent of their genes, while fraternal twins share only 50 percent of their genes. This suggests that the genes that identical twins share make them more likely to form fibroids, since both are identical and nonidentical twins have equal exposure to environmental factors. This difference between identical and fraternal twins has been observed in a general population of women undergoing hysterectomy and a population of women with fibroids leading to hysterectomy.

There is also evidence that women who have close relatives, such as a mother or sister, with fibroids are much more likely to have fibroids themselves. This propensity is called familial aggregation. Just as with breast cancer, if you have many relatives affected by fibroids, your risk of disease is likely to be increased.

## Molecular Genetics and Genome Wide Scan for Fibroid Genes

Understanding which genes are involved in fibroids does not automatically tell us why fibroids develop or how to control them. From our understanding of fibroid behavior, we would guess that genes involved in estrogen or progesterone production, metabolism, or action would be involved. Unfortunately, science is seldom that straightforward. Most guesses regarding these "candidate genes" turn out to be wrong, and much study is usually required to find out how these genes lead to disease.

There are also small variations called polymorphisms in genes that may play a role in influencing the risk of fibroids. Both polymorphisms and mutations are changes in the sequence of genes, but the difference is in the degree of change. A mutation makes a major change in the gene that leads to a change in the protein the gene is coding for. It changes the amino acid from alanine to glycine, for example, or causes the protein to be prematurely cut off.

Finally, in the age of molecular genetics, we can look for genes involved in a disease which are not marked by chromosome breaks, effectively looking for a needle in a haystack. This process is called a genome-wide scan. This is a common approach to finding genes in complex diseases, such as diabetes, asthma, and heart disease. With a genome-wide scan, women who are sisters and both have fibroids (an affected sibling pair) are recruited to participate in the study. Their DNA is studied for common genes. If hundreds of women are studied, each region of every chromosome can be examined, and it can be determined which genes are shared by the sisters who share the fibroid phenotype but are different in many other respects. This approach often produces novel genes that were not previously thought to be involved in the disease process.

## MICROSCOPIC FACTS AND FIBROID VIABILITY

Fibroids are composed primarily of smooth muscle cells. The uterus, stomach and bladder are all organs made of smooth muscle. Smooth muscle cells are arranged so that the organ can stretch, instead of being arranged in rigid units like the cells in skeletal muscle in arms and legs that are designed to "pull" in a particular direction. In women with fibroids, tissue from the endometrium typically looks normal under the microscope. Sometimes, however, over submucosal fibroids there is an unusual type of uterine lining that does not have the normal glandular structures. The presence of this abnormality, called aglandular functionalis (functional endometrium with no glands), in women having bleeding disorders is sometimes a clinical clue for their doctors to look more closely for a submucosal fibroid. A second pattern of endometrium, termed chronic endometritis, can also suggest that there may be a submucosal fibroid, although this pattern can also be associated with other problems such as retained products of conception and various infections of the uterus. Once we move beyond hysterectomy as a one-size-fits-all solution to fibroids, distinctions in size, position, and appearance will likely be important for treating fibroids. Once we understand these issues, we may be able to tell why some women have severe bleeding and other women with a similarly sized fibroid have no problem.

## COSTS OF FIBROIDS

In fact, accurately capturing all the costs attributable to uterine fibroids will help us move toward more, and more effective, innovative therapies. When deciding whether or not to launch a new concept, companies typically look at the amount currently spent for other treatments. The economics of fibroids has chiefly been discussed in terms of the healthcare costs of hysterectomy. This in itself is a huge amount of money. According to a recent estimate, in the United States, more than $2 billion every year is spent on hospitalization costs due to uterine fibroids alone. Additionally, one study estimates that the healthcare costs due to uterine fibroids are more than $ 4,600 per woman per year.

When you incorporate all the costs of fibroids, however, the total is even more significant.

- The costs of myomectomy, uterine artery embolization (UAE), and other minimally invasive therapies.
- The costs of birth control pills and other hormonal treatments to control bleeding.
- The costs of tampons, pads, and the adult diapers many women require to contain the bleeding.
- The costs of alternative and complementary therapies.
- The cost of doing nothing (for many women this means missing work or working less productively during their period).

Why should a patient have a hysterectomy today when so many alterative treatment structures are given? Firstly, up to a certain size of the enlarged uterus, laparoscopic subtotal hysterectomy completely solves the problem and if women want to eliminate every risk of recurrent fibroids, hysterectomy is their only choice. Of course, hysterectomy also eliminates coexisting problems such as adenomyosis, endometriosis and endometrial polyps or cervical dysplasia.

## WILL THE OVARIES BE REMOVED OR LEFT IN PLACE?

The ovaries generally are not removed when a hysterectomy is performed for uterine fibroids. Removing the uterus alone will cure the bleeding and the size-related symptoms caused by the fibroids. Removing the ovaries is thus not required in treating fibroids as it is sometimes for other diseases like endometriosis or gynecologic cancers.

Many physicians were taught that at a set age (which varies between 35 and 50) women should be told that removal of the ovaries is recommended as part of the surgery, with the speculation of "while we are there, we may as well." The general teaching had been that ovaries do not have any function after menopause and the risk of ovarian cancer increases with increasing age, so removing the ovaries near the time of menopause was a no-lose proposition. This was especially true if hormone replacement therapy could be used to help younger women transition to the time when they would naturally go through menopause.

However, more recent research suggests that although after menopause the ovaries do not make much estradiol (the major estrogen in premenopausal women), they make a tremendous amount of androgens (usually thought of as male hormones). It is thought that these androgens may be important in maintaining mood and sex drive. In addition, the risks of hormone replacement have become clearer, and many women choose to use hormones following menopause. (Most women are aware that there has been research from the women's health initiative demonstrating significant complications with postmenopausal hormone replacement therapy. However, it is not widely known that the risks are lower for women without a uterus, who are able to take estrogen alone. Recently the association of premature loss of ovarian function and the increasing risk of heart disease has also been explored.

Considering all these factors, there are good reasons to retain the ovaries if possible. The major reason to remove them at the time of fibroid surgery is if the woman has a high risk of ovarian cancer.

### Resection of Fallopian Tubes in Cases of Hysterectomy

Once the reproductive function is completed, the tubes of a female should be removed within the reproductive age while ovaries, as said above need to stay to support the female wellbeing. Beyond the reproductive age, tubes should always be removed with the uterus while ovaries, as previously discussed are routinely removed only above the age of 65 years.

According to new research presented today at the Annual Clinical Meeting of The American College of Obstetricians and Gynecologists, bilateral salpingectomy, the removal of both Fallopian tubes during hysterectomy while preserving the ovaries, is considered a safe way of potentially reducing the development of ovarian serous carcinoma, the most common type of ovarian cancer. Increasing evidence points toward the Fallopian tubes as the origin of this type of cancer. Removing the Fallopian tubes does not cause the onset of menopause, as does the removal of the ovaries.

Prophylactic removal of the Fallopian tubes during hysterectomy or sterilization would rule out any subsequent tubal pathology, such as hydrosalpinx, which is observed in up to 30% of women after hysterectomy. Moreover, this intervention is likely to offer considerable protection against later tumor development, even if the ovaries are retained. Thus, we recommend that any hysterectomy should be combined with salpingectomy. Women undergoing hysterectomy with retained Fallopian tubes or sterilization have at least a doubled risk of subsequent salpingectomy. Removal of the Fallopian tubes at hysterectomy, should therefore, generally be recommended.

## LAPAROSCOPIC SUBTOTAL HYSTERECTOMY

### General Aspects

There is an opinion that the cervix absolutely does not need to be removed to cure the symptoms caused by uterine fibroids. The advantage of the cervix left in place is that cardinal and uterosacral ligaments remain in place.

Until we have long-term outcome studies, every patient will need to make an informed decision along with her doctor to be executed based on individual needs and availability. A woman who routinely undergoes preventive medical care is a better candidate for a LSH than a woman who is unlikely to go for a PAP smear annually following LSH. Likewise, if pressure against the cervix is a critical part of a woman's sexual response-very few women are aware of this—an LSH may be a better choice. We counsel woman that there is a chance of formation of cervical fibroids following a subtotal/supracervical hysterectomy although this is really a small risk. Sometimes, the cervix needs to be removed surgically later in separate procedure. Being aware, however, of a less invasive procedure in the beginning, this is accepted easily. For patients that want to really minimize their chances of later surgeries, a laparoscopic total hysterectomy (LTH) may be preferable. Furthermore, suspicion of adenomyosis uteri is an important factor for the decision towards LTH as we know that the risk of persisting bleeding and dysmenorrhea is higher after LSH with the detection of adenomyosis.

### Preoperative Preparation

The exclusion of any cervical pathology or infection is important. Endometriotic lesions around the cervix require cervical resection along with the uterus as a part of LTH. The patient has to be ready for regular gynecologic screening twice a year.

### Instruments and Equipment

The instrument set consists of trocars, a uterine manipulator (for LTH only), needle holders, a cutting electique loop, sutures and a morcellator in addition to the basic set of laparoscopic instruments, there is a requirement of a coagulation or thermofusion device with integrated knife, graspers, scissors, biopsy forceps and window forceps and a suction irrigation unit. If a robotic set up is available the instruments have to be adjusted.

In details:
- 1 10 mm trocar
- 2 -4 5 mm trocars
- 2 atraumatic forceps
- 1 traumatic forceps
- 1 claw forceps
- 1 scissor
- 1 bipolar or thermofusion instrument
- 1 monopolar hook, needle and cutting loop
- 1 uterine manipulator or myoma screw (for LTH only)
- 1 pair of needle holders, sutures.

## PREREQUISITES

Stable health condition, indication for myomectomy-hysterectomy, full consent of the patient after detailed explanation of the operative procedure. A large uterus or a uterus with multiple myomas is no contraindication for a laparoscopic procedure. Solely, the placement of the trocars might be set higher in the abdominal wall and there might be a need of more than the usually used two ancillary trocars.

## STEPS OF SURGERY

### Port Placement

According to the size of the uterus with the fibroids, the trocar placement points are selected.

Once the cutaneous region has been determined from the outside with the aid of diaphanoscopy, the safe distance to the plica umbilicalis lateralis can be verified by palpation. The correct point of insertion is usually about two thumbs medial of the anterior superior iliac spine. Being distant to the plica, the trocar is placed at a 90° angle and pushed forward until the tip of the trocar can be seen with the laparoscope.

Precondition for safe trocar insertion is the elevation of the abdominal wall by means of a sufficient pneumoperitoneum (excluding blind entry without pneumoperitoneum). Therefore, an extensive insufflation pressure up to 20 mm Hg can be tolerated.

For correct handling, the trocar and sheath are held between the middle and index finger with the hub of the trocar against the palm of the hand.

### Optic Trocar

Insertion of the optic trocar is performed in two steps. During the first step, a 5 mm optic trocar and laparoscope are inserted to confirm the correct pneumoperitoneum and the absence of local adhesions. In the second step dilation to 10 mm occurs, either under sight or blindly, which guarantees an optimal overview during all operations. In low-risk operations and short operations that do not require a maximal light source, a 5 mm optic trocar and laparoscope may be sufficient.

**1st Step:** Entry is performed by a Z *technique* in the following manner: After proceeding with the trocar forward horizontally for about 1.5 cm, the tip of the trocar is moved to the right at a 90° angle for about 1.5 cm. After lifting the abdominal wall in the same manner as when inserting the Veress needle, the trocar is screwed with the dominant hand straight into the abdominal wall at a 90° angle, towards the hollow of the os sacrum. The index finger is extended under tension along the shaft of the trocar so that excessive penetration of the trocar through the abdominal wall can be prevented.

The sign for correct placement of the trocar is the hissing sound created when gas escapes through the open valve of the trocar. The obturator is then removed and the trocar is held in place. Insertion must be stopped immediately once the intra-abdominal position has been attained. Before dilating to 10 mm, a 5 mm laparoscope is introduced and rotated through 360° to check visually for any bleeding, intra-abdominal abnormality and adherent bowel loops. If there is concern that the bowel might be adherent in the umbilical region, the primary trocar site needs to be visualized from a secondary port site, e.g. in the lower abdominal wall with a 5 mm laparoscope.

**2nd Step:** (only if required): A blunt palpation probe is placed in the 5 mm trocar and the shaft is pulled over the palpation probe and taken out. A 10 mm trocar is then screwed into the abdominal cavity using the palpation probe as stylet. It is important to screw the trocar as the sheath is a nuance shorter, and therefore, needs high exertion of force. The risk of abrupt excessive penetration with injury of intra-abdominal organs is increased. It demands a lot of patience depending on the strength of the abdominal wall and its thickness to screw the 10 mm trocar inside.

### Ancillary Trocars

All ancillary trocars must be inserted with an intra-abdominal pressure of 15–20 mm Hg under direct vision. The inferior epigastric vessels are visualized laparoscopically whereas the superficial vessels can be visualized by diaphanoscopy. By this means, it can be ensured that the entry points are away from the vessel. It has to be kept in mind that in some cases an extension of the incision is needed during the operation.

Once the tip of the trocar has pierced through the peritoneum, it should be angled in the direction of the uterine fundus under visual control until the port is placed correctly and the sharp tip can be removed.

Before any ancillary trocars are inserted, the patient is moved into the Trendelenburg position. Premature Trendelenburg position can also increase the risk of retroperitoneal vascular injury as the iliac vessels lay right in the axis of a preconceived 45° insertion angle, especially in thin patients with minimal retroperitoneal fat. In the *Trendelenburg position,* the patient is on an elevated and inclined plane, usually at about 15°, with the head down and legs and feet over the edge of the table. The number of ancillary trocars is variable but they all must be inserted under direct view. If two working trocars are needed, they should be placed in the lower quadrant above the pubic hairline lateral to the deep epigastric vessels from the interior view. From the exterior view, the trocars are placed two fingers medial of the spina iliaca anterior superior. For safe insertion, the two major superficial vessels in this region have to be avoided. These are the superficial epigastric artery and the superficial circumflex iliac artery. These two superficial vessels can be visualized by diaphanoscopy. If a third ancillary trocar is needed, the suprapubic midline is the most common site. Diaphanoscopy cannot be relied upon to locate the deep vessels, especially in obese patients (Figs 16.2 and 16.3).

Finger-tapping from the outside can identify the right area of trocar placement, and a small skin incision should be made before the trocar sleeve is inserted. The trocars must be inserted by the shortest route at a 90° angle to the skin surface so that the risk of injuring structures on the way to the abdominal wall is minimized. Once the trocar tip is seen under the peritoneum, the pressure on the trocar should be released and the trocar twisted until it enters the abdominal cavity. For the use of trocars in the midline, the Foley catheter must be identified to avoid accidental bladder perforation. By this means, a false route in the sub-peritoneal tissues or damage to the large pre-vertebral vessels can be avoided.

## Subtotal Hysterectomy

1. Inspection of the pelvis tracing of the ureters and planning of the surgery (Figs 16.4A to D.)
2. Pushing the uterus into the opposite direction of separating the adnexas or the ligaments from the pelvic side wall with the assistance of the intrauterine manipulator or by traction (Fig. 16.5).
3. Division of the infundibulopelvic ligament and round ligament from the pelvic side wall or in cases the adnexas remain division of the adnexas from the uterus (Figs 16.6 to 16.10).
4. Dissection of broad ligament: The broad ligament is opened and each leaf separately coagulated (Figs 16.11 and 16.12).
5. Separation of the bladder from the uterus by opening the vesicouterine ligament and pushing the bladder downwards for about 1-2 cm (Figs 16.13A to D).
6. Presentation of the ramus ascendens of the uterine artery and division of uterine pedicles (Figs 16.14A to D)
7. The same stepwise dissection of the left adnexas (Figs 16.15 and 16.16) opening of the bladder peritoneum and broad ligament (Figs 16.17A to D) and dissection of uterine vessels (Figs 16.18 to 16.20) is performed on the left side. Thorough inspection all around the cervix.
8. Considering LTH, by pushing the intrauterine manipulator upwards the bladder is sliding down (Figs 16.21A to D).
9. Separation of cervix from the uterus with the help of the electric cutting loop (Figs 16.22 to 16.24).
10. Coagulation of the cervical canal and remaining cervical stump for adhesion prevention (Fig. 16.25).
11. Closure of the peritoneum over the cervical stump with help of a purse string or figure of eight suture (Figs 16.26 to 16.29).
12. Morcellation of the uterine body, if adnexas are also resected, they should be put into an endobag for extraction (Figs 16.30 and 16.31).

## Post LSH Inspection

Under a continuous irrigation with Ringer's lactate or Adept (Baxter), a careful inspection of pedicles, bladder, ureters and bowels has to be performed

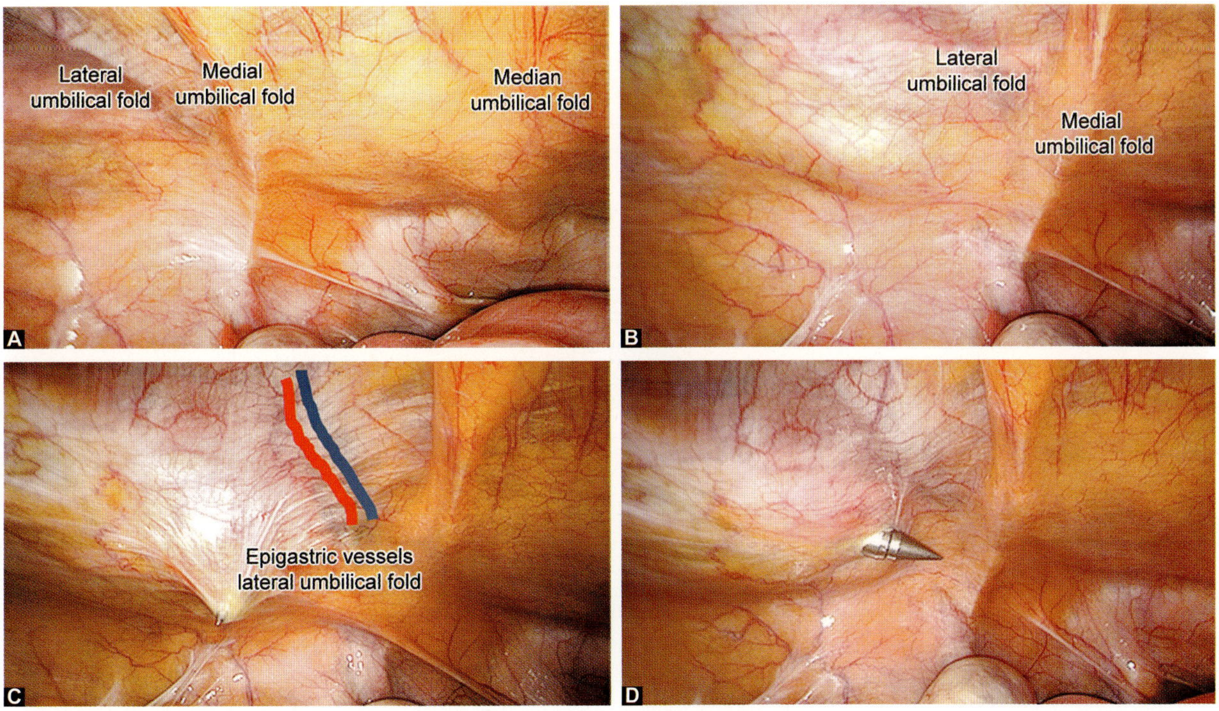


**Figs 16.2A to D:** Secondary trocar placement, left lower abdominal entry. From A–D, the Z-like abdominal insertion through the layers of the abdominal wall is demonstrated

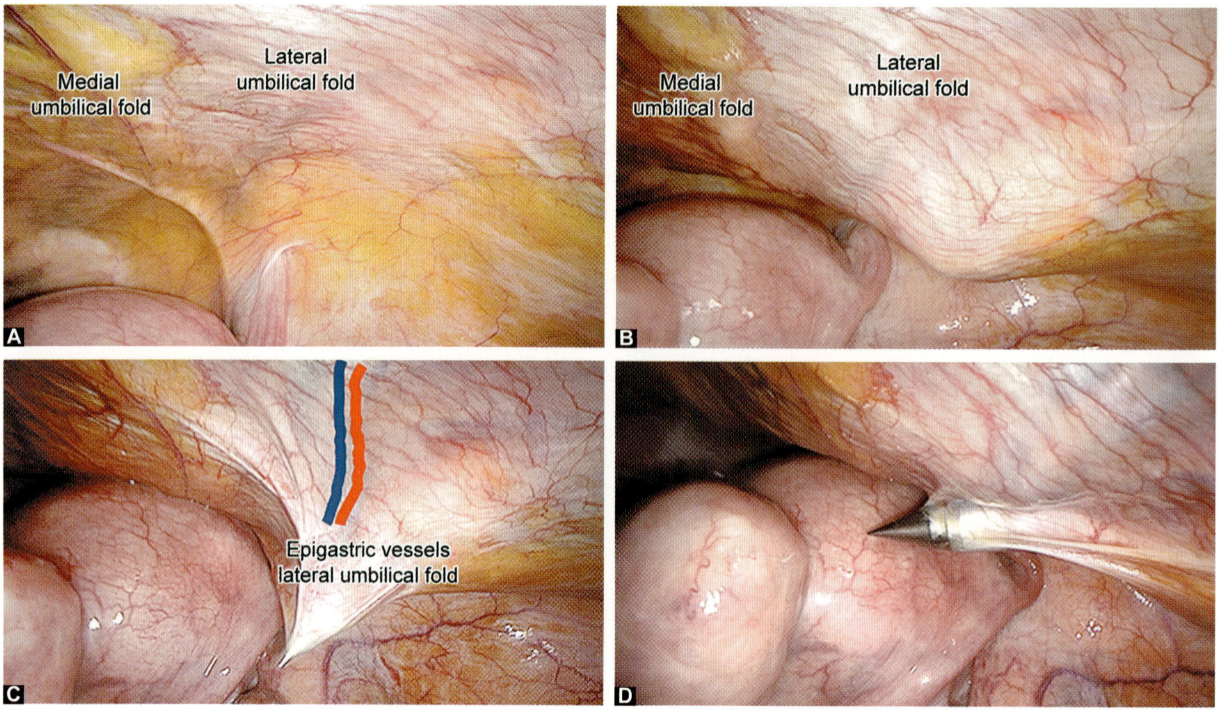


**Figs 16.3A to D:** Secondary trocar placement, right lower abdominal entry. Z-like abdominal insertion through the layers of the abdominal wall is demonstrated

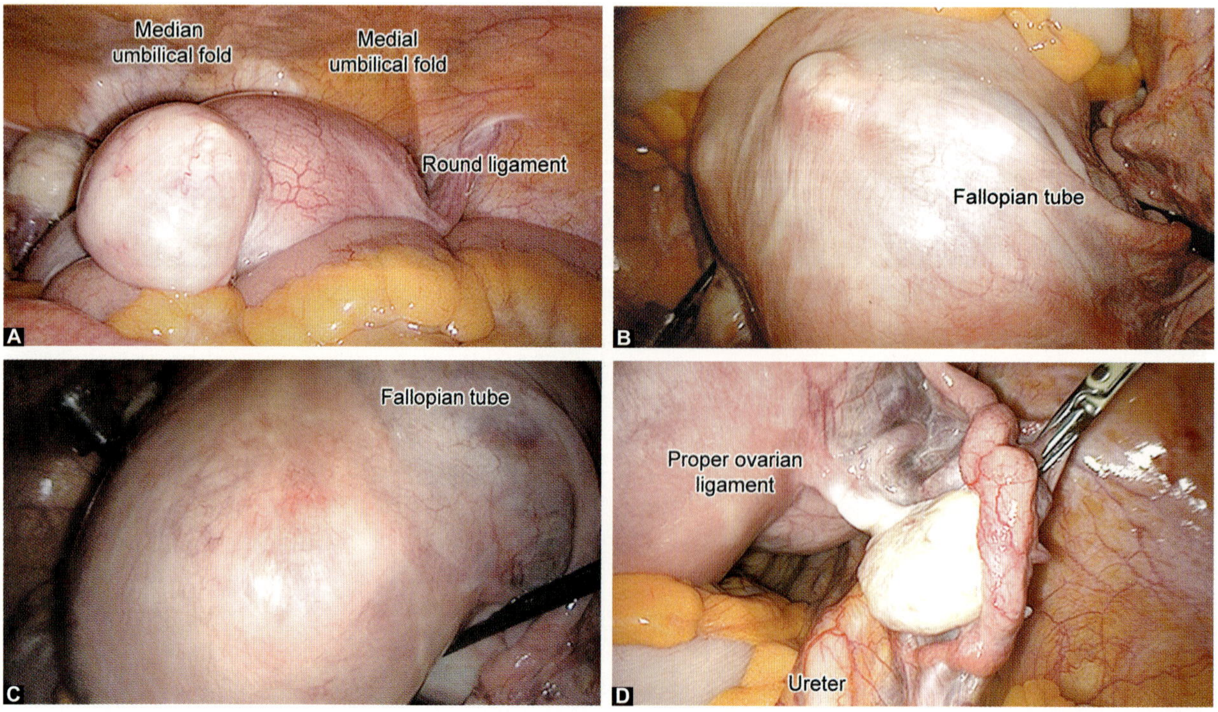


**Figs 16.4A to D:** First inspection and positioning of uterus with the help of the intrauterine manipulator

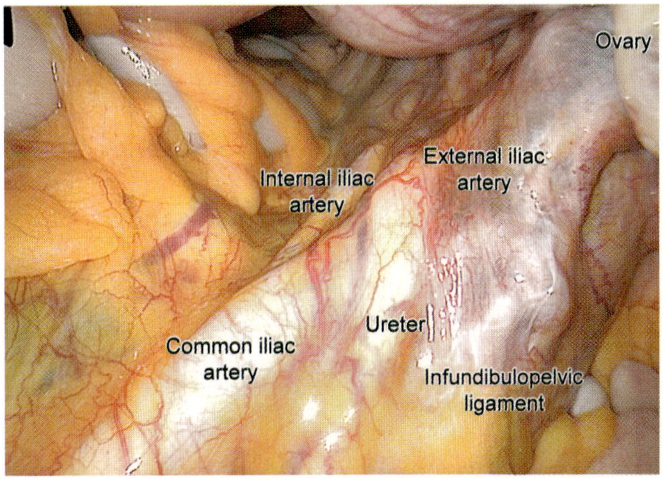


**Fig. 16.5:** Anatomical site recognition

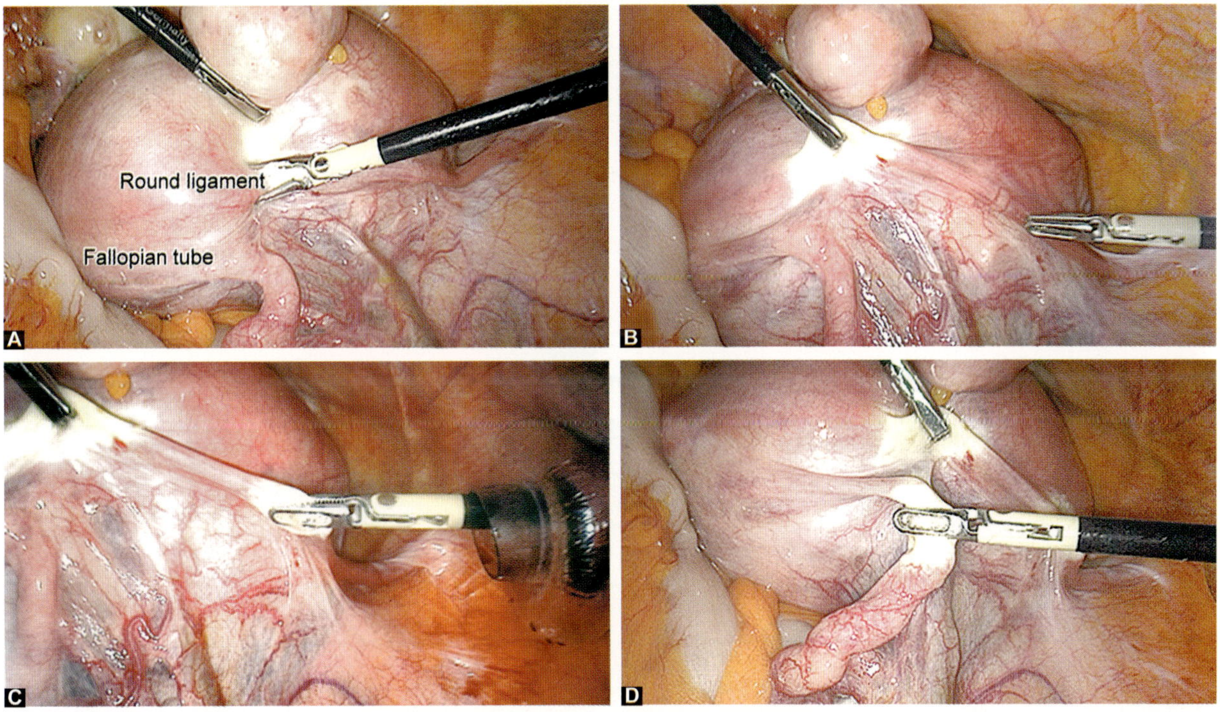


**Figs 16.6A to D:** Stepwise bipolar coagulation of right tube and right round ligament

## Postoperative Management

Retraction of urinary catheter which only in specific cases remains. A postoperative cystoscopy is rarely performed. Early ambulation after a few hours postsurgically is a good practice. Clear liquids can be started 6 hours postsurgically followed by a light diet. The patient can be discharge after 8–12 hours, can perform normal light activities and can get back to work after 4–5 days.

## Anticipated Problems

The vital symptoms, pain and temperature have to be meticulously controlled over the first 8 hours. A patient who is discharged early must have a phone number to call back in case of distress and pain.

# LAPAROSCOPIC TOTAL HYSTERECTOMY (LTH)

## General Aspects

Laparoscopic total hysterectomy today is an easy procedure and can be performed by using suture techniques alone, a combination of suture and coagulation techniques or by applying bipolar coagulation or any of the modern thermofusion, ultrasound and combined instruments for hemostasis.

## Preoperative Preparation

The patient is placed in lithotomy position with the buttocks at the end of the table. A uterine manipulator, like the HOHL or the Mangeshikar manipulator is fixed to the

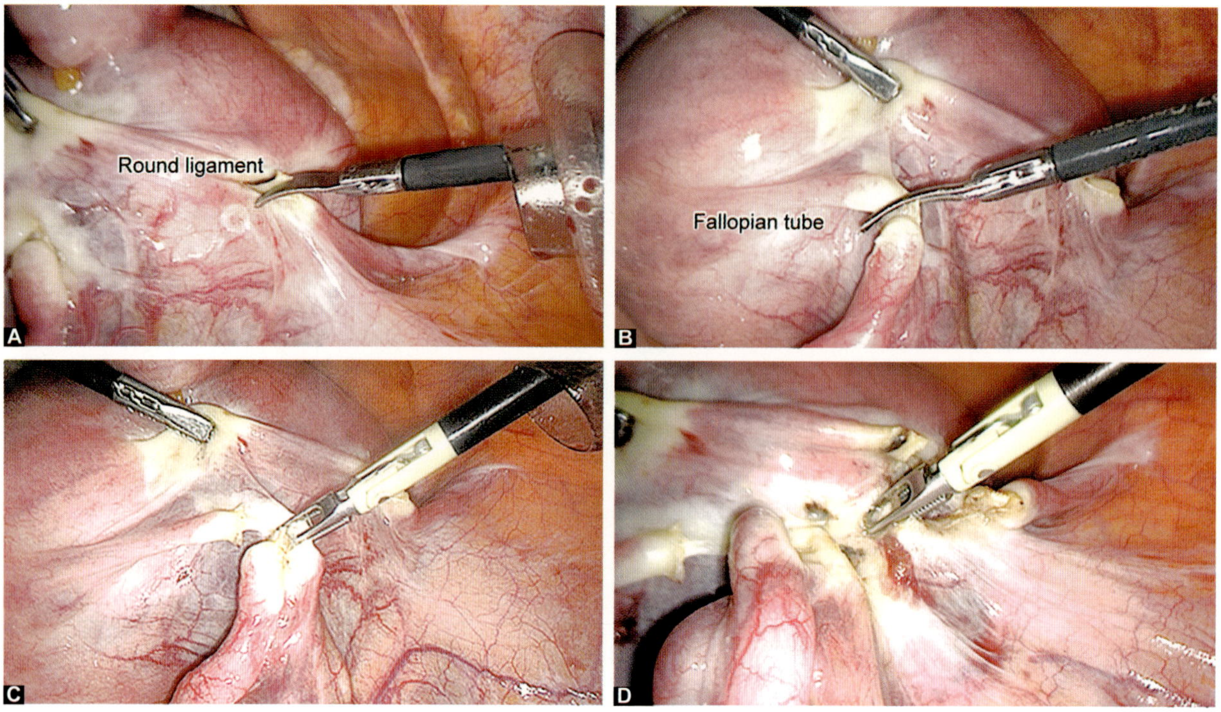


**Figs 16.7A to D:** Stepwise dissection of right tube and round ligament

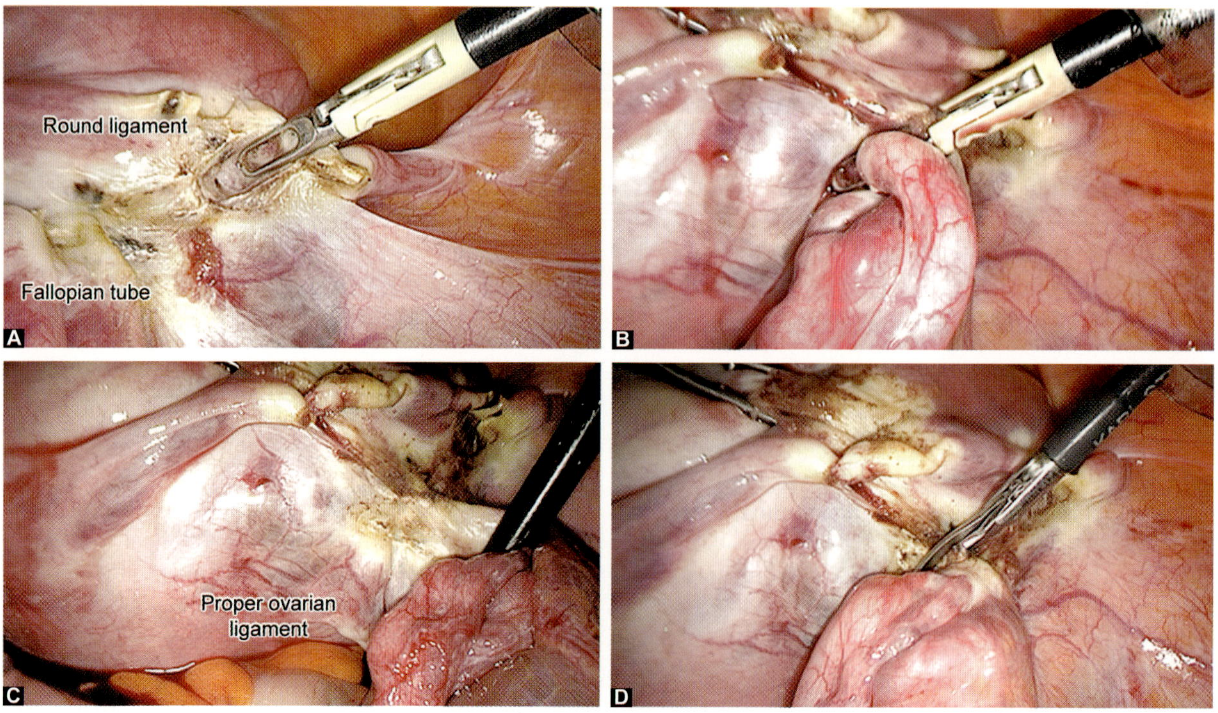


**Figs 16.8A to D:** Continuous stepwise dissection and beginning of opening the broad ligament

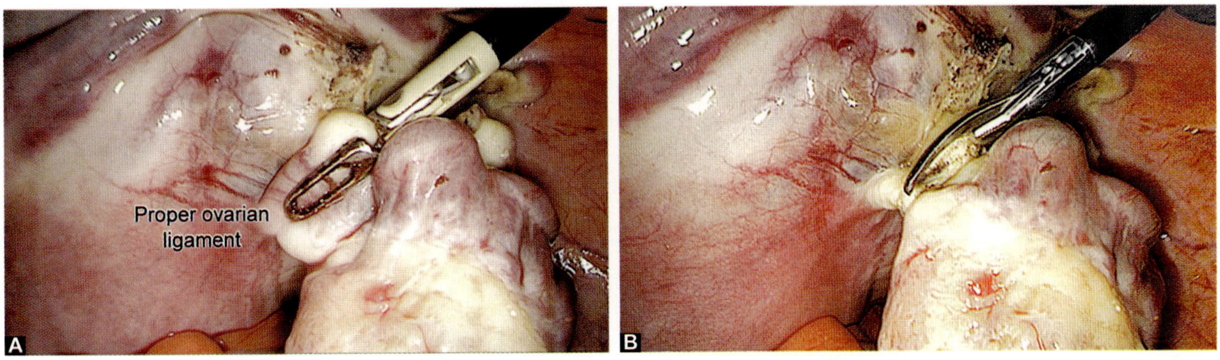


**Figs 16.9A and B:** Coagulation of the ovarian ligament

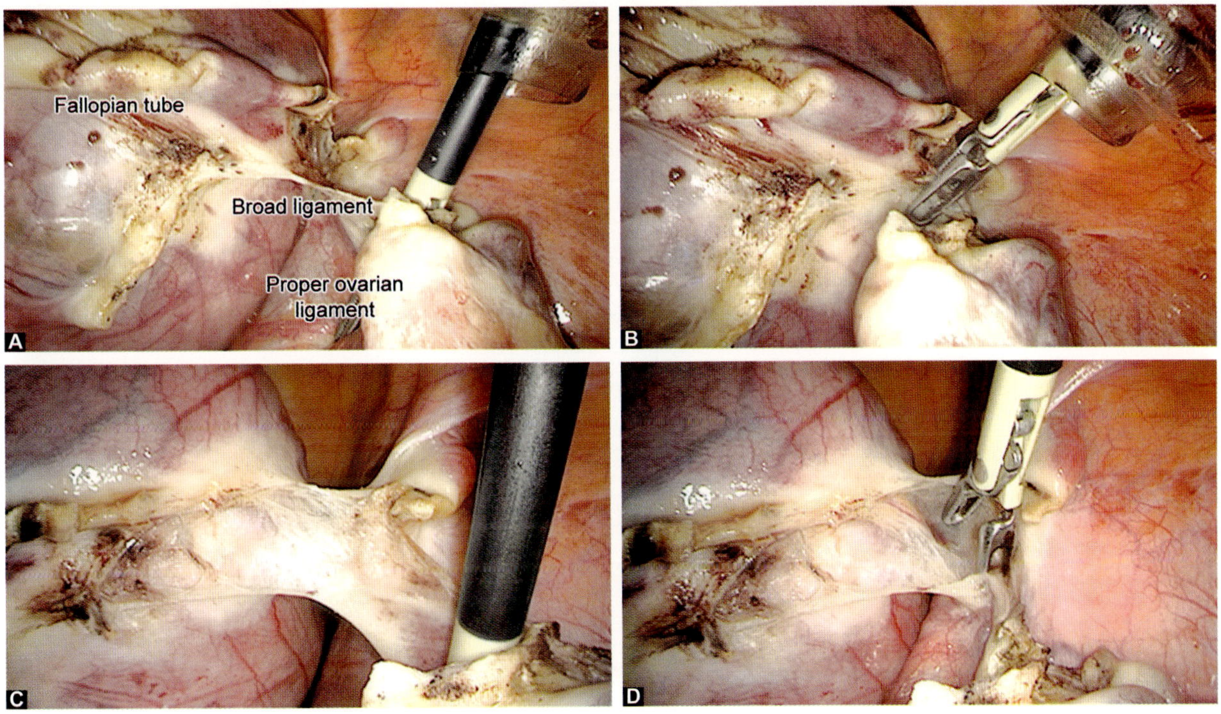


**Figs 16.10A to D:** Dissection of the proper ovarian ligament and opening of the broad ligament

cervix after a standard Foley's catheter is placed into the bladder. The purpose of the manipulator is to move the uterus in the abdominal cavity for better exposure for its resection.

## Instruments and Equipment

The uterine manipulator is used as a third hand of the surgeon in cases of hysterectomy for multiple fibroids. We do not insist on its use in cancer surgery. The vagina has to be closed after the necessary colpotomy at LTH either by a continuous suture, interrupted sutures, barbed sutures, or by sutures for extracorporeal knotting after they have been prepared. The prepared needle holders should be well-known to the surgeon. In addition to these, the instruments detailed under LSH are necessary.

## Prerequisites

The indication for total hysterectomy in the case of fibroids must be at hand. The full consent of the patient of removing her uterus with or without removal of tubes or/and ovaries must be given. In cases of large and multiple fibroids, an intravenous pyelogram or CT scan may be indicated.

## Steps for Surgery

1. The first five steps for surgery are identical to the five steps mentioned under subtotal hysterectomy in this chapter (Figs 16.2 to 16.21).
2. At separation of the bladder from the uterus, the bladder is pushed and dissected down 2–3 cm to clearly visualize the rim of the cervical cap. In cases of postcesarean section, a careful and gentle blunt and intermediate sharp dissection has to be carried out (Fig. 16.32).
3. While lateralizing the ureter by pushing up the manipulator, the uterine artery and vein with its collaterals is totally coagulated near the cervix and dissected.
4. Resection of the vagina from the cervix with the monopolar hook by stretching the manipulator firmly cranially, carefully performing an intrafacial dissection

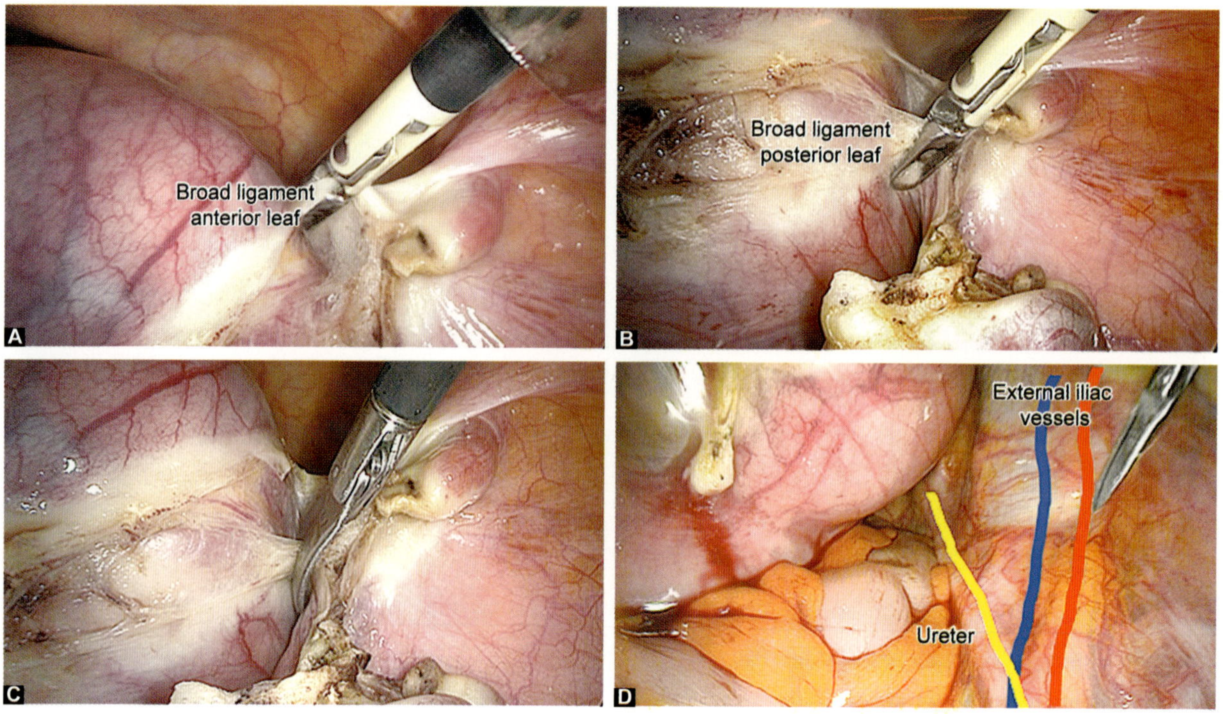


**Figs 16.11A to D:** (A to C) Separation of the anterior and posterior leaf of the broad ligament; (D) In relation to the ureter and pelvic vessels

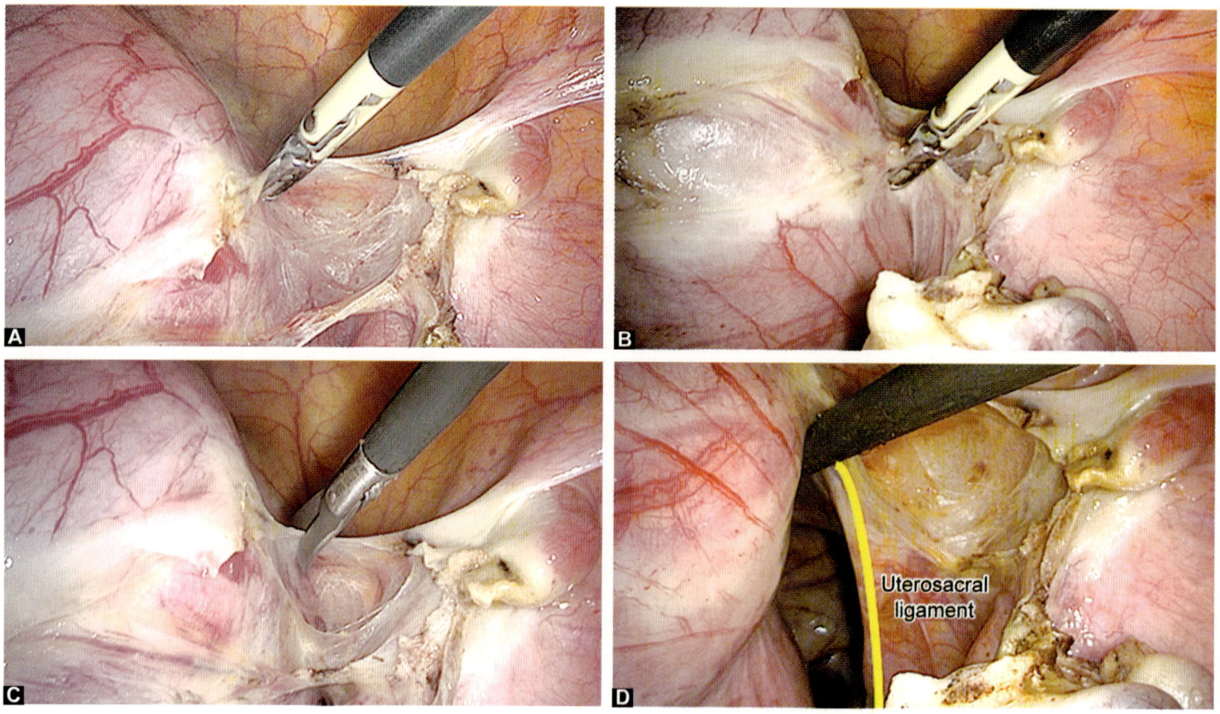


**Figs 16.12A to D:** (A to C) Final separation of the leafs of the broad ligament; (D) Up to the uterosacral ligament

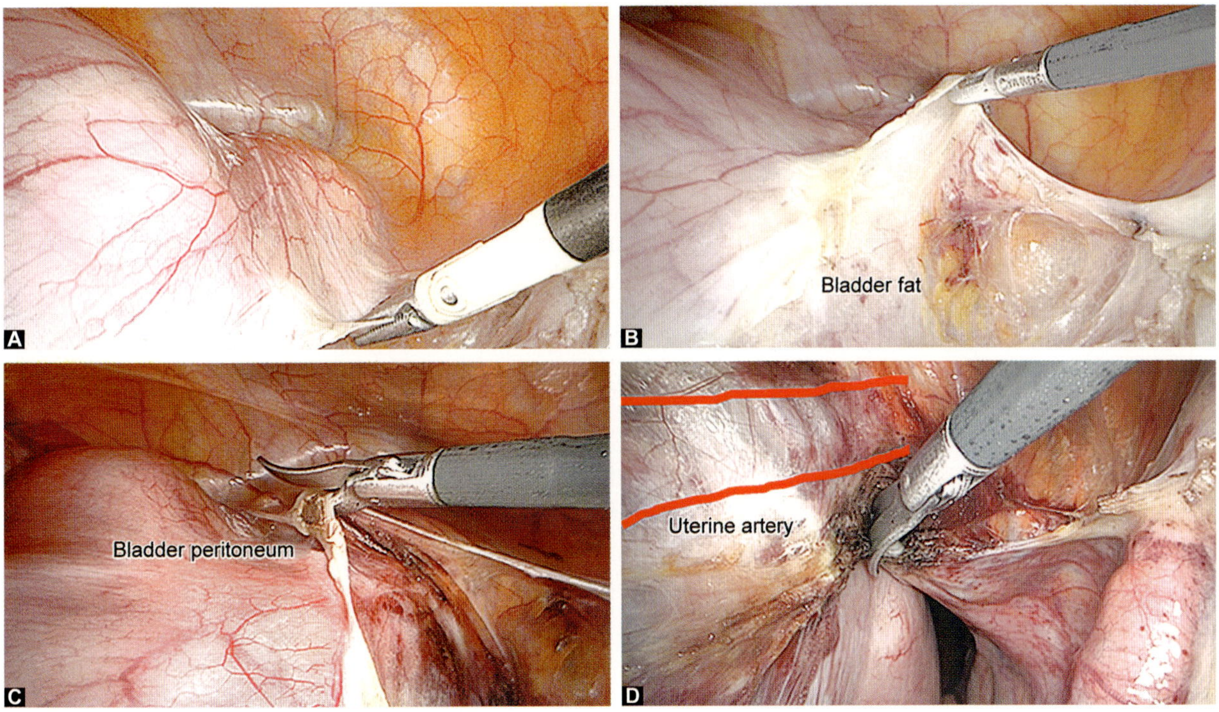


**Figs 16.13A to D:** (A to C) Opening of the bladder peritoneum from the right side; (D) Freeing the uterine vessel bundle

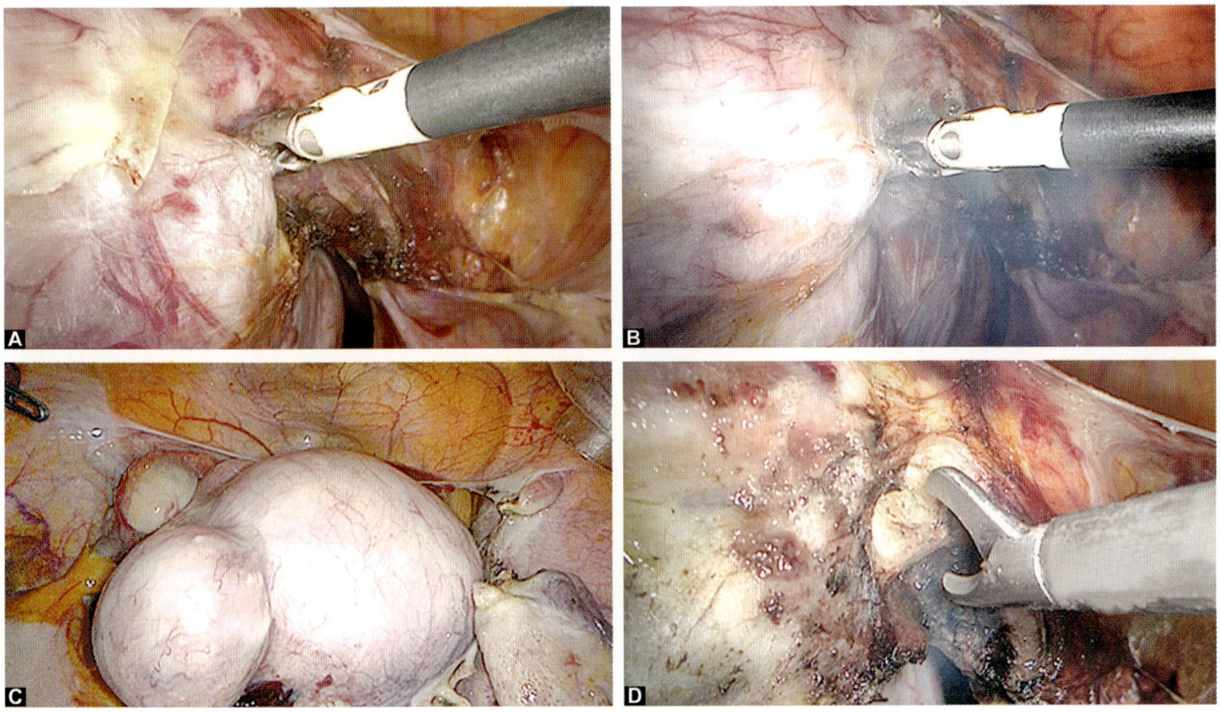


**Figs 16.14A to D:** Bipolar coagulation and dissection of the uterine vessels

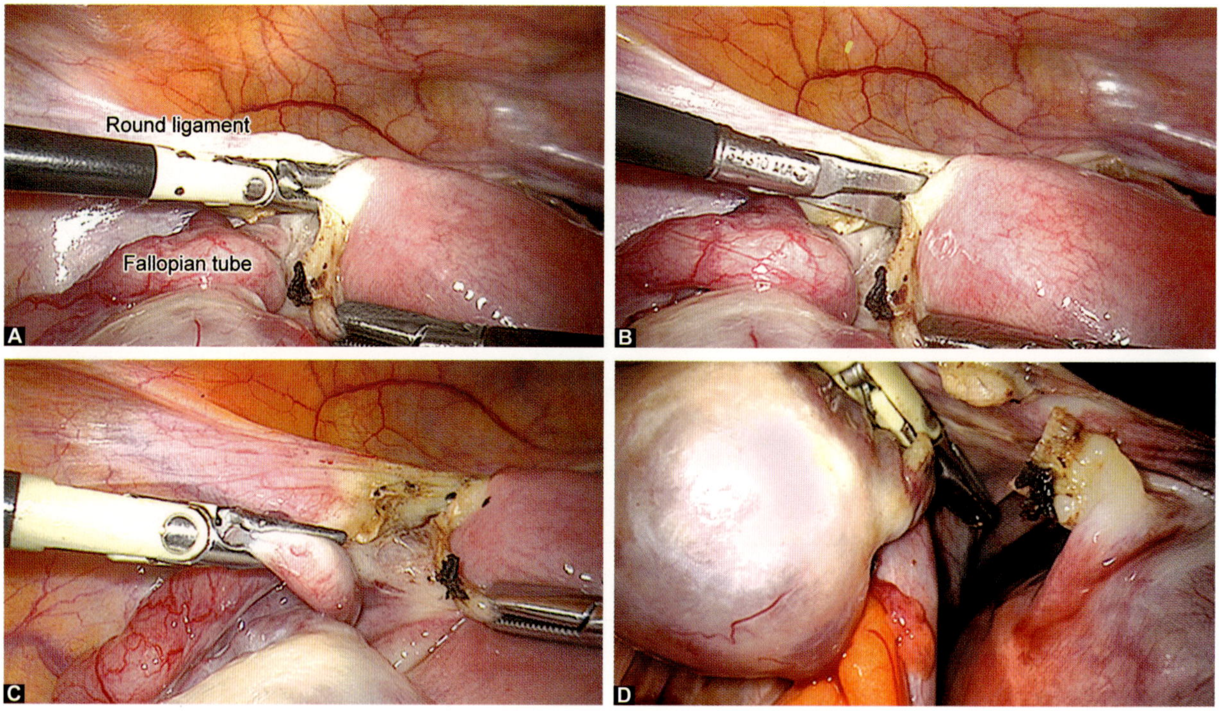


**Figs 16.15A to D:** (A to C) Stepwise coagulation and dissection of left round ligament and tube; (D) Ovarian ligament

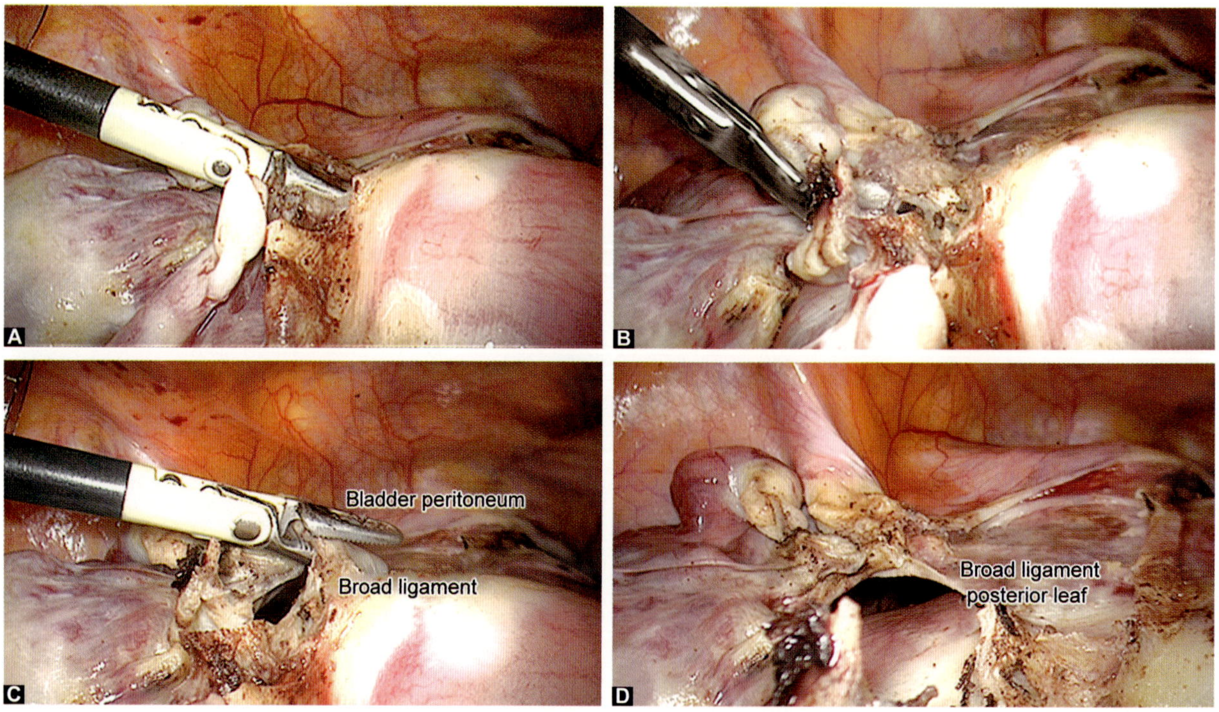


**Figs 16.16A to D:** Dissecting of the bladder peritoneum as well as the anterior and posterior leaf of the broad ligament of the left side

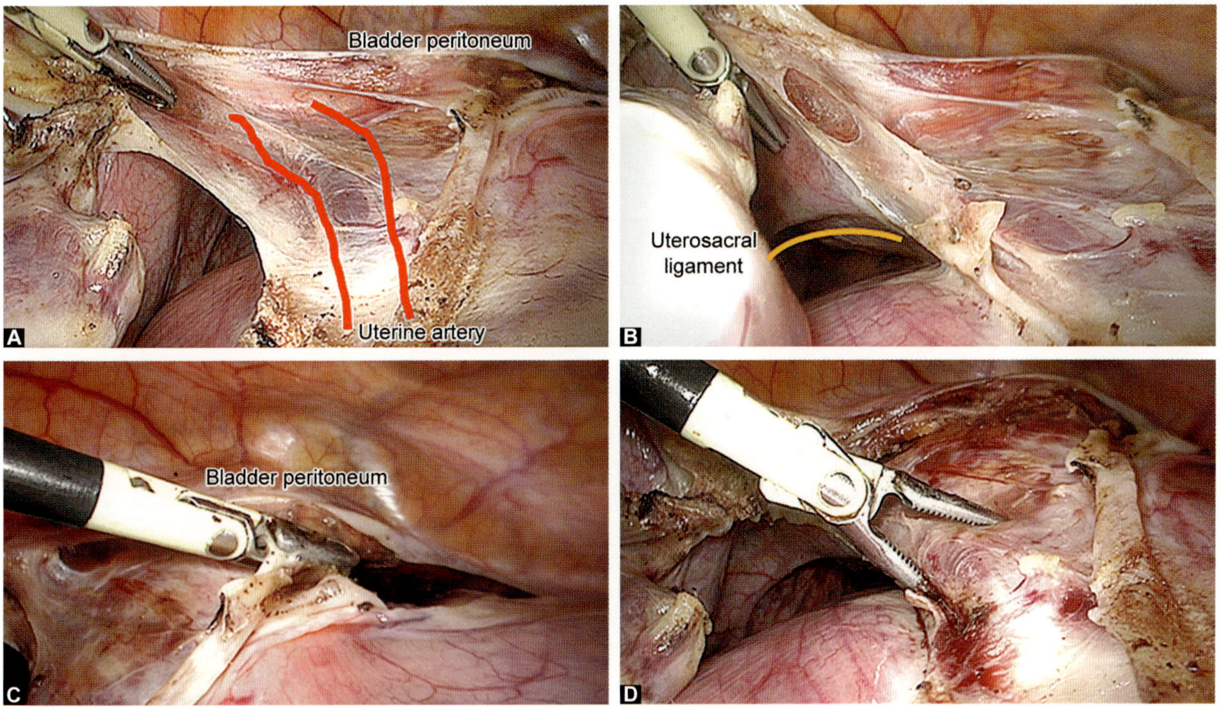


**Figs 16.17A to D:** (A and C) Further opening of the bladder peritoneum; (B) Opening of the broad ligament; (D) Beginning coagulation of the left uterine vessels

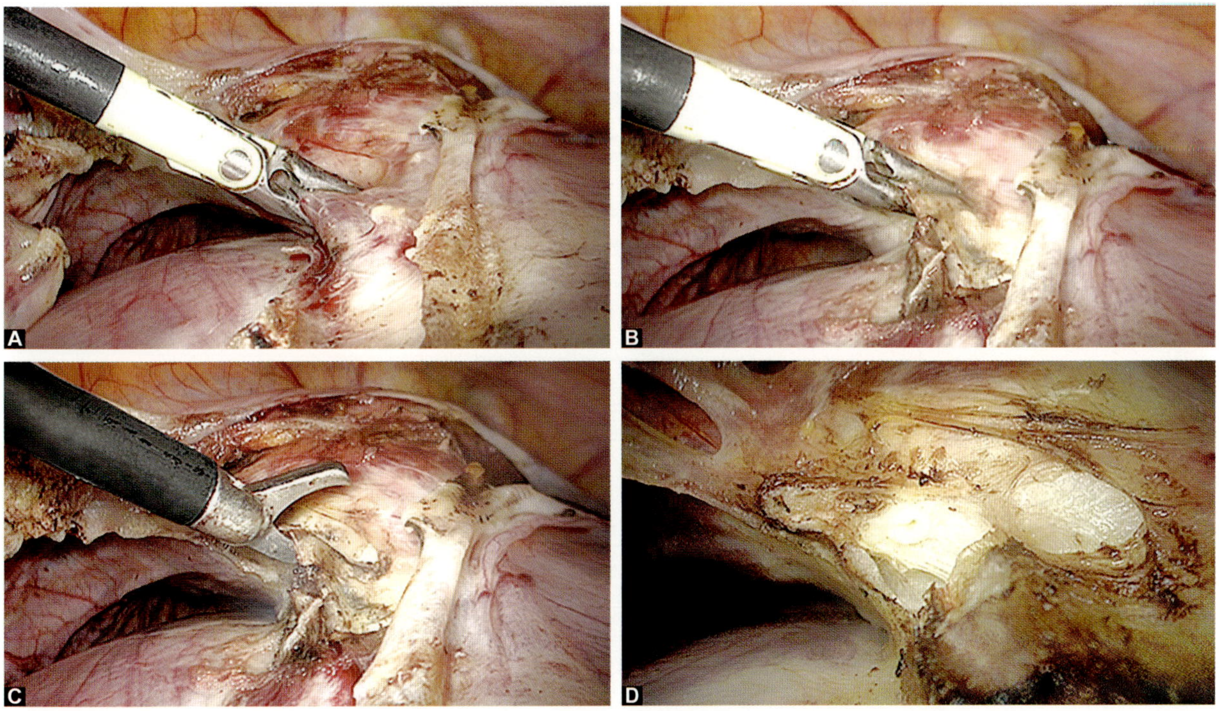


**Figs 16.18A to D:** Coagulation and separation of the uterine vessels on the left side

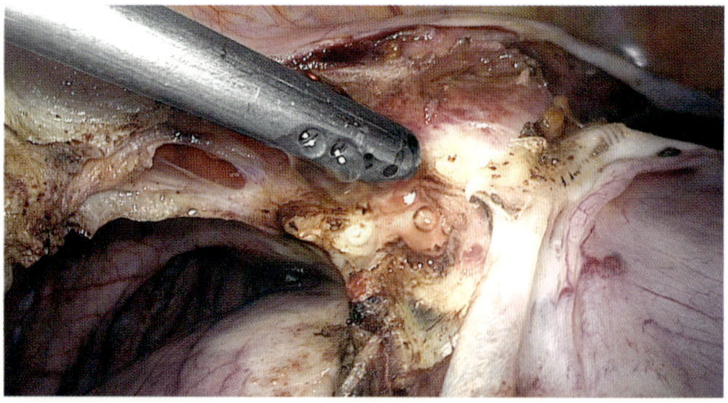

**Fig. 16.19:** Visualization of the separated left uterine pedicles

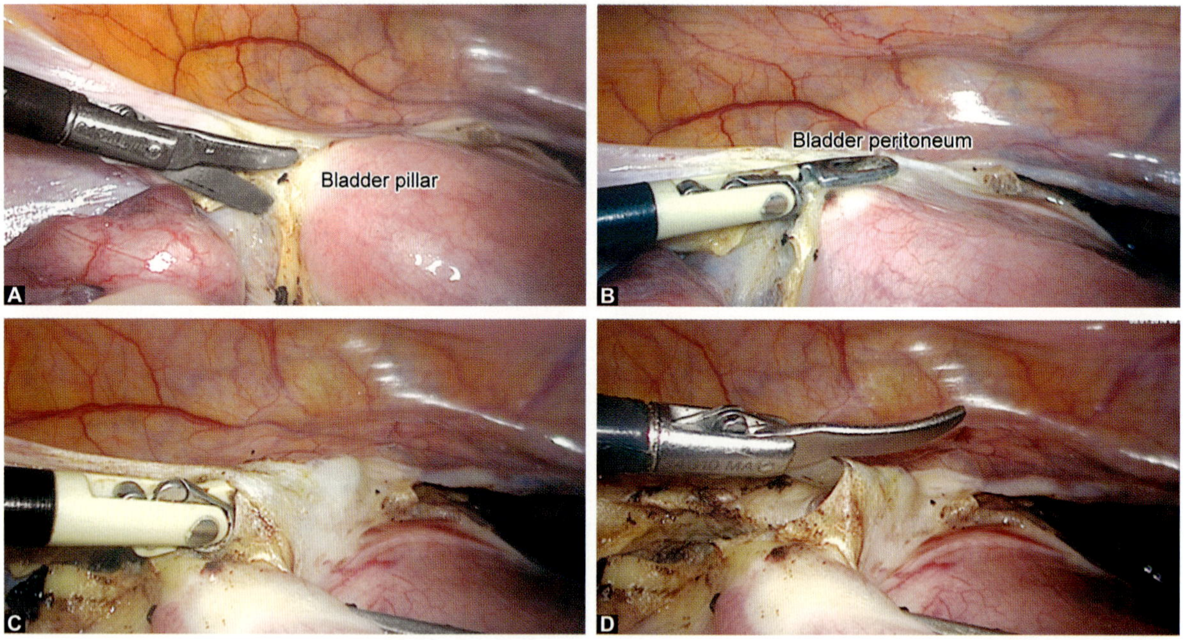


**Figs 16.20A to D:** Final dissection of the bladder pillar and the bladder peritoneum from left to right, letting the $CO_2$ distension medium lead the path

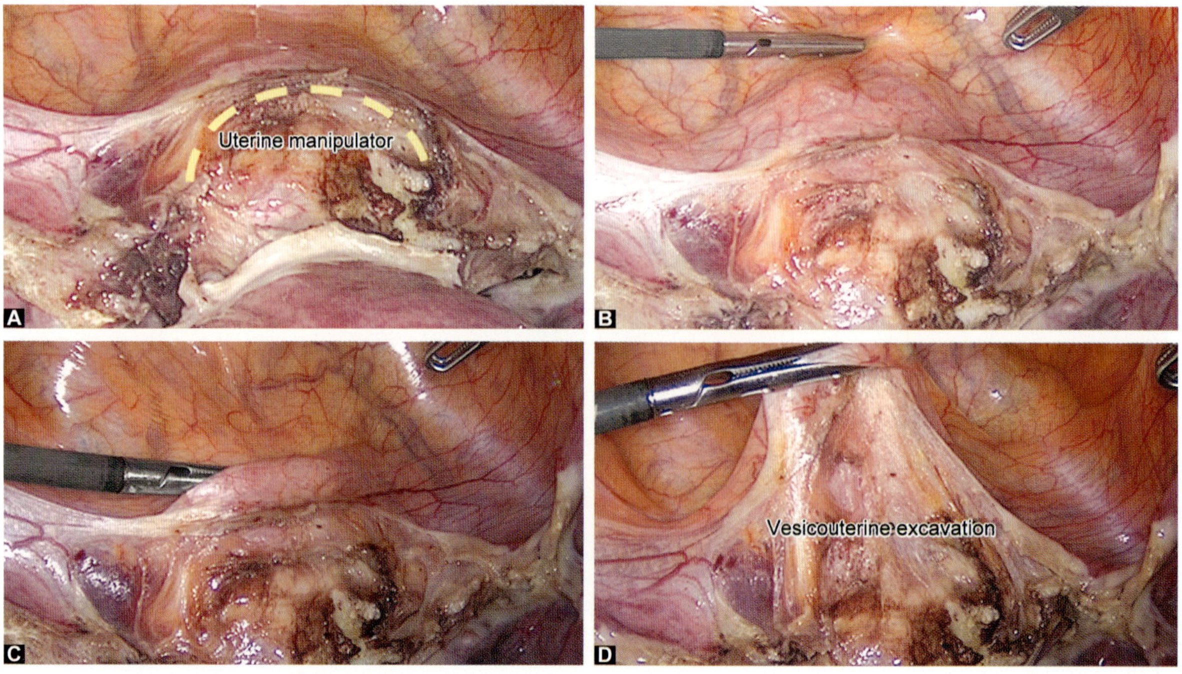


**Figs 16.21A to D:** Visualization of the intrauterine manipulator, elevation of the bladder peritonium

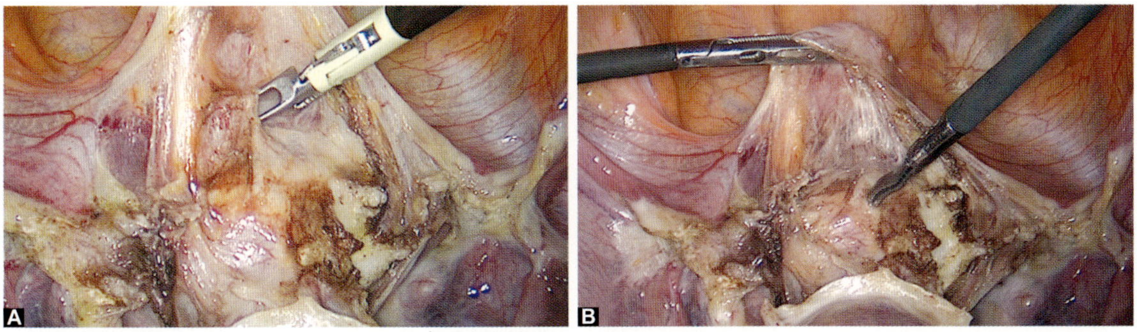


**Figs 16.22A and B:** Minimal dissection of the bladder peritoneum of about 1cm for LSH and 2–3 cm for LTH

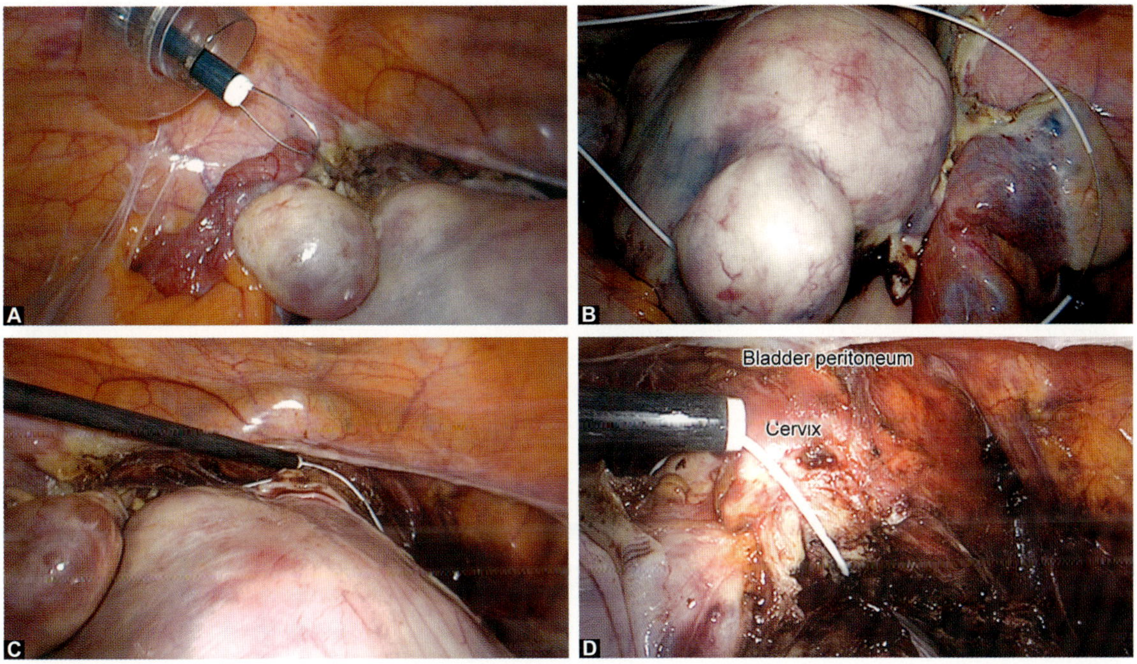


**Figs 16.23A to D:** Introduction of the Storz cutting loop for the cervix and exact placement prior to activation

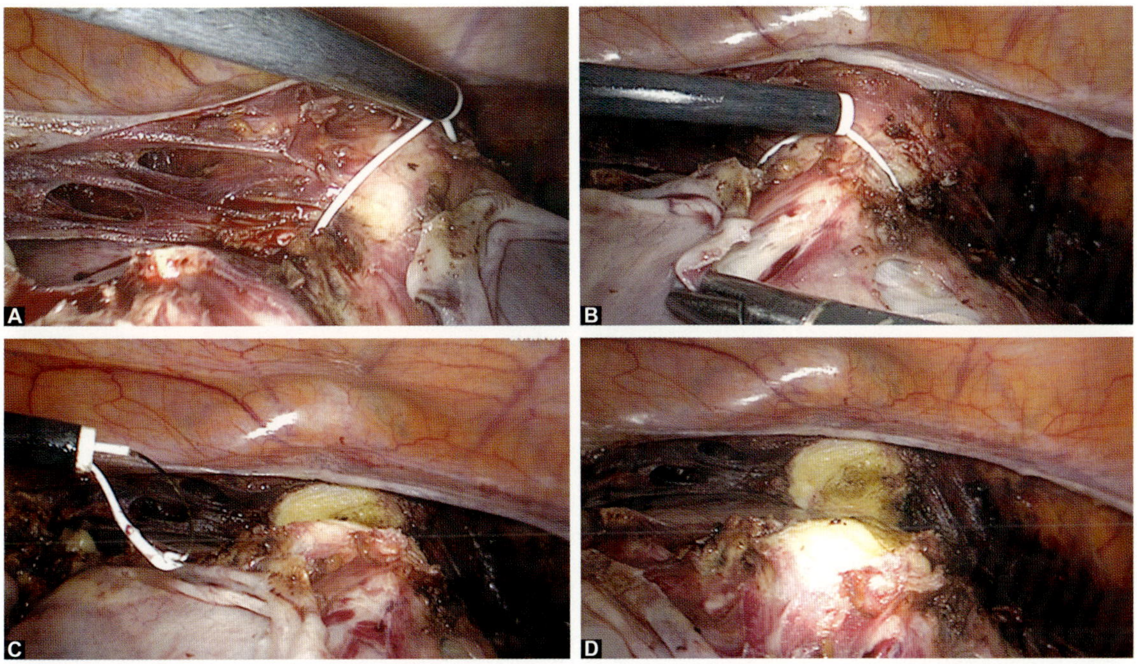


**Figs 16.24A to D:** (A and B) Resection of vagina from cervix after placing the cutting loop with the cutting point on the posterior cervix; (C and D) performing the dissection of cervix and uterus; in this case of LSH

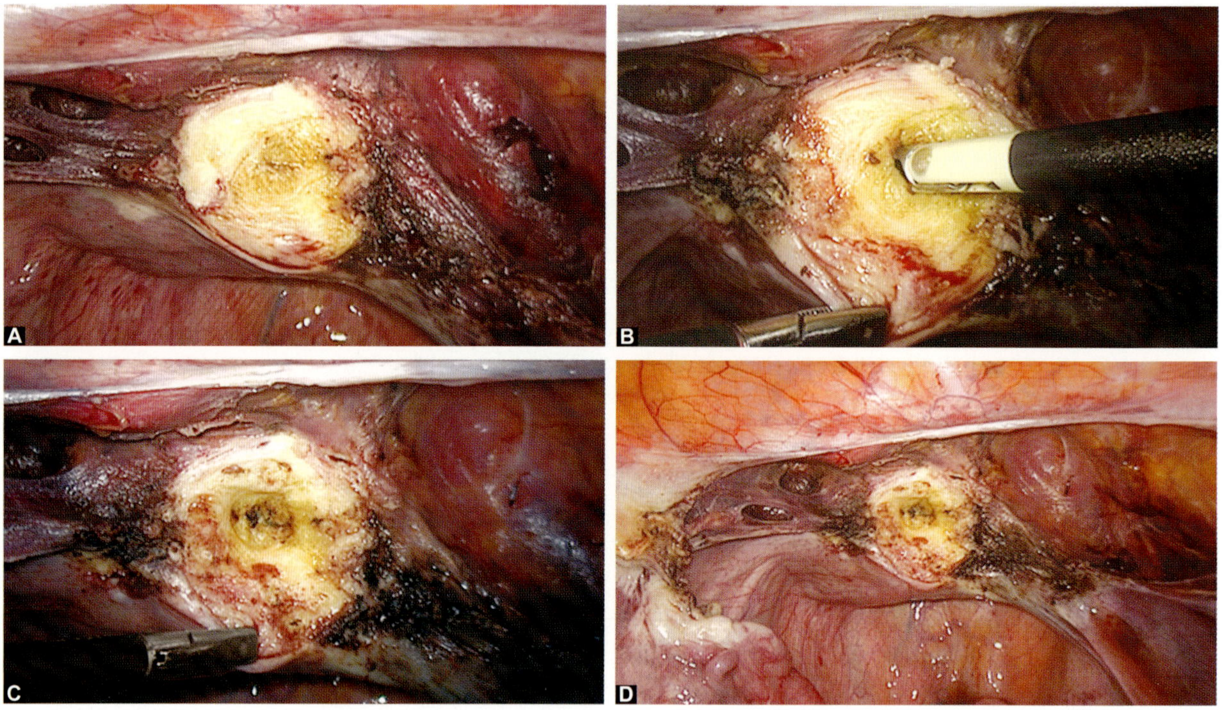

**Figs 16.25A to D:** LSH. (A) After separation of uterus from cervix; (B) coagulation of inner cervical canal; (C and D) Final inspection

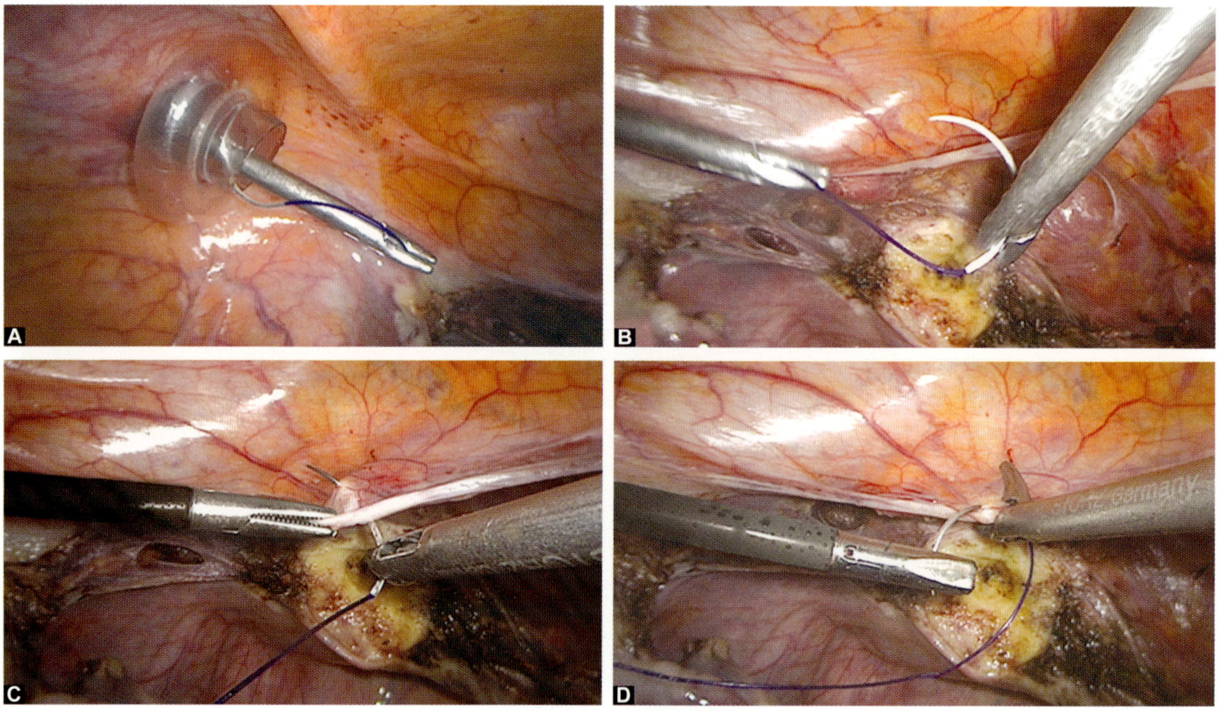

**Figs 16.26A to D:** LSH. (A) Introduction of peritoneal suture; (B to D) Closure of visceral peritoneum over the cervical stump with a continuous PDS suture

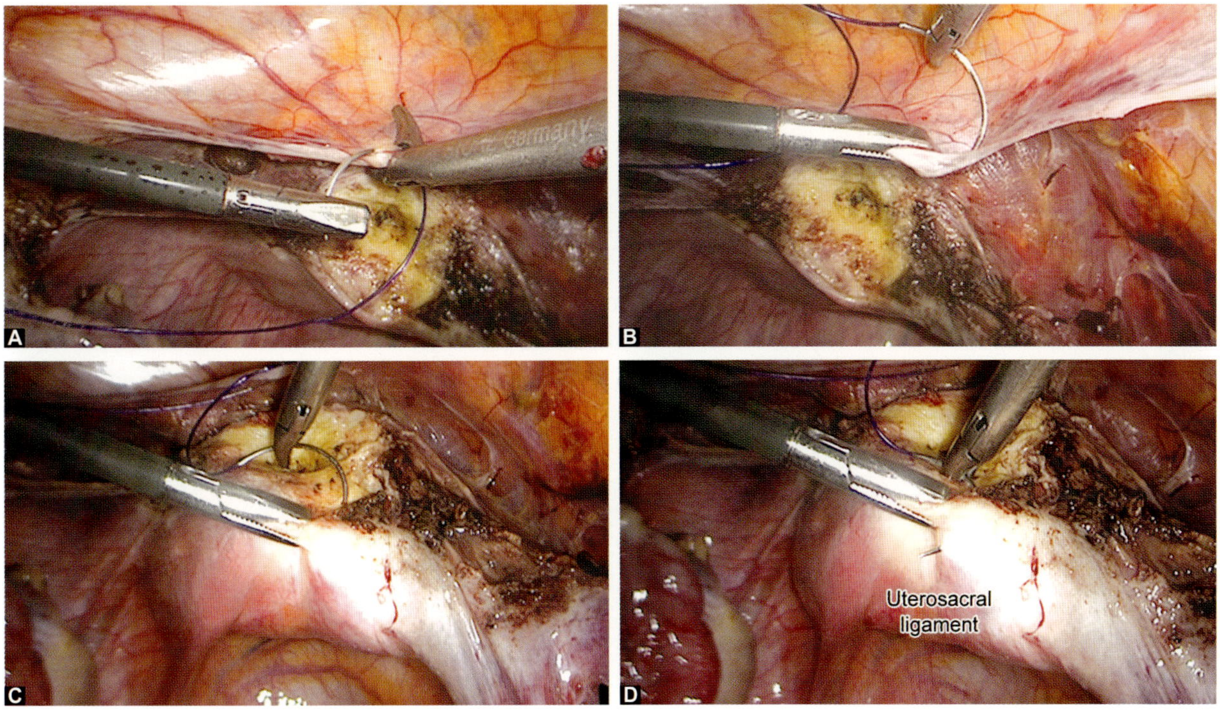


**Figs 16.27A to D:** LSH: Continuous suture covering the entire cervical stump

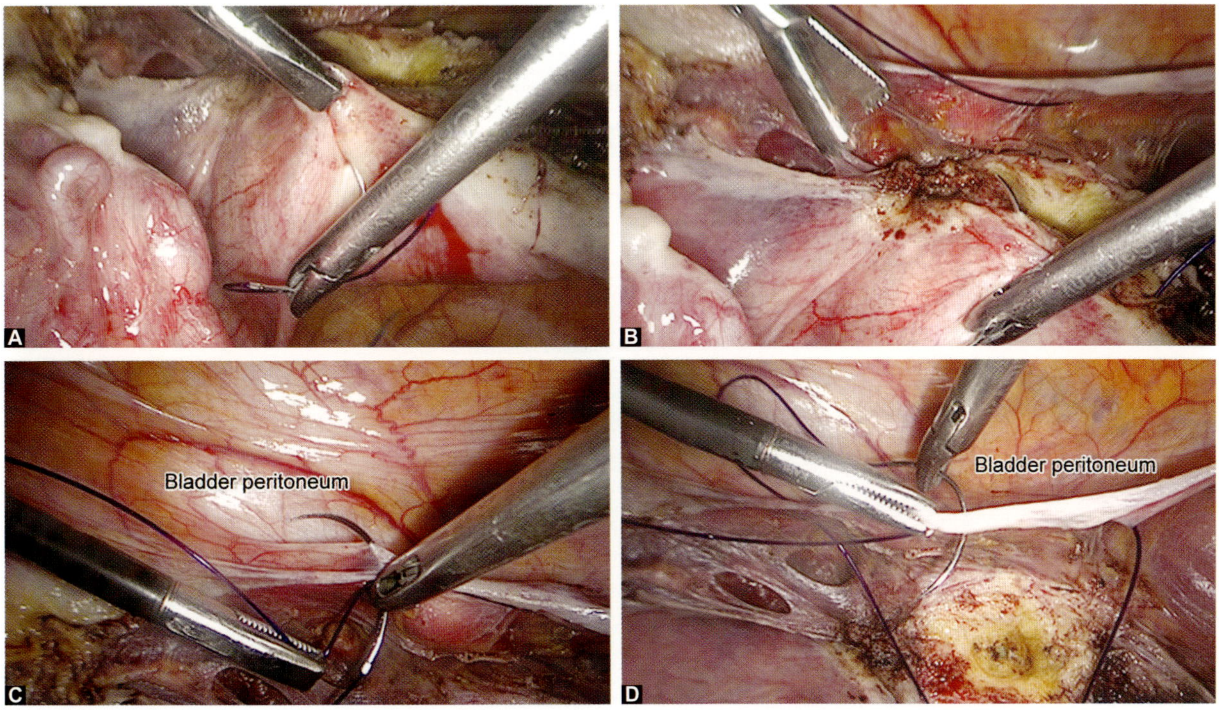


**Figs 16.28A to D:** LSH: Connecting the bladder peritoneum to the posterior peritoneum

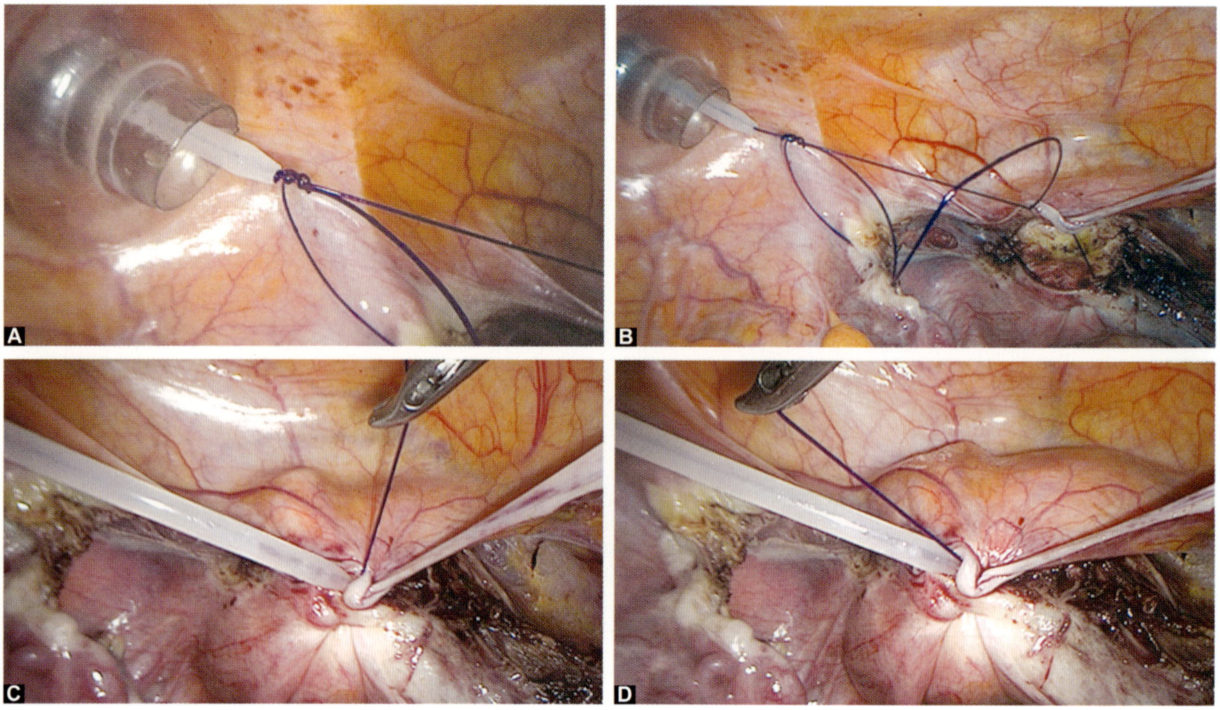

**Figs 16.29A to D:** LSH: Finalizing the extra corporal knot of the PDS suture

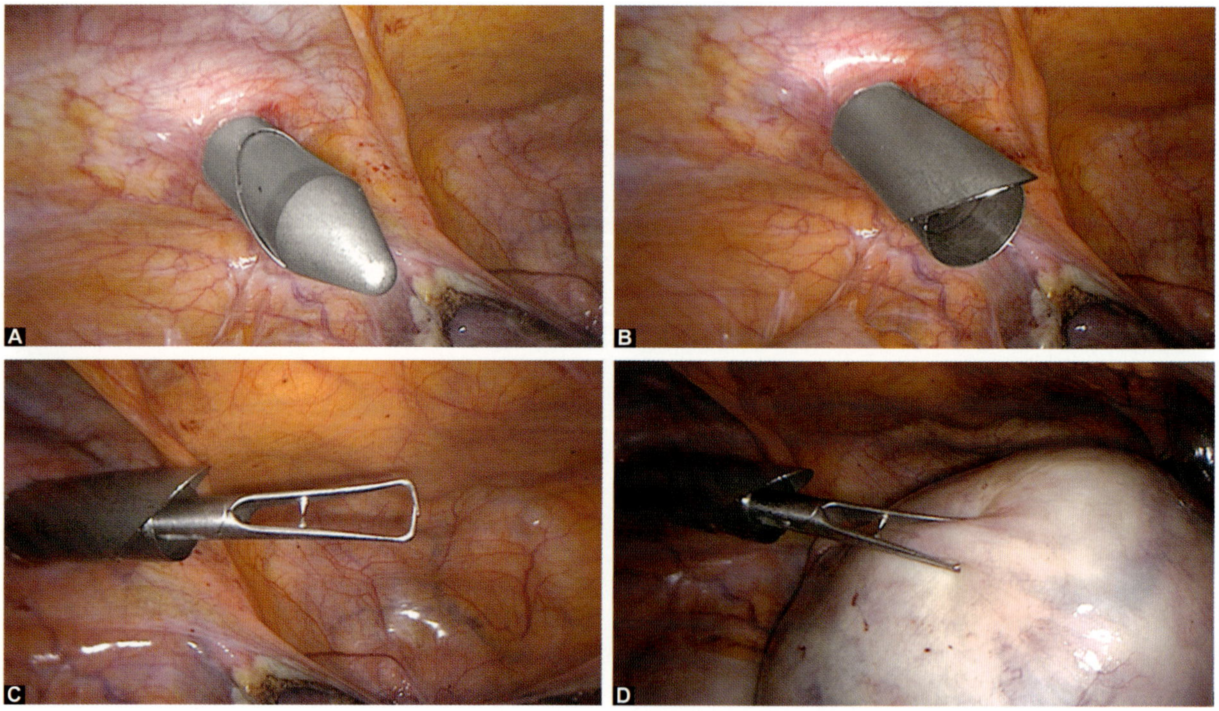

**Figs 16.30A to D:** LSH: Introduction of Rotocut morcellator from the left pelvic side wall and grasping of the uterus with a claw forceps

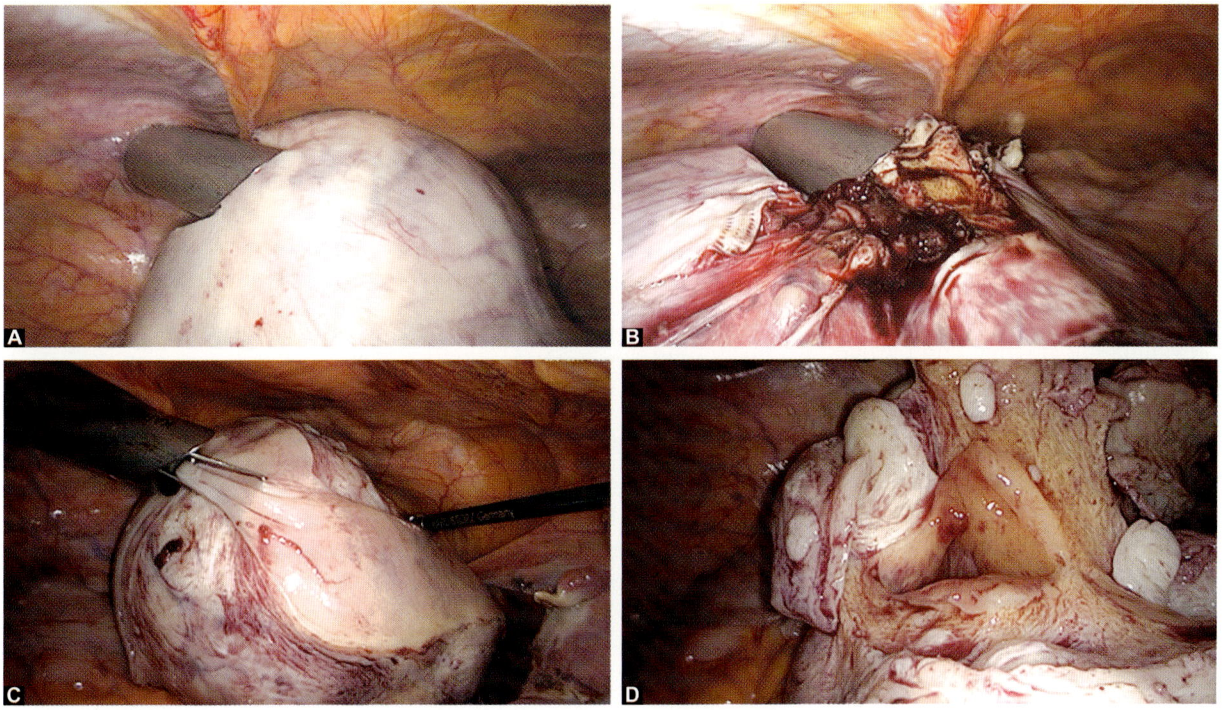

**Figs 16.31A to D:** LSH: Morcellation of the myomatous uterus (850 g) under continuous observation of the rotating cutting edge and protection shield of the morcellator

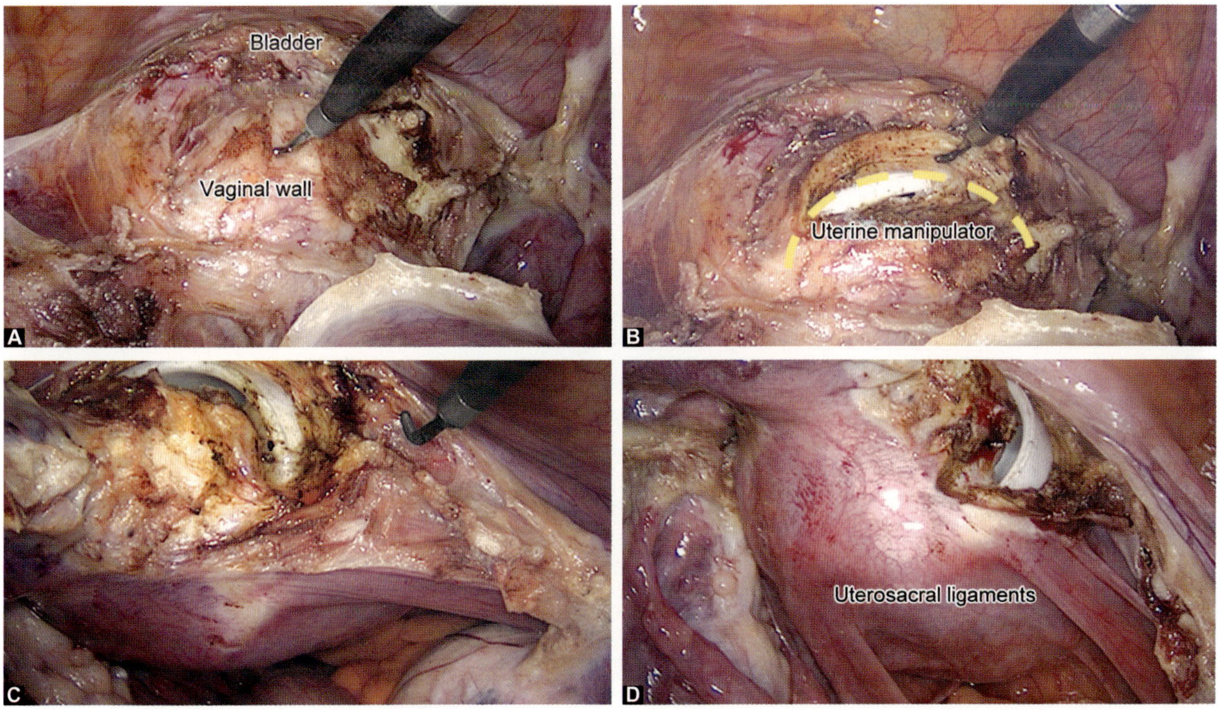


**Figs 16.32A to D:** (A) In this case of LTH, the distance between the vagina and bladder is increased; (B to D) The intrauterine manipulator is firmly pressed into the abdomen and the uterine dissection from the vagina is performed stepwise

leaving the sacrouterine ligaments nearly completely in place (Fig. 16.33).

5. The uterus is retracted through the vagina while still fixed to the manipulator. If the uterus is too big, it has to be morcellated either intra-abdominally or trans-vaginally. While morcellating the cutting edge of the morcellator must be continuously visible (Fig. 16.34).
6. Control of pedicles under continuous irrigation.
7. Closure of the vagina with 2 corner sutures and 1 or 2 figure of 8 sutures in between with both corner sutures. The sacrouterine ligaments and the middle portion of the vagina are stitched and elevated for prevention of vaginal prolapse or enterocele formation at a later time (Figs 16.35 to 16.44).
8. Final inspection (Figs 16.45 and 16.46). Peritonealization and drainage is not required.

## Postoperative Inspection

After LTH, a cotton-filled glove that had been introduced into the vagina after colpotomy or the part of the uterine manipulator like the Mangeshikar tube have to be taken out of the vagina. Manually, the strength of the vaginal closure can be tested. At suction and irrigation, all pedicles are checked.

## Postoperative Management

Sometimes a cystoscopy is indicated in longer lasting procedures. Think of antibiotic coverage and thrombo-prophylaxis (mechanical and medical) in appropriate cases. The urinary catheter is removed or may stay for 24 hours. Early ambulation and discharge on the same day or after 24–48 hours.

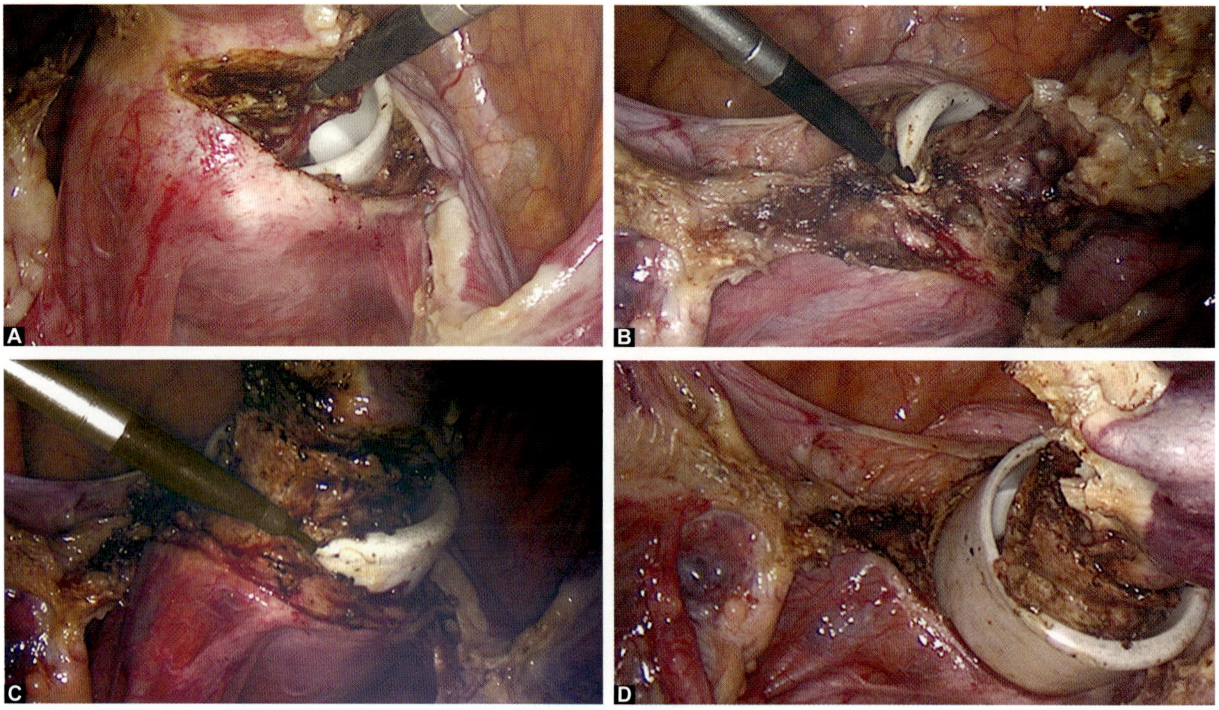


**Figs 16.33A to D:** (A to C) Completion of the dissection of the vagina from the cervix; (D) Beginning retraction of the uterine cervix still grasped by the manipulator forceps transvaginally

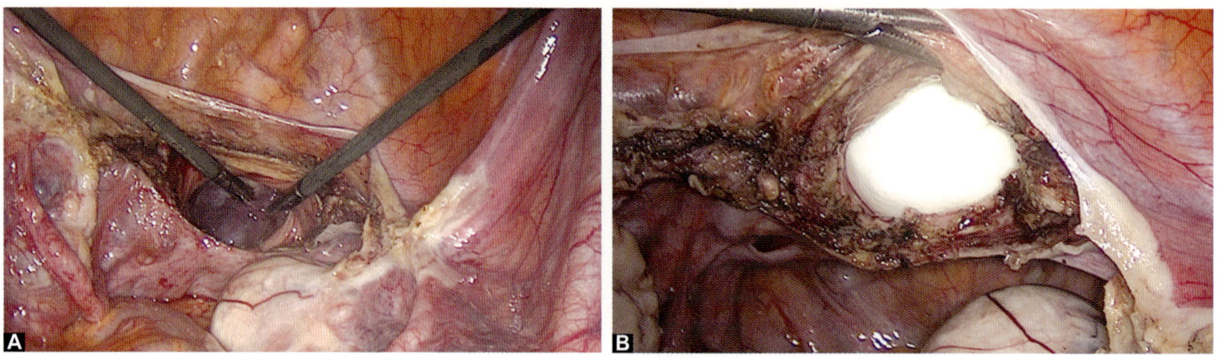


**Figs 16.34A and B:** (A) Retraction of uterus through the vagina; (B) Introduction of a cotton swab filled glove trans-vaginally to hinder the breakdown of CO2 pneumoperitonium

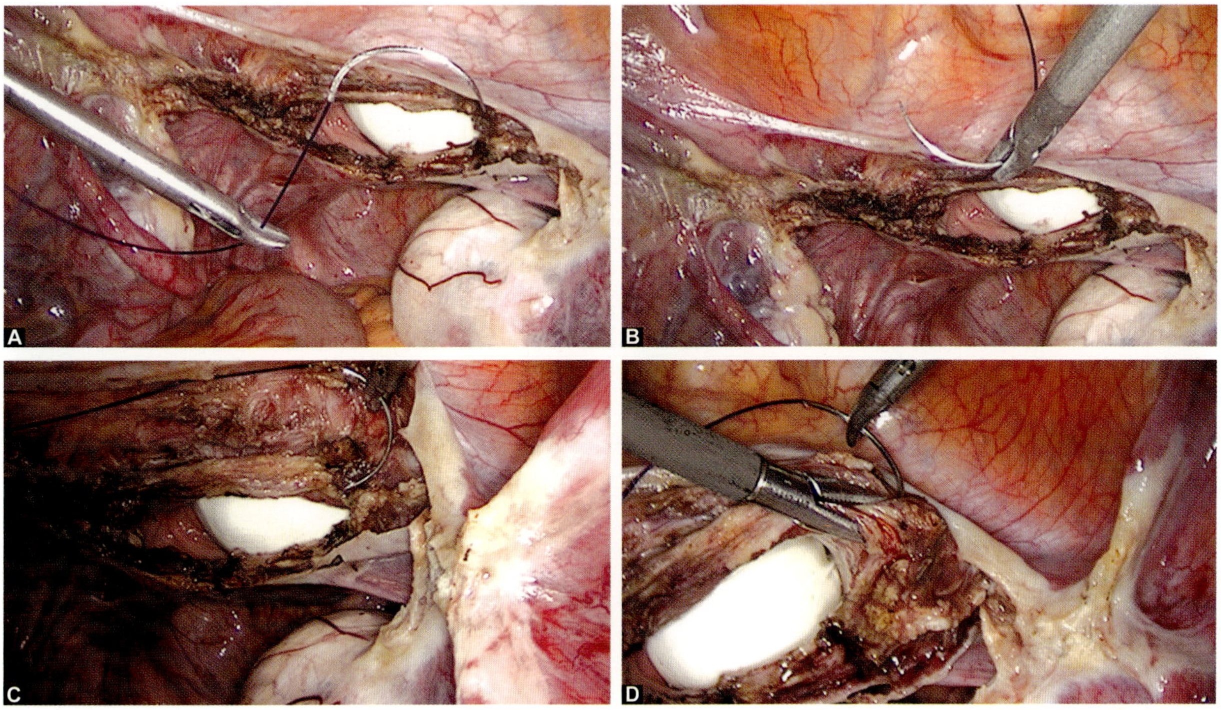

**Figs 16.35A to D:** LTH: Right corner suture uniting the vaginal anterior and posterior wall, bladder and posterior peritoneum as well as right sacrouterine ligament

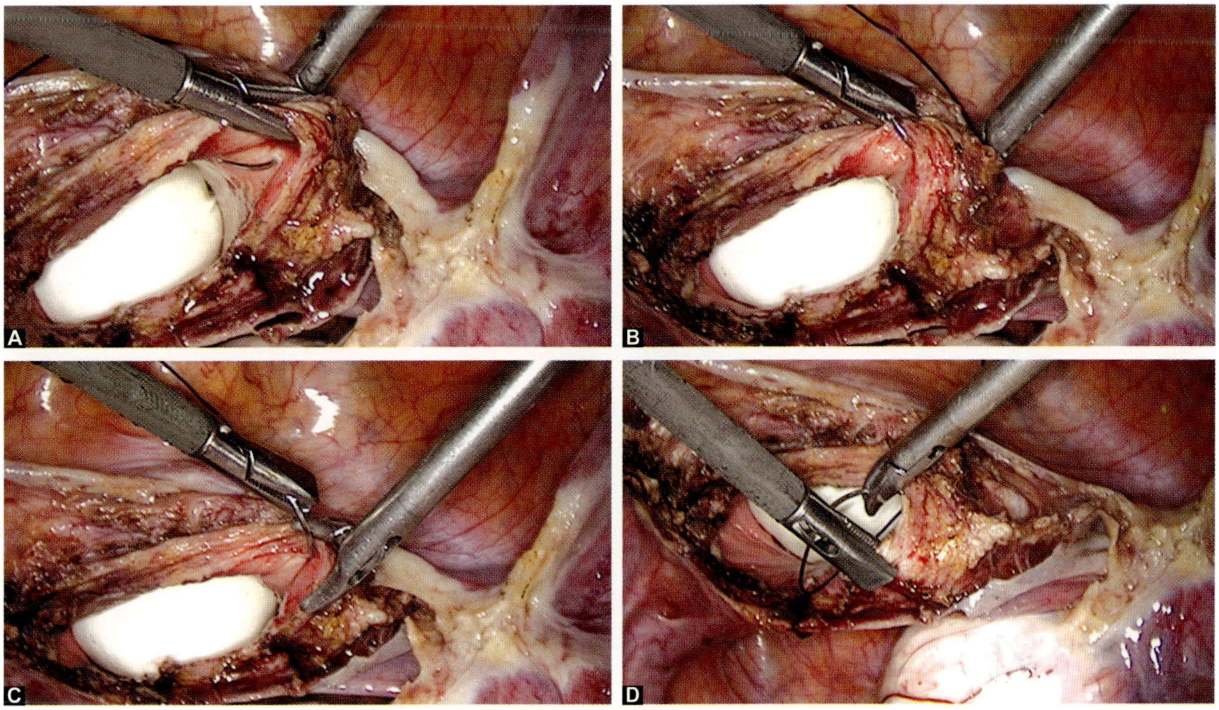

**Figs 16.36A to D:** LTH: Continuing the right corner suture

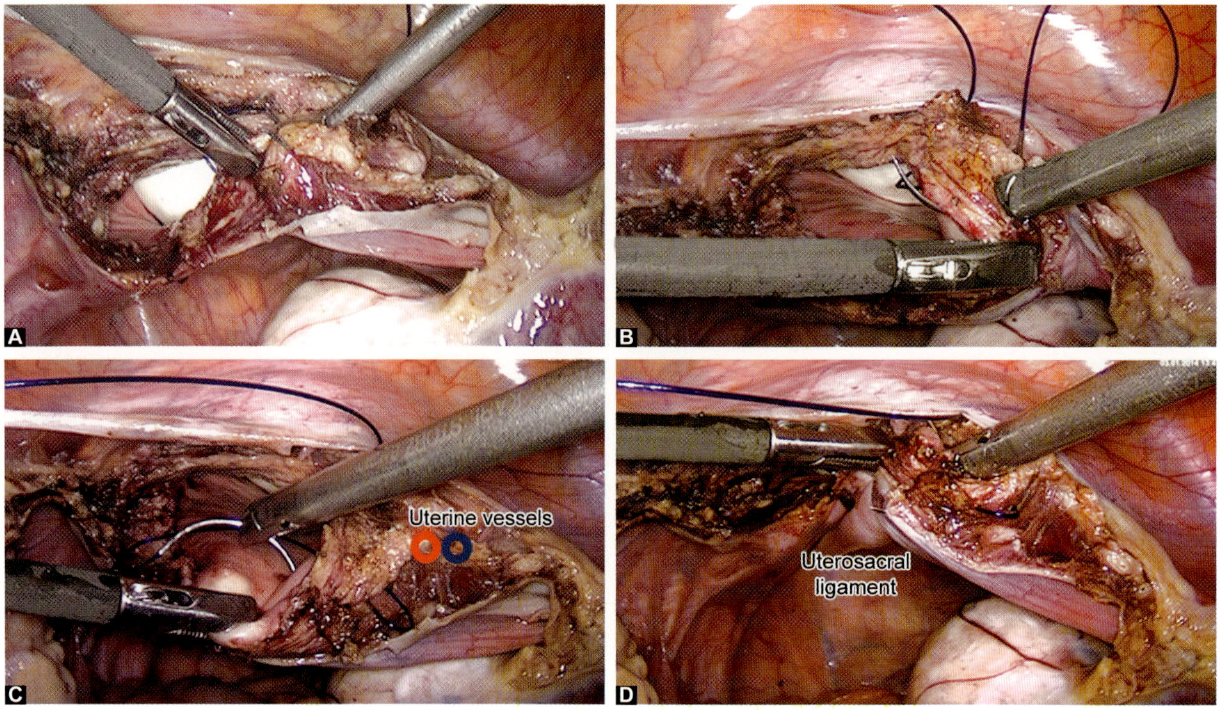


**Figs 16.37A to D:** LTH: Continuing the right corner suture while grabbing the right sacrouterine ligament

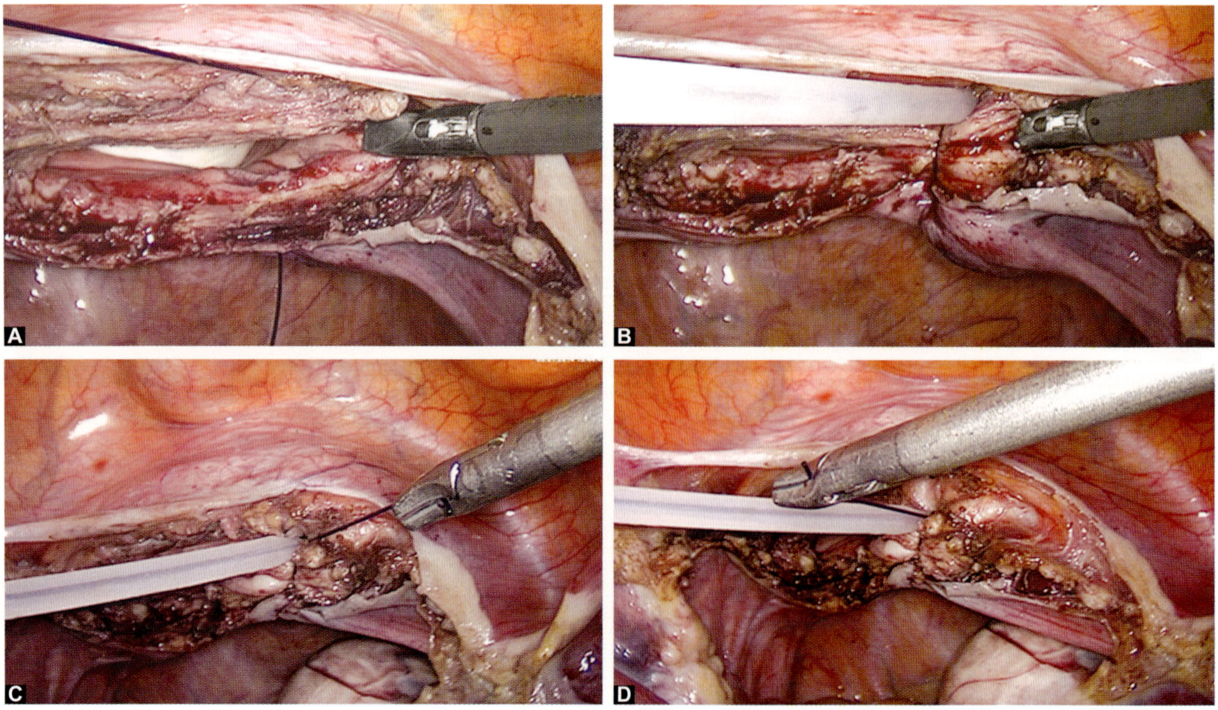


**Figs 16.38A to D:** LTH: Completing the extracorporal Roeder knot and pushing it down with a plastic push rod (B-D)

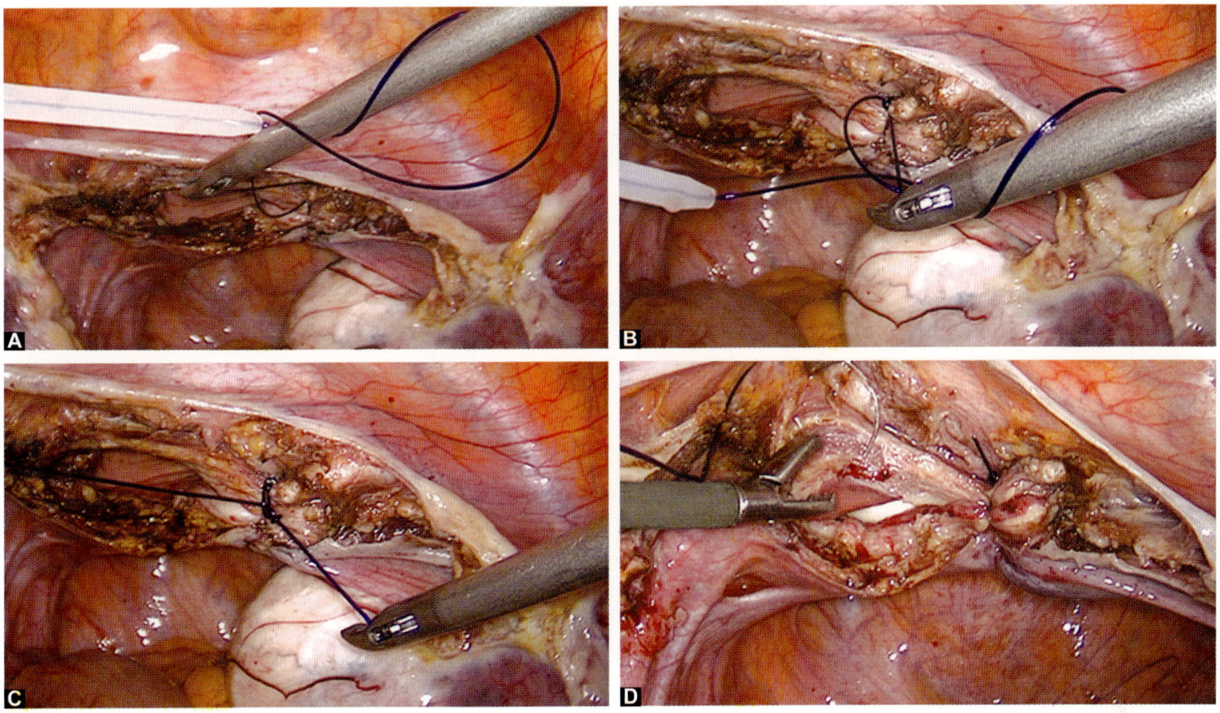

**Figs 16.39A to D:** LTH: Putting a security knot on the right corner stitch and cutting of the thread

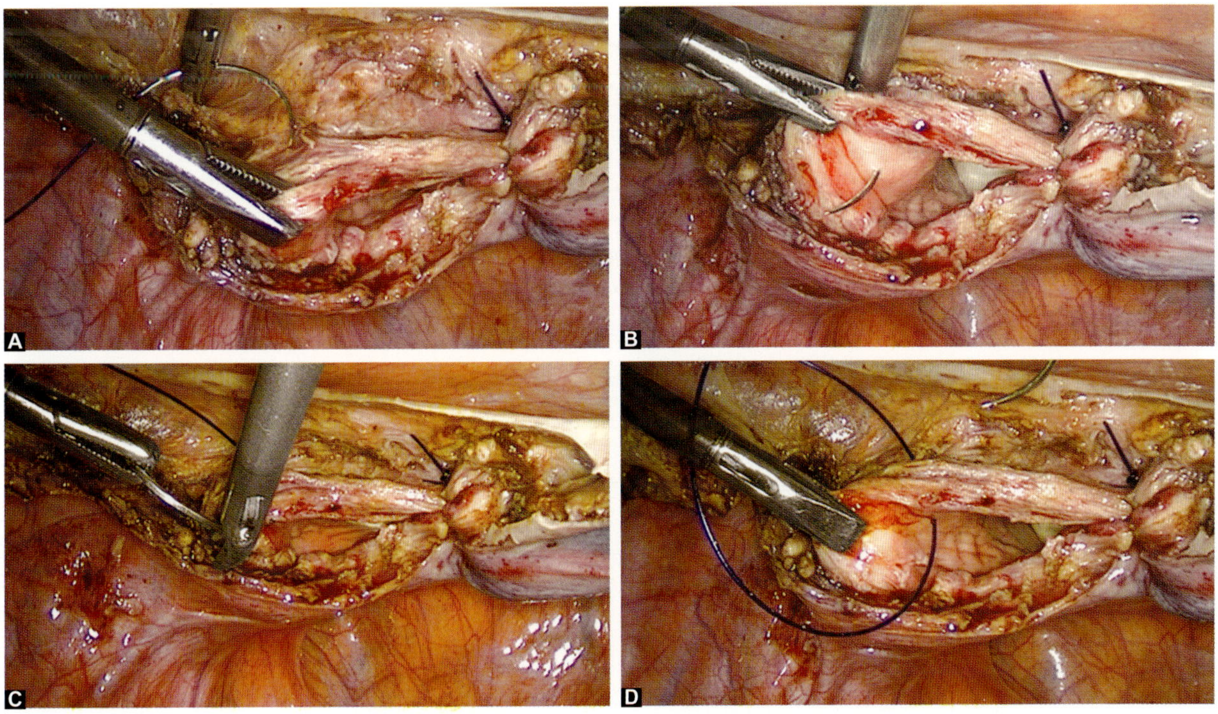

**Figs 16.40A to D:** LTH: Left corner suture uniting the vaginal anterior and posterior wall, bladder and posterior peritoneum as well as right sacrouterine ligament

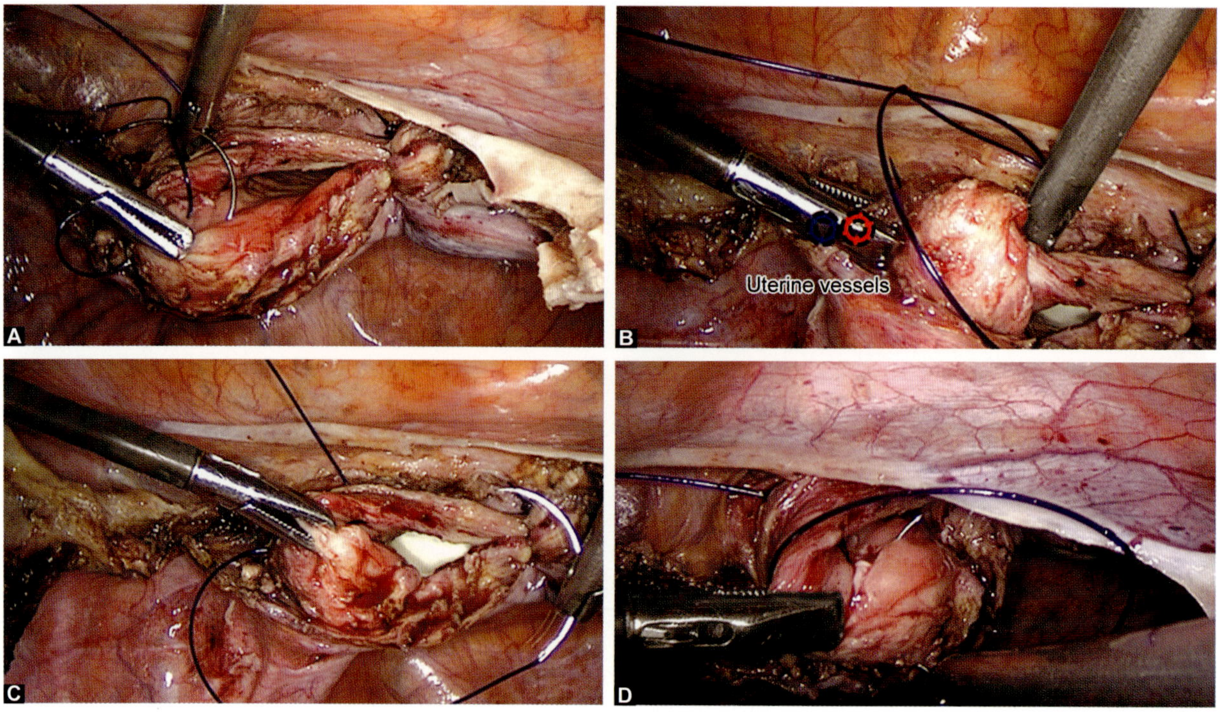


**Figs 16.41A to D:** LTH: Continuing the left corner suture

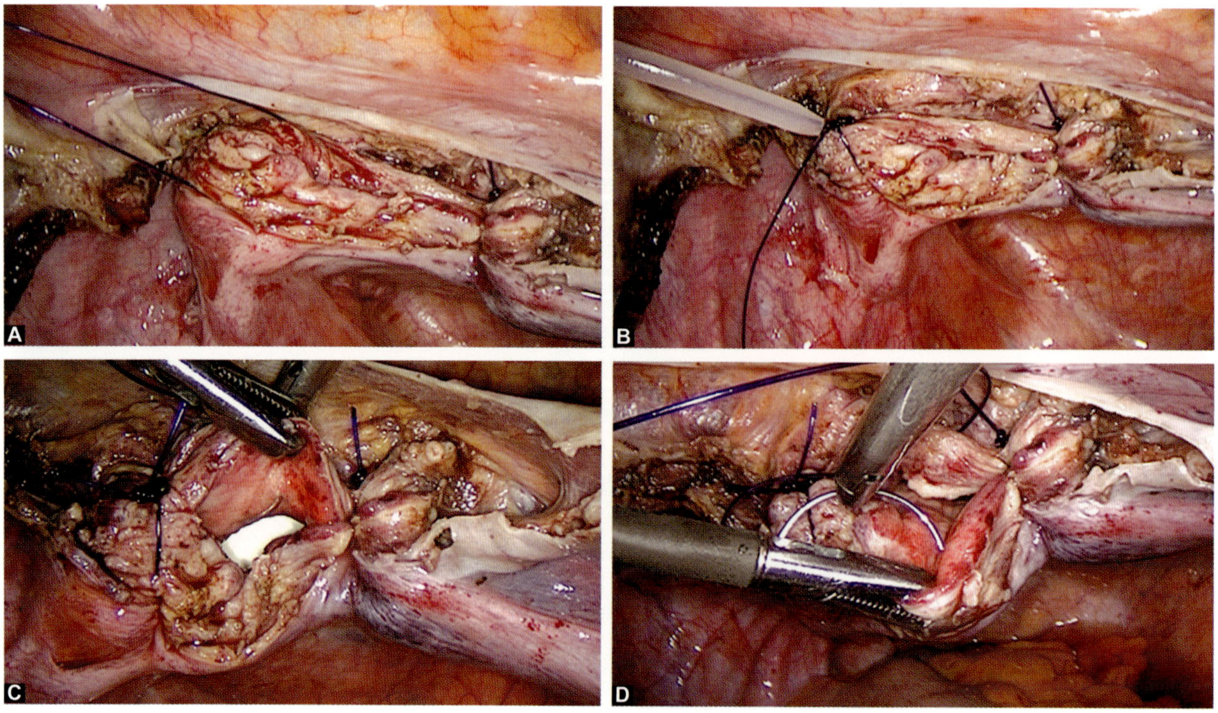


**Figs 16.42A to D:** LTH. (A to C) Completion of left corner suture and extracorporeal knot pushed down by the push rod; (D) Starting the in-between figure of 8 suture

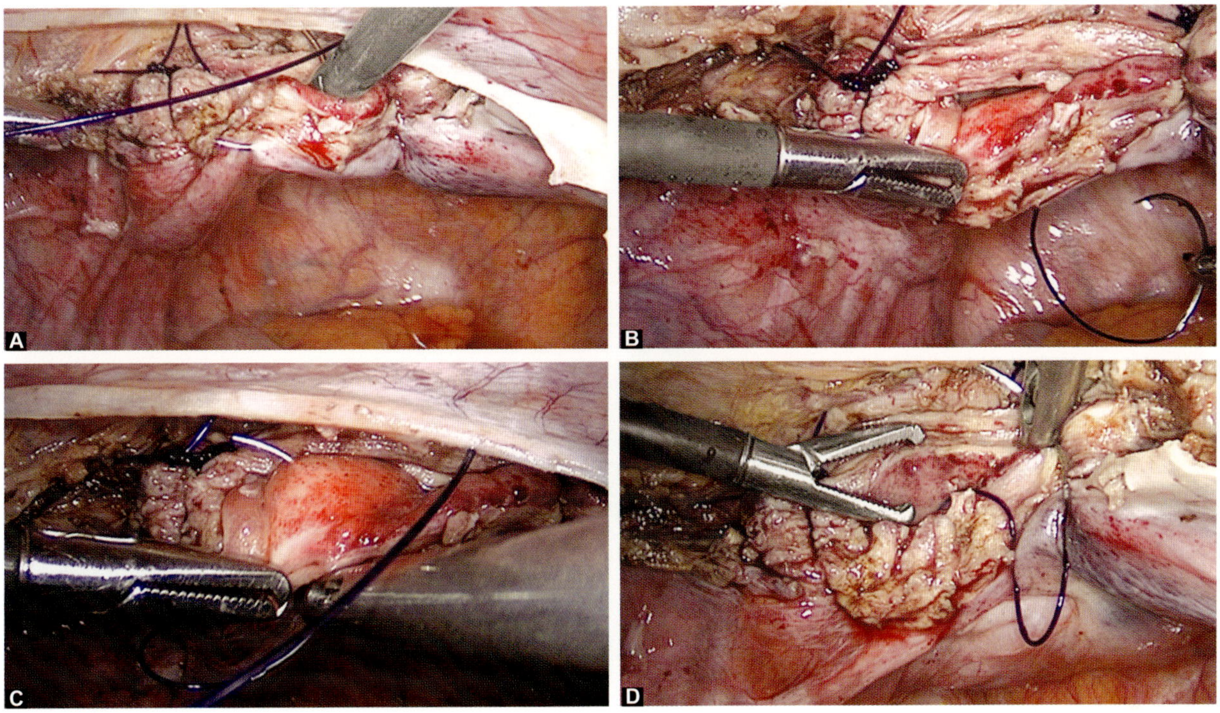


**Figs 16.43A to D:** LTH: Final closing of the remaining vaginal opening by figure of 8 suture

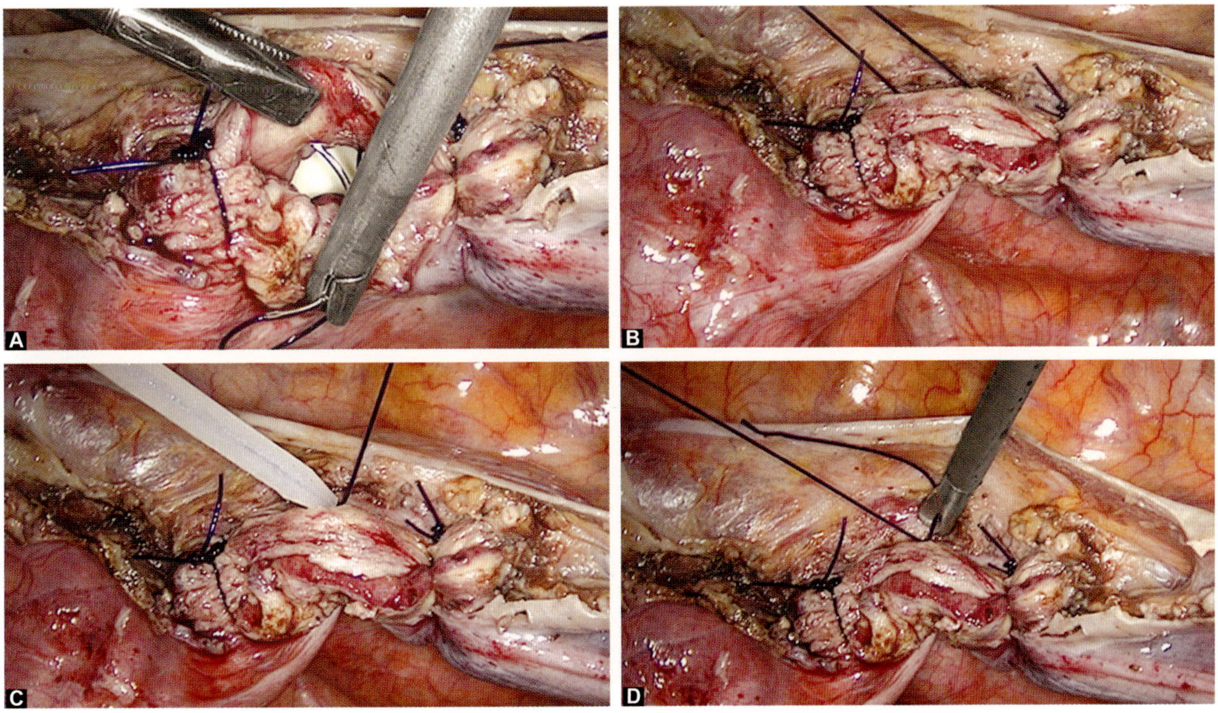


**Figs 16.44A to D:** LTH: Completion of the central suture

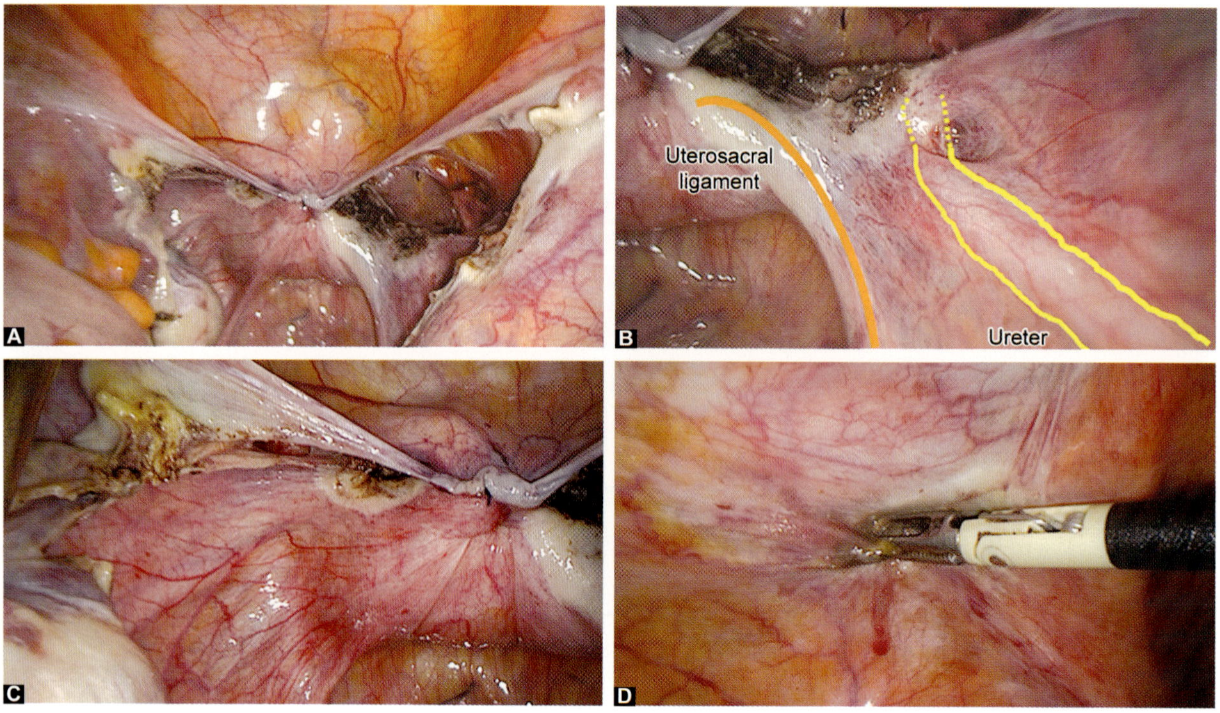


**Figs 16.45A to D:** LSH. (A to C) Observation of ureteric integrity by observing the peristalsis; (D) Coagulation of the right trocar entry point

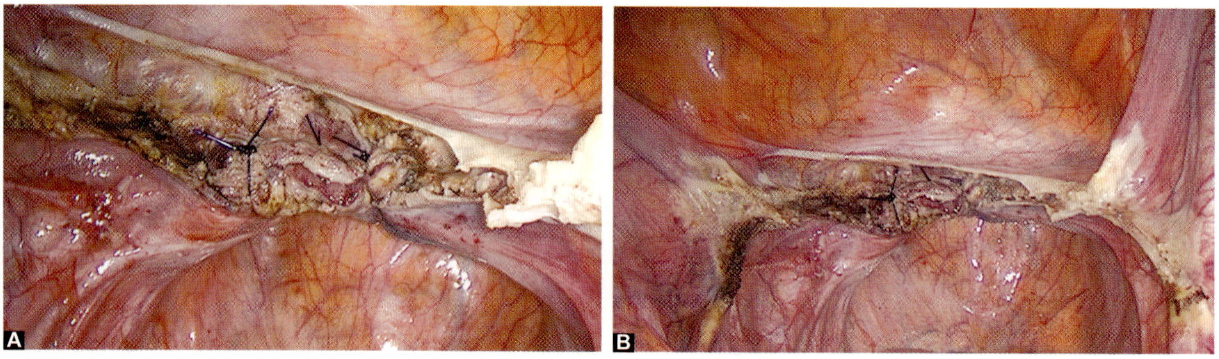


**Figs 16.46A and B:** LTH: Final situs after closure of vaginal stump and elevation of sacrouterine ligaments by 2 corner sutures

### Anticipated Problems

Fever, early pain situations, abdominal distension, delirious situations, decreased urine output and shock index with hypotension, must be recognized and attended to immediately.

## SUMMARY AND CONCLUSION

Besides the well-known laparoscopic techniques for myomectomies, as well as the hysteroscopic techniques for submucous fibroidectomy, laparoscopic subtotal and total hysterectomy are surgical choices to be taken in a combined decision between patient and doctor for the treatment of multiple fibroids. The individual steps described in this chapter help to perform a satisfying surgery to finish the serious burden of multiple fibroids in a patient that has completed her family planning.

### Acknowledgement

We acknowledge the secretarial help of Nicole Guckelsberger.

Chapter

17

# Laparoscopic Hysterectomy in Case of Large Uteri

*Bruno J van Herendael, Lisbeth Jochems*

## INTRODUCTION

When dealing with large uteri, there are some specific aspects of endoscopic surgery to be taken into consideration. The surgeon has to deal with the way of access and ponder the pros and cons of the different access routes. The main concerns are enough space to complete the operation, positioning of the secondary trocars as to be able to complete the complete operation laparoscopically, maneuverability of the uterus as to be able to access the vascular pedicles. It is also mandatory to evaluate if the adhesions are present in the specific patient due to previous interventions. Considering all of the above, it becomes clear that the large uterus is to be operated by the experienced endoscopist. The main danger for the patient is the IEE (Inexperienced endoscopist).

A uterus is considered to be large as its weight is estimated to be over 500 (five hundred) grams.

## PREPARATION OF THE SURGERY

### Placing the Uterine Manipulator

This is the a critical manipulation, even before the operation has started. The manipulator will give the assistant, between the legs, the opportunity to present the uterus to the surgeon. The best manipulator is the one that allows the assistant to push the uterus into the abdomen whilst presenting the side to be operated upon with relative easy to the surgeon so that the surgeon is able to concentrate on the spot. When the uterus has been fried from its attachments the optimal manipulator is the one that allows for vaginal extraction—or bringing the cervix to the level of the spina ischiadica so that it can be morcellated vaginally. The author, therefore, uses the Mangeshikar manipulator (Karl Storz Gmbh & Co, Tuttlingen, Germany). The reason is that this manipulator had grasping teeth that grasp the cervix so that rotation of the uterus can be performed whilst pushing the uterus into the abdomen and at the end, the uterus can be pulled down (Fig. 17.1). The only difficulty with this manipulator is that the cervix has to be dilated up to Hegar 6–7 to allow for the passage of the working element of the jaws (Fig. 17.2).

### Creating a Pneumoperitoncum

In most cases, introduction of the Veress needle into the umbilicus will still be possible in case of large uteri. This is still the recommended spot as the two layers of the peritoneum fuse in the umbilicus leaving only two pops for the Veress, one of the fascia and one of the peritoneum.

In case of possible adhesions, it is wise to insert the Veress needle in the Palmer point, midclavicular some 4 cm (two fingers with) under the last rib. Here, the surgeon has to hear three pops, one each when the needle passes through the two fascias and one of the peritoneum (Fig. 17.3).

Direct entry with the trocar can be performed but carries a greater risk of traumatizing the posterior aspect of the fundus of the uterus provoking unnecessary bleeding.

### Placing the Optical Trocar

A bimanual palpation of the abdomen is recommended in the patients with BMI under 25. The fundus of the uterus is delineated when the patient is under general anesthesia and in the position to bring in the optical trocar. In our theater this means in lithotomy position with the buttocks some 15 cm over the edge of the table and the body of the patient, not the table, in horizontal position. This latter fact is important to secure that the trocars are brought in as far as possible away from the main abdominal vessels.

For patients with a BMI over 25, the ideal solution is to have an MRI scan as to visualize the whole of the uterus in comparison to the rest of the organs and the total volume of the abdomen.

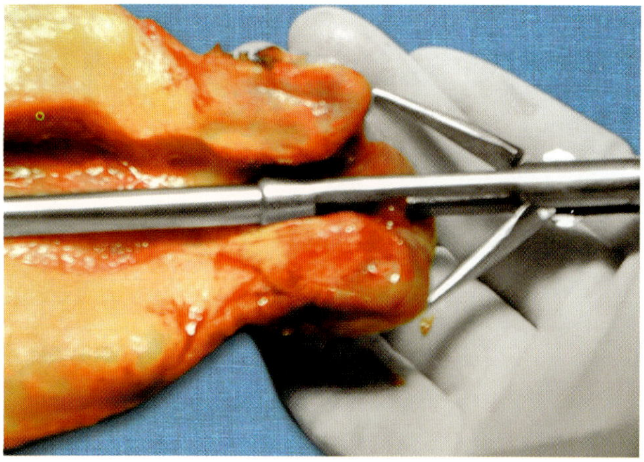

**Fig. 17.1:** The Mangeshikar trocar is seen to grasp the cervix. This allows the assistant to push the uterus into the abdomen, to turn the uterus in the desired position and to pull the uterus into the vagina

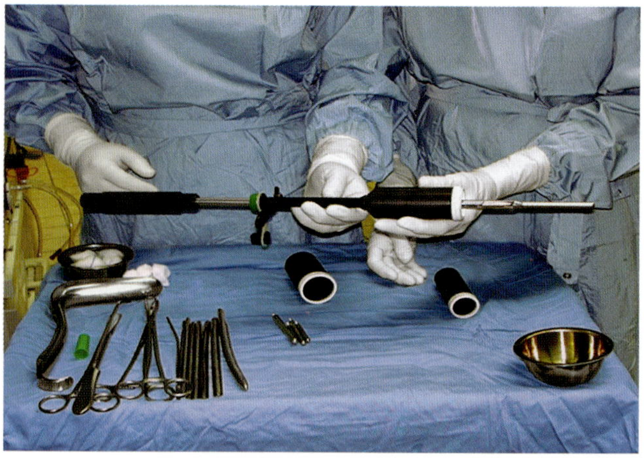

**Fig. 17.2:** Illustration of the different cup sizes and the different lengths of intracavitary sounds. The dilators on the table indicate that the cervix has to be dilated to allow for the grasping movement

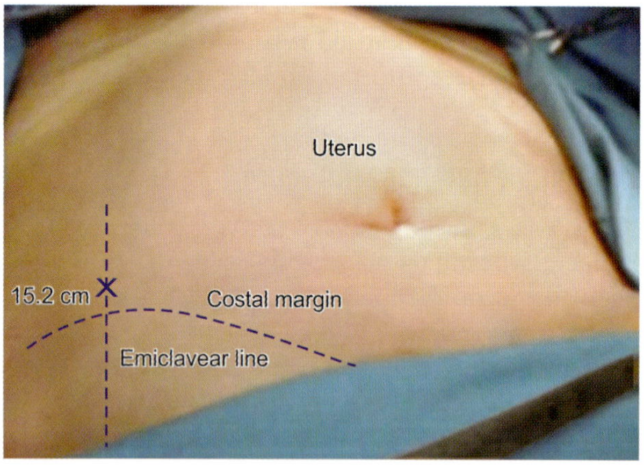


**Fig. 17.3:** Palmer's point. The Veress needle is brought in mid-clavicular and some 1.5–2 cm under the rib

If the uterus reaches the height of the umbilicus, the solutions are twofold:

1. The surgeon switches immediately to the Lee Wang point some 10 cm in the midline under the sternum after having asked the anesthetist to bring in a naso-gastric tube in the stomach to prevent ballooning of the stomach.
2. The surgeon chooses for the Palmer point (Fig. 17.3). In this adhesion-free zone of the abdominal cavity, the uterus can be visualized even in cases of suspicion of adhesions, due to previous interventions.

The aim is to reduce the visual seize of the uterus. As scopes give the surgeon an enlargement of up to 20 times, it becomes important for the final lens to positioned away from the target zone in a way to assure maximal functionality for the operator.

The size of the optical trocar used by the authors is 12 mm with reduction to 10 mm as a High Cap

(Karl Storz Gmbh & Co, Tuttlingen Germany) trocar allowing for 30 L of preconditioned $CO_2$ per minute are used to compensate the pneumoperitoneum when the vagina is opened.

### *What optic to use?*

Nowadays, most classical hysterectomies are performed with a 0°–30° 3 mm optic.

In the case of the large uterus, it is advisable to use a 0°or 30° 10 mm optic. As most gynecologists work preferably with 0° optics, this can be used in most instances. The 30° optic can come in handy is the posterior aspect of the uterus is bulky as it becomes easier to work around the mass of tissues.

Industry has made optics that can be used as 0° up to 180°, i.e. the EndoCameleon (Karl Storz Gmbh & Co Tuttlingen, Germany). These can come in handy when operating on large structures.

### *Where to Place the Secondary Trocars and How Many?*

The placement of these trocars is done under direct vision, the usual way. The location depends mainly on two considerations:

1. Instruments confined in these trocars should be able to deliver energies perpendicular to the vessels, artery and veins, at the level of the isthmus.
2. The way the surgeon wants to suture the vaginal vault when the uterus has been delivered through the vagina.

The authors suture with a reduced triangulation—one needle holder in the midline and one lateral. For surgeons using the ipsilateral or minimal triangulation technique two ancillary trocars have to be brought in from the lateral side—left or right—of the patient. In this case there still has to be one additional trocar in the other side of the patient to deliver the energies safely.

The conclusion is that in the surgery of the large uterus at least four trocars are used: The optical trocar, the side trocars—two in number—and the central of side trocar to suture.

It goes without saying that in case of need additional trocars have to be used and placed so that instruments can reach the particular spot causing the problems.

Mostly 5 mm trocars are used as ancillary trocars. In case larger instruments or mechanical or bipolar morcellation is needed trocars of 10 mm or larger diameter have to be used. In cases of morcellation, these are preferably placed is the side of the patient.

## THE TEN STEP LAPAROSCOPIC HYSTERECTOMY

Keep to the rules, know the anatomy and get experience.

1. Start at the round ligament 2/3 away from the uterus. To make it easier and keep the ureter out of the dissection plane, fenestrate the broad ligament when possible.
   i. Parallel to the uterus when the ovaries stay in place
   ii. Parallel to the infundibulo-pelvic (IP) ligament when the ovaries are taken.
2. Transect the anterior and posterior leaf including the round ligament, the tubes and the ovarian ligament after desiccation.
3. Open the broad ligament anteriorly.
4. Open the broad ligament posteriorly.
5. Grasp the bladder not the peritoneum and open the uterovesical space. Take care of the vessels in the bladder pillars.
6. Coagulate the uterine artery, if it is a fibroid uterus, try not to include the veins in the first coagulation to drain the large uterus.
7. Transect the uterine artery and veins inside the cup of the uterine manipulator.
8. Transect the sacro-uterine ligaments as high on the posterior aspect—torus uterinus as possible.
9. Open the vagina and morcellate the uterus through the vagina.
10. Suture the vagina starting with reconnecting the paracervical ring and use prophylactic suturing to prevent future descent.

**1. Start at the round ligament:**

Energy is applied to the round ligament, the latter has to be brought under tension by a grasping forceps and stretched medially. The forceps applying the energy is brought in perpendicular on the round ligament. This last maneuver means that the energy applying forceps is brought in from the left for the left round ligament and from the right for the right round ligament. This implies that the forceps has to be given. Too many surgeons try to control the whole operation and in doing so expose themselves to unnecessary accidents, in the case of the round ligament mainly bleeding.

Take the round ligament as far from the uterus as possible towards the pelvic wall.

The kind of energy does not really matter. The author uses mainly bipolar energy both with the classical forceps or the sealers. This implies cutting with scissors when classical forceps are used. When cutting with scissors the ideal way is to bring in the scissors through the same ancillary trocar as the energy as to cut the tissues in the same way these have been desiccated. Ultrasound energy is a favorite with other surgeons although in difficult cases—such as the large uterus—the desiccation effect is less reliable due to the interference of the energy of the vessels.

If at all possible considering the volume of the uterus it can be wise to get the ureter out of the working field by the fenestration of the broad ligament. The fenestration is performed in the transverse way if the ovaries are preserved and in the antero-posterior way when the ovaries are taken. The main advantage is that in performing this fenestration the surgeon has a good vision, through the opening, on the aspect of the uterus deeper in the pelvis. The other advantage is that, if the ovaries are taken out, the infundibulo pelvic ligament is isolated and can be lifted very easily out of the vicinity of the ureter.

**2. Transect the Round Ligament**

The round ligament is transected after desiccation of the vessels as to gain access to the vascular pedicle at the level of the isthmus.

As more and more evidence is gathered that a very important percentage of the carcinoma's of the ovary are diagnosed to have an ampullary origin, the tube should be removed during this phase of the hysterectomy.

If the ovaries are taken, the IP ligament is transected and the broad ligament is opened completely.

At this stage, the ovarian ligament is desiccated and transected if the ovaries remain in situ.

Be aware that in the large uterus, it is in most of the cases, depending on the bulk of the uterus if these steps can be carried out in parallel the one side after the other or if the surgeon has to finish the steps first on one side and then on the other.

**3. Open the anterior leaf of the Broad ligament.**

The anterior leaf can be opened with cold scissors or with energy. The use of energies avoids bleeding although the bleeding of the small vessels in the peritoneum is seldom the cause of further difficulties during the operation.

The aim is to reach the vascular pedicle formed by the uterine artery and veins at the isthmus of the uterus.

In specific cases where the vascular pedicle is difficult to reach it can be of interest to get to the uterine artery at its origin off the obliterated umbilical artery when it crosses the ureter. Here the artery can be desiccated and cut. This maneuver can be of help during the further sequence of the operation.

**4. Open the posterior leaf of the broad ligament.**

The posterior leaf can be opened in the same way as the anterior. Here the aim is to get to the insertion of the sacro-uterine ligament just above it insertion into the uterus.

Again the surgeon stays very superficial as not to open the ascending branch of the uterine artery situated on the lateral aspect of the uterus. The surgeon has to have in mind that in the large uterus, the exact anatomical location of this artery can vary case by case and that the surgeon has to be careful at this stage of the operation as opening this artery may hamper the vision during the rest of the operation.

**5. Grasp the bladder.**

As now the anterior leaf of the broad ligament has been opened, it is time to dissect the bladder peritoneum without entering the bladder.

It is, therefore, mandatory that the assistant grasps the bladder with an atraumatic forceps. The surgeon pushes the bladder from the lateral side and the assistant grasps the latter not the peritoneum. As the bladder is not fixed to the cervix, except in cases of previous cesarean section, it is movable under the peritoneum to be cut. If the edge of the peritoneum is grasped, the surgeon can easily inadvertently enter the bladder.

In cases of a fixed bladder due to previous surgery a sharp dissection is to be carried out. In these cases, it is wise to fill the bladder with 100 mL of methylene blue to diagnose immediately possible small holes.

The bladder is mechanically pushed out of the reach. It is best to have the cup of the manipulator in place so that the position of the cup indicates the exact location of the incision. The bladder has not to be moved further down as this specific spot as to avoid nerve damage and consequent functional bladder problems for the patient.

The bladder pillars are identified and desiccated. Here again, be aware of the nerves running on the posterior aspect along with the pillars.

**6. Desiccate and cut the vascular pedicle at the level of the isthmus.**

In the large uterus, try to desiccate the uterine artery at its origin or skeletonize the artery near the uterus but avoid to desiccate the veins in the same motion this to allow the uterus to drain most of the blood before desiccating and cutting the veins. This avoids back bleeders to the maximum when the uterus has to be manipulated during the rest of the operation.

**7. Transect the vascular pedicle within the confines of the cup of the manipulator.**

If coagulating the vascular pedicle near the uterus try and stay within the confines of the cup of the manipulator. The assistant sitting between the legs of the patients and holding the manipulator has to push the manipulator up into the abdomen to the maximum of his or her ability at this stage of the operation. In doing so you will be sure to be far enough away from the ureter as to avoid thermal damage to the latter.

**8. Transect the sacrouterine ligaments high just above the insertion into the uterus.**

When transecting the sacrouterine ligaments at this level the surgeon keeps part of the pericervical ring intact so that it becomes easier to repair this ring at the time of the vaginal closure.

The surgeon has to try and use as less energy to desiccate as possible at this stage but has to be aware of the artery and veins within the sacrouterine ligaments. It is, therefore, wise to desiccate and cut these structures as high as possible again to stay away as far as possible from the ureters.

Here again, the pushing into the abdomen of the uterus by the assistant sitting in between the legs is of importance to delineate this zone as clear as possible for the surgeon.

**9. Open the vagina and morcellate the uterus through the vagina.**

In this phase again, the cup of the manipulator plays an important part. The assistant between the legs of the patients has to push the manipulator as far as possible into the abdomen delineating the specific area to be cut by the surgeon and has to follow or rather to foresee where the surgeon will cut and present this particular area.

The surgeon uses in preference monopolar energy between 80 and 120 pure cut (undamped ) wave form delivered through a hook or a spatula. A bipolar forceps has to be ready to secure bleeding vessels in most of the hysterectomies at this stage of the operation the ramus vaginalis of the uterine artery can be cut. A simple short application of the bipolar current is sufficient to master this problem.

In this step, care is taken to avoid unnecessary use of energies as not to overd desiccate the vaginal wall as to prevent dehiscence in the postoperative phase.

Morcellation of the uterus can be left to the surgeon as charge as far as the technique of morcellation is concerned. In exceptional cases, morcellation can be performed from the abdominal side by using a long number 11 knife or a laparoscopic morcellator. Only very experienced endoscopic surgeons, however, should undertake these maneuvers.

**10. Suture the vagina starting with restoring the para-cervical ring.**

To prevent vaginal dehiscence in the postoperative phase, it is mandatory to restore the paracervical ring. The author has adapted the vaginal closure of Te Linde's suture for laparoscopy called the van Herendael Omega suture (Prashant Mangeshikar personal communication).

A large needle with a braided suture (the author uses Vicryl 1) is used to transfix the sacrouterine ligament from the abdomen towards the vagina securing the ligament on the posterior aspect of the vagina. The needle is regrasped to penetrate the vaginal wall from the vagina towards the parametrium taking care to let the needle emerge under the uterine artery. The needle is grasped again and passed in between the vagina and the uterine artery from posterior to anterior. The needle is grasped and is now again passed through the vaginal wall from the abdominal side towards the vagina. The needle is grasped a last time now to be brought through the vaginal wall from posterior to anterior and in this movement the Fascia Pelvica is transfixed and fixed to the vagina in the knot that follows.

When this sequence is followed on both sides there is no need for a second layer of sutures as all the possible bleeders residing in the paravaginal tissues between the uterine artery and the vagina are closed. A simple suture or two to close the vaginal dome is all what is needed to finish the operation.

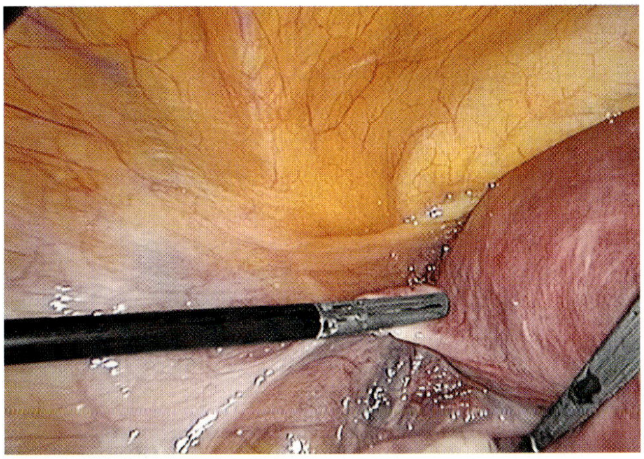

**Fig. 17.4:** Step 1: The round ligament is grasped. The authors use the Ligature sealer (Covidien Boston USA) as the tissue separator acts in the same plane as the seal—bipolar coagulation of tissues

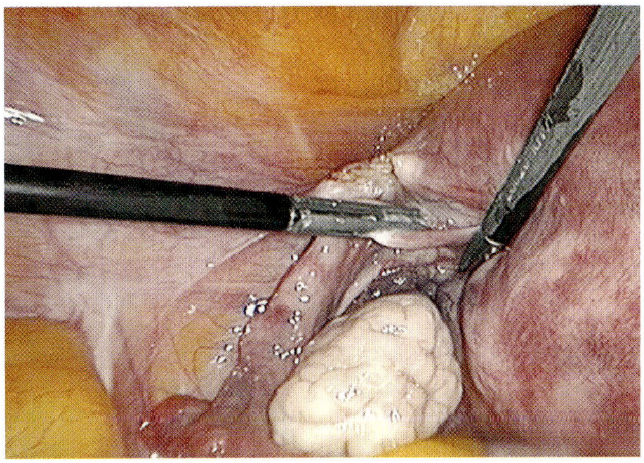

**Fig. 17.5:** The tube is coagulated and cut. The energy is applied in a perpendicular plane to the tissues. This implies that the sealer has to be given to the assistant to separate the planes on the right side in this case as the surgeon here stands on the left of the patient

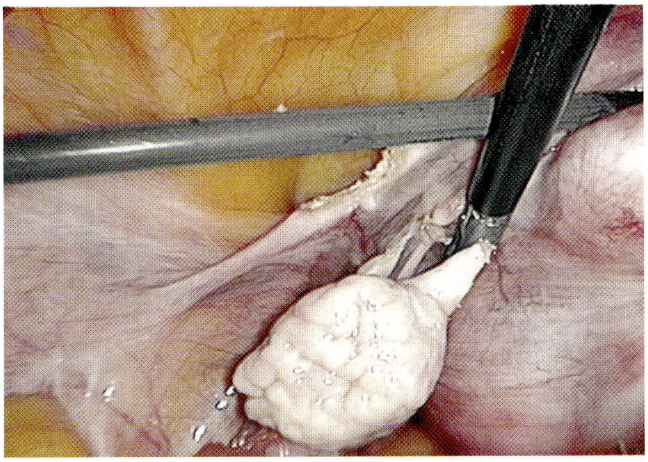

**Fig. 17.6:** When the uterus is big it is advisable to work step-by-step to avoid unnecessary bleeding. Here the ovarian ligament is coagulated and transected separately before opening the parametrium

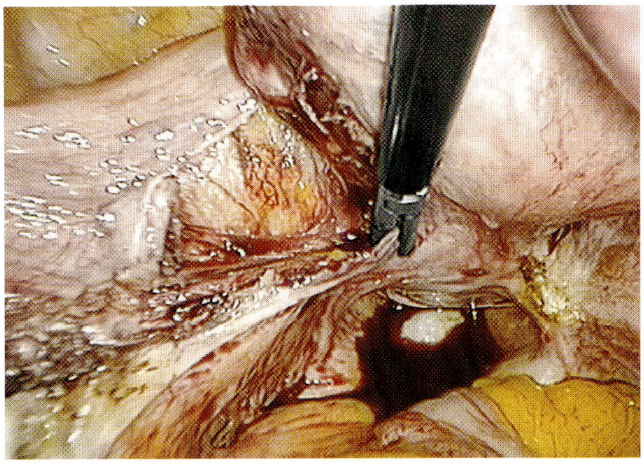

**Fig. 17.7:** The parametrium is opened and the coagulation and transection proceeds upto the sacrouterine ligament before the uterine artery and veins are tackled

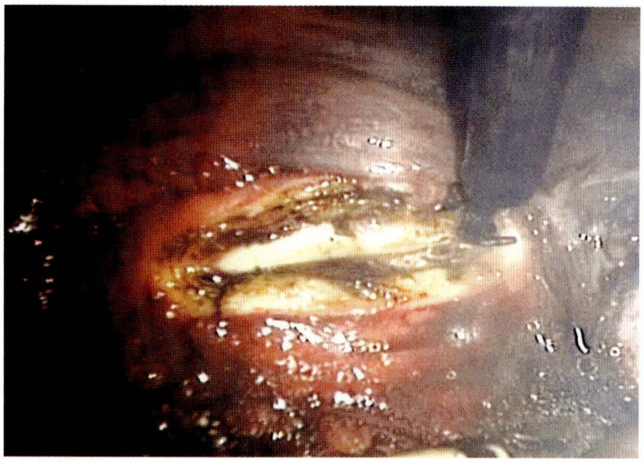

**Fig. 17.8:** The vagina is cut with unipolar energy at terminal wattage of 120 W over the cup of the uterine manipulator. This cup has been around the cervix in the vagina since the beginning of the operation as to delineate the vagina and to push the ureters aside out of the field.

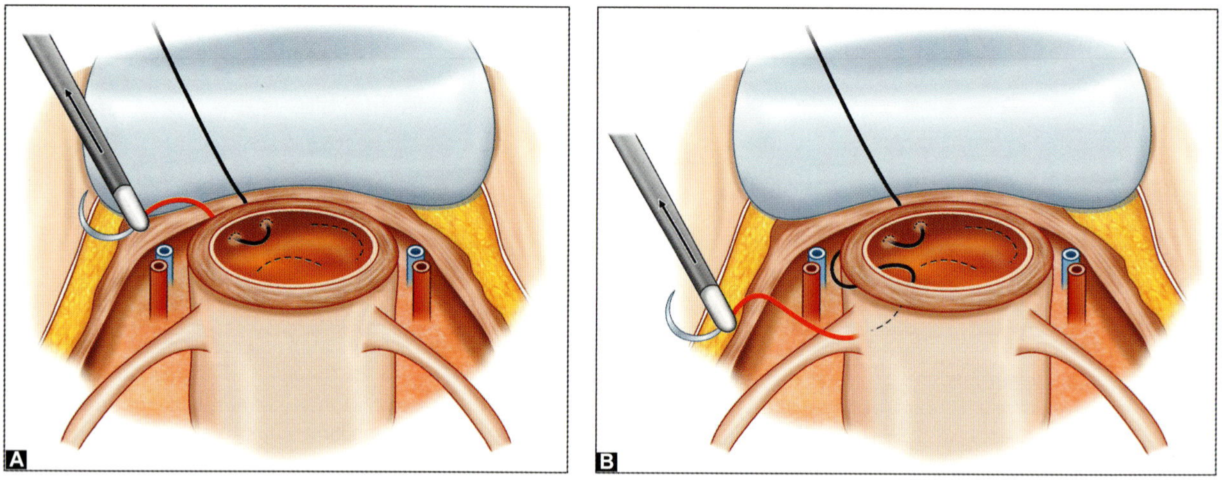

**Figs 17.9A and B:** The Te Linde repair of the paracervical ring adapted by B van Herendael called Omega Suture (As advertised at the university of Schleswig, Holstein campus, Kiel, Germany). *Note* that here the surgeon starts anteriorly

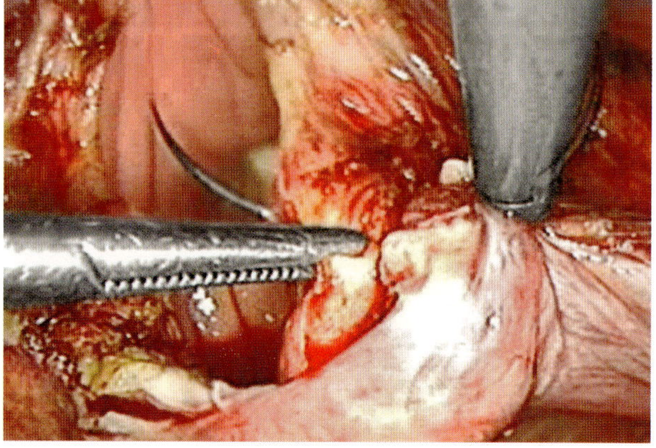

**Fig. 17.10:** The author starts at the posterior side and transfixes the lateral border of the sacrouterine ligament so that the needle emerges into the vagina 1 cm under the cut edge

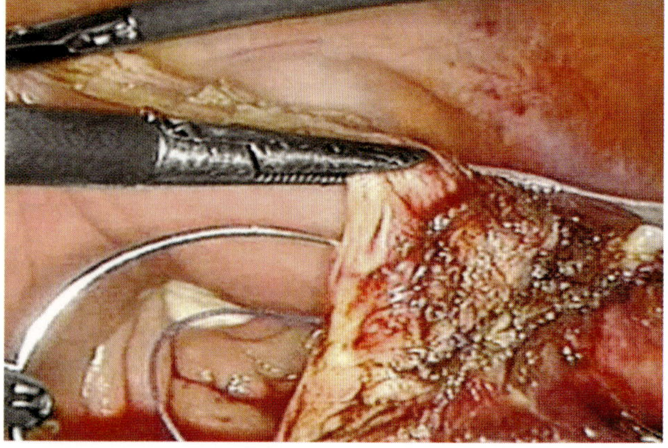

**Fig. 17.11:** The needle is grasped to be able to orient it towards the vaginal wall to emerge between the outer vaginal wall and the uterine artery. This as a precaution not to interphere with the ureter. *Note* also the swab—in a glove—to close the vagina to stop the $CO_2$ gas escaping from the abdomen

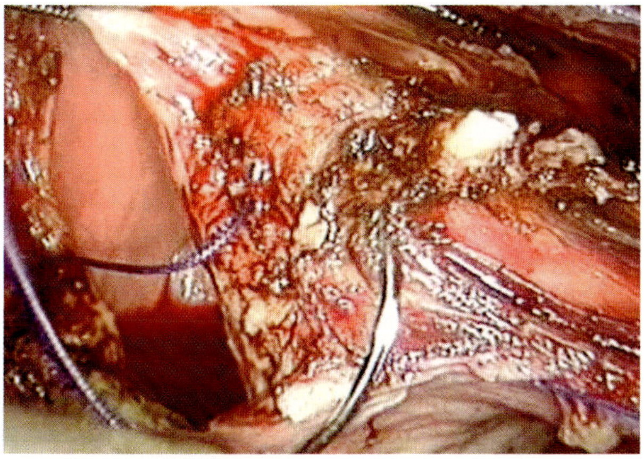

**Fig. 17.12:** The needle is grasped again and transfixes the lose areolar tissues, consisting of blood vessels, nerves and fibers, as to secure the small vessels to avoid hematoma. This is the reason why a large needle is used so that these tissues can be secured in one bite. *Note* the coagulated uterine artery—the white structure to the right in the parametrium

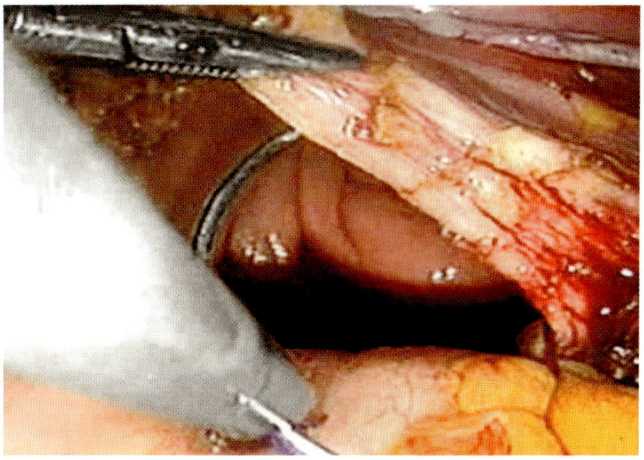

**Fig. 17.13:** The needle is regrasped when it emerges in the vaginal lumen and is now turned to transfix the vaginal wall anteriorly some 2 cm from the lateral edge. In this bite, the fascia pelvis is also taken as to complete the restoration of the paracervical ring

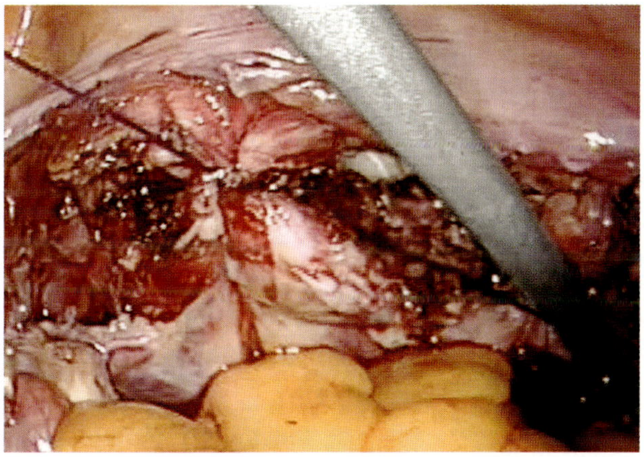

**Fig. 17.14:** The end result is the restoration of the cervical ring on both sides to prevent future descent. The closure of the vagina is performed making a simple figure of eight stidge to approximate the anterior and the posterior vaginal wall. Using the van Herendael Omega suture, there is no need for a second layer of sutures.

Chapter

18

# Laparoscopic Hysterectomy for Previous Cesarean Sections

*Ornella Sizzi, Giuseppe Florio*

## PREOPERATIVE EVALUATION

Thorough patient examination is essential. It usually gives the surgeon the idea of presence of adhesions and uterus ventral fixation.

Ultrasound examination can confirm the suspects. Bladder US can also be useful. Ventral fixation could be diagnosed by US using both transabdominal and transvaginal view. In the first case, a pronounced anteflexion could be identified as a possible symptom whereas precise indications performing transvaginal US could be obtained only by a dynamic approach, using the probe as a palpator. Looking for the sliding sign of the anterior compartment is the gold standard in diagnosing this pathology: A positive slide sign automatically excludes ventral fixation; on the contrary, negative sliding sign could be considered a reliable marker of uterus fixation thus ventral fixation should be considered after excluding other pathologies of the anterior compartment.

## PREOPERATIVE PREPARATION

### Bowel Preparation

Diet: One day prior to surgery soft diet till dinner. No intake of food or fluids after midnight.

Enema in the morning of surgery.

### Position of Patient

The patient is positioned with arms tucked at her side to allow free movements for the surgeons and to avoid brachial plexus injury in a low lithotomy position on the Allen stirrups with adjustable and padded leg rest. The legs are abducted at 90°. The bladder is catheterized and the uterus mobilized by a manipulator. A pad with a blockage keeps the shoulders in place to avoid sliding on the patient on the operating table with the Trendelenburg position and uterine manipulator pushing upwards.

## EQUIPMENT

Bipolar coagulation forceps, monopolar hook, scissors, grasping forceps, suction-irrigator probe, suturing set and uterine manipulator complete our basic set for hysterectomy. All the instruments are reusable (Table 18.1). The new sealing vessels bipolar systems (Ligasure®, Gyrus®, Thunderbeat® or the BiClamp® ERBE reusable system) could be handy, especially in case of varicosities.

### Uterine Manipulator

The role of the uterine manipulator is extremely important in cases of very enlarged uteri (Figs 18.1A to F). Many functions are required from the uterine manipulators (whether LAVH or total or supracervical laparoscopic hysterectomy is performed): (a) to suitably mobilize the uterus. This is obtained by allowing three kinds of movements: Anteversion and retroversion, lateral and, very important for TLH, elevation movements; (b) to clearly identify and distend the vaginal fornices to enable a circular section of the vaginal fornices; (c) to elevate and define the cervicovaginal junction to enable a safer dissection of the vesicouterine fold and fascia; (d) to enable the elevation of the uterus upwards in the abdomen, in order to obtain a good visualization of the uterine artery and its removal from the ureter; (e) to maintain a regular pneumoperitoneum (Table 18.2).

## TECHNIQUE

### Standard Technique

LH is nowadays a standardized procedure (Table 18.3). Lateral suprapubic trocars are inserted higher than usual (Fig. 18.4).

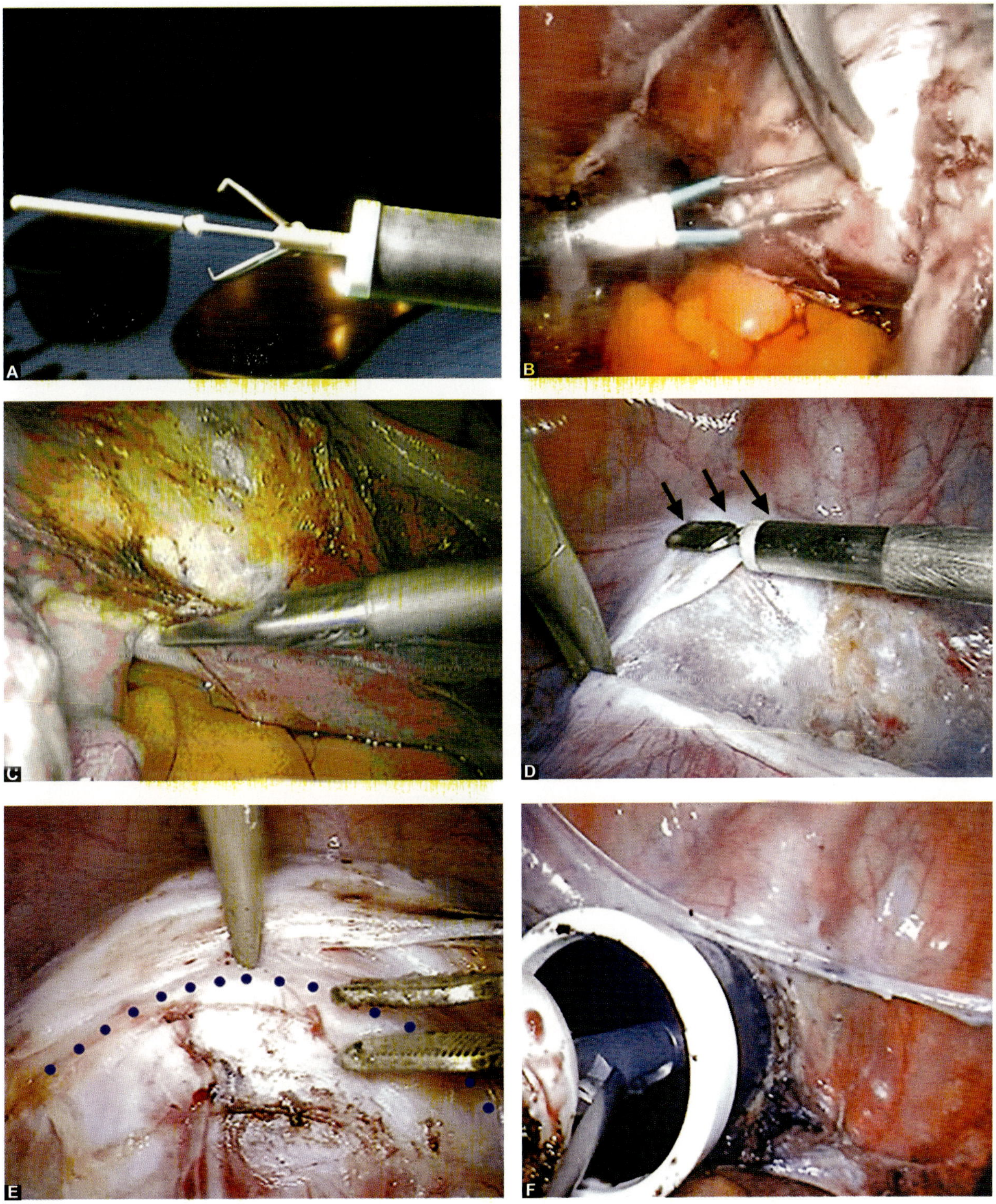


**Figs 18.1A to F:** Standard technique for usage of reusable and user-friendly uterine mainiplator

Round ligaments and infundibulopelvic or ovarian ligaments are coagulated and dissected with bipolar scissors. The round ligament should be coagulated in its middle part far from the uterine horn. A fenestration is performed, if space allows it, in the posterior leaf of the broad ligament to move the ureter laterally and downwards before coagulation of the infundibulopelvic or ovarian ligament. The vesicouterine fold, elevated with EndoClinch or Manhes forceps, is incised by EndoShears starting from the round ligament: This lateral approach

**Table 18.1:** Basic set for (Fig. 18.2) total laparoscopic hysterectomy (TLH)

*Operative Set-up*

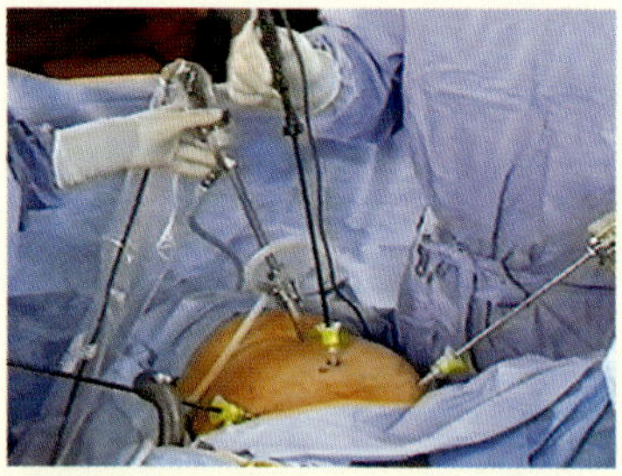

**Fig. 18.2:**

- Lithotomy, abducted legs, general anesthesis
- 2 TV monitors at the feet of the patient
- Surgeon left, 1st assistant right, 2nd assistant between the patient's legs
- 1 optical trocar, 3 suprapubic 5 mm trocars
- Foley catheter

- 1 Curved scissors
- 2 Grasping forceps
- 1 Bipolar forceps
- 1 Monopolar hook
- 1 Washing-suction device
- 2 Needle holders
- 1 Tenaculum
- 1 Uterine manipulator (Fig. 18.3)
- Set for vaginal surgery

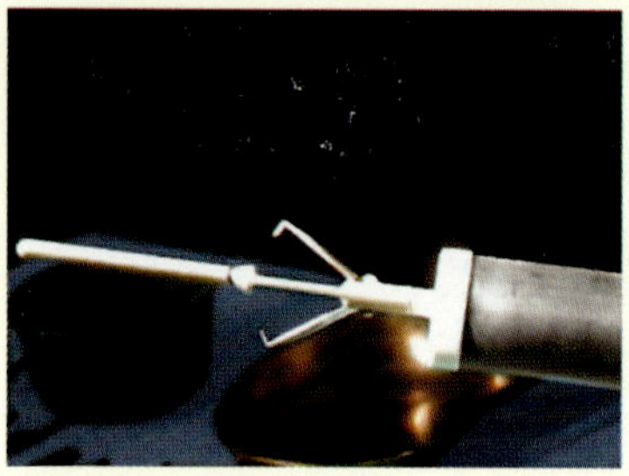

**Fig. 18.3:**

**Table 18.2:** Uterine manipulator essential requirements

**Main functions required of the uterine manipulators**:
(whether LAVH or total or supracervical laparoscopic hysterectomy is performed)

- To suitably mobilize the uterus: This is obtained by allowing three kinds of movements:
  - Anteversion and retroversion movements
  - Lateral movements
  - Elevation movements (whether total laparoscopic hysterectomy is performed)
- To clearly identify and distend the vaginal fornices to enable a circular colpotomy
- To elevate and define the cervicovaginal junction to enable a safer dissection of the vesicouterine fold and fascia
- To enable the elevation of the uterus upwards in the abdomen, in order to obtain a good visualization of the uterine artery and its removal from the ureter to maintain a regular pneumoperitoneum to be nonconductive of electricity

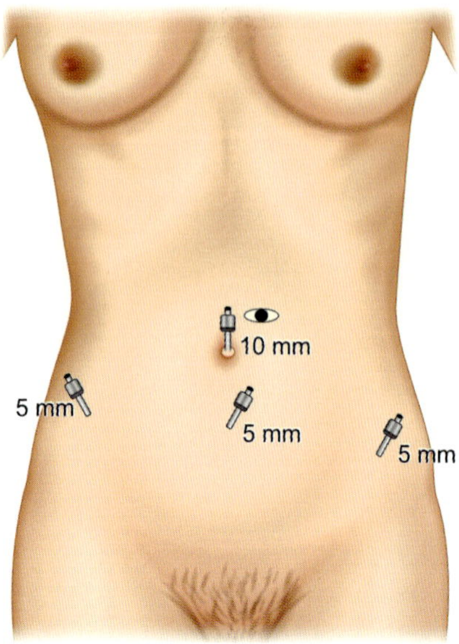


**Fig. 18.4:** Illustration to depict the points to insert the lateral suprapubic trocars

makes the dissection easier in cases of adhesions due to previous cesarean sections. While pushing on the uterus, the valve of the uterine manipulator highlights the anterior fornix and allows the vesicovaginal dissection plane to be entered. Internal pillars of the bladder are coagulated and sectioned upto the uterine pedicles. Thereafter, the uterus is anteverted and anteflexed to show and elevate the uterosacral ligaments. The uterus is pushed upwards into the pelvis and the valves of the uterine manipulator delineate the rectovaginal septum more clearly. The ligaments are intrafascially coagulated and sectioned, so that lateralization of the ureter from the uterus is obtained and ureteral injuries are avoided. The uterine vessels are exposed, skeletonized, and only then coagulated and transected. A coagulation is applied on the ascending branch of the uterine artery to avoid back blood flow. Suture-ligating uterine vessels give the surgeon a referential lateral landmark beyond which coagulation should occur, but it can be difficult to perform in a narrow space. An intrafascial dissection of the vagina with circular

**Table 18.3:** Operating steps

1. Coagulation and section of the round ligaments
2. Opening of the anterior peritoneum of the broad ligaments
3. Fenestration of the broad ligaments
4. Bipolar control of the adnexal vessels
5. Vesicouterine dissection
6. Uterine vessels dissection (ureter identification)
7. Coagulation of the uterine vessels
8. Opening of the vagina
9. Uterine extraction (+/– morcellation)
10. Vaginal closure

colpotomy is carried out using monopolar hook or scissors. The uterus is removed vaginally.

## CHANGING OF TECHNIQUE FOR PREVIOUS CESAREAN SECTIONS

### First Entry Technique

In case of suspect of adhesions, the entry technique should be changed. The option of open abdominal entry should be considered to minimize the risk of lacerating the uterus, if it reaches or exceeds the midline, but it is not recommended in case of adhesions. The visual entry technique using the Ternamian EndoTip Cannula could be a choice.

Using the Palmer point to insert the Veress needle is the best option, especially if adhesions are suspected.

### Port Placement

#### *Trocar Placement and Ergonomics*

Obviously, there is a physical limit to the space of maneuver of our instruments and to the angle of vision represented by the space between the distended abdominal wall and the uterus. The goals are better exposure and handling of the instruments without the hindrance of the uterus.

In cases with larger uteri, the optic trocar should be placed up to 10 cm above the umbilicus (Fig. 18.6).

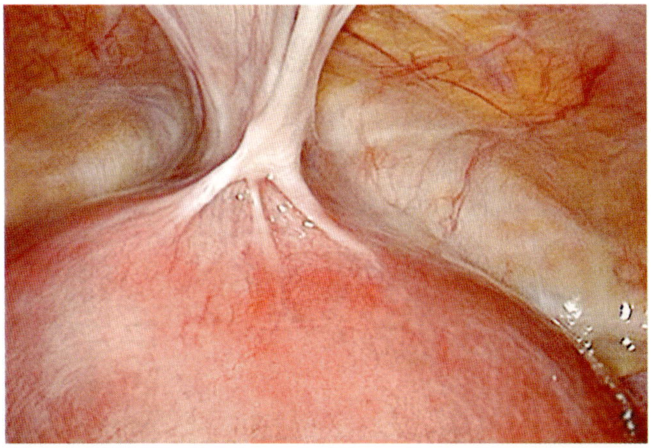

**Fig. 18.5:**

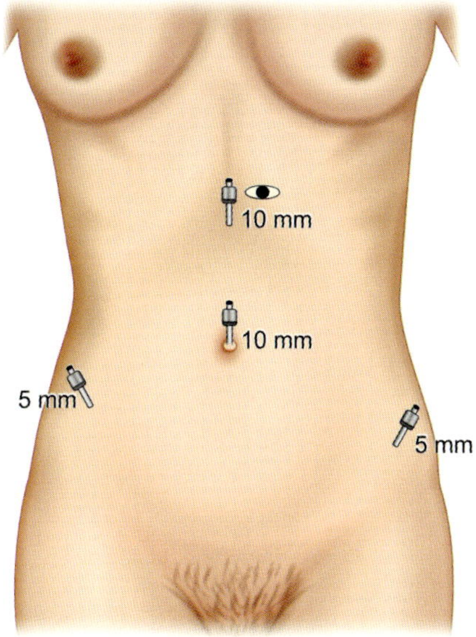


**Fig. 18.6:** Points of insertion of optic trocar in case of adherion

The middle trocar should be placed through the umbilicus or even higher. The other two lateral trocars should be placed according to uterine size and location of myomas. The higher the uterus, the higher the ancillary trocars should be inserted, at umbilical line or even some centimeters further up. Therefore, instruments that are inserted in lateral trocars will approach the uterine vessels anteriorly and posteriorly to the uterus and above. With these modifications, a larger intraperitoneal manipulation space can be achieved. Or alternatively, the left ancillary trocar should be placed lower to reach better the anterior structures and the right ancillary trocar should be placed higher to reach the posterior structures. When the surgeon is working on the left side, he/she uses the bipolar forceps in the left lateral port and the scissors in the midline. The assistant has a grasping forceps to mobilize the adnexa, showing the operative field or applying traction on the uterus in the opposite direction to allow better exposure of the uterine vessels and cardinal ligaments. On the right side, the surgeon is holding the grasping forceps with the left hand, to allow exposure of the right side and the scissors in the central port. The assistant is using the bipolar forceps. In this way, most of the time, the surgeons do not need to continuously change the instruments during the procedures and all the structures are approached from the best angle (Figs 18.7A to E).

## STEPS IN CASE OF ADHESIONS AND UTERUS VENTROFIXATION

Adhesiolysis is performed to allow a better exposure of the pelvic structures and of the uterus. If the omentum is attached to the abdominal wall, the use of harmonic scalper energy can make the procedure faster.

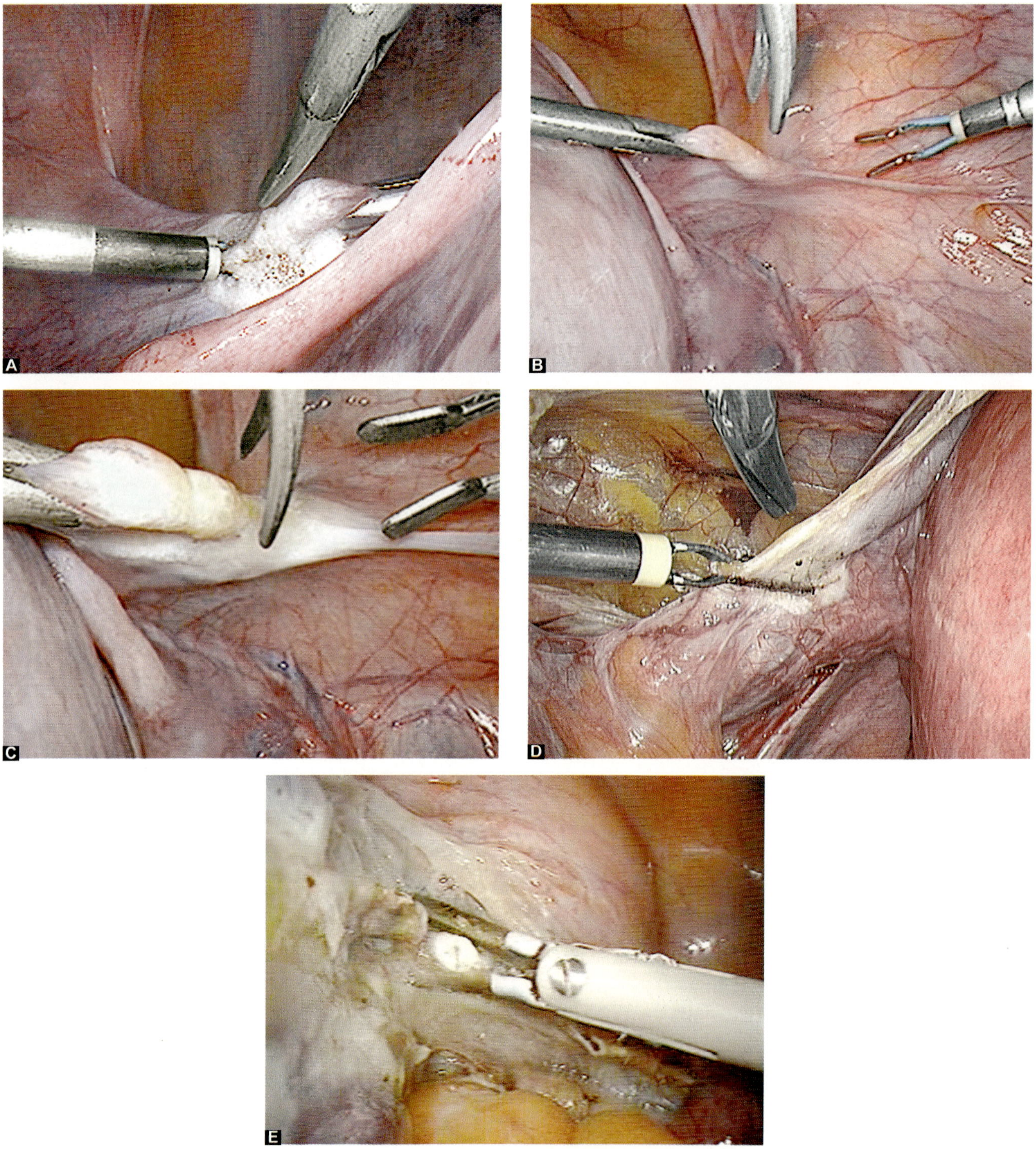

**Figs 18.7A to E:** Port placement technique. *Note* that both surgeon and assistant operate in their own side caution is taken to approach the structures at the right angle

If the uterus is stuck to the abdominal wall, a thorough cold dissection with bipolar coagulation is the best way for detaching it or again we recommend the use of the harmonic scalpel.

After freeing the uterus from the abdominal wall and having separated the adnexa and ligaments from the adhesions, in many situations the bladder is adherent to the uterus.

In all these situations, the procedure starts at the round ligaments, using or bipolar and scissors or vessel sealing systems. From the cut round ligament, the dissection is directed towards the anterior aspect of the uterus, always starting laterally and moving centrally. At this point, the use of cold scissors and bipolar instead of the vessel sealing system is preferable.

When possible, the anterior flap of the bladder is coagulated and cut.

In many cases, this is not immediately possible, so the dissection slowly proceeds from medial to central, finding fiber after fiber, using bipolar and scissors, always staying closer to the uterus.

The goal is to dissect the peritoneum, being able to find the percervical/vesicovaginal fascia and pull down the bladder.

Starting laterally usually help to more easily find the S. Sheth space from where an easier dissection of the fascia is possible.

The uterus is cranially displaced with the help of the uterine manipulator, pushed laterally at the beginning of the dissection and later midpositioned and pushed in to visualize the fascia and bladder margins. Once the bladder

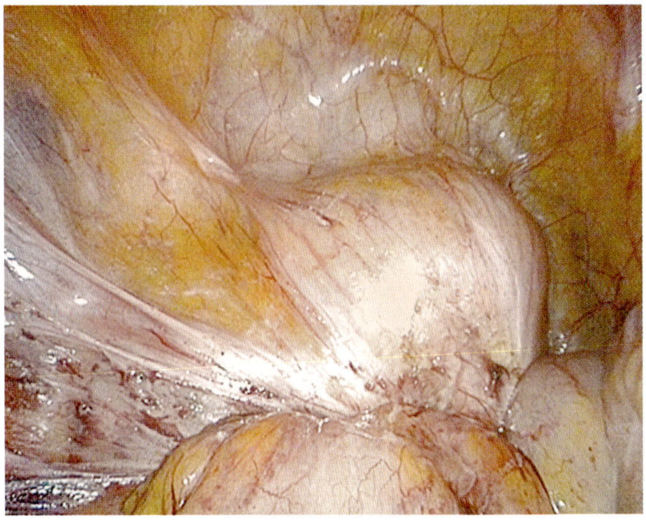

Fig. 18.8

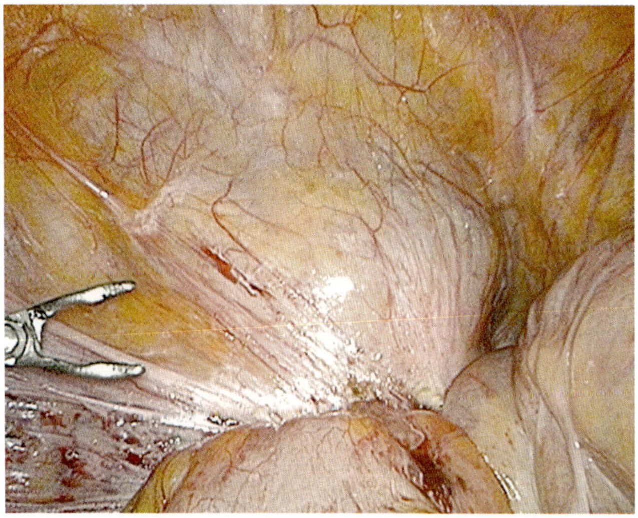

Fig. 18.9

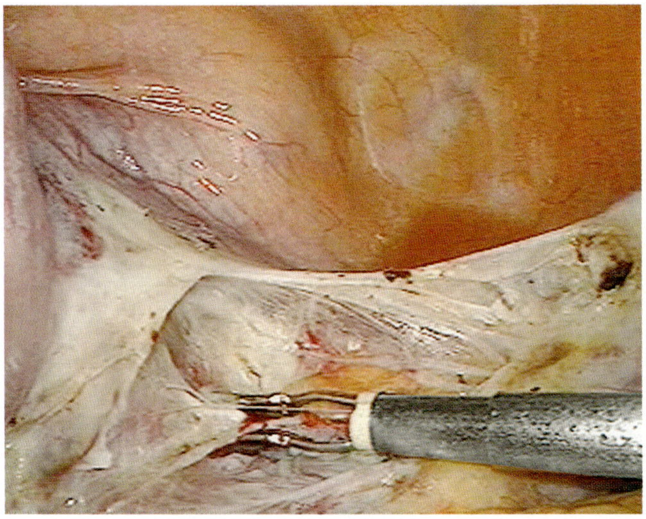

Fig. 18.10

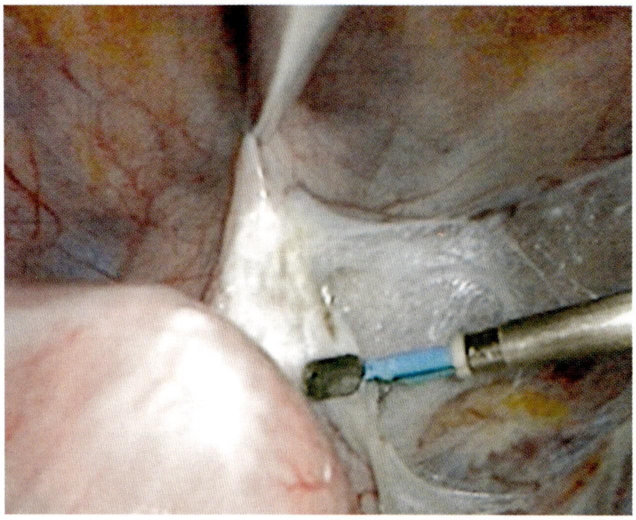

Fig. 18.11

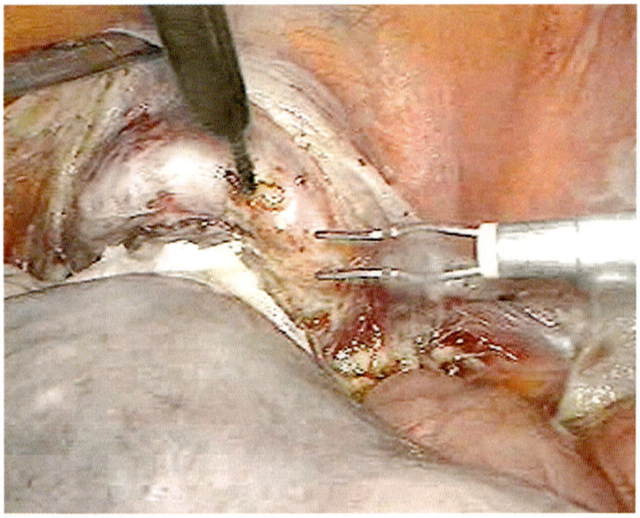

**Fig. 18.12**

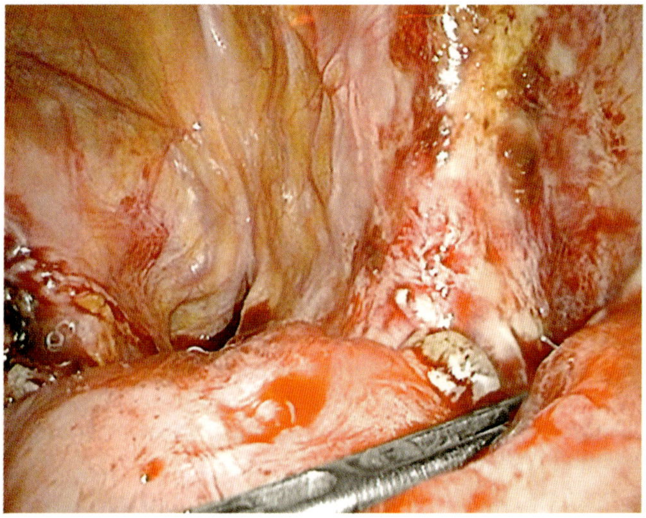

**Fig. 18.13**

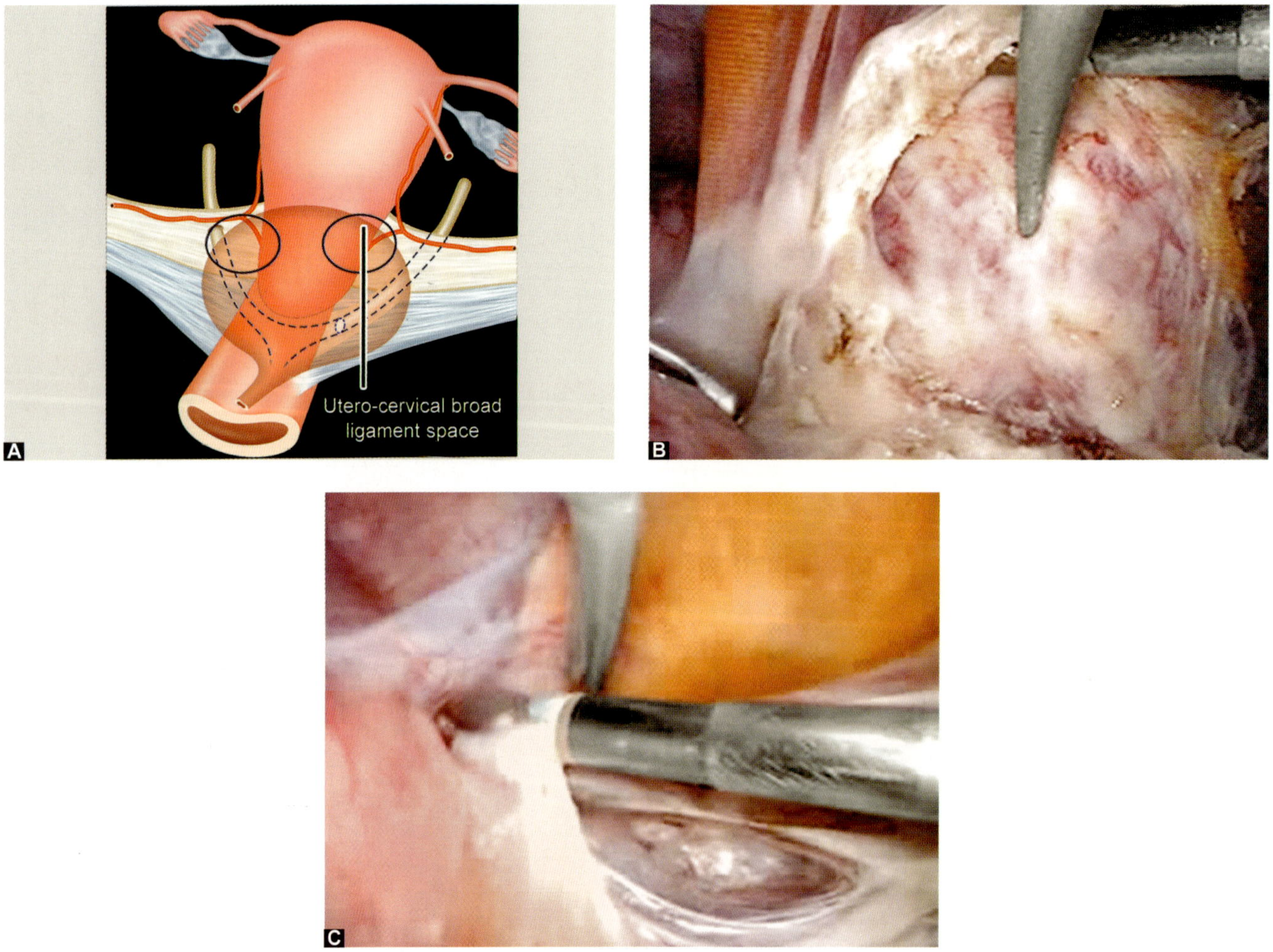


**Figs 18.14A to C:** Lateral access to the vesicouterine space in case of thick abhesions from previous C-sections of anterior myomas

has been visualized, pushed down and the fascia has been dissected and divided the hysterectomy continues with the usual steps and techniques.

## Post Hysterectomy Inspection

After closing the vaginal cuff, a peritoneal washing is carried out and the pedicles are inspected.

Bladder, ureters and bowel are also thoroughly checked. The bladder can be filled with blue dye to check for injuries and a cystoscopy can be performed.

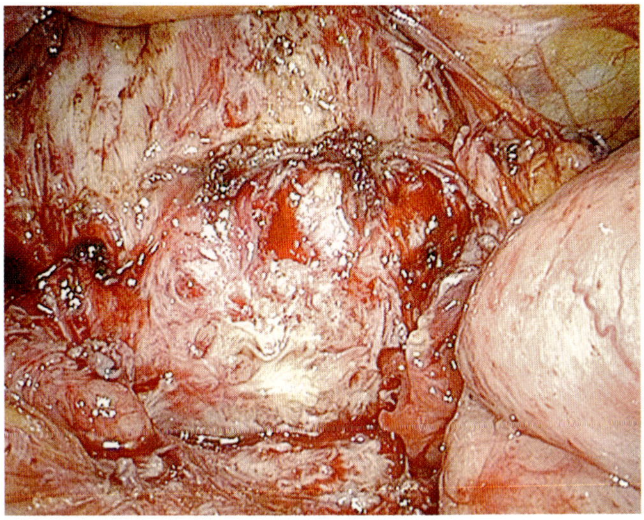

Fig. 18.15

## Postoperative Management

The Foley's catheter is postoperatively kept in place until the day after. Liquid intake is started after bowel mobilization.

The patient can be discharged after 24 to 48 hours and can resume her normal activities, within a week's time.

## Problems Anticipated and How to Avoid Them?

In case of uterine ventral fixation, attention has to be given to not to cut into the uterus (which will lead to bleeding of the muscle difficult to control without the use of suturing) or into the abdominal cavity (which will lead in increase of $pCO_2$).

In difficult cases, it could be useful at the beginning of the bladder dissection, to fill in the bladder with 240 cc of saline to be able to recognize its margins and avoid injuries. Once the bladder has been visualized, it is easier to void it again to avoid encumbrance of the surgery.

Bladder injury can always happens despite precautions taken. In this situation, the major issue is not making an intraoperative diagnosis and facing a later problem of urine leakage or vesicovaginal fistula.

At the end of the procedure, fill in the bladder again with very diluted blue dye, perform a cystoscopy to evaluate ureter integrity and location. In case of bladder injury, apply a single or running suture with PDS, 3-0. In this case the Foley catheter has to be kept in place for at least 10 days. If a thermal injury is suspected, the leakage will not be evident immediately. It is good practice in this situation to oversew the damaged tissue.

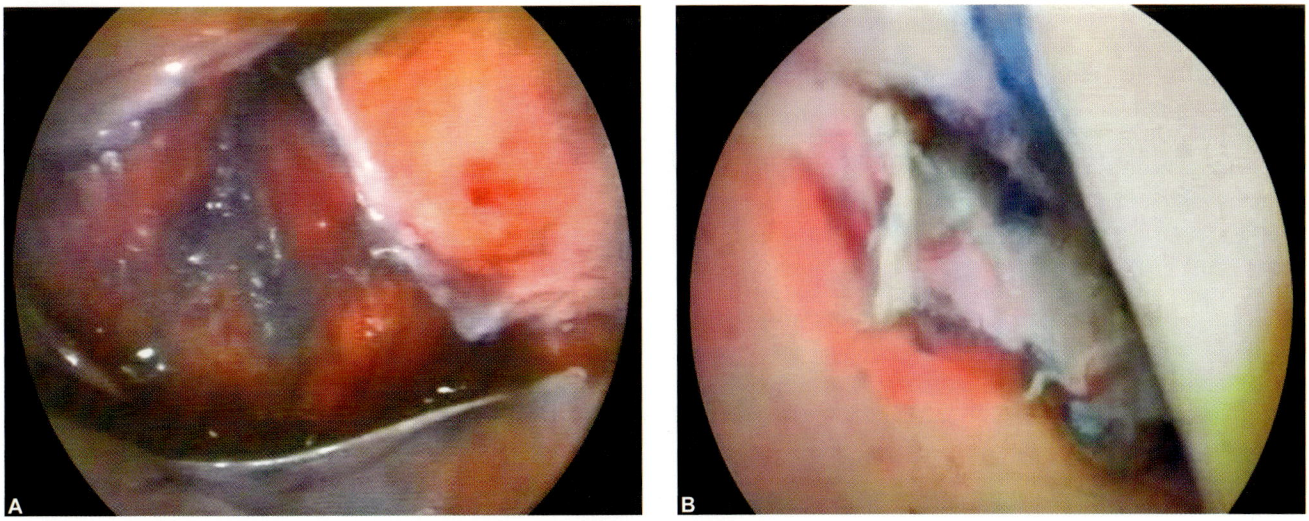



Figs 18.16A and B

Chapter

19

# Laparoscopic Hysterectomy in Endometriosis

*Sanjay Patel, Yogendra Jhala*

## HYSTERECTOMY IN ENDOMETRIOSIS WITH FROZEN PELVIS

### Preoperative Investigations

- Transvaginal sonography is a must.
- MRI pelvis should be done to know colorectal nodule and the extent of the disease.
- CT-IVP may be required if there is hydronephrosis or one suspects ureteric stricture due to cardinal ligament involvement by endometriosis (Fig. 19.1).
- In patients complaining of per rectal bleeding, colonoscopy should also be done to see for rectal involvement in endometriosis.

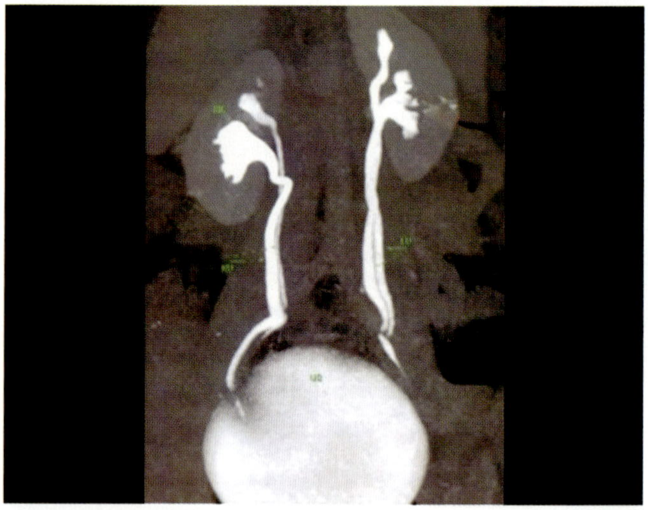

**Fig. 19.1:** CT-IVP should be done preoperatively in every case of endometriosis with frozen pelvis to identify exact course of ureter, to see for hydroureter and hydronephrosis as well as any congenital anomaly of the ureter. This picture shows bilateral double ureter system

### Preoperative Bowel Preparation

- Diet—One day prior to surgery, soft diet till afternoon followed by clear liquid diet and then nil by mouth for 8 hours prior to surgery.
- Peglec powder—dissolve the pack in 2 liter of water, to be given over 2–3 hours on previous evening.

### Important Equipment

Apart from routine equipment, following instruments are required:

- Rectal probe.
- Laparoscopic good scissors.
- Harmonic scalpel for good dissection.
- Vessel sealing system for better hemostasis.
- Cystoscope and ureteric stents.

### Position of Patient

Patient is placed in Lloyd-Davies position (Fig. 19.2).

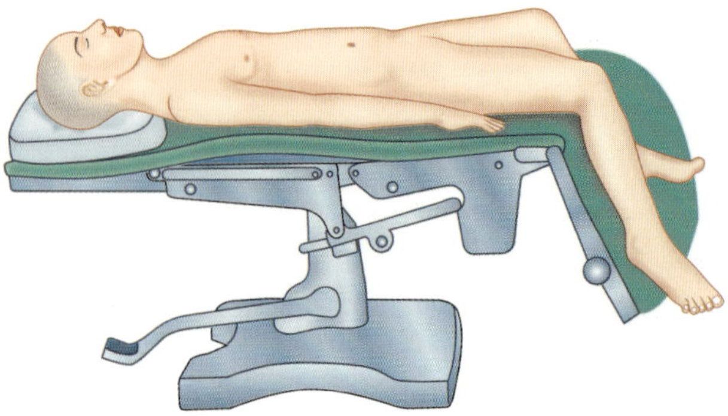

**Fig. 19.2:** Patient in Llyod-Davies position

## Technique

Manipulator: We use either Prashant Mangeshikar's uterine manipulator or Clermont-Ferrand uterine manipulator.

### *Port Placement*

Primary 10 mm port intra-umbilically.

- Three secondary 5 mm port which are at left iliac fossa, right iliac fossa (both lateral to mid-clavicular line) and in midline as shown in the Figure 19.3. Middle port is very versatile port as it is helpful for dissection on both sides in cases of frozen pelvis in endometriosis.

## Steps of Laparoscopic Hysterectomy

1. Thorough inspection of pelvis should be done in cases of frozen pelvis (Figs 19.4 and 19.5).
    i. In cases of previous surgery, small bowel adhesions to anterior abdominal wall and to uterus are present. Sharp dissection should be done with scissors for small bowel adhesions. We do not use any energy sources for the small bowel dissection. Also in advance cases, rectosigmoid colon is densely adherent to the posterior wall of uterus.
    ii. In advance endometriosis, ureters are displaced medially.
    iii. Apart from pelvis, abdominal cavity should also be inspected. In some cases, appendix is low and adherent to right adnexa (tubo-ovarian mass). Some time tip of appendix is involved by endometriosis (Fig. 19.6).
    iv. Small intestine, large intestine, omentum, diaphragm should also be inspected for endometriotic implants. Also we look liver for liver bed adhesions.
2. Aim of dissection is to start from virgin (retroperitoneal area) to non-virgin area (pathological site posterior to the uterus, adnexal area and both paracolic gutters).
3. Injection pitressin (1:200 mL dilution) is injected posteriorly in the uterus to reduce bleeding and avoid the staining of the tissue with blood. So it indirectly facilitates dissection. (Fig. 19.7).
4. We usually start laterally by mobilizing mesentery of sigmoid colon on left side and entering retroperitoneal space (Fig. 19.8).
5. Commonest site to identify ureter is at the level of pelvic brim as it crosses external iliac and internal iliac vessels. So retroperitoneal spaces are opened at the level of pelvic brim and ureters are mobilized laterally and dissected till it enters ureteric tunnel. This step helps to avoid injury to the ureter. Dissect parallel to the ureter as it is more easy to dissect the ureter. Sometime, we use fiberoptic ureteric catheter to exactly see the course of the ureter. Then tubo-ovarian mass excision or salpingo-oophorectomy is done (Figs 19.9 to 19.15).
6. Then we enter the retroperitoneal space where we identify origin of the uterine vessels. It is easy to identify uterine vessels which are the only tortuous vessels in the pelvis traversing the para-rectal space. Uterine vessels are ligated at their origin using vessel sealing system, taking care of avoiding injury to the ureter (Fig. 19.16).
7. Round ligaments are then coagulated and cut using 5 mm ligature.
8. After making the uterus retroverted, bladder is mobilized either using harmonic scalpel or by sharp dissection in cases of previous cesarean section (Fig. 19.17).
9. Posteriorly sharp dissection is done flush to the uterus inside the colorectal nodule using scissors to separate rectum from the posterior wall of the uterus. Care should be taken to remain inside the colorectal nodule to avoid injury to the rectum. Energy source should not be used to avoid thermal injury to the rectum. Colorectal nodule should be left on the rectum and should be excised after completion of hysterectomy (Fig. 19.18).

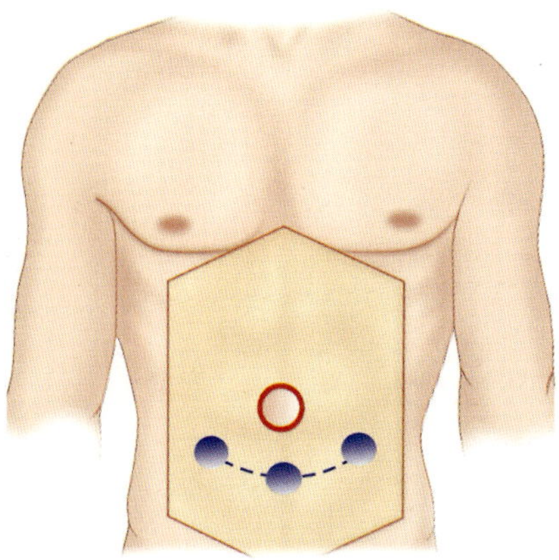

**Fig. 19.3:** Port placement in patient

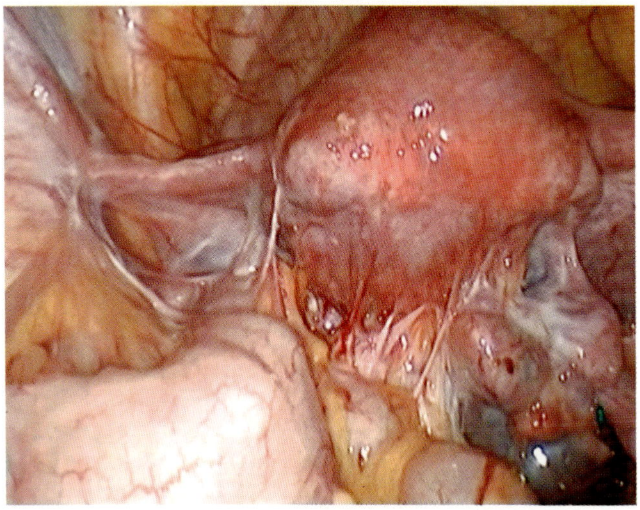

**Fig. 19.4:** Laparoscopic panoramic view of endometriosis with frozen pelvis

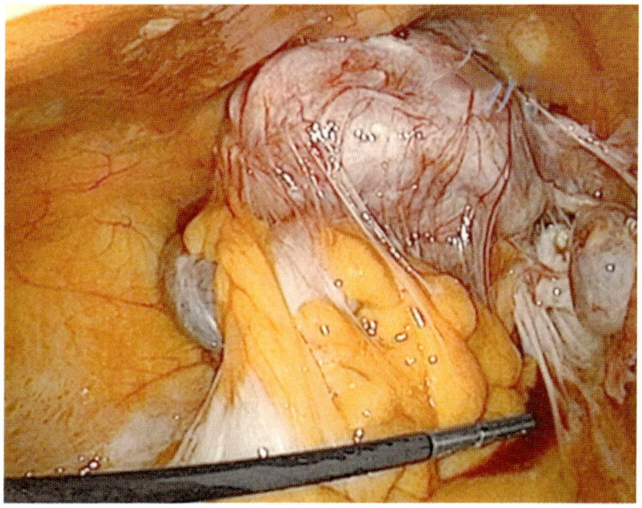

**Fig. 19.5:** Laparoscopic panoramic view of endometriosis with frozen pelvis

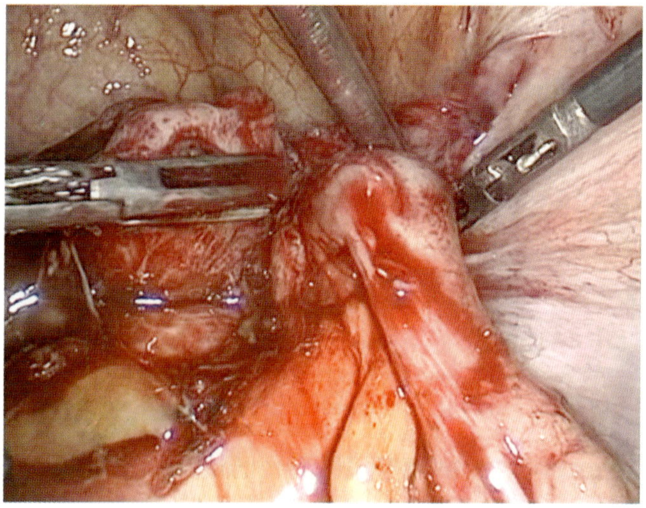

**Fig. 19.6:** Sometimes appendix is adherent to right adnexa

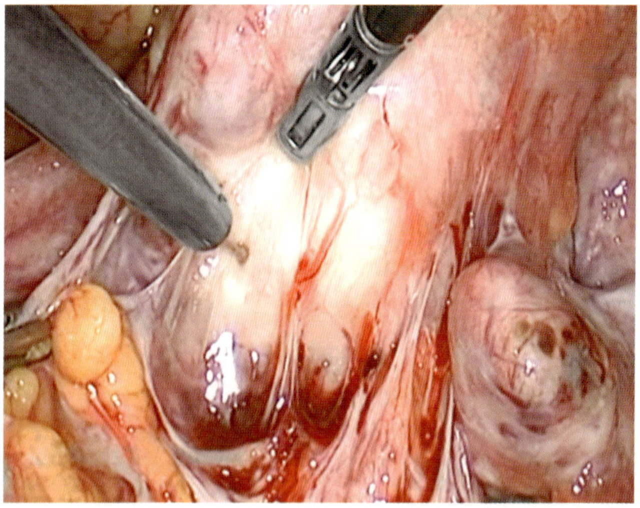

**Fig. 19.7:** Vasopressin (1:200 mL dilution) injected in the uterus to reduce bleeding to avoid staining of the tissue during dissection

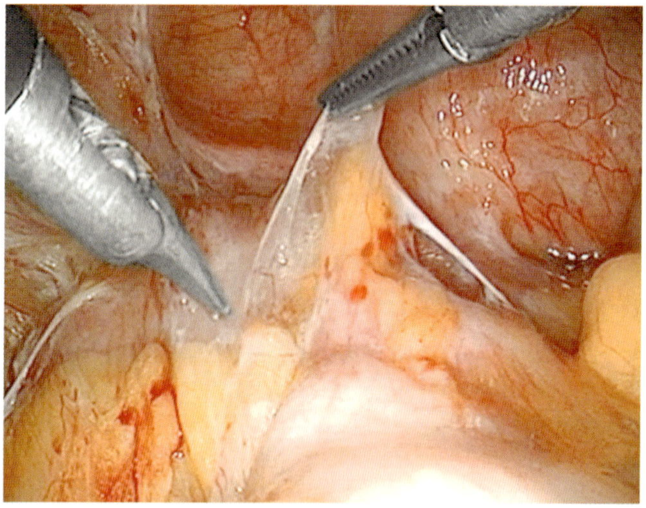

**Fig. 19.8:** Lateral mobilization of sigmoid colon should be commenced by sharp dissection

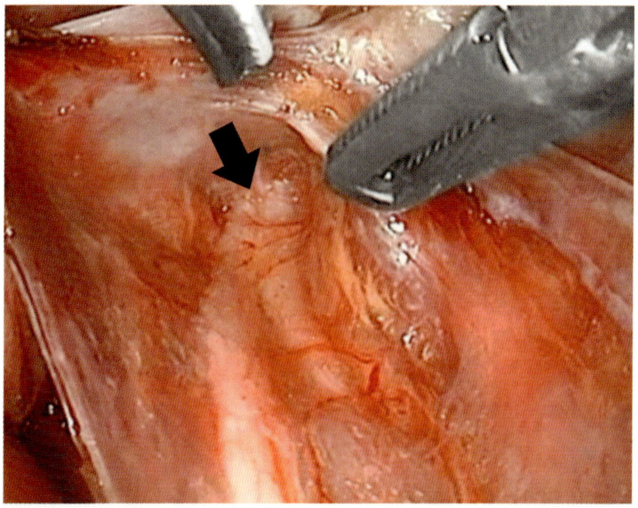

**Fig. 19.9:** Always start dissection laterally by opening retroperitoneal space (virgin area). Identify the course of ureter at the site of pelvic brim

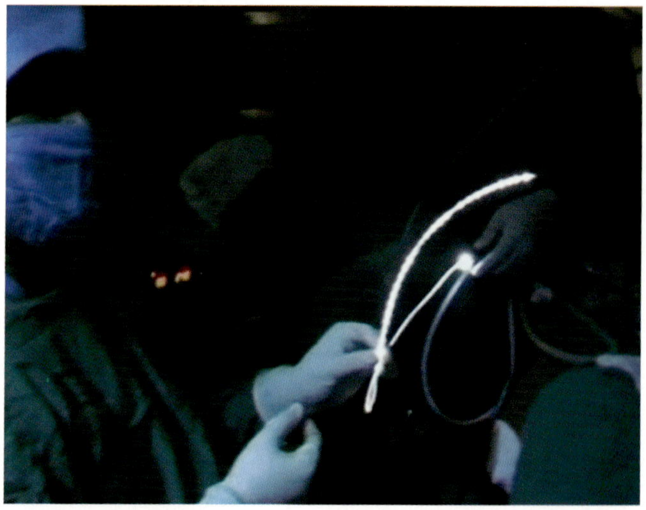

**Fig. 19.10A:** Fiberoptic ureteric catheter—Illumination effect of the catheter helps to find the pathway of the ureter

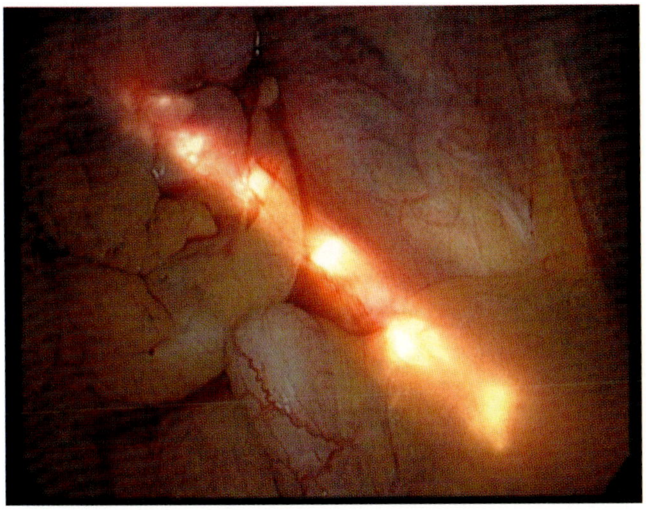

**Fig. 19.10B:** Fiberoptic ureteric catheter—Illumination effect of the catheter helps to find the pathway of the ureter

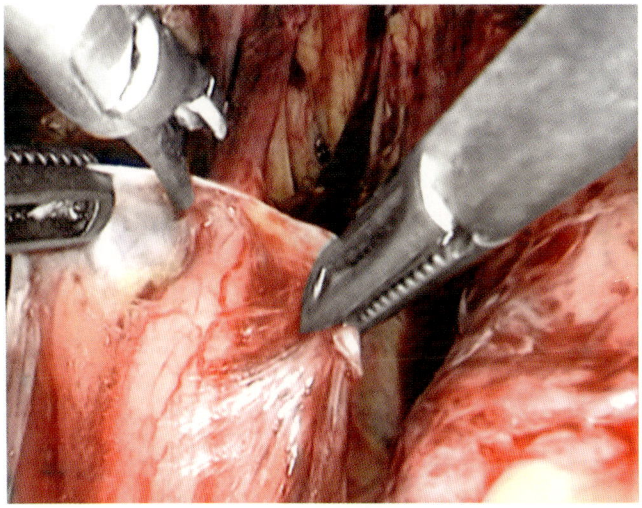

**Fig. 19.11:** Mobilization of the ureter in retroperitoneal space. Do dissection parallel to the ureter

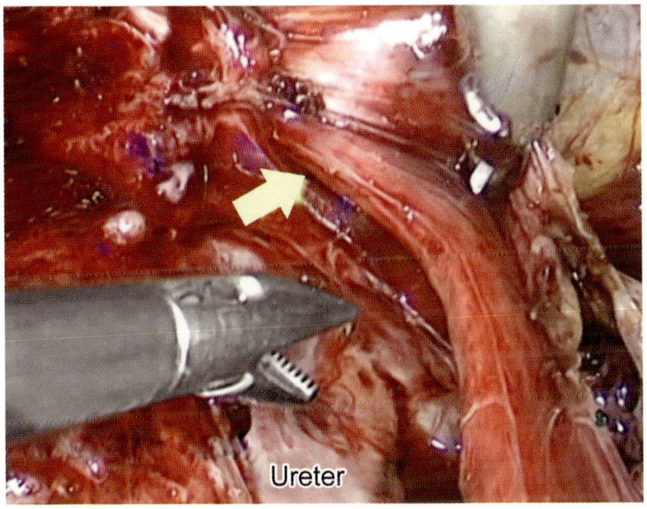


**Fig. 19.12:** Ureter should be mobilized after which salpingo-oophorectomy should be performed

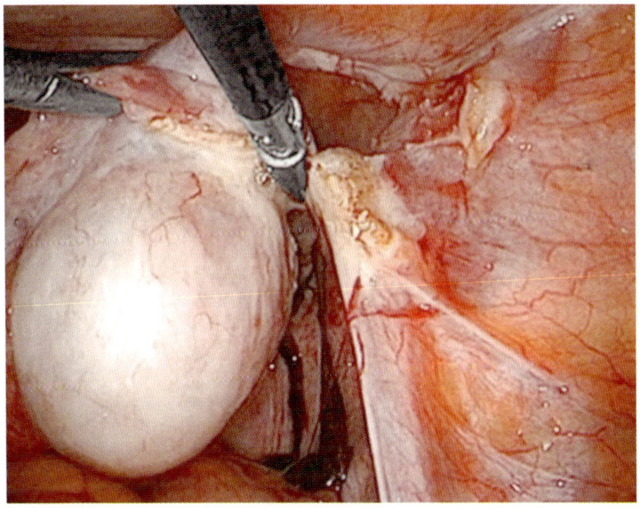

**Fig. 19.13:** Salpingo-oophorectomy should be done after ureter mobilization

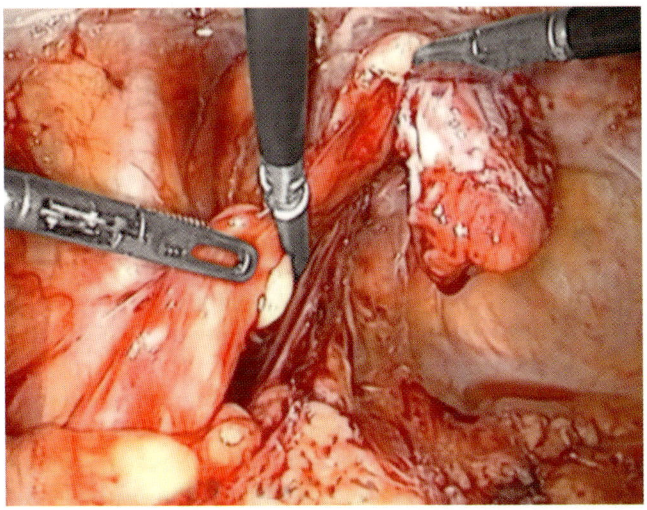

**Fig. 19.14:** Left tubo-ovarian mass excision after ureter mobilization

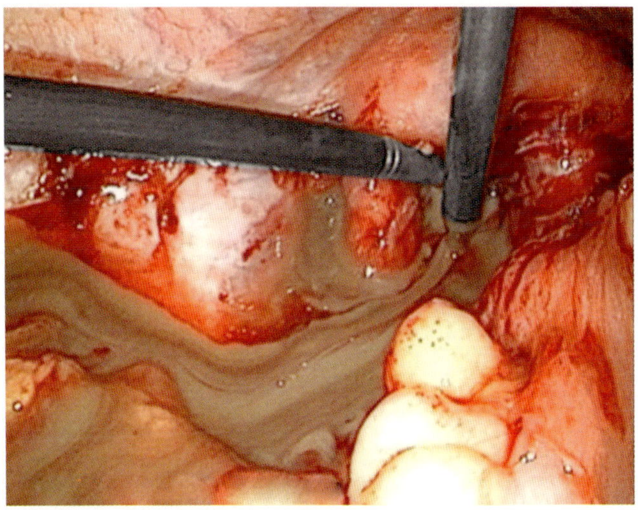

**Fig. 19.15:** Left tubo-ovarian abscess following ovarian endometrioma aspiration. Salpingo-oophorectomy should be done

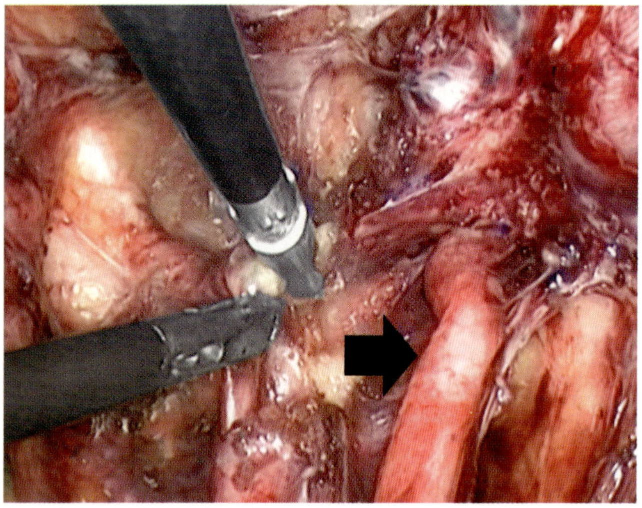

**Fig. 19.16A:** Uterine vessels ligated at their origin using 5 mm ligasure after doing ureteric dissection. They are only tortuous vessels crossing the para-rectal space. This figure arrow shows hydroureter (dilated ureter) due to stricture at the site of cardinal ligament in ureteric tunnel

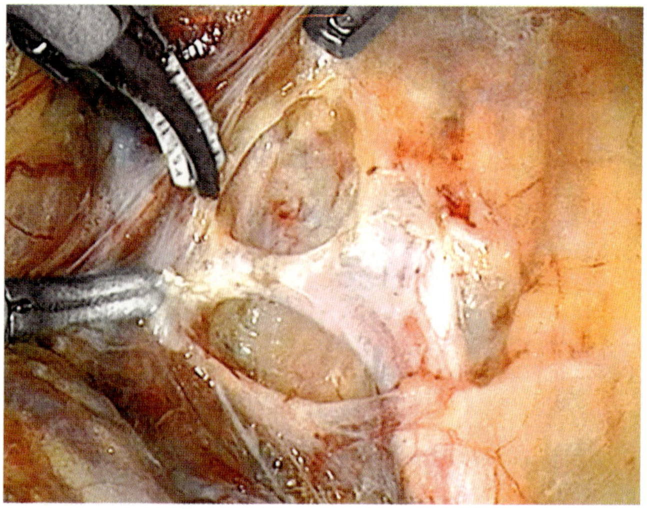

**Fig. 19.16B:** Uterine vessels ligated at their origin

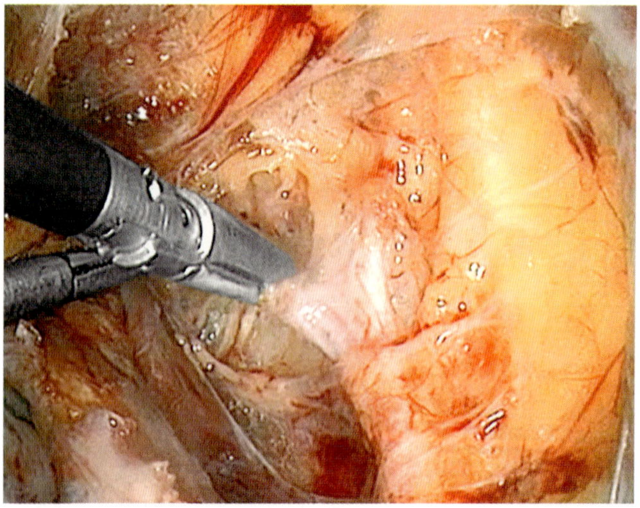

**Fig. 19.16C:** Uterine vessels ligated at their origin

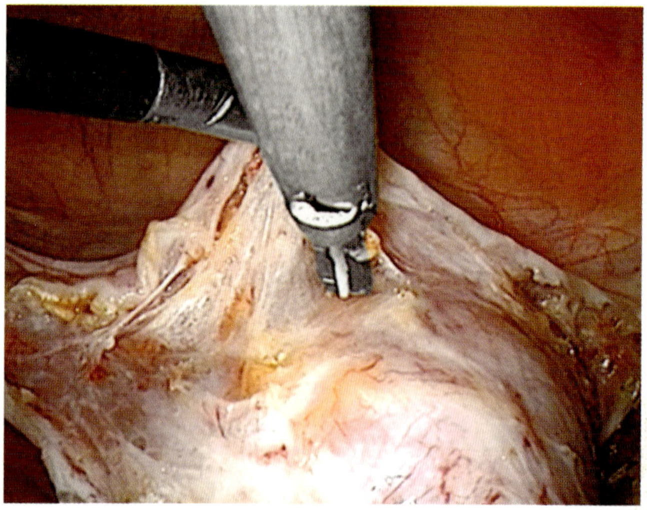

**Fig. 19.17:** Bladder mobilization

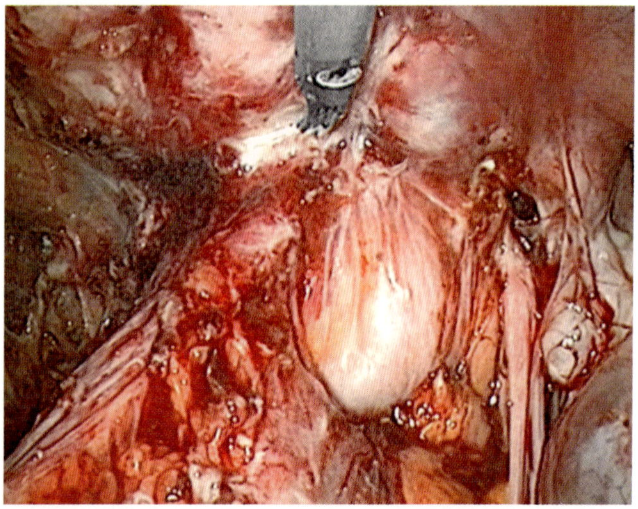

**Fig. 19.18:** Posteriorly dissection done flush to the uterus to avoid colorectal injury. Try to bring nodule on the colon. Colorectal nodule is removed after completion of hysterectomy

10. Subsequently we follow steps of intrafascial hysterectomy. Due to axis rotation of the uterus, uterine vessels get displaced anteriorly. Uterine vessels are again cut flush to the uterus on both sides after proper skeletonization. Cardinal ligament and uterosacral ligament are also coagulated and cut subsequently (Fig. 19.19).
11. Colpotomy (Fig. 19.20) is done using 5 mm harmonic scalpel or harmonic hook after inserting Prashant Mangeshikar's uterine manipulator (Fig. 19.21A) or Clermont Ferrand uterine manipulator (Fig. 19.21B) and specimen removed vaginally.
12. Colorectal nodule is excised after completion of intrafascial hysterectomy. Two techniques are recommended for excision of colorectal nodule: Either shaving of the nodule after inserting rectal probe or circular stappler is recommended to completely excise the nodule. We prefer shaving

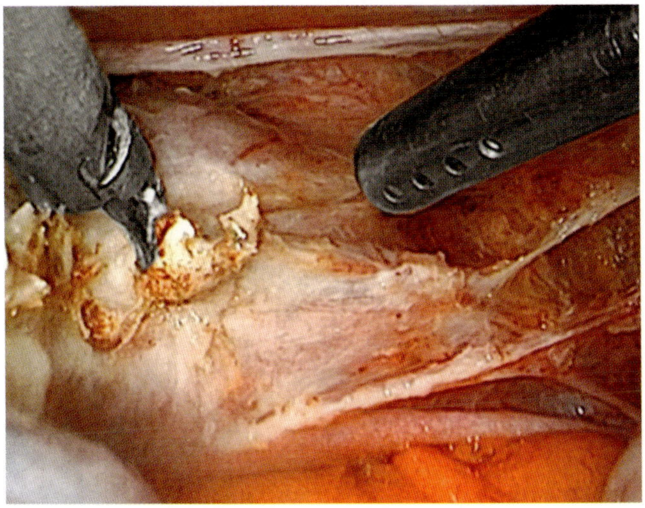

**Fig. 19.19:** Uterine vessels ligated and cut using harmonic scalpel flush to the uterus

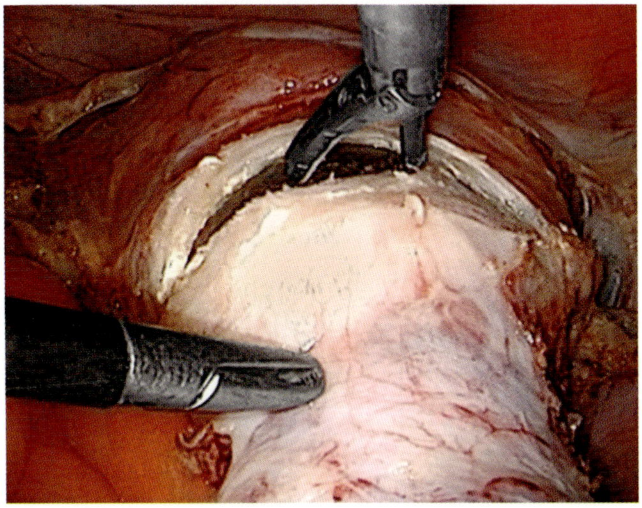

**Fig. 19.20:** Colpotomy with 5 mm harmonic salpel or harmonic hook

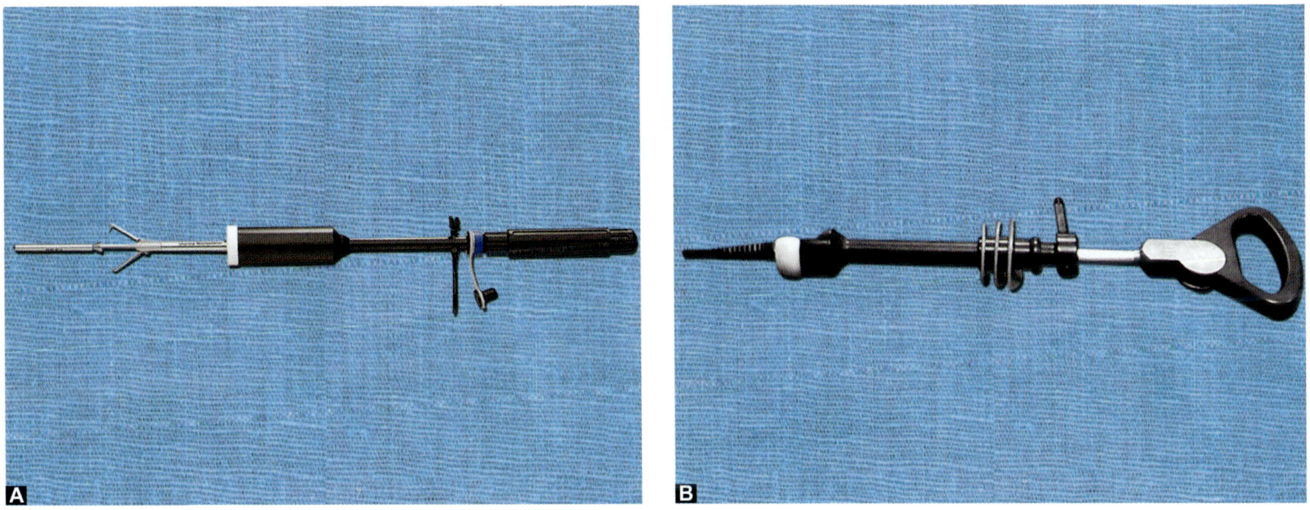

**Figs 19.21A and B:** (A) Prashant Mangeshi kar's uterine manipulator; (B) Clermont Ferrand uterine manipulator

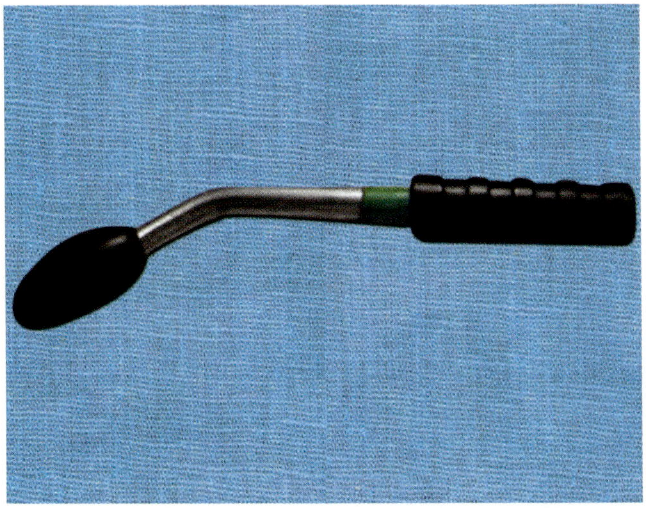

**Fig. 19.22:** Rectal probe should be introduced before shaving of the colorectal nodule

technique with scissors as it gives less morbidity post-operatively (Figs 19.22 to 19.25).

13. In some cases, ureteric stricture is present due to involvement of cardinal ligament by endometriosis. Ureteric tunnel dissection is done to excise the endometriotic nodule to relieve external compression over the ureter. In few cases due to severe ureteric stricture, excision of the disease portion of the ureter and uretero-ureter anastomosis is done. Ureteric stenting should be done post-procedure and stent should be kept for 6 weeks (Figs 19.26 to 19.30).
14. Vault is closed laparoscopically by contra-lateral intra-corporeal suturing using Vicryl no.1 (Fig. 19.31).
15. Colorectal integrity test is done (air-enema test) (Fig. 19.32). Pelvis is filled up with normal saline and air is pushed from below inside the rectum to see bubbling of the air in the pelvis to rule out rectal injury. As we prefer sharp dissection with scissors, we do primary

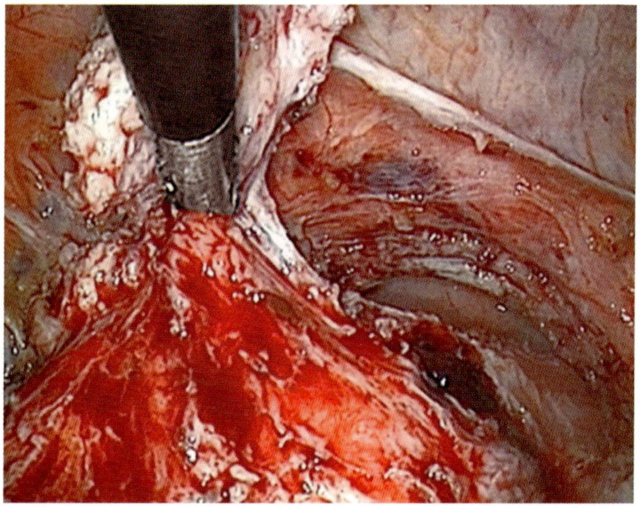

**Fig. 19.23:** Shaving of the colorectal nodule should be done after colpotomy

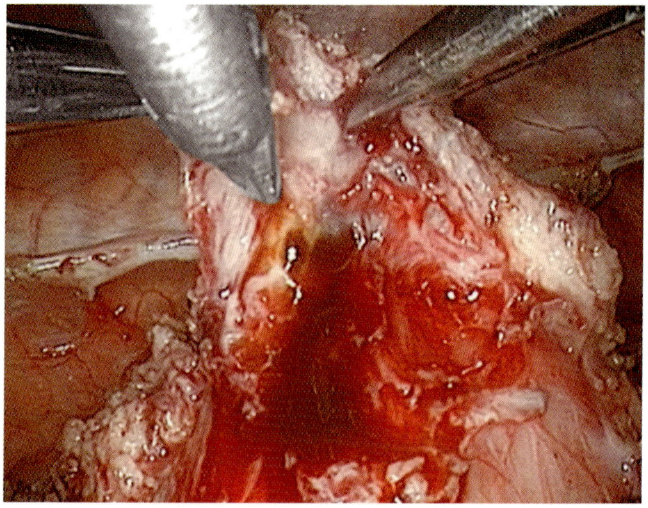

**Fig. 19.24:** Shaving of the colorectal nodule with scissors. Sometimes we find choky material coming out from the nodule (lacunae of colorectal nodule)

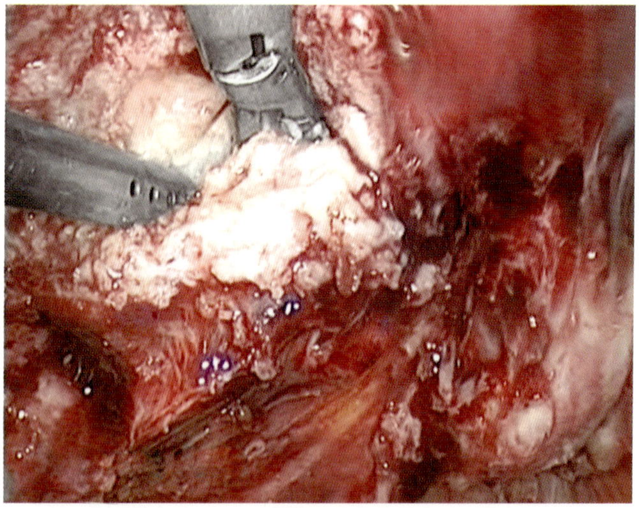

**Fig. 19.25:** Shaving of the colorectal nodule with harmonic scalpel

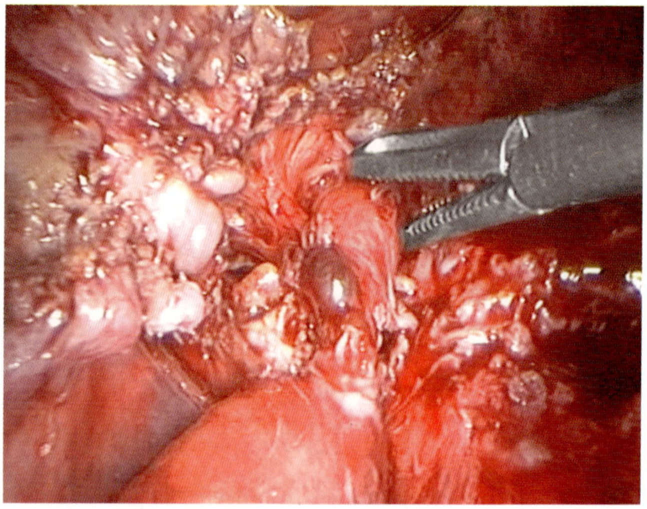

**Fig. 19.26:** Ureteric stricture at the level of the cardinal ligament. Ureteric tunnel dissection is done to excise the endometriotic nodule

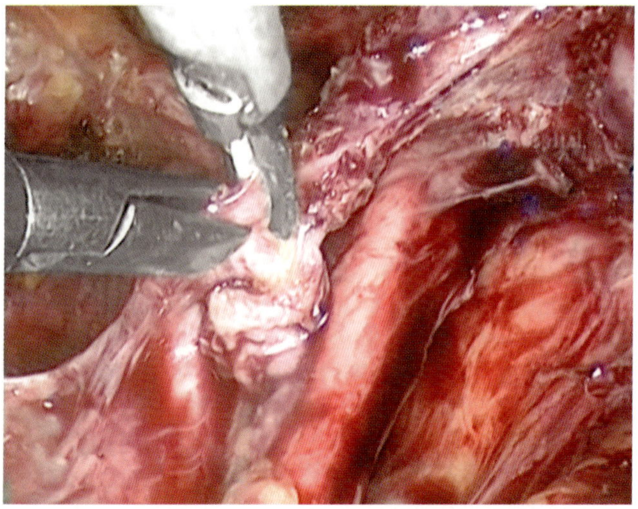

**Fig. 19.27:** Endometriotic nodule causing ureteric structure excised at the level of the cardinal ligament

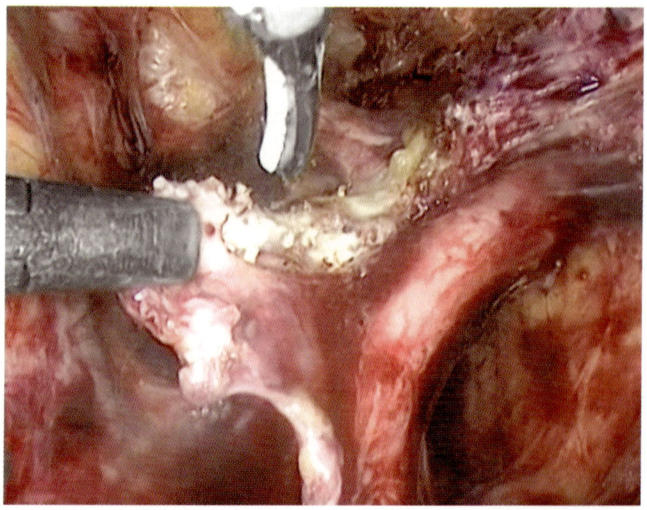

**Fig. 19.28:** Endometriotic nodule causing ureteric structure excised at the level of the cardinal ligament

suturing with vicryl 2-0 for rectal injury. But if we use any energy source which leads to injury of the colon, primary suturing along with colostomy is required.

16. Similarly cystoscopy is must to see for bladder mucosal involvement in endometriosis as well as to see urine spurts from both ureteric orifices. If bladder mucosal involvement is present, we prefer to excise the bladder mucosa and resuturing of the bladder wall with vicryl 3-0.
17. Hemostasis is confirmed. If still oozing is present from the raw surfaces in POD, we prefer to do laparoscopic bilateral internal iliac artery ligation. It reduces pulse pressure by 85% which helps in blood clot formation distal to ligation (Figs 19.33 and 19.34). Sometimes surgicel snow (J&J) is kept over the raw area to achieve hemostasis.
18. We prefer to keep intra-peritoneal drain and Foley's catheter in each case.

## Postoperative Management

- We prefer to keep patient nil by mouth till she passes flatus as we have done extensive dissection for colo-rectal nodule.
- Glycerine syringe may be required per-rectally to relieve the gaseous abdominal distension.
- We routinely do CBC, S. electrolytes and S. creatinine post-operatively next day.
- Patient is usually discharged 48–72 hours once she passes urine and stool normally.
- We give GnRH analogues post-operatively to treat micro-implants of endometriosis especially in cases where we have preserved the ovaries.

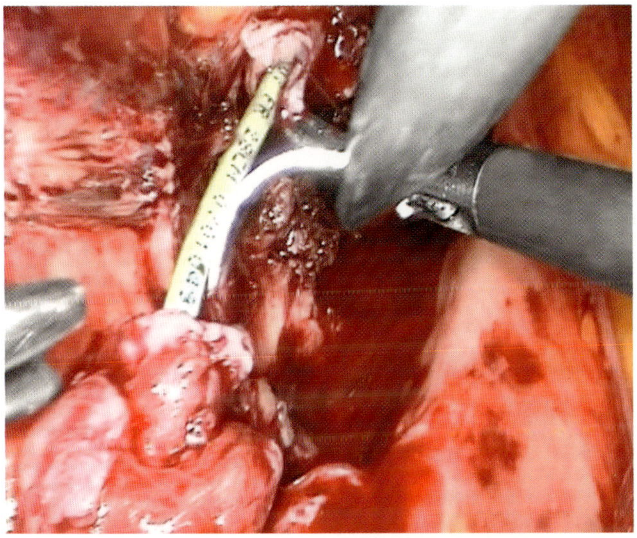

**Fig. 19.29:** Severe ureteric stricture with large area of ureter involvement along with mucosa, resection followed by uretero-ureteral anastomosis should be done

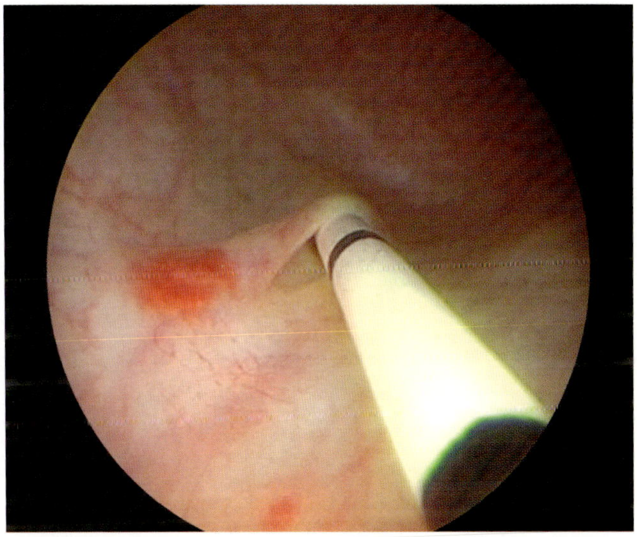

**Fig. 19.30A:** Ureteric stenting should be done after the procedure and stent should be kept for 6 weeks

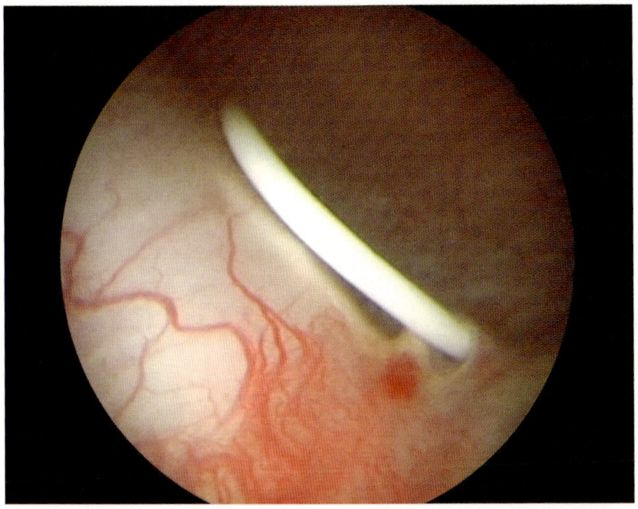

**Fig. 19.30B:** Ureteric stenting should be done after the procedure and stent should be kept for 6 weeks

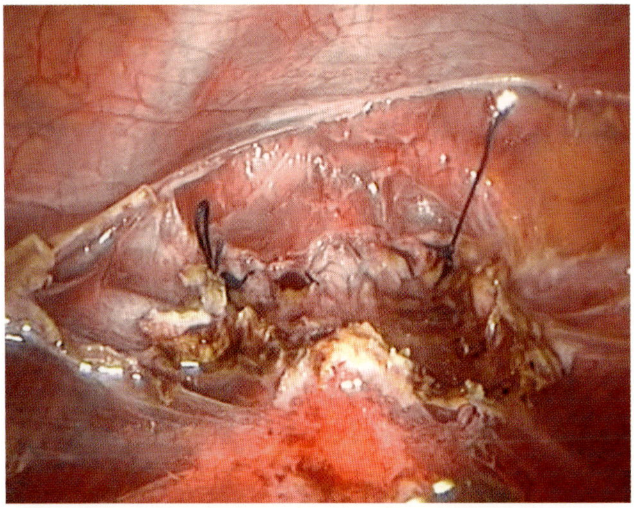

**Fig. 19.31:** End result: Vault suturing by contralateral intracorporeal suturing technique using Vicryl no.1 after excision of the colorectal nodule

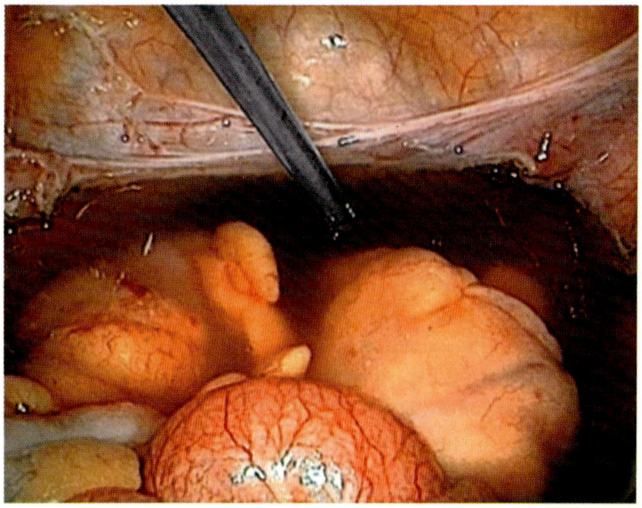

**Fig. 19.32:** Colorectal integrity test

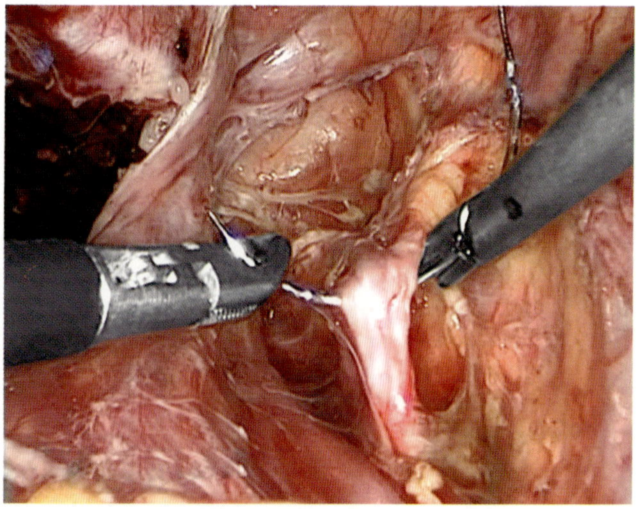

**Fig. 19.33:** Bilateral internal iliac artery ligation may be required if bleeding persists from raw surfaces. It reduces pulse pressure by 85% which helps in blood clot formation

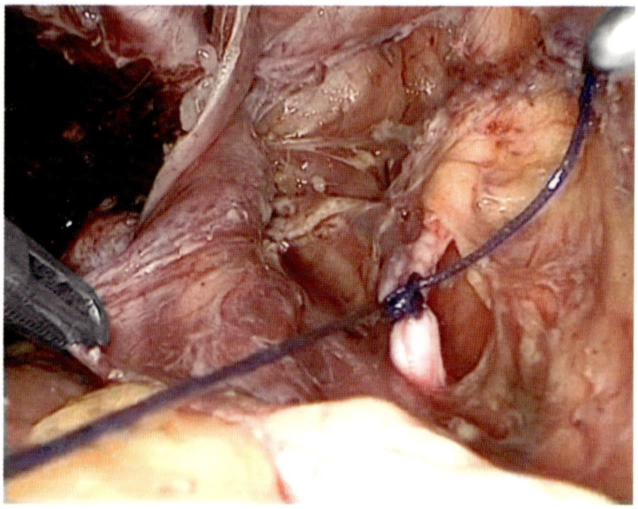

**Fig. 19.34:** Bilateral internal iliac artery ligation may be required if bleeding persists from raw surfaces. It reduces pulse pressure by 85% which helps in blood clot formation

*Note:* This method has been popularized by author as 'Mayflower Technique' of hysterectomy for endometriosis.

Chapter 20

# Laparoscopic Radical Hysterectomy

*Shailesh Puntambekar*

## PREOPERATIVE PREPARATION

- FIGO staging
- Mechanical bowel preparation
- Preoperative antibiotics.

## INSTRUMENTS AND EQUIPMENT

- Myoma screw
- Two non-traumatic graspers
- One needle holder
- One Maryland dissector
- Harmonic scalpel
- Bipolar forceps
- Allis' forceps
- Suction cannula
- 0 degree telescope.

## TECHNIQUE

1. Regional anesthesia, either spinal or epidural preferred in combination with general anesthesia.
2. Patient is placed in modified Lloyd Davis position at approximately 30- to 45-degree angle.
3. The ports taken are as follows:
   - A total of 5 ports are used.
   - A 10 mm camera port at the umbilicus.
   - A 10 mm working port at the McBurney's point on the right side.
   - A 5 mm port pararectally at the midclavicular line.
   - A set of 5 mm ports in the mirror image on the left side.

The surgeon is on the right side, the assistant and camera surgeon on the left side. The surgeon need not change the position during the contralateral dissection.

## PROCEDURE

A myoma screw is introduced from the upper left port and inserted into the fundus for uterine manipulation.

The following standardized steps are followed:

1. Step 1: **Anterior U cut**

   The dissection is begun by taking an anterior U cut, cutting the round ligament on the right side with harmonic shears.

   This cut is then extended into the uterovesical fold and is carried downward up to the urinary bladder. The uterus is pulled cranially and the assistant lifted the bladder. The peritoneum is then incised and the fascial plane between the bladder and the uterus is developed. The bladder when dissected with harmonic shears and then blunt dissection is done with gauze. This dissection is carried downward to achieve a good vaginal cuff and is facilitated by carbon dioxide insufflations. The peritoneal cut then extended on the left side up to the round ligament. This ligament is cut with the harmonic shears.

2. Step 2: **Posterior U cut**

   The peritoneal cut is further extended up to the left infundibulopelvic ligament. The uterus is anteverted and the assistant pushes the rectum to the right side. This stretched the peritoneum medial to the left infundibulopelvic ligament. The ureter is then visualized

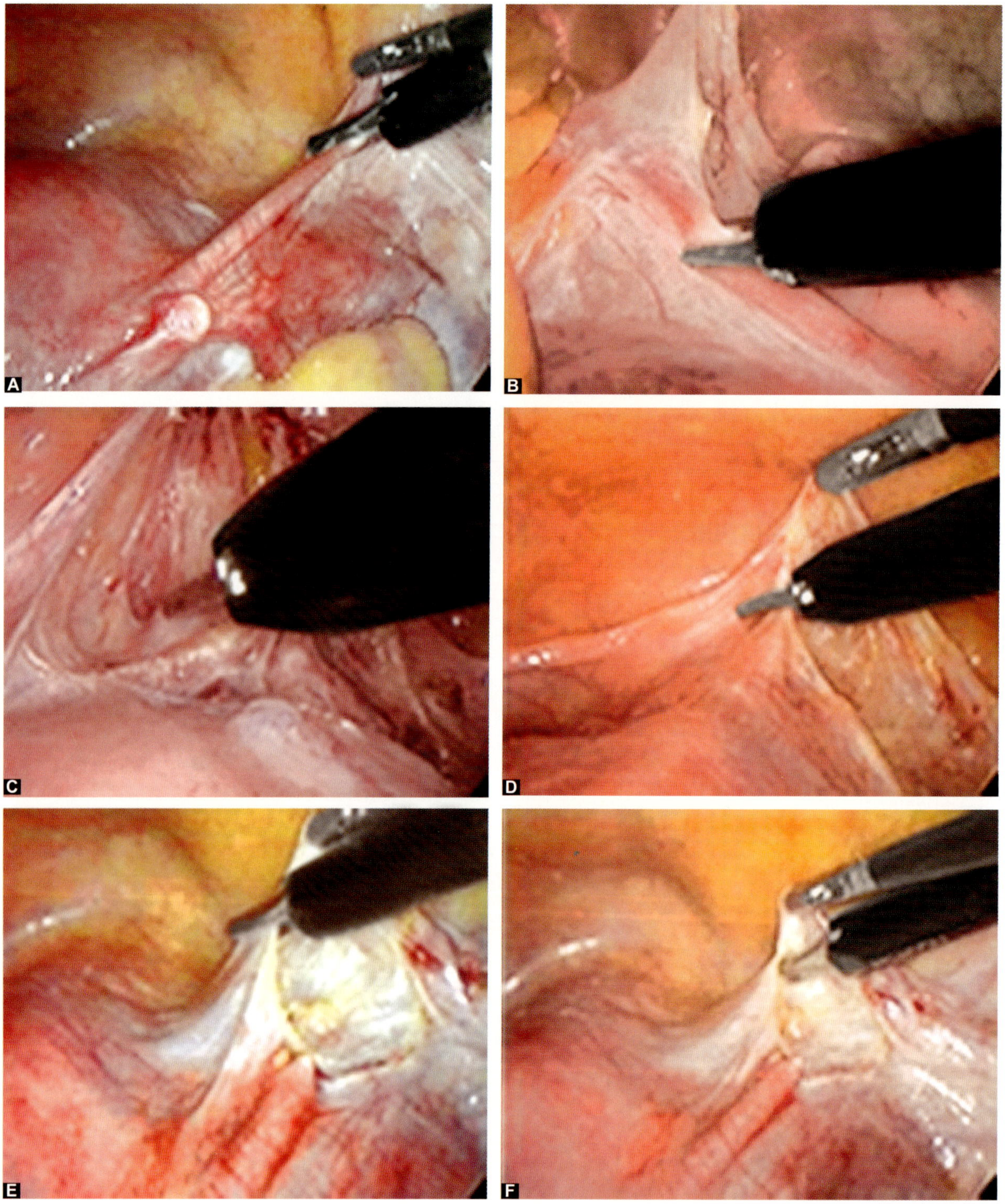

**Figs 20.1A to F:** Anterior U-cut taken on the right side and round ligament is cut

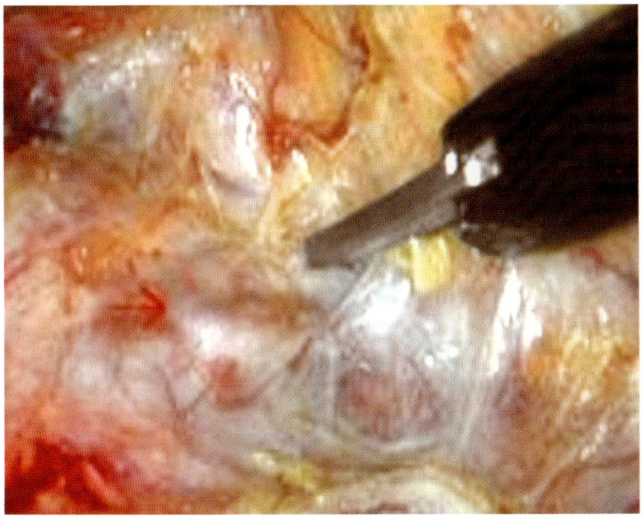

**Fig. 20.2:** Uterovesical fold is cut and bladder dissection done. Dissection done till exposure of good vaginal cuff

underneath the peritoneum at the level of sacral promontory.

The peritoneum medial to the infundibulopelvic ligament is incised with the harmonic shears to expose the ureter, which is then pushed laterally. The peritoneal cut (Posterior U cut) is extended down into the pouch of Douglas keeping the ureter constantly under vision. The same step is repeated on the right side and the right ureter is pushed laterally. The ureteric dissection is always done parallel to the ureter.

3. Step 3: **Dissection of rectovaginal space**

The assistant pulls the rectum cranially so as to stretch the peritoneum in the pouch of Douglas. This peritoneum is incised with harmonic shears. The insufflation of carbon dioxide gas opens the lose areolar planes between the two layers of Denonvilliers fascia.

The rectum is dissected off the posterior vaginal wall up to the levator ani. The trick of the trade is to retain the fat

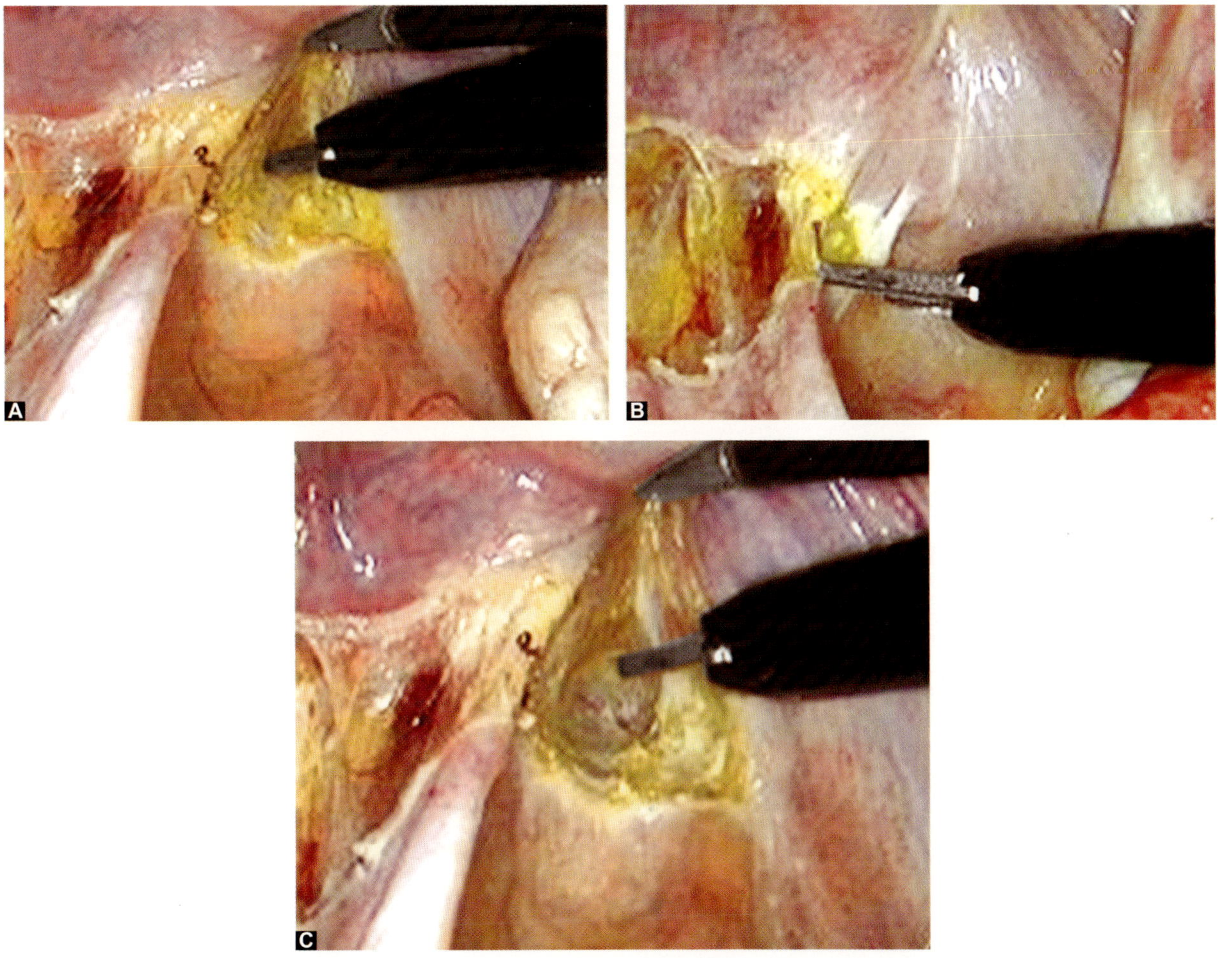


**Figs 20.3A to C:** Posterior U cut: The peritoneal cut is extended to the infundibulopelvic ligament. The ureter is exposed and pushed laterally. Ureteric dissection is done parallel to the ureter

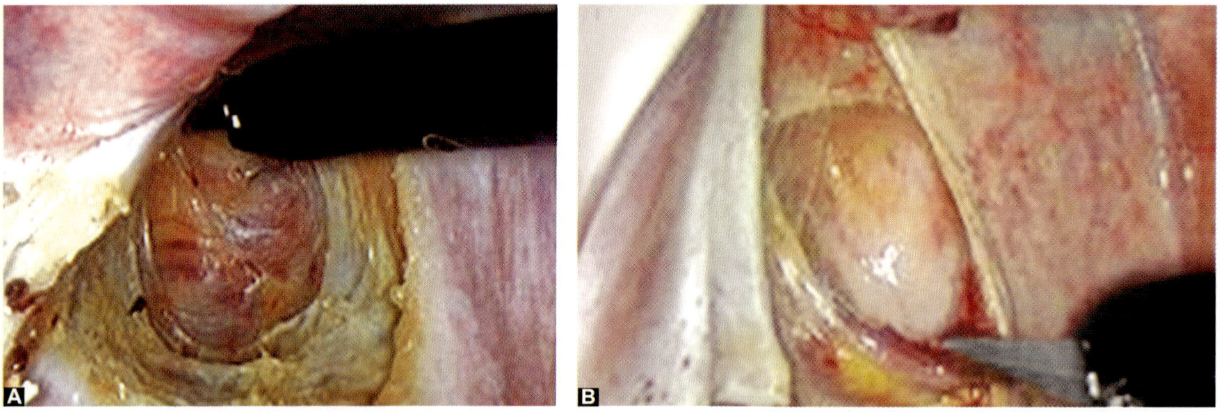

**Figs 20.4A and B:** Dissection of rectovaginal space, by opening up the loose areolar tissue between the two layers of Denonvilliers' fascia

on the rectum. One has to remember that the fat belongs to rectum and so the dissection should be between this fat and the posterior vaginal wall. No rectal wall fibers should be visualized.

4. Step 4: **Dissection of pararectal space**

The left ureter is retracted medially and the posterior leaf of broad ligament above the ureter is cut. This cut is extended downward toward the bladder so that a window in the broad ligament is created. The ureter is again retracted medially and the harmonic is swept parallel to the ureter to open the pararectal space. The internal iliac artery which forms the lateral boundary of this space is immediately seen. The only structure which crosses the pararectal space transversely is the uterine artery.

This can be traced to its origin from the internal iliac artery. This artery is then clipped or ligated and cut. The pararectal space dissection is extended caudally up to the levator ani muscle.

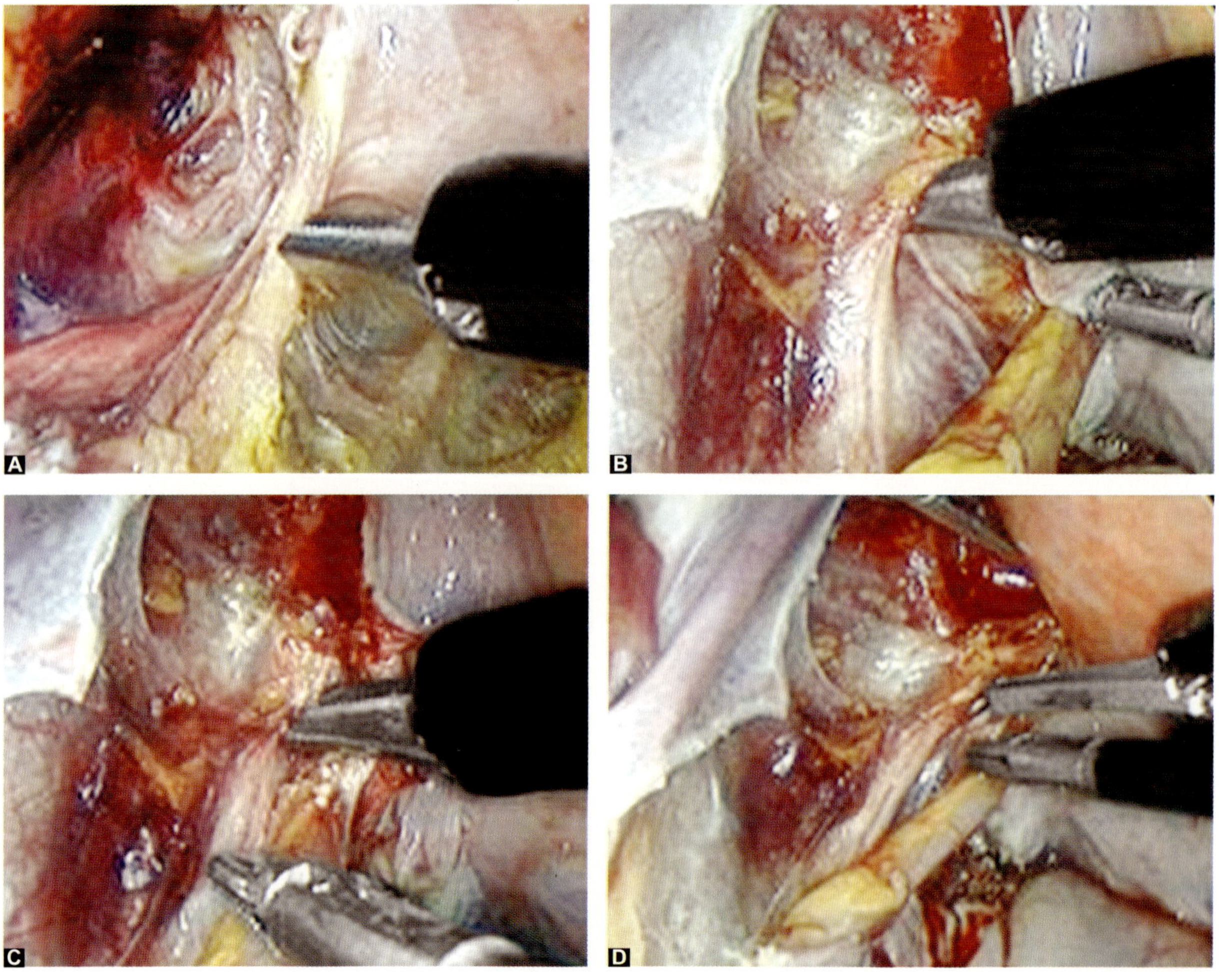

**Figs 20.5A to D:** Dissection of the pararectal space: The posterior leaf of broad ligament is opened up and ureter is retracted medially and the pararectal space is opened

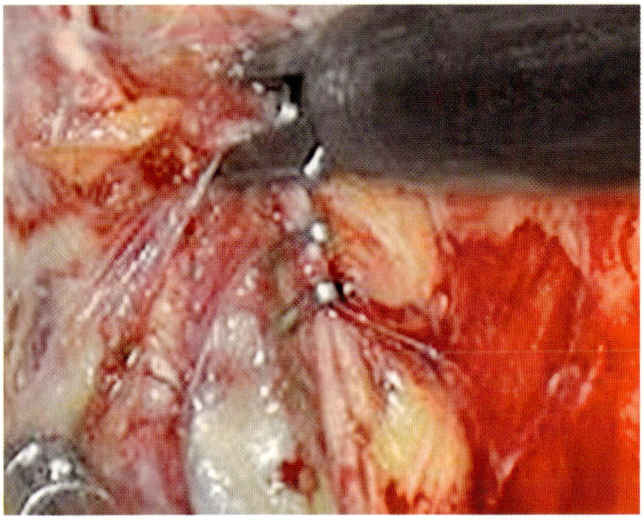

**Fig. 20.6:** Uterine artery is traced to its origin from the internal iliac artery and the artery is clipped/ligated and cut

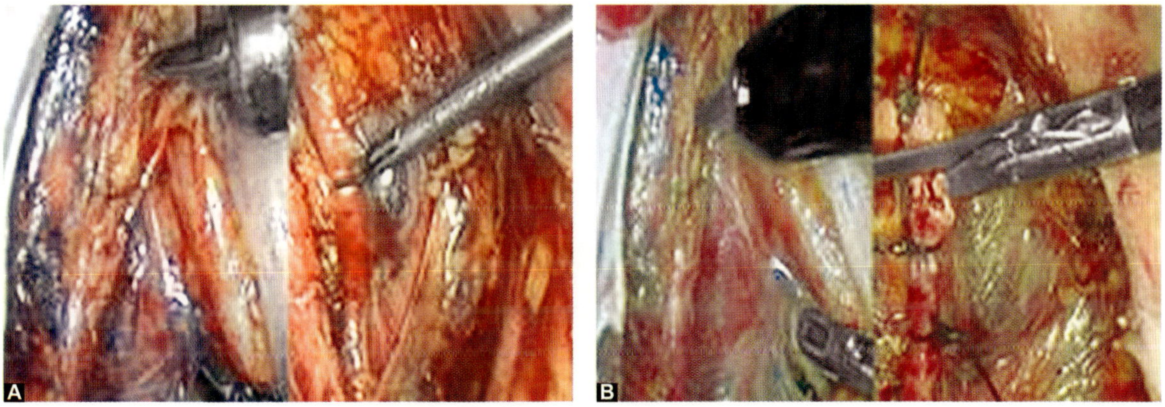

**Figs 20.7A and B:** Fused uterosactal and Mackenrodt ligaments are cut

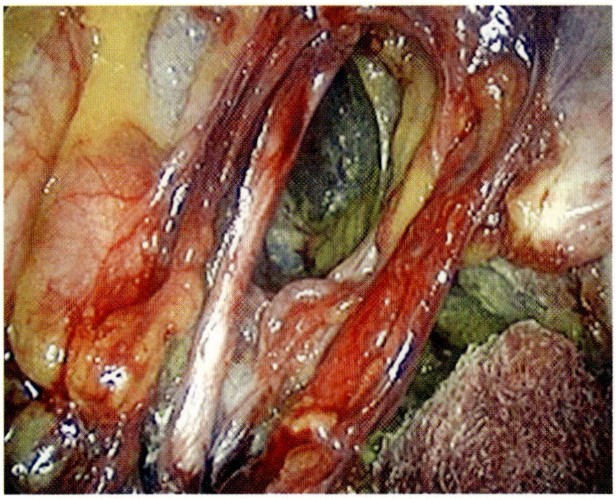

**Fig. 20.8:** Cut is extended to the levator ani

The uterosacral and Mackenrodt's ligament's were thus seen as a single fan-shaped structure. These ligaments were cut with ligature. This cut is extended up to the levator ani.

5. Step 5: **Lateralization of ureter**

The ureter is then retracted laterally and the uterine vein is seen coming from below the ureter. This vein is either clipped or ligated or cut with harmonic shears or with ligature similar steps are taken on the right side. The uterus is pulled cranially and then to the right. This exposes the ureter from the top. The ureter is then traced along its course toward the urinary bladder. At this point, the bladder is held stretched upward by the assistant surgeon. Thus, the ureteric tunnel could then be visualized along with small veins.

This tunnel is either dissected with Maryland forceps or with harmonic shears. This helps in pushing the ureter further laterally. The ureter could be seen as it enters the bladder at the uterovesical junction. The bladder is then pushed further down to achieve a good vaginal cuff. The ureteric dissection exposes the paracolpos, which is then cut as laterally as possible. The same steps are repeated on the right side. Finally a good length of vagina below the growth is exposed. The vagina is opened with harmonic shears.

This kind of dissection usually achieves about 2.5 to 3 cm of vaginal cuff. Lastly, the infundibulopelvic ligaments are cut and the entire specimen is separated.

This is then removed through the vagina and the vagina is again packed to prevent carbon dioxide leak. The length of the parametrium and vaginal margin of the specimen are measured.

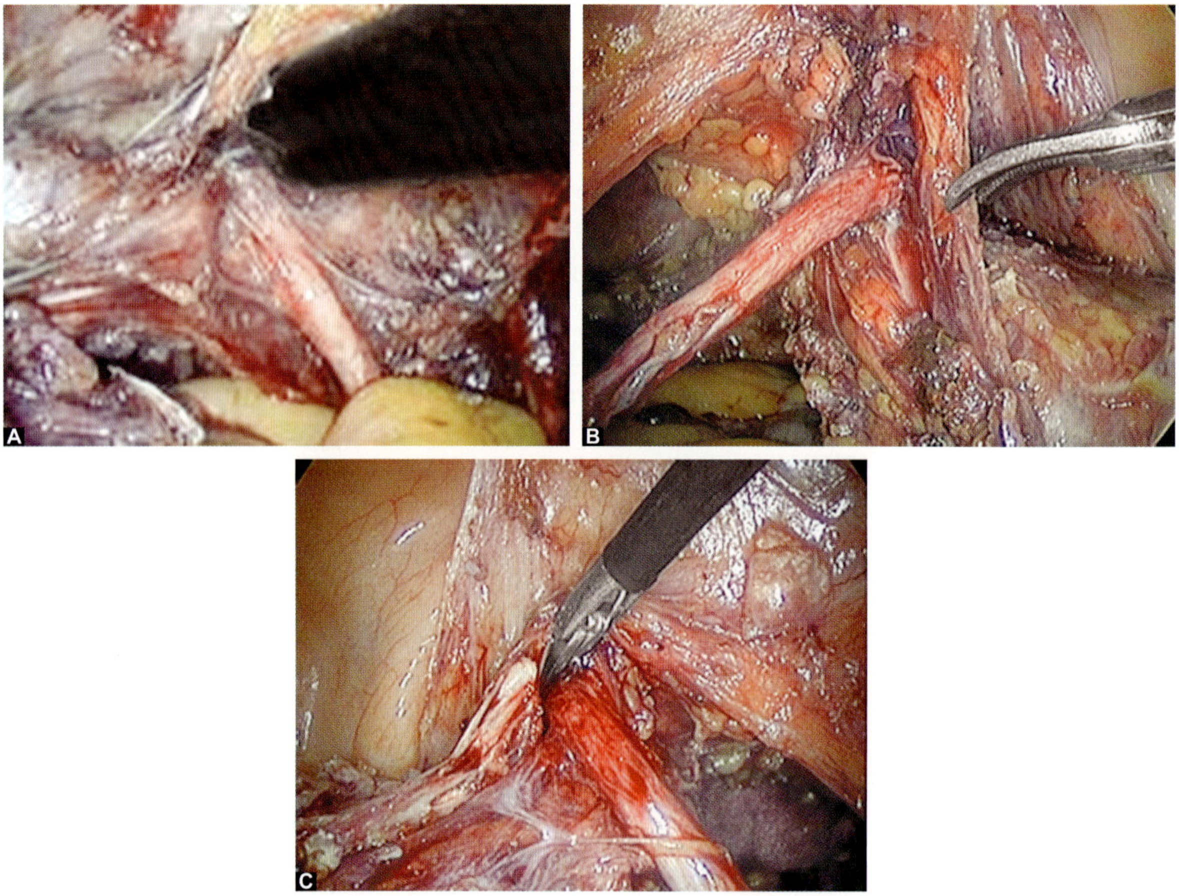


**Figs 20.9A to C:** Lateralization of the ureter and clipping the uterine vein

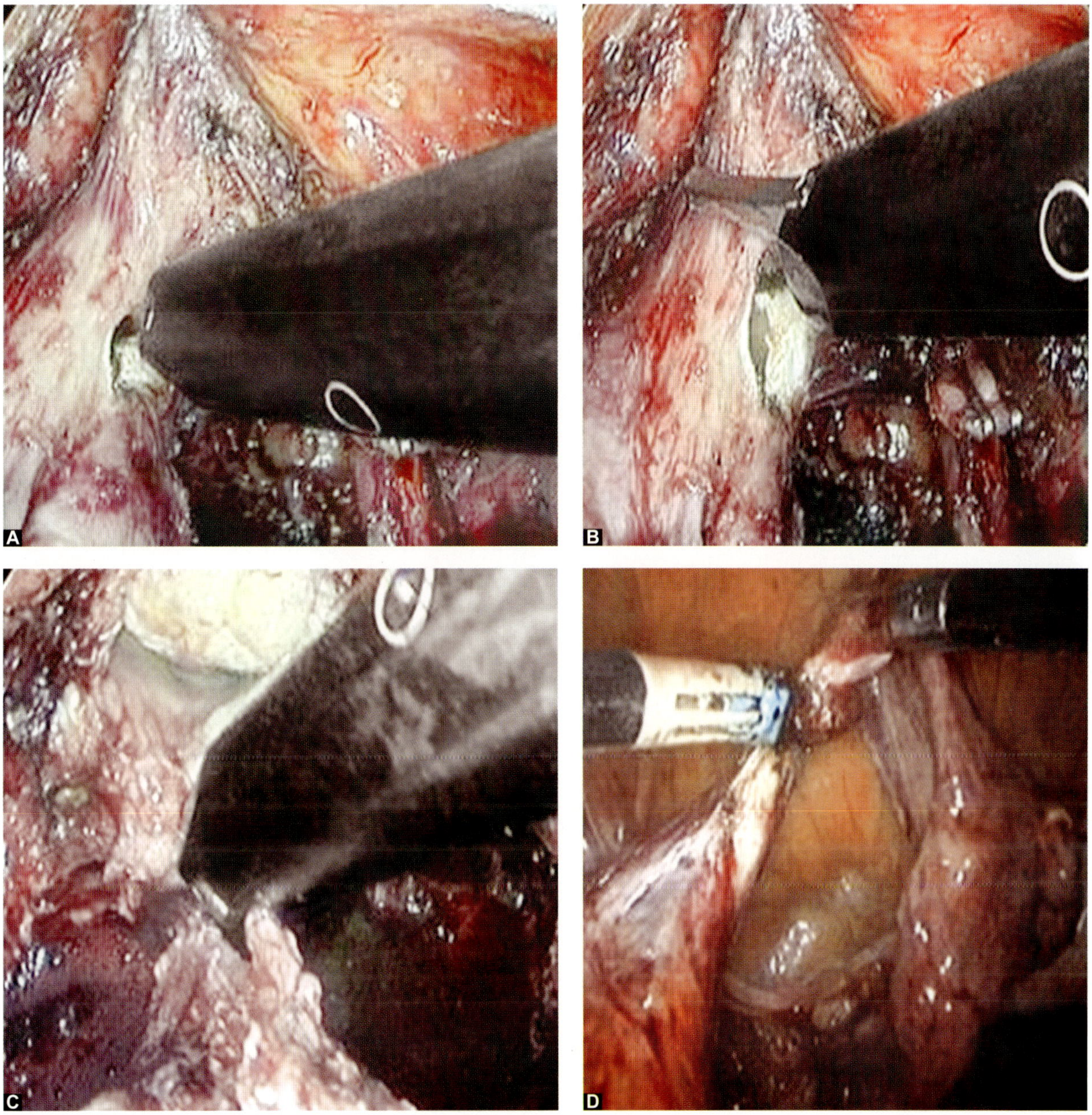

**Figs 20.10A to D:** Finally the infundibulopelvic ligament is cut and specimen is delivered vaginally

6. Step 6: **Lymph node dissection**

The lymph node dissection is started at the bifurcation of common iliac artery. The suction cannula is the preferred instrument for dissection. The lose areolar tissue along the external iliac artery is swept till the inguinal ligament. All the fibrofatty tissue along the external iliac vein are dissected. At this point, the iliac bone is exposed which is the lateral limit of dissection. The nodes in the obturator fossa are visualized by stretching the peritoneum by the assistant. The nodes are swept from the pubic bone cranially. The obturator nerve is exposed and all the nodes above the nerve are cleared. This dissection is done right up to the bifurcation of the iliac vein. The entire fibrofatty tissue is then dissected medially till the internal iliac artery is exposed and cleared off the fibrofatty tissue. This is the medial limit of dissection. At the end of dissection, the external iliac artery, vein and the obturator fossa should be devoid of any fibrofatty tissue. The psoas muscle along with the ilioinguinal nerve is the lateral limit of dissection. The same dissection is done on the other side. The entire nodal tissue is removed through the vagina.

Hemostasis is achieved and the wound is irrigated with normal saline. The vaginal closure is done abdominally with a 30 mm 2-0 vicryl introduced through the 10 mm working port and continuous interlocking sutures are taken. A nasogastric tube No. 16 is introduced through one of the 5 mm ports and is kept as a drain. The posterior peritoneum is not closed. The ports are removed under vision and the 10 mm port sites are sutured.

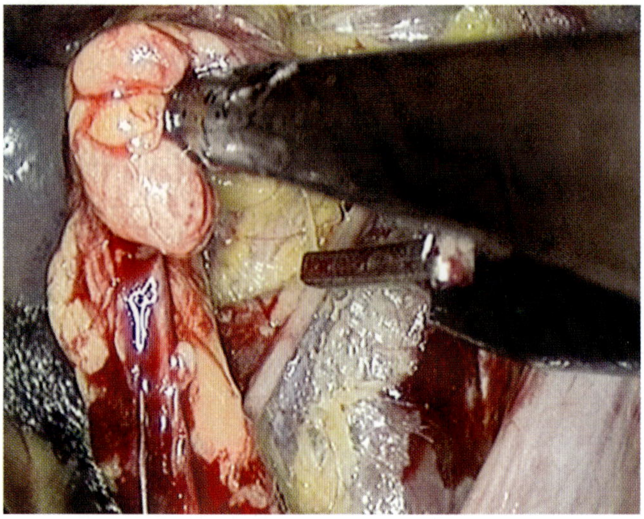

**Fig. 20.11:** Lymph node dissection

Chapter

21

# Laparoscopic Myomectomy

*Sunita R Tandulwadkar, Nirzari Mangeshikar*

## PREOPERATIVE EVALUATION OF THE PATIENT

- History examination.
- Ultrasound for location, number of fibroids, any associated organic pathology like endometriosis, adnexal mass, etc. (Transvaginal ultrasound is preferable). An abdominal ultrasound can be performed, especially in fundal fibroids.
- Color Doppler to rule out uterine malignancy or a sarcomatous fibroid.
- Limited MRI for uterus.
- Routine investigations.
- A hysteroscopy is always done before starting laparoscopy to exclude a submucous myoma. Submucous myomas more than 50% projecting into the cavity should preferably be removed hysteroscopically.

## PREOPERATIVE PREPARATIONS

Usually no preparation. In cases of large fibroids or multiple fibroids, bowel preparation can be done.

## INSTRUMENTS AND EQUIPMENT

The following are the additional laparoscopic instruments required for different types of myomectomy:

- 10 mm claw/tenaculum forceps
- 5 mm or 10 mm myoma screw
- Unipolar diathermy needle
- Two 5 mm toothed graspers
- Two needle holders
- Motorized morcellator
- CCL vaginal extractor—optional

## BOWEL PREPARATION

- Diet—one day prior to surgery, soft diet till afternoon followed by liquid diet and then, nil by mouth for 8 hours prior to surgery.
- Peglec powder—dissolve the pack in 2 liters of water to be given within 2–3 hours on previous evening.

OR

- Exelyte solution 90 mL to be added in 300 mL of limca/fruit juice to be given on previous evening.

## PREREQUISITES

- Skilled laparoscopic surgeon; especially skilled in laparoscopic suturing and morcellation.
- Anesthetist, skilled and trained assistant, nursing staff.
- A complete set of operative laparoscopy instruments, 5/10 mm myoma screw, and electromechanical morcellator.
- Both monopolar and bipolar cautery, harmonic if available.
- Proper suturing set with needle holders, knot pushers for extracorporeal knots and scissors.
- Injection vasopressin—20 units in 100 mL normal saline.

*Position of the patient*—same as laparoscopic hysterectomy.

## PROCEDURE

1. Placement of primary and secondary trocars depends upon the size and site of fibroid.
2. Relation of fibroid with the uterus and fallopian tube should be carefully assessed after inserting primary trocar and then site of secondary trocars to be decided.
3. Vasopressin 1 in 100 dilution is injected into fibroid at 3 to 4 sites to minimize bleeding (action will remain only for 20–30 minutes).
4. Careful planning of incision is done.
5. Incision is usually taken with a monopolar hook/spatula over the most bulging part of the myoma.
6. Most preferred incision is transverse incision, as it will cut fewer vessels.
7. Incision should be of sufficient depth, so that capsule of fibroid is visualized.

8. With 2 Allis′ forceps, cut edges are pulled apart so as to expose capsule of fibroid wall and make space for myoma screw insertion.
9. Once the myoma screw is inserted, myoma is pulled outward and upward keeping countertraction on uterus downward with 2 Allis′ forceps applied on the anterior lip of the cervix.
10. If one is in the right plane, myoma is usually extracted easily and there is minimal bleeding.
11. Position of myoma screw is changed from time-to-time so that traction is applied next to cleavage line.
12. Usually the base of myoma will have large feeding vessels, which should be cauterized and cut.
13. Only active bleeders of the bed are cauterized which can be easily identified by underwater inspection.
14. Undue cautery should be avoided, as it will give defective healing.
15. Myoma after removal is parked at right paracolic gutter.

## CLOSURE OF UTERINE FLAP

1. Reconstruction of myoma bed is performed with vicryl no. 1 suture.
2. Whether single or multiple layer closure is individual's decision but the ultimate aim is to obliterate the dead space completely so as to avoid hematoma formation, which is another cause of weakening of scar.
3. Start from one angle, first stitch is placed beyond angle either with intracorporeal or extracorporeal suture and then rest of defect is closed by taking deep continuous locking sutures and the end suture should be again beyond the angle of opposite side.
4. If it is a single layer closure, ensure that stitches are deep enough to obliterate the dead space.
5. We do not advocate multiple layer closure neither closure of endometrial layer.

## EXTRACTION OF MYOMA

1. Myomas are extracted by electronic morcellation. Smaller myomas can be extracted by colpotomy.
2. A meticulous lavage is given and hemostasis is checked.
3. End result should be a clean pelvis.
4. To keep a drain in the postoperative period is again an individual's choice.

## MYOMECTOMY IN DIFFICULT SITUATIONS

### Pedunculated Fibroid with a Broad Base

1. Instead of transverse incision, circular incision should be taken at the base of fibroid in a circumferential manner.
2. With myoma screw, myoma is pulled up and enucleated after cauterizing base of the pedicle.

### Broad Ligament Myomas

1. Majority of broad ligament myomas are removed by a posterior incision unlike at laparotomy where division of round ligament and removal by anterior route is preferred.
2. The oblique incision is made in the broad ligament parallel to the vessels.
3. A myoma screw is now inserted and traction is applied slowly while a grasper is used for retracting the broad ligament.
4. Any bleeding vessels are coagulated then and there.
5. After complete enucleation, broad ligament is inspected for complete hemostasis.
6. A drain is kept in the pelvis and observed.
7. There is no need to suture the broad ligament back.

**TIPS**

- In case of multiple fibroids where the shape of the uterus is distorted, round ligaments help in identification.
- As far as possible, incision should be taken anteriorly than on posterior wall. Self pre-operation USG always helps to enhance surgical performance on table especially in cases of multiple myomas. One can decide the number of myomas that can be taken out through a single incision. There is no tactile sensation in laparoscopy, so small myomas hidden under large myomas, if known beforehand, can be removed successfully.
- We do not advocate use of preoperative GnRH analogues to reduce the size of myoma but is practiced by few endoscopic surgeons.
- Traction on uterus downward with Allis′ forceps applied to anterior lip of cervix and upward countertraction on myoma with myoma screw, next to cleavage line will facilitate dissection.
- Myomas up to 5–6 cm can be delivered with colpotomy.
- Proper serosal approximation, hemostasis, clean pelvis at the end, early mobilization will help in prevention of postoperative adhesions.
- Instillation of vasopressin, speedy surgery, skillful and rapid suturing, good knot tying techniques will help to minimize bleeding.
- Occassionally, one can encounter excessive bleeding from vasopressin injection so one should keep in instilling vasopressin even while withdrawing the needle as shown.
- Hematoma, infection and tissue necrosis are the triad which can weaken the myomectomy scar.
- Avoid hematoma formation by proper obliteration of the dead space after myoma excision.
- Tissue necrosis can be avoided by not using excess cautery at the myoma bed. Instead the assistant can compress the tissue with non-traumatic grasper, till the surgeon inserts the suture material. This will help in stopping oozing from small veins and capillaries.
- Avoid infection by giving good antibiotic coverage and ensuring thorough lavage at the end of procedure.

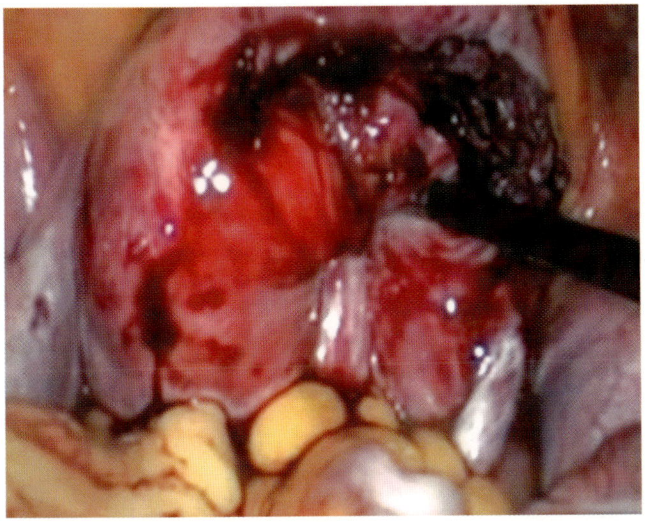

**Fig. 21.1:** The assistant can compress the tissue with nontraumatic grasper till the surgeon inserts the suture material: This willl help in stopping oozing small veins and capillaries

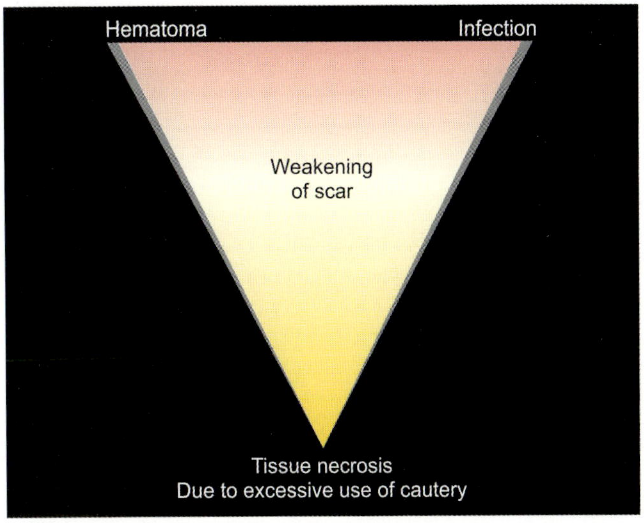


**Fig. 21.2**

## TIPS

- Incision for myomectomy- Vertical versus horizontal:
  - Those who perform suturing from ipsilateral port, prefer horizontal incision, whereas those who perform suturing from contralateral port prefer vertical incision.
  - In infertile women, we recommend assessing the size and site of myoma and then planning incision in such a way that it does not cause cornual damage.
    - In case of multiple myomas, incision should be planned in such a way that through one incision many myomas can be removed.
- Single versus multi-layer closure:
  - Whenever uterine cavity is opened, we suggest multi-layer closure: 1st Subendometrial-myometrial tissue (never to take endometrium), 2nd layer of myometrial tissue and 3rd layer of myometrial-serosal layer.
  - When the endometrial cavity is not opened, one can go for a single layer or multi-layer closure depending upon the size of the myoma bed. The aim here should be obliteration of the dead space and thus prevention of hematoma formation as seen in Figures 21.3A and B.
- To avoid opening of cavity:
  - For any intramural myoma causing depression of the cavity, we recommend enucleation of the myoma up to 60-70% and then irrigating with 100-200 cc of normal saline all around in the space beneath the myoma, so as to create a plane between the endometrium and myoma capsule.
  - The morbidity in pregnancy definitely differs when the cavity is opened, versus when it is not opened.

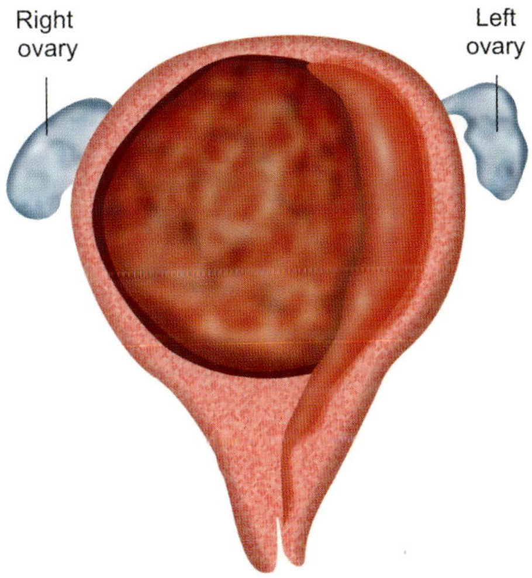


**Fig. 21.3A:** Diagrammatic representation of myoma abutting the endometrium

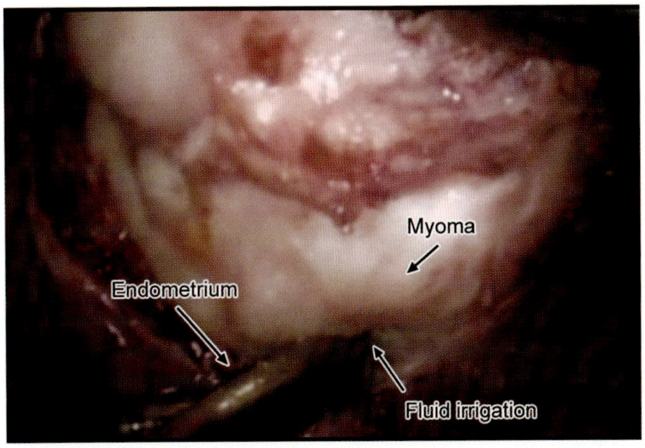


**Fig. 21.3B:** Hydrodissection technique to avoid opening of endometrial cavity in such cases

***The technique of laparoscopic myomectomy has to be modified according to the size, type, location, number and degenerative changes undergone by the myoma. It also has to be modified according to the experience of the surgeon and instruments available.***

## Laparoscopic Myomectomy

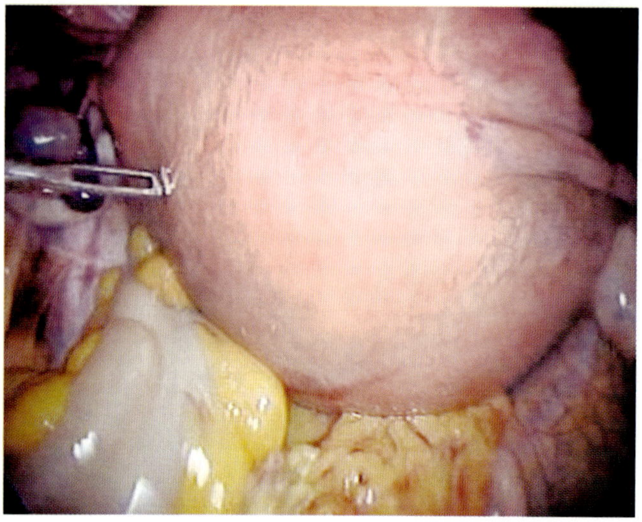

**Fig. 21.4:** Intramural myoma

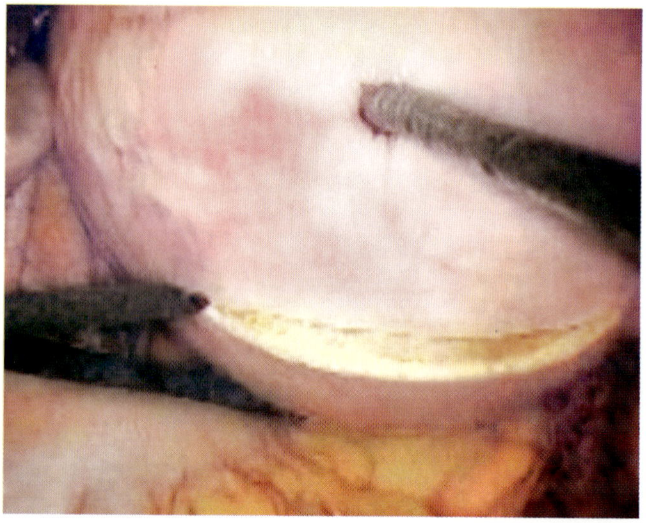

**Fig. 21.5:** Incision with monopolar hook after vasopressin instillation

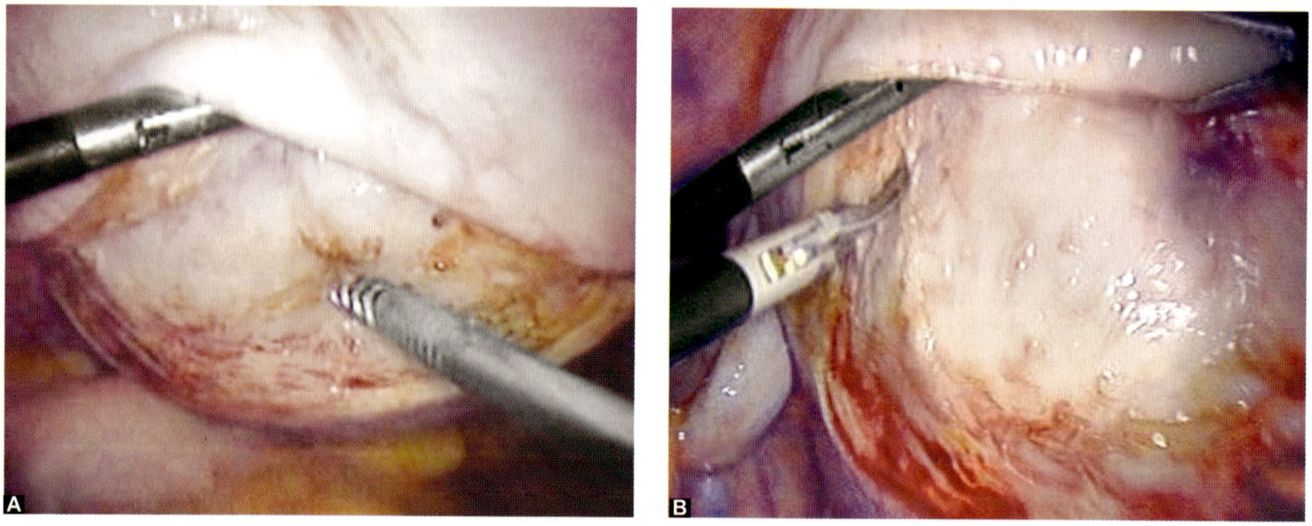



**Figs 21.6A and B:** Enucleation in process

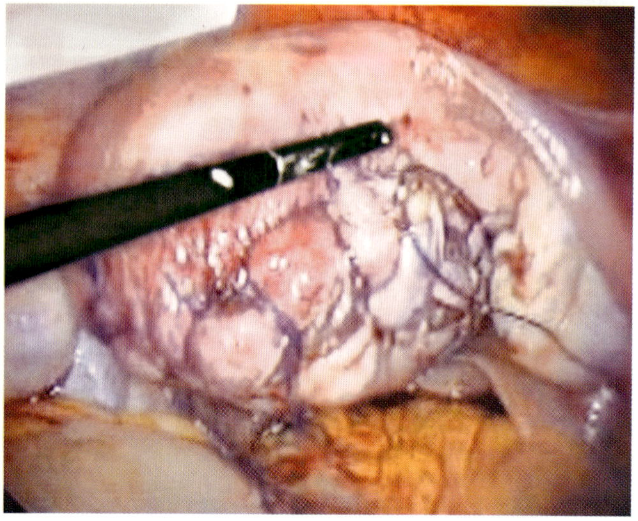

**Fig. 21.7:** End result

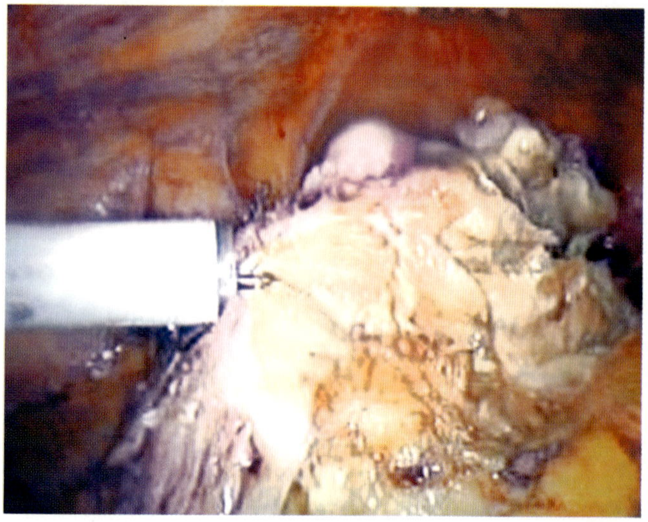

**Fig. 21.8:** Morcellation

## Removal of Large Posterocervical Fibroid

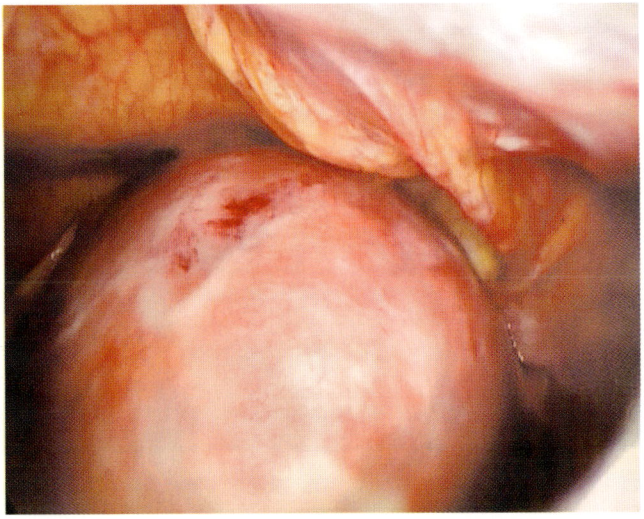

**Fig. 21.9:** Panoramic view

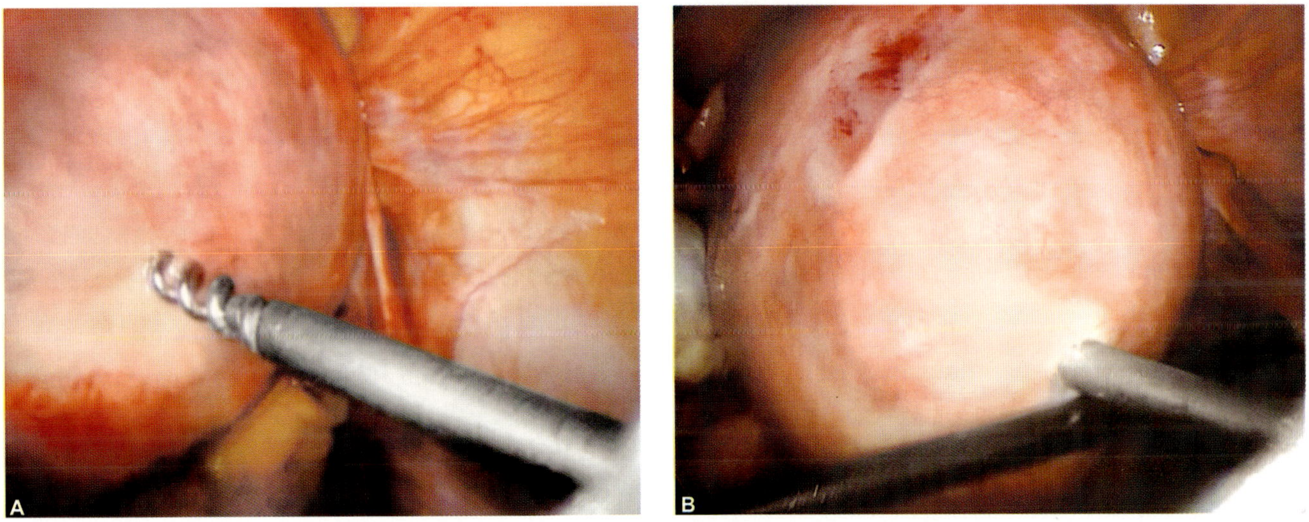

**Figs 21.10A and B:** Myomectomy made easier by deimpacting myoma with myoma screw. This step makes myoma accessible and easier for further extraction in routine way

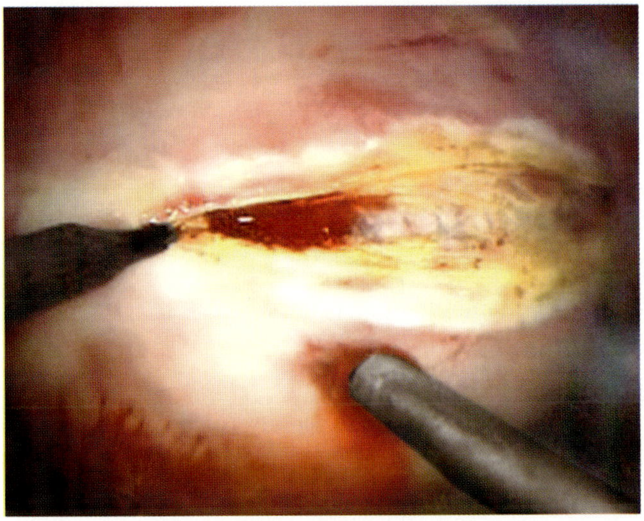

**Fig. 21.11:** Incision with monopolar hook

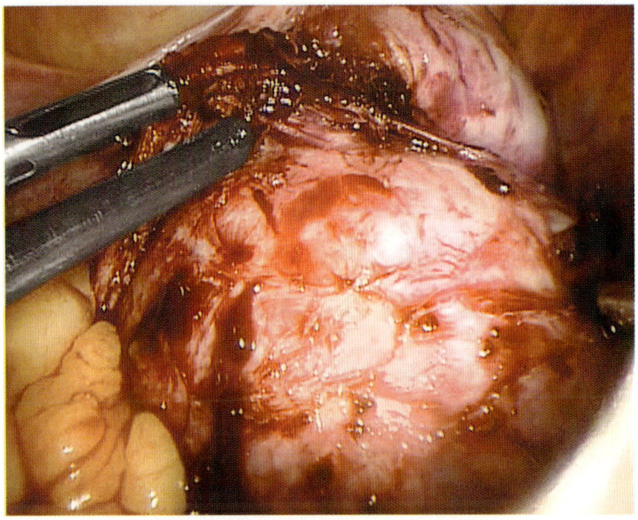

**Fig. 21.12:** Enucleation in process

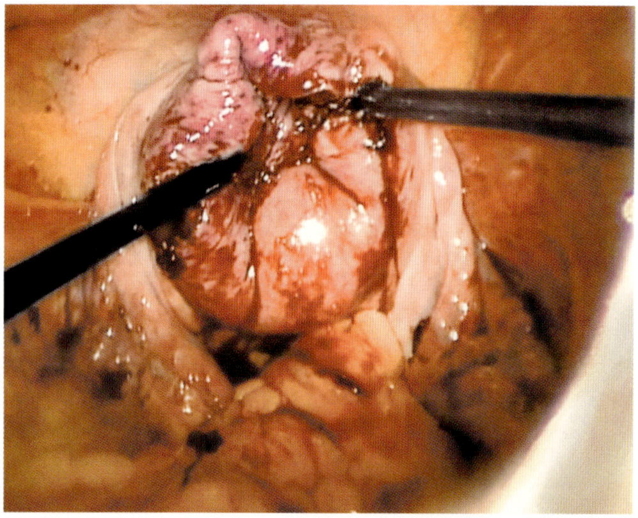

**Fig. 21.13:** Myoma bed compressed to allow stoppage of capillary oozing

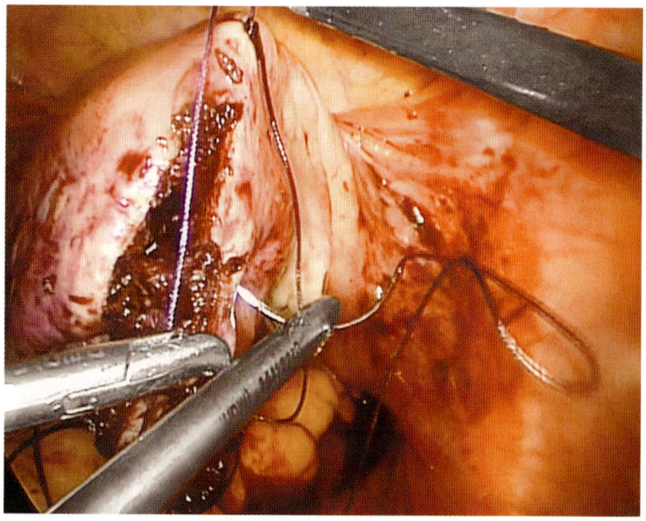

**Fig. 21.14:** Right angular stitch

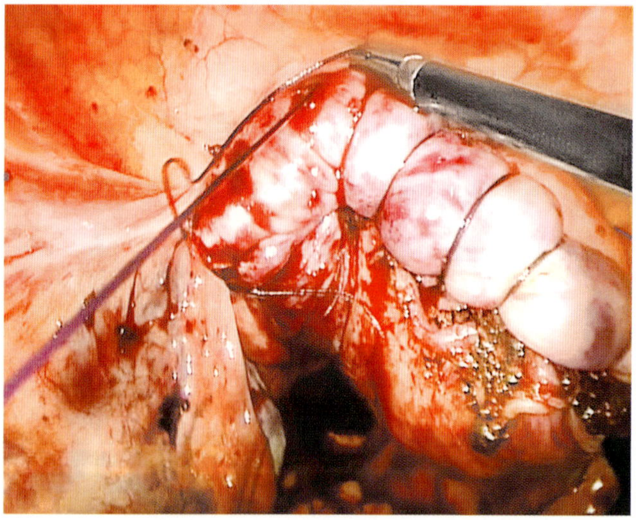

**Fig. 21.15:** Continuous locking sutures

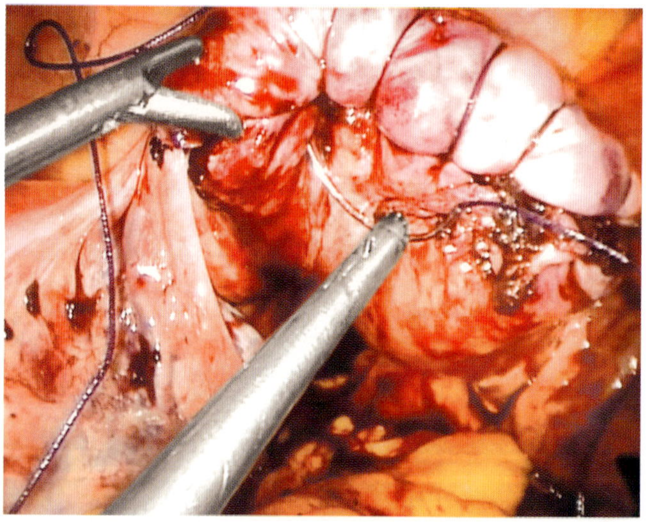

**Fig. 21.16:** Left angular stitch

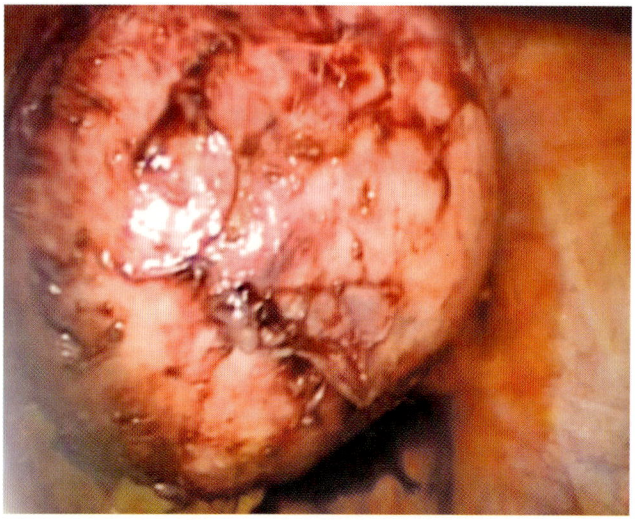

**Fig. 21.17:** Enucleated large myoma

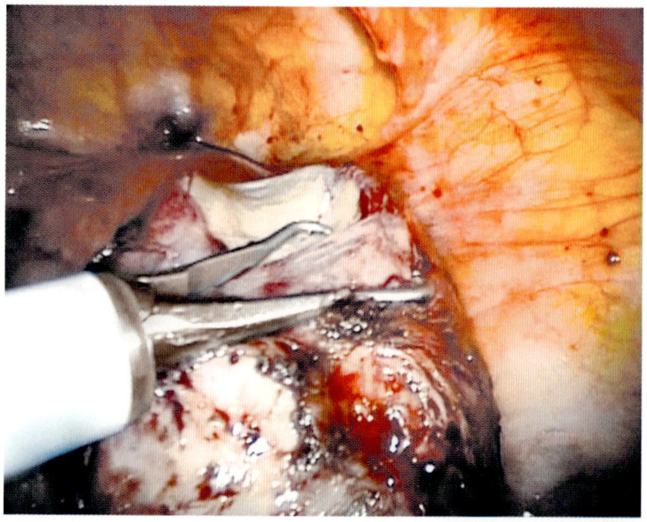

**Fig. 21.18:** Morcellation in progress

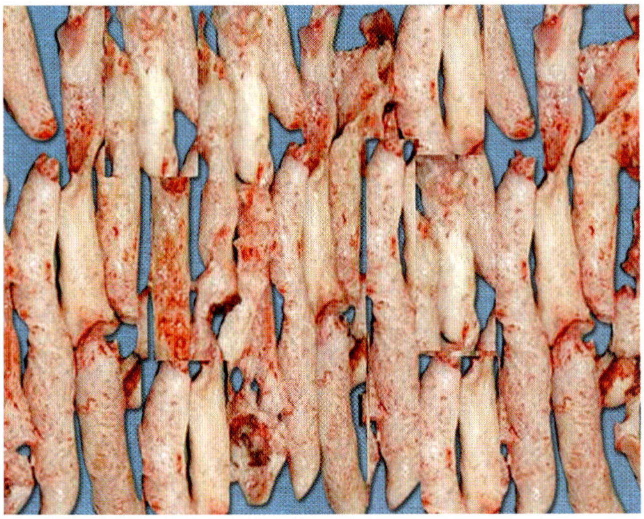

**Fig. 21.19:** Morcellated pieces

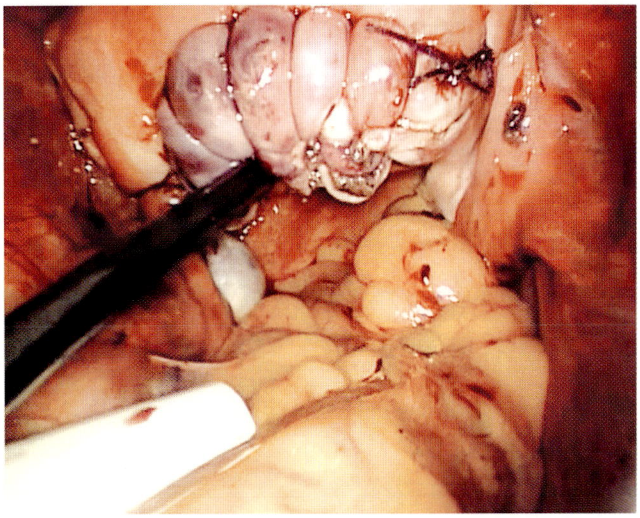

**Fig. 21.20:** End result has to be clean pelvis with good hemostasis

## Removal of Small Posterocervical Fibroid

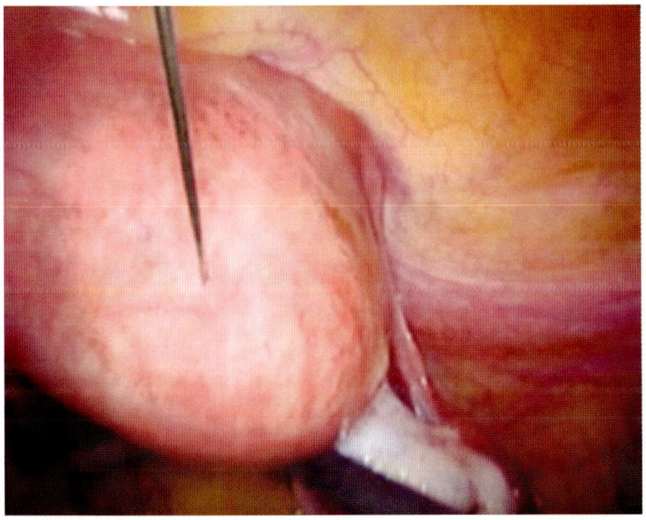

**Fig. 21.21:** In case of smaller posterior cervical fibroid accessibility can be achieved by just lifting and supporting myoma with grasper for vasopressin injection

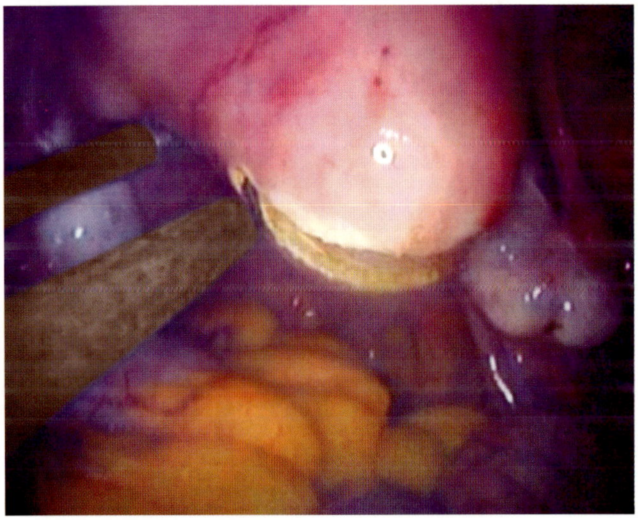

**Fig. 21.22:** Incision with monopolar hook

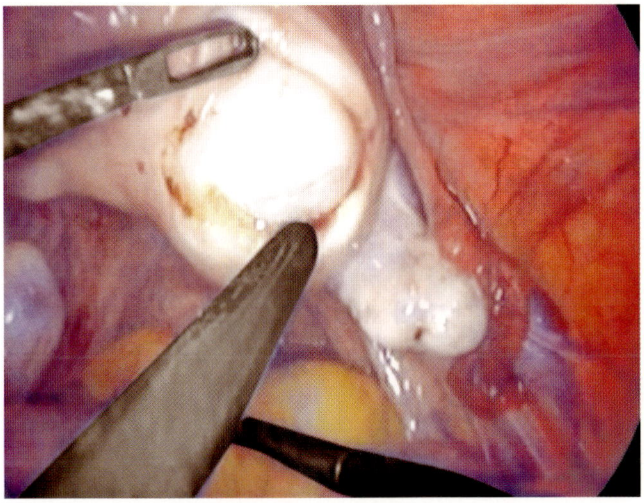

**Fig. 21.23:** Separation of capsule of fibroid

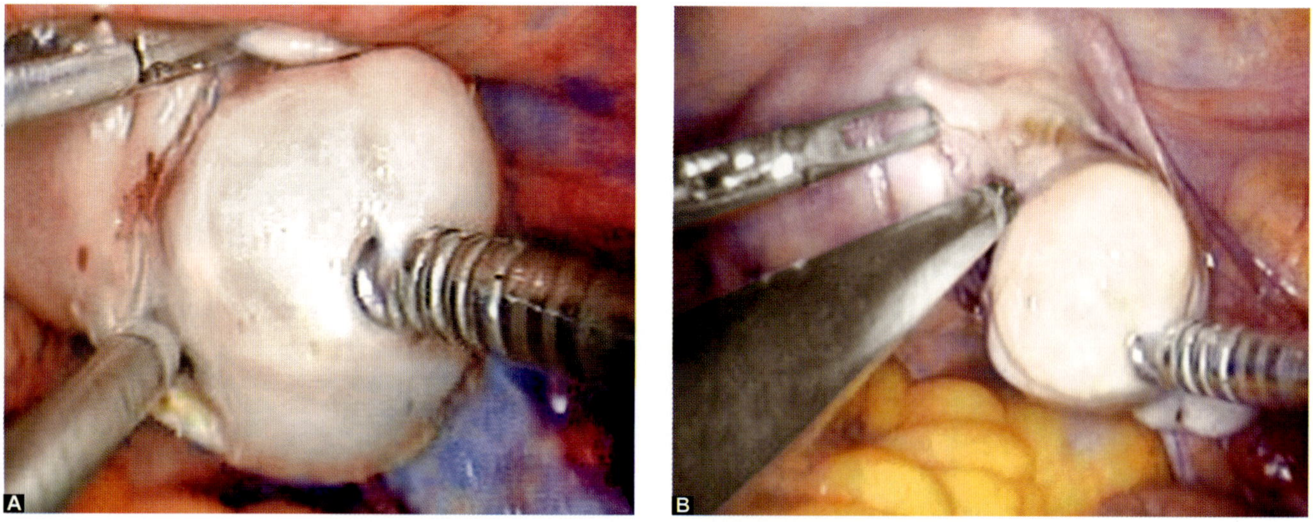

Figs 21.24A and B: Enucleation in process

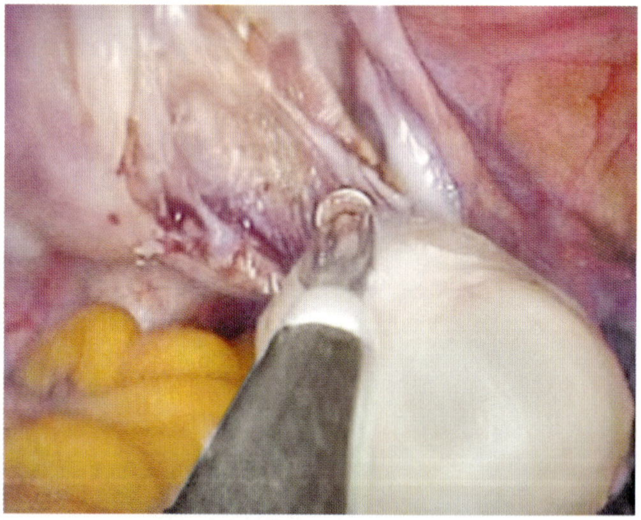

Fig. 21.25: Enucleation completed

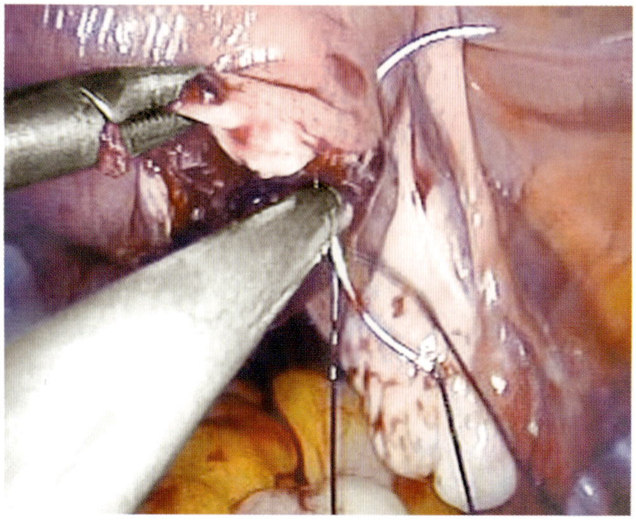

Fig. 21.26: Suturing

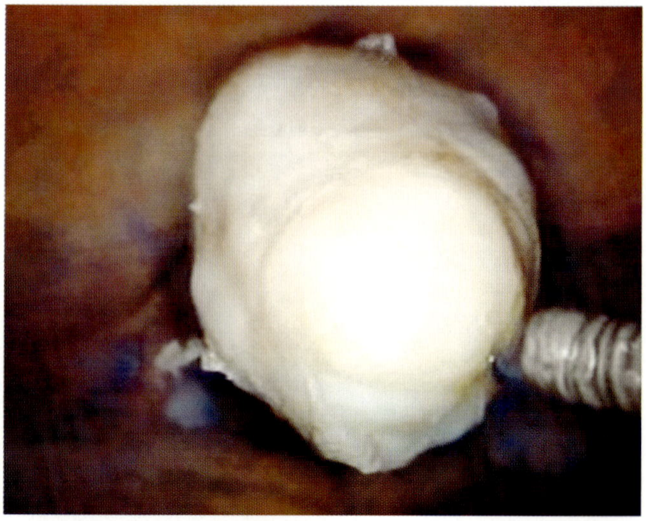

Fig. 21.27: Enucleated myoma of this size can be removed through colpotomy

## Myomectomy with Vertical Incision

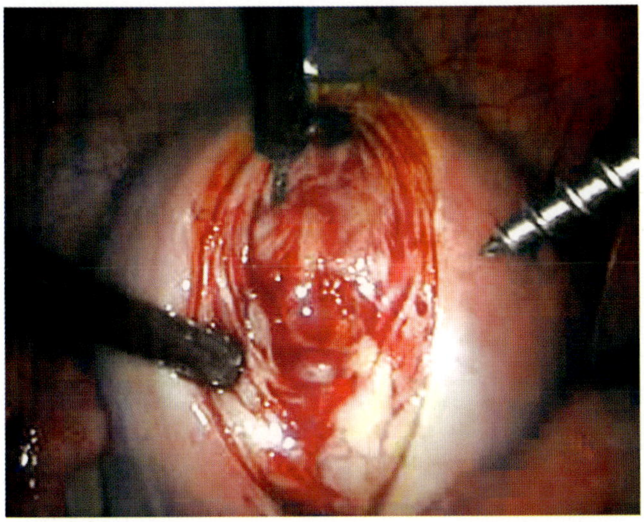

**Fig. 21.28:** Incising the myometrium

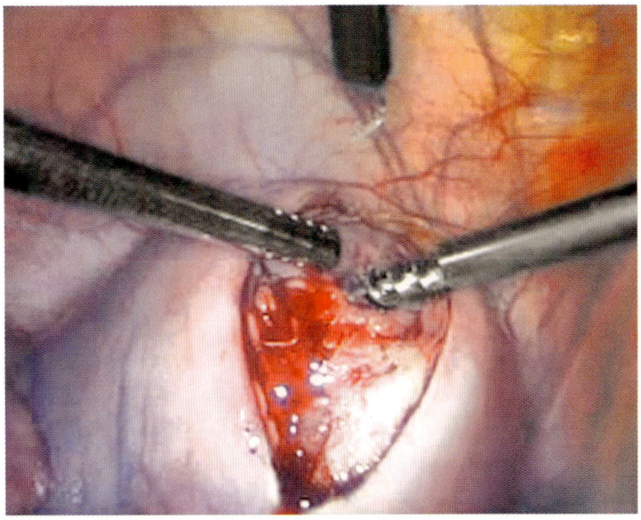

**Fig. 21.29:** Enucleating the myoma

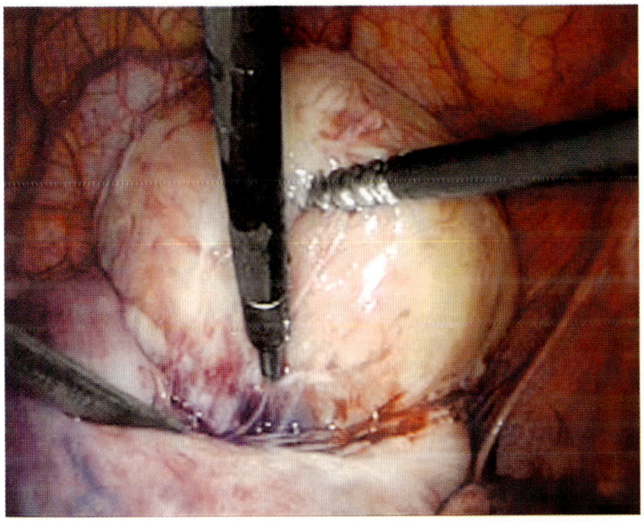

**Fig. 21.30:** Coagulation of vessels of myoma bed

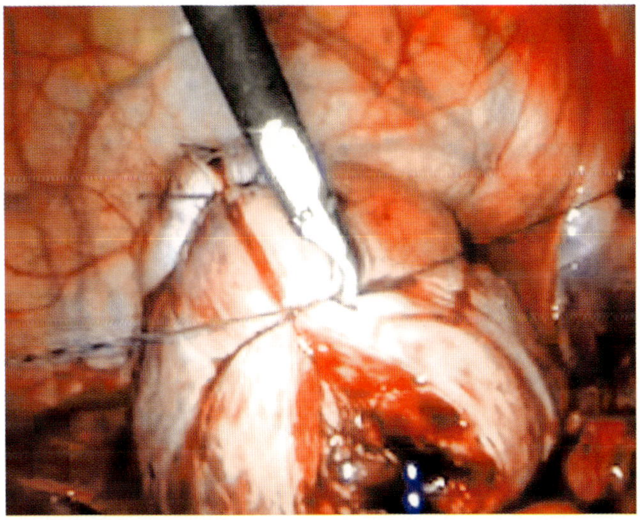

**Fig. 21.31:** Re-approximating the myometrium using intracorporeal sutures

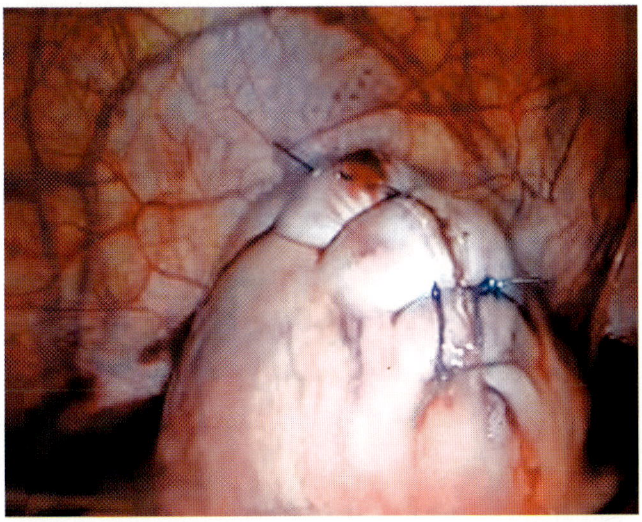

**Fig. 21.32:** End result

# Various Myomas

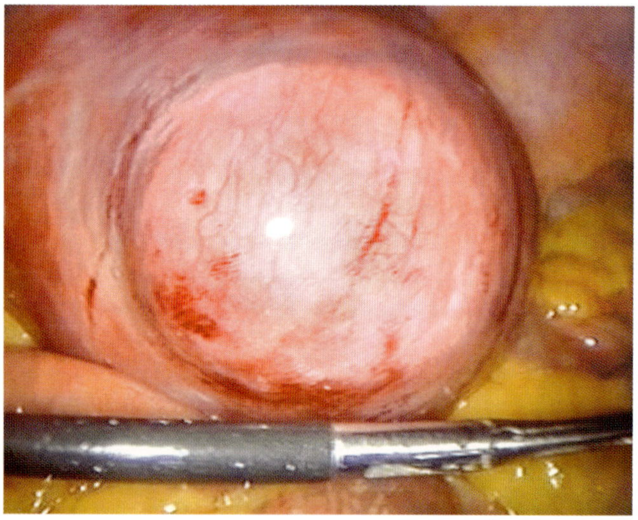

**Fig. 21.33:** Myoma above myoma

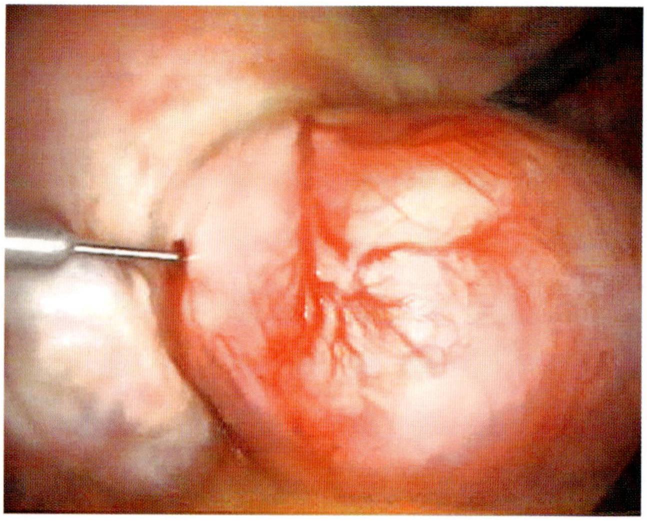

**Fig. 21.34:** Vascular myoma

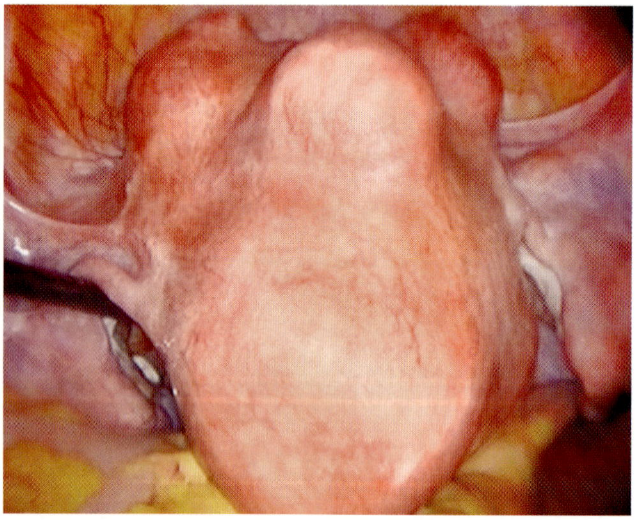

**Fig. 21.35:** Multiple myomas

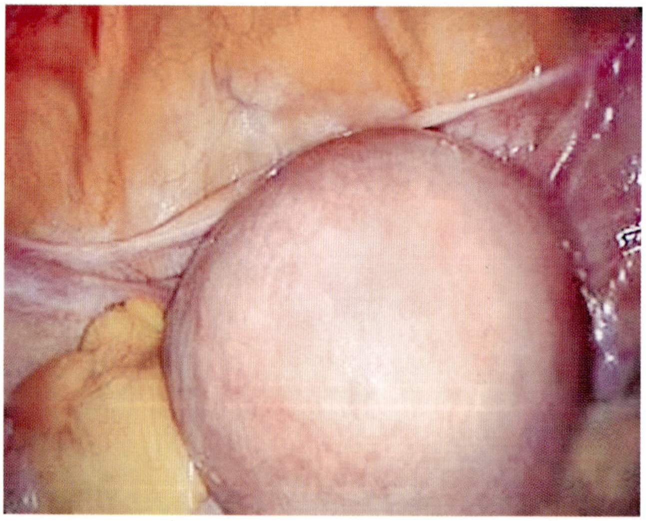

**Fig. 21.36:** Fundal intramural globular myoma

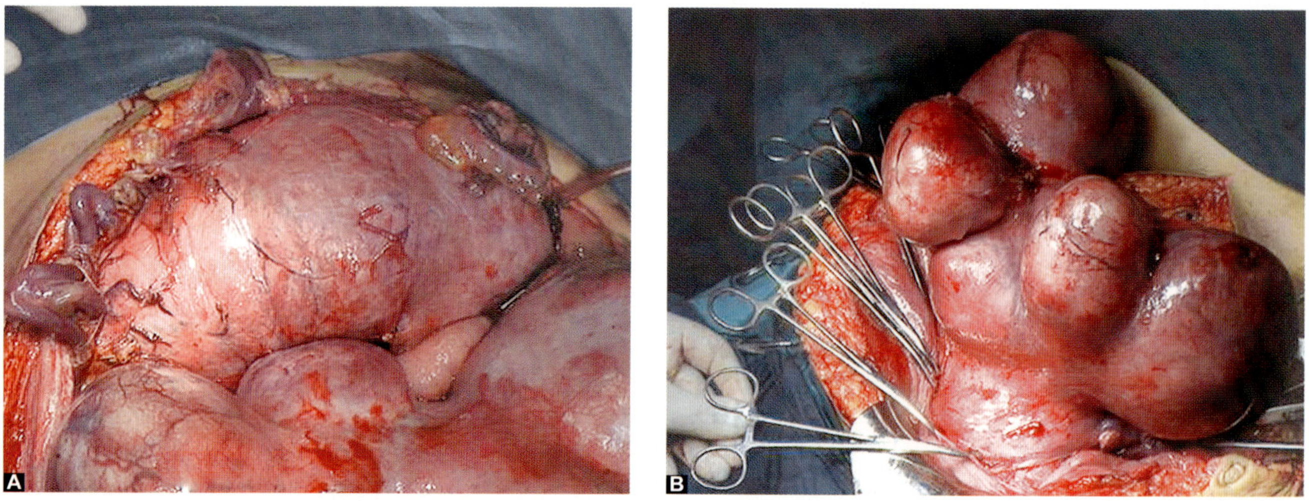

**Figs 21.37A and B:** Few myomas can not be tackled by laparoscopy

Chapter 22

# Laparoscopic Myomectomy for Intramural Fibroids

*Rafique Parkar*

## DEFINITION

- Procedure to extract a uterine fibroid from its pseudocapsule and bed.
- Extra-abdominal retrieval of the fibroid either by morcellation, enlargement of the abdominal port site incision, a posterior colpotomy or a "minilap incision".
- Adequate apposition, repair and restoration of the uterine defect.

## INTRODUCTION

Laparoscopic myomectomy has been a subject of considerable debate over the decades. Semm and Mettler first reported the laparoscopic removal of a subserous myoma in 1977. In the 1990s, the laparoscopic removal of intramural myomas was standardized. The challenging procedure required advanced laparoscopic skills and expertise.

Laparoscopic myomectomy is now the accepted norm and is regarded as the" gold standard" and valid option for approaching uterine fibroids that are related to menorrhagia or compromised fertility provided the surgical team has acquired significant skills in suturing.

## INDICATIONS

- Preservation of fertility and future child bearing.
- Menorrhagia, menstrual abnormalities including inter-menstrual bleeding.
- Pressure symptoms in large fibroids resulting from compression of the bowl, bladder or ureters (with renal backflow changes).
- Poor obstetric performance.
- Abdominopelvic pain and distortion.
- Dysmenorrhea, dyspareunia.

## CONTRAINDICATIONS

- Laparoscopic myomectomy is a safe and feasible procedure in adequately trained and experienced hands.
- Innially the number, size and location of fibroids were considered as limiting factors.
- The success of the laparoscopic approach is generally related to the level of expertise attained in suturing, microsurgical techniques and the development of efficient electric morcellators.
- The absence of significant coexisting adenomyosis enhances success of the procedure.
- Dissection of the fibroids should be performed ideally without opening the uterine cavity.
- Myomectomy in obese patients or with previous surgeries and large multiple fibroids require significant experience.
- Anesthetic contraindications and the presence of co-morbid conditions would be limiting factors especially if a prolonged procedure is anticipated.

## ADVANTAGES

- Short hospital stays, quick postoperative recovery, faster return to work.
- Reduced postoperative discomfort and pain requiring rescue analgesia.
- Reduced postoperative febrile morbidity.
- Reduced hemoglobin drop and postoperative transfusion rates.
- Decreased postoperative peritubal and periovarian adhesion formation.
- Significantly higher fertility rates and outcomes.

## PRINCIPLES FOR A GOOD LAPAROSCOPIC MYOMECTOMY

- Gentle and atraumatic handling of the uterus, respect all surgical planes.
- Adequately plan uterine incisions avoid multiple incisions and excising any redundant serosa and myometrium.
- Dissect, develop and extend the cleavage plane separating the myoma from adjacent myometrium.
- Sparing use of electrocoagulation for hemostasis, should be site specific and not global.
- Meticulous obliteration of the dead space using full thickness sutures with good approximation or a multi layered closure so as to avoid any secondary constitution of deep myometrial hematomas.

## PREOPERATIVE EVALUATION/PREPARATION

1. Routine blood works along with a good ultrasound, pelvic or TVS and a MRI (during the early secretory phase) to determine the location, size and number of the myomas adequately mapping them. A hysterosalpingogram is advised.
2. The use of preoperative GnRH agonists to reduce the intraoperative blood loss, to facilitate the myomectomy and shorten the operating time is not advisable as this may cause the myomas to degenerate, render the cleavage plane to be obscured and more adherent hence increasing the operating times, blood loss, transfusion and conversion rates significantly. The increased recurrence of myomas have also been implicated.
3. Soft to liquid diet on the day prior to surgery then nil orally 8 to 12 hours prior to surgery
4. Laxatives (Peglec, Exelyte, Picolax) taken on the previous evening.
5. Prior anesthetic and cardiac evaluation, if indicated.
6. Admission on the day of surgery.

### Position of Patient

- Patient is placed flat with a modified lithotomy position at the time of trochar entry which is then converted to a deep Trendelenburg position once safe entry has been achieved.
- Allen stirrups with adjustable and padded leg rests are advised.
- Bladder catheterization.
- Intraoperative hysteroscopy is advised.

### Specific Equipment and Instrumentation

- Complete laparoscopic tower with camera, high flow insufflator, light source, electrocautery unit and aquapurator.
- Morcellator.
- Two to three 5 mm trochars, one or two 10 mm trochars, one to two 15 or 20 mm trochars with their relevant reducers.
- Atraumatic graspers, claw forceps, tenaculums (5 mm and 10 mm).
- Scissors (tissue cutting and suture cutting).
- Bipolar forceps, monopolar spatula or hook, harmonic scalpel.
- Uterine manipulator (optional), myoma spiral.
- Pair of needle holders, adequate sutures.
- Suction/irrigation cannula.
- Laparoscopic injection needle.

## SURGICAL PROCEDURE

### Port Placement

1. Port placement depends on the surgeon's preference particularly in relation to their suturing abilities.
2. Veress needle, direct trocar entry or Hasson's open technique at Palmer's or Lee-Huang's point or intra-umbilical depending on the size and number of fibroids.
3. A general rule is to have the camera port at least 4 to 5 fingers breadth above the dominant fibroid.
4. The secondary ports (5 mm) are placed under direct vision, 2 to 4 as preferred by the surgeon.
5. One of the secondary ports is subsequently converted to a 10 mm trochar at the end of the procedure to accommodate the morcellator.

### Surgical Steps

1. Once the laparoscope is inserted, the abdominal cavity is scanned for adhesions and any coexisting pathologies.
2. The uterus is examined for the number, location and size of the fibroids.
3. A laparoscopic ultrasound probe is beneficial to locate deep seated fibroids.
4. Interventions on the uterine arteries such as laparoscopic uterine artery dissection, clipping, ligation or cauterization, uterine artery embolization or the placement of a pericervical mechanical tourniquet have been advocated. Some authors advise the temporary occlusion of the uterine arteries at their origin with clips, especially for large and multiple fibroids.
5. The use of a vasoconstrictive agent (POR 8 solution [8, ornithine vasopressin]: 5 IU in 50 mL of saline, Pitressin [8, Arginine vasopressin]: 20 U in 10–40 mL of saline or glypressin (triglycyl-lysine vasopressin) followed by instillation of copious amounts of normal saline (400 to 600 mL) into the serosa overlying the prominant dominant fibroid until significant blanching is attained, is effective as this facilitates hydrodissection, provides a clear view of the plane and allows for a faster and easier enucleation of the fibroid with significantly less blood loss.

6. The solution should be injected into the area of least resistance as this signifies the correct plane between myoma and its psuedocapsule.
7. Instillation is undertaken through one puncture only as this enables a good tamponade effect and allows the solution to spread adequately between the fibroid and pseudocapsule thereby enhancing this plane clearly.
8. This limits the use of bipolar electrocautery, reduces the intraoperative blood loss and the subsequent need for transfusions.
9. The use of bupivacaine hydrochloride 0.25% with 0.5 mL of epinephrine injected into the uterosaccral or round ligaments has been shown to reduce intra-operative blood loss, operating times and post-operative pain by facilitating myoma enucleation. However the effect wears off only after 5 to 6 hours reducing accurate hemostasis and may cause delayed postoperative bleeding and tissue necrosis due to prolonged hypo-oxygenation.
10. A transcervical chromotubation is performed before initiating the myomectomy.
11. Identify the dominant fibroid and carefully plan the uterine incisions. As a general rule, anterior fibroids are approached through a vertical or oblique incision and posterior fibroids through a transverse or vertical incision since this facilitates effective suturing.
12. Elliptical incisions are preferred for large fundal fibroids. Advocates of transverse incisions claim that these incisions cause less bleeding and better healing with less adhesion formation since the main arterial vessels of the myometrium which run horizontally are avoided.
13. Uterine incisions can be achieved by sharp dissection, monopolar hook or spatula (30 to 60 W unblended cutting current), a harmonic scalpel or spatula or laser and are made generously over the serosa and myometrium up to the pearly white surface of the myoma along its entire dominant dome length.
14. The myoma is then gently teased along the inside of the avascular plane between the pseudocapsule and the surrounding myoma creating a significant space and progressively increasing the same retracting the myometrium away from the fibroid.
15. The myoma is then grasped and stabilized as low as possible close to the bed by a strong grasping forceps (claw or tenaculum) or the myoma spiral and is pulled and rotated away from the floor of the uterine bed (as opening a sardine can).
16. At the same time, the uterine incision is pushed away from the fibroid using a rigid instrument like the suction irrigation cannula, progressively increasing the the depth of the defect and at the same time gently lifting the fibroid off its bed.
17. It is a good trick to tackle the fibers within the bed of the myoma with a bipolar forceps or the harmonic scalpel so as to promptly control and avoid any undue hemorrhage from feeder vessels at the base of the fibroid.
18. Once the fibroid is delivered, the bed is inspected for any obvious hemorrhage. Cauterization should be site specific and not global or indiscriminate so as to enable good scar integrity. Avoid excessive charring of the myometrium as this compromises scar healing and integrity and may be a risk factor for scar dehiscence in future pregnancies.
19. Any residual fibroids should be tunneled through the primary incision since this avoids a hematoma formation.
20. Avoid trimming off any redundant or excessive serosa or myometrial tissue since spontaneous involution is evident within a week and scar integrity is maintained and strength enhanced.

## Suturing

1. Most challenging part of the procedure and is highly surgeon specific.
2. Single plane by full thickness vertical mattress interrupted or continuous vicryl, PGA or PDS sutures by the intracorporeal or extracorporeal method. These sutures are applied as a vertical "purse string" or figure of "8" sutures taking adequate bites of the walls and including deep sutures in the bed of the defect.
3. Two layered or multilayered closure using the barbed sutures.
4. The sutures are placed sufficiently close to each other approximating the edges adequately without any excessive tension. Inadequate repair of the defect compromises scar integrity and may result in future dehiscence or uteroperitoneal fistulae.
5. When the cavity has been breeched or the defect is deep, suturing in two planes with deep interrupted and superficial sutures is advised.
6. A transverse U-shaped transfixing stitch that runs through the uterine serosa taking the full thickness of the myometrium, with a vicryl 1 suture on a large curved needle provides additional hemostasis (Hason's stitch)
7. The most important factor for a successful laparoscopic myomectomy is to avoid any dead space which would invite a hematoma formation, invert the edges and restore uterine wall and suture line integrity so as to minimize subsequent adhesion formation and scar dehiscence.
8. Suturing can be ipsilateral or contralateral depending on the surgeon's preferences.
9. Avoiding sutures along the endometrium prevents prolonged bleeding, synechiae formation, and iatrogenic adenomyosis.

## Morcellation

Several techniques have been described to extract the fibroids. These include:

- Direct port extraction.

- Intra-abdominal morcellation using scissors, cold knife or electric morcellators.
- Posterior colpotomy with or without cold knife morcellation or debulking.
- Mini-laparotomy.

### Conversion

At any point during the procedure conversion should be considered in the best interest of the patients especially in the presence of excessive hemorrhage. With increased surgical experience and confidence, these rates usually decrease over a period of time.

### Adhesion Barriers

- Copious irrigation, evacuate obvious clots.
- Relook at suture lines, trim exposed sutures lengths.
- The risk of postoperative adhesions is reduced in laparoscopic myomectomy by the use of adhesion barriers, Interceed, Gore Tex, Seprafilm and may be regarded as an adjuvant.
- This does not replace good surgical technique and adequate hemostasis.

### Postoperative Management

#### *Routine Observations*

- Postoperative Misoprostol (Cytotec) 4 tablets rectally facilitates a reduction in blood loss or postoperative hematoma formation and maintains a firmly contracted uterus.
- Routine antibiotics and analgesia.
- There are many risk factors proposed for scar dehiscence and rupture during pregnancy and labor.
- Pregnancy rates after laparoscopic myomectomy are significantly higher when compared to myomectomy by laparotomy.

### Tips and Tricks to Optimize Results

- Appropriate patient selection in keeping with one's level of expertise.
- Good surgical technique, develop and respect the planes of surgical dissection.
- Achieve good hemostasis.
- Avoid overzealous use of cautery.
- Good tissue approximation, obliterate the dead space and prevent any hematoma formation.

### Recurrence Rate of Myomas

The recurrence rates following laparoscopic myomectomy are difficult to ascertain but should be considered when symptoms are not alleviated or desired fertility has not been achieved. The systematic use of the ultrasound, color Doppler or a second look laparoscopy to determine scar integrity and possible recurrence is advisable.

### Modifications of Techniques of Laparoscopic Myomectomy

- Laparoscopically-assisted myomectomy.
- Laparoscopically-assisted vaginal myomectomy.
- Single incision laparoscopic myomectomy.
- Robotic myomectomy.

## CONCLUSION

Laparoscopic myomectomy has always been a subject of great debate.

Has the reputation of being technically long, difficult and is associated with excessive blood loss along with a high risk of conversion to laparotomy.

The scars during subsequent obstetric performance have been subjected to minute scrutiny. However, the risk of uterine rupture is low and many studies have now proved that good quality scars can be obtained with minimal use of electrosurgery and sound endosuturing techniques.

The use of hormonal tourniquets and methods to control the uterine artery have reduced the risk of hemorrhage.

The size of the myomas tackled has increased with surgical expertise and good team coordination.

Advances in electric morcellators have helped achieve to reduce operating times.

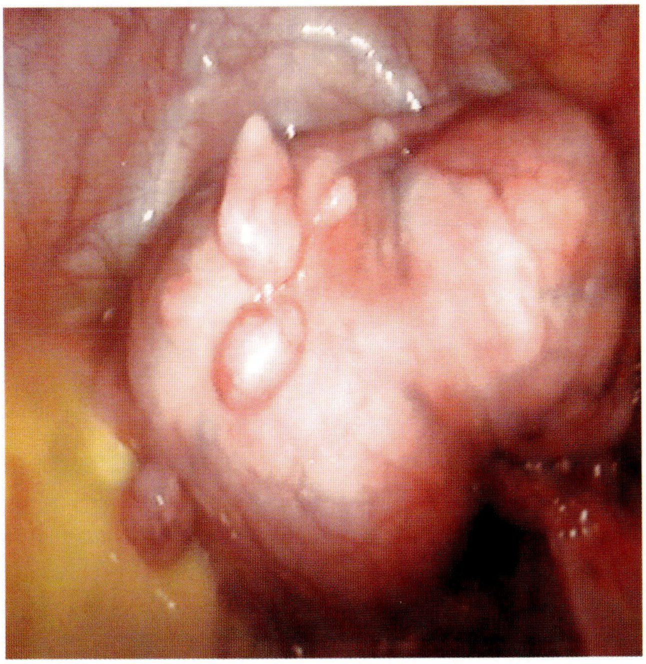

**Fig. 22.1:** Appearance of the uterus with fibroids before myomectomy

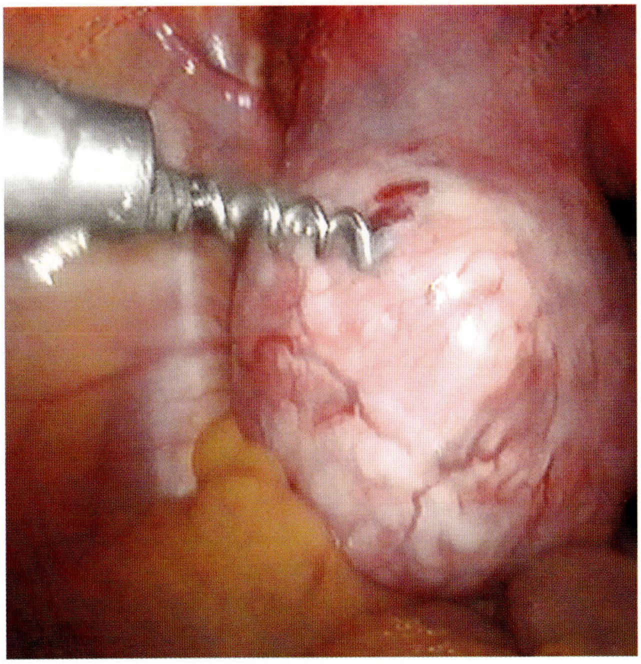

**Fig. 22.2:** A posterior wall fibroid approximately 6 cm held with a myoma spiral

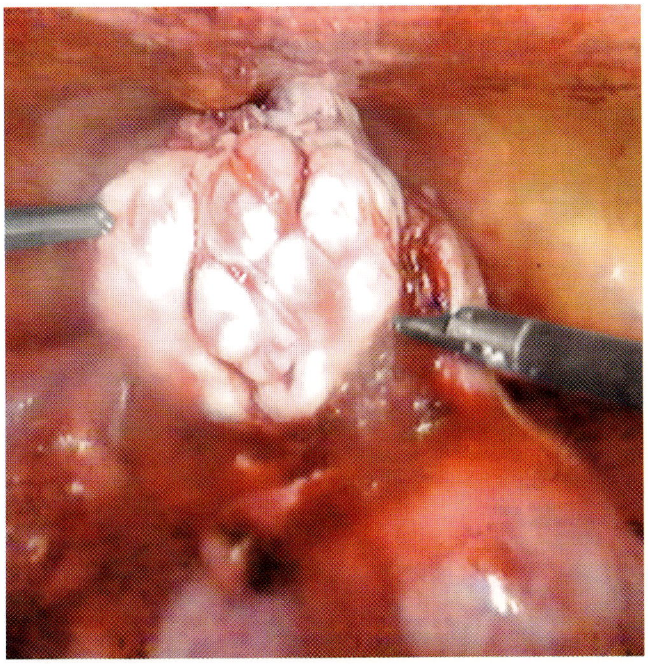

**Fig. 22.3:** Removal of an intramural fibroid with breach of the uterine cavity

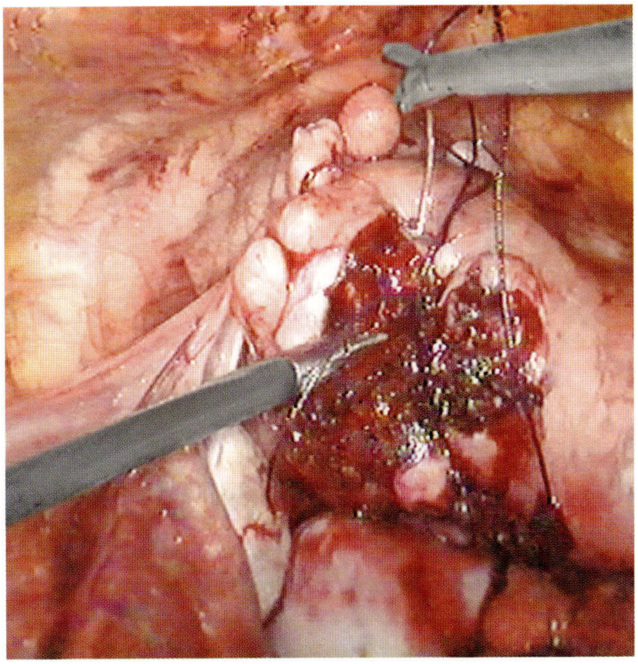

**Fig. 22.4:** Suturing of the of the myomectomy site

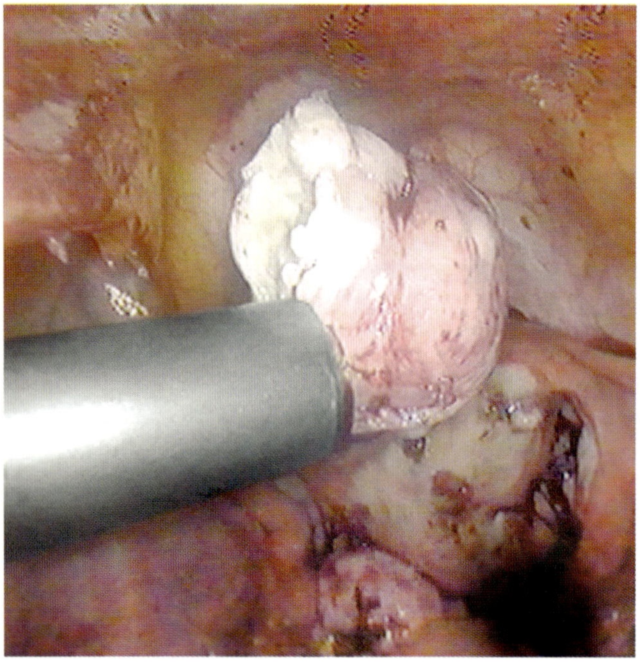

**Fig. 22.5:** Morcellation of the myomas

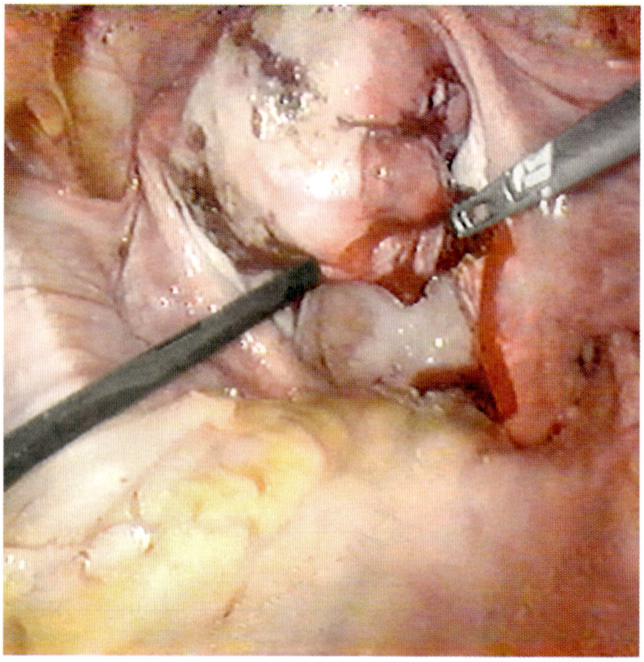

**Fig. 22.6:** Appearance of the uterus after myomectomy

## Laparoscopic Myomectomy for Intramural Myoma

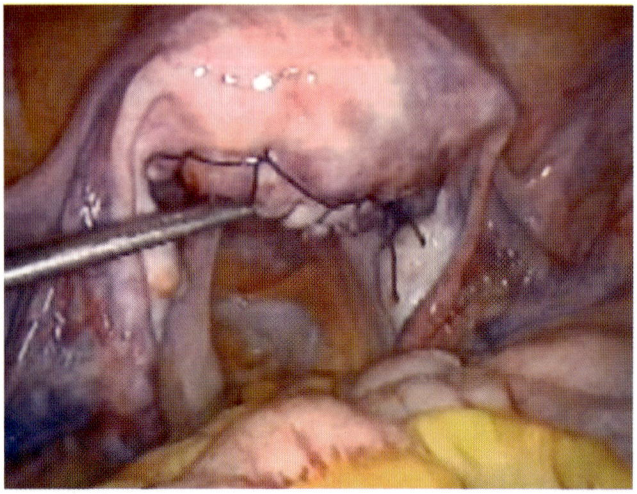

**Fig. 22.7:** Posterior wall intramural myoma

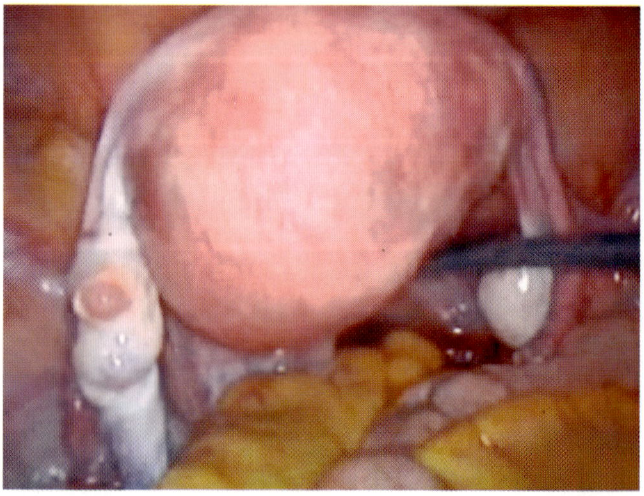

**Fig. 22.8:** Horizontal incision taken over the myoma

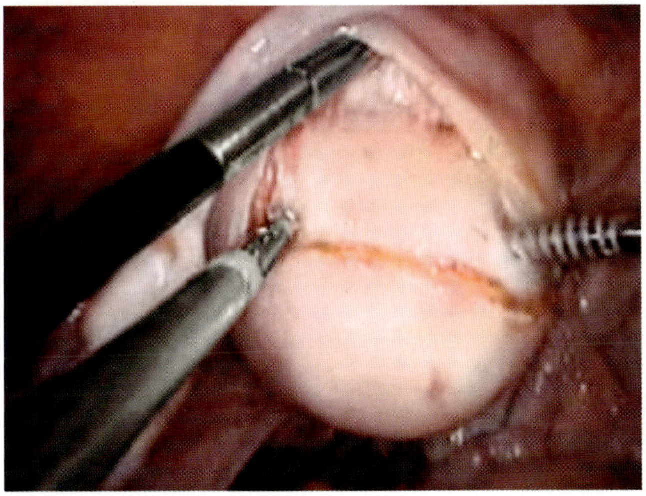

**Fig. 22.9:** Enucleation of myoma by traction and countertraction

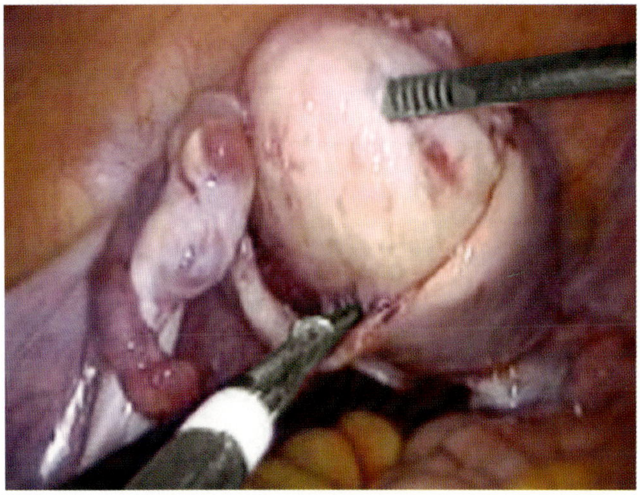

**Fig. 22.10:** End result

Chapter 23

# Laparoscopic Management of Benign Ovarian Mass

*Prakash Trivedi*

## PREOPERATIVE EVALUATION

- Diagnosis with a thorough history and clinical examination (per vaginal, per rectal).
- Routine blood investigation.
- Tumor markers—Ca125/CEA/alpha fetoprotein/beta hCG.
- Transvaginal sonography .
- Color Doppler to rule out malignancy.

After confirming that the ovarian cyst is benign, laparoscopic ovarian cystectomy can be done.

## PREOPERATIVE PREPARATION

No specific preparation is required.

## LAPAROSCOPIC OVARIAN CYSTECTOMY

A standard 10 mm laparoscope is introduced with 3 side ports, 2 on the left side and one on the right side.

Intraoperatively, cell washings from the pelvis and upper abdomen should be collected and sent for evaluation to rule out malignancy.

Characteristics of the mass, age of the patient should be seen and decision taken, whether to do oophorectomy or cystectomy.

In ovarian cystectomy, it is necessary to remove the cyst intact with minimal trauma to the residual ovarian tissue.

1. If a cyst is larger than 10 cm in size, then first with 18-gauge needle fluid in pouch of Douglas is aspirated and sent for cytologic examination.
2. Cyst wall is identified and separated from ovarian tissue by applying two claw forceps on the cyst wall and ovarian wall each and pulled apart.
3. Claw forceps are advanced from time-to-time next to the cleavage line for proper dissection and to avoid tearing of healthy ovarian tissue.
4. Cyst is punctured and opening is increased so as to accommodate suction irrigation cannula. Fluid is sucked out and inner cyst wall is examined. Bipolar forceps is used to control the bleeding at the base of the capsule.
5. A densely adherent cyst may require sharp dissection to completely free the cyst wall.
6. After removing or excising the cyst, the cyst can be removed intact by following methods:
   i. Removal in Endobag/Lapsac
   ii. Removal in a probe cover or nonlubricated sterile condom
   iii. Colpotomy.

## POLYCYSTIC OVARIAN DRILLING

- Ovary is stabilized by holding its ligament with nontraumatic grasper.
- Insulated PCOD needle is passed through left upper port and placed perpendicular to ovarian surface with power set at 20–40 watt in cutting mode.
- Ovary at prominent follicle is then punctured with 4–6 punctures for 2 seconds, 1 cm away from each other in each ovary at the depth of 2–3 mm to prevent deep penetration.
- Then ovaries are lavaged with ringer lactate solution. Any bleeding points at punctured site are seen under water flow and tackled.

Thorough lavage at the end, will avoid postoperative adhesion.

**TIPS**

- During drilling, area close to the ovarian pedicle should be avoided to prevent jeopardizing ovarian blood supply.
- 4–6 holes are sufficient for achieving hypoandrogenism.
- Hysteroscopy should be done in all the cases since fair number of PCOS have concomitant uterine septum.

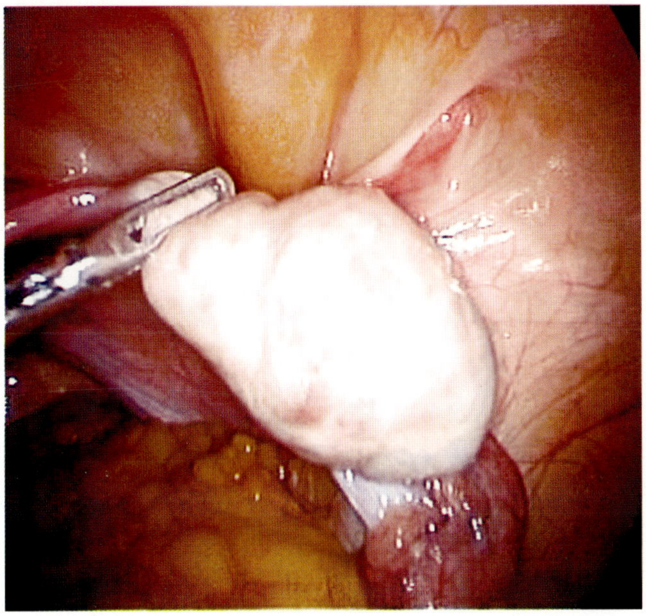

**Fig. 23.1:** Right polycystic ovary

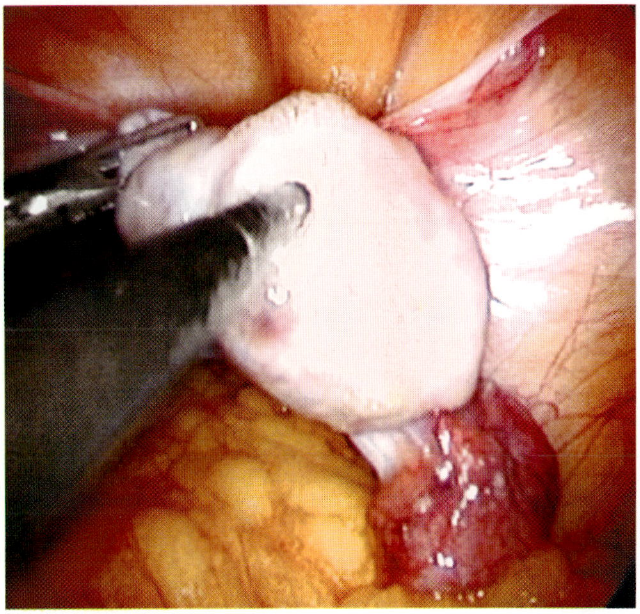

**Fig. 23.2:** Cysts punctured with insulated PCO drilling needle

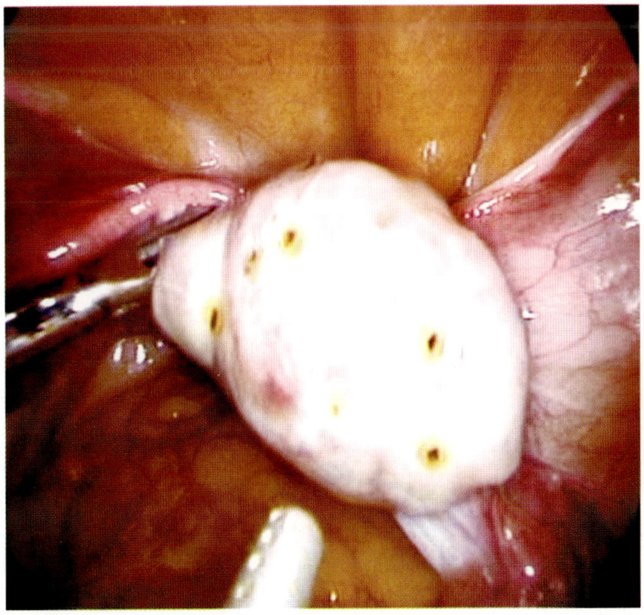

**Fig. 23.3:** End result

## Simple Ovarian Cystectomy

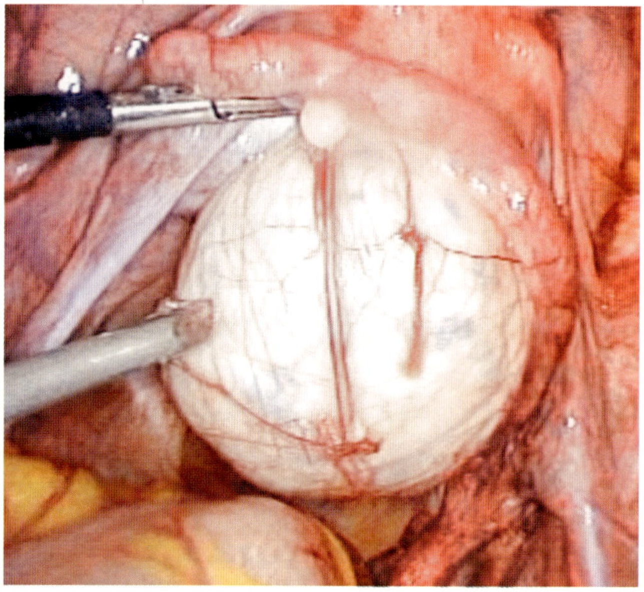

**Fig. 23.4:** A 30-year-old-female with left ovarian cyst ~ 7 cm not responding to oral contraceptive pills. Tumor markers and Doppler normal

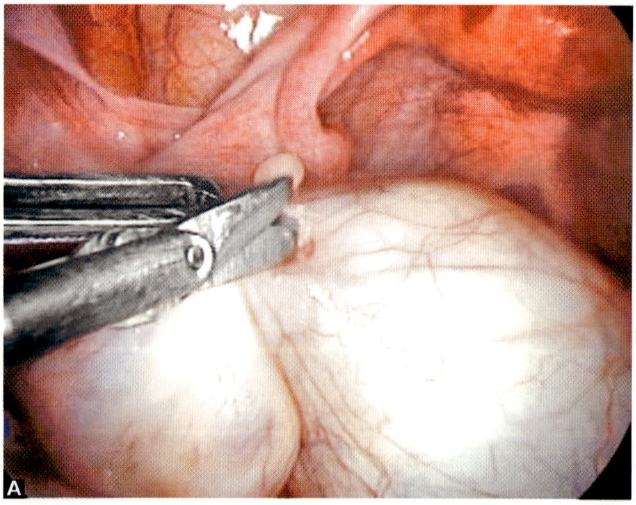

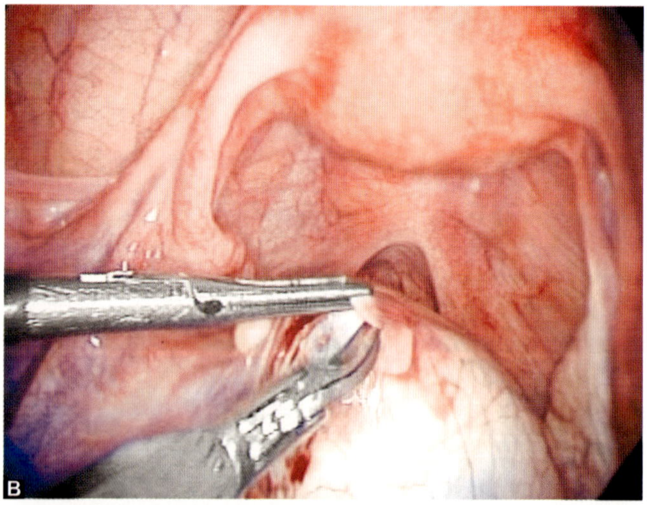

**Figs 23.5A and B:** Cyst wall incised with scissors and dissected

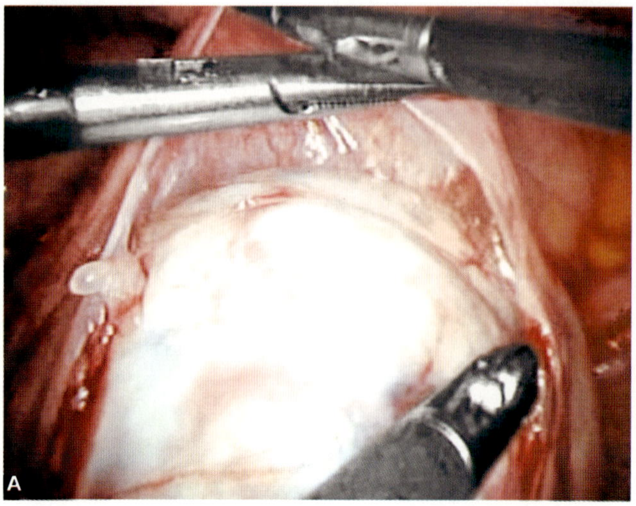

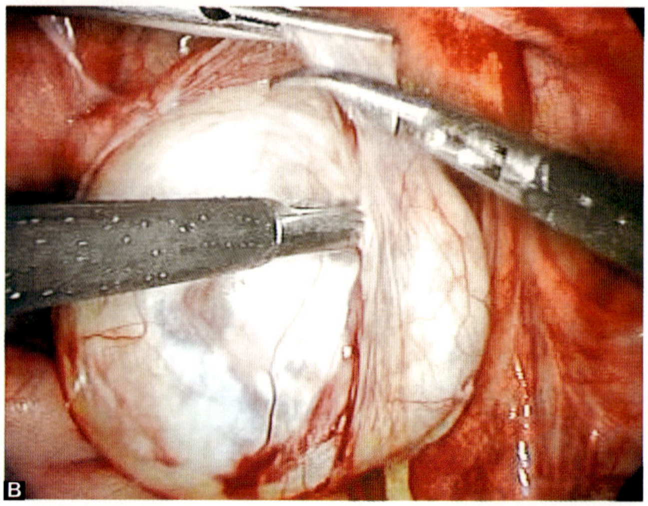

**Figs 23.6A and B:** Enucleation of cyst in toto in endobag without puncturing

# Excision of Benign Adnexal Mass and Extraction in Endobag

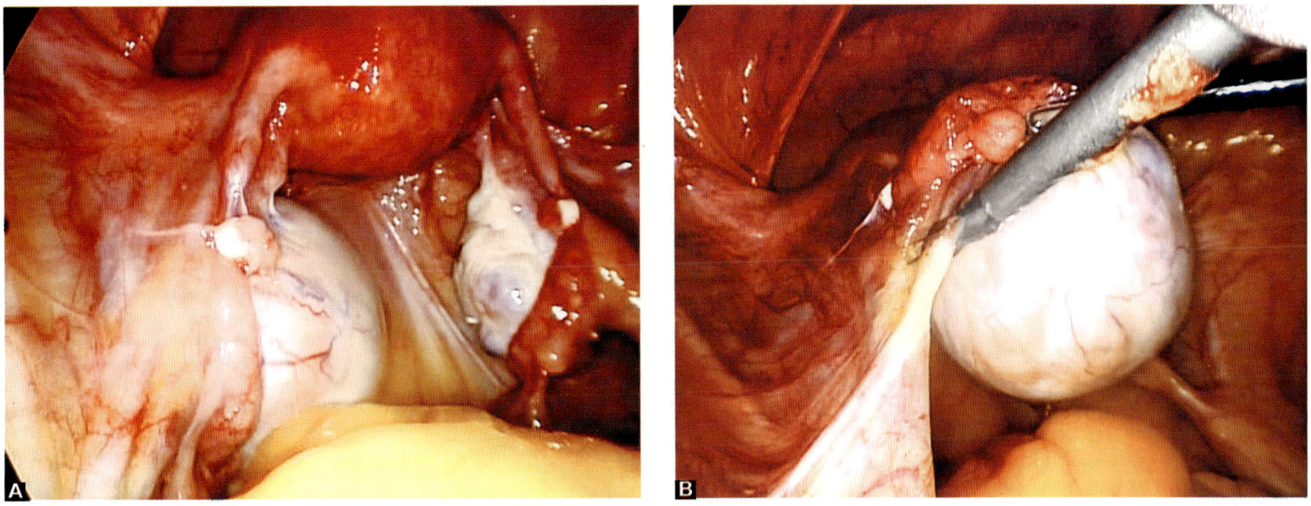


**Figs 23.7A and B:** No adhesions with lateral pelvic wall and pouch of Douglas

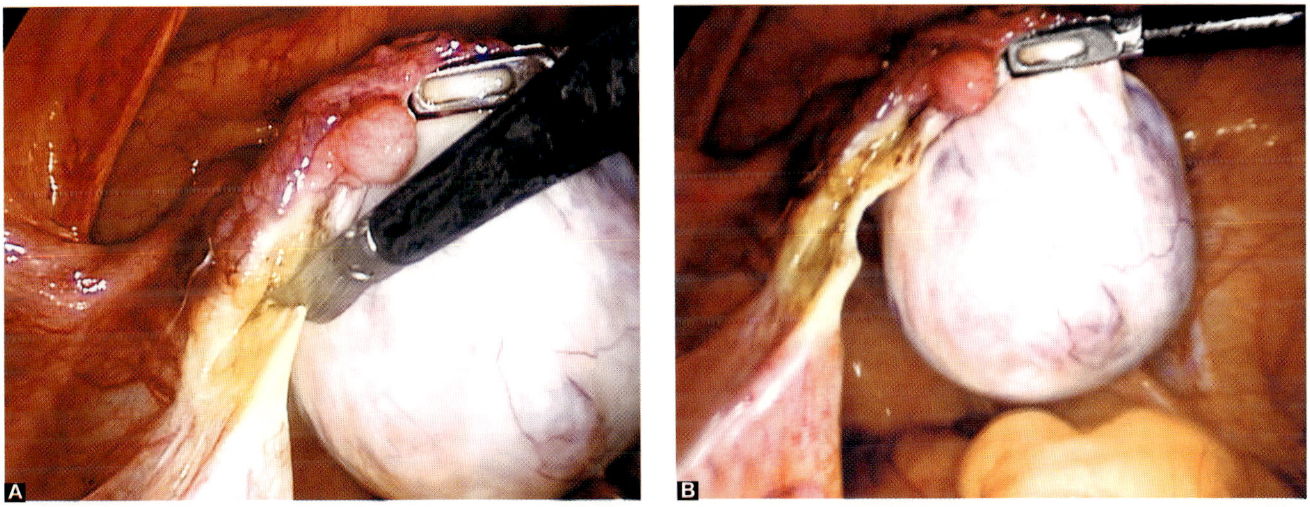


**Figs 23.8A and B:** Infundibulopelvic ligament cauterized and cut

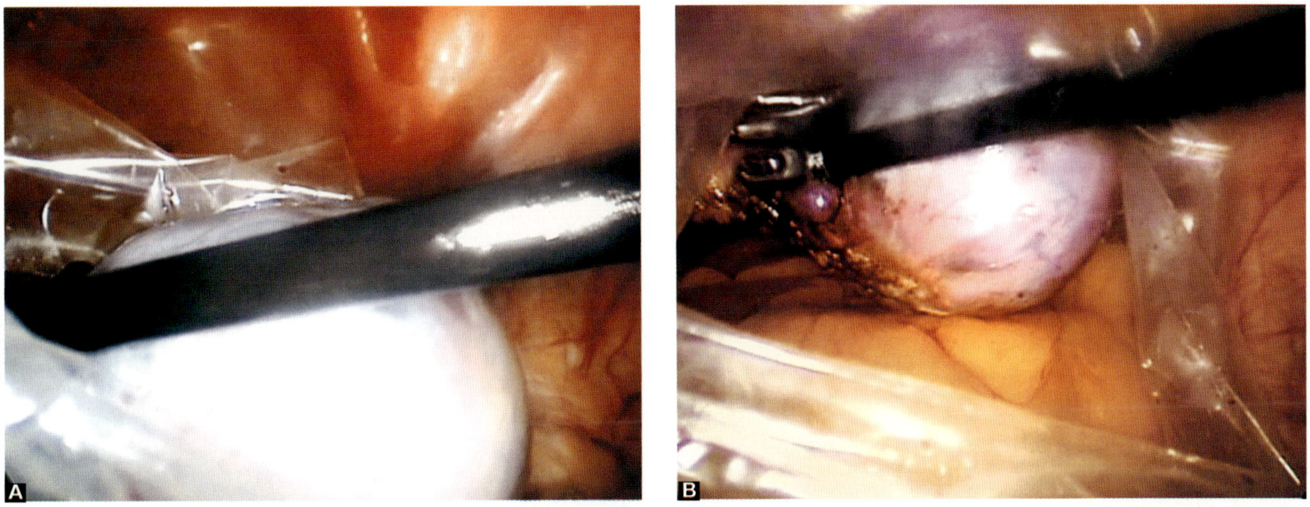


**Figs 23.9A and B:** Adnexa removed in endobag

A 42-year-old female with huge multicystic right ovarian cyst. Tumor markers and color Doppler studies show benign cystadenoma.

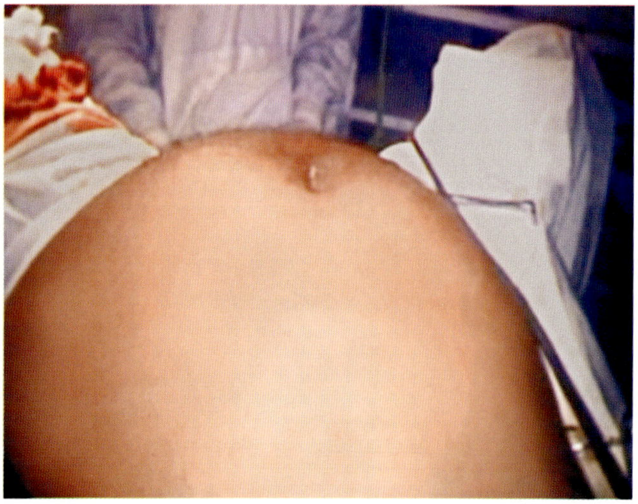

**Fig. 23.10:** Patient on table–obvious distension of lower abdomen with huge ovarian cyst

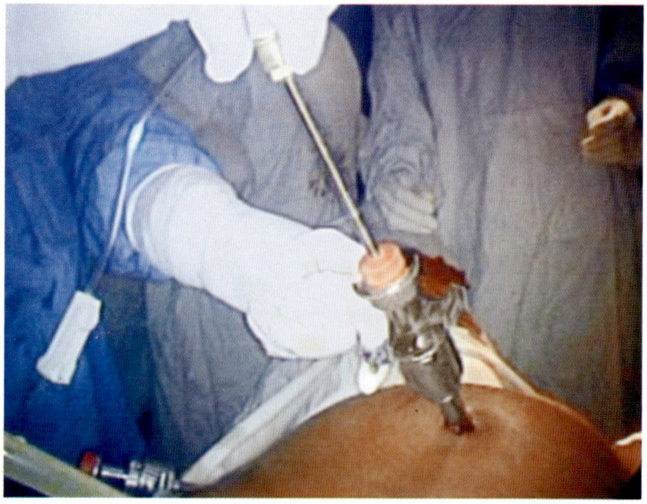

**Fig. 23.11:** Direct trocar entry into the ovarian cyst under vision through video telescope at palmer's point

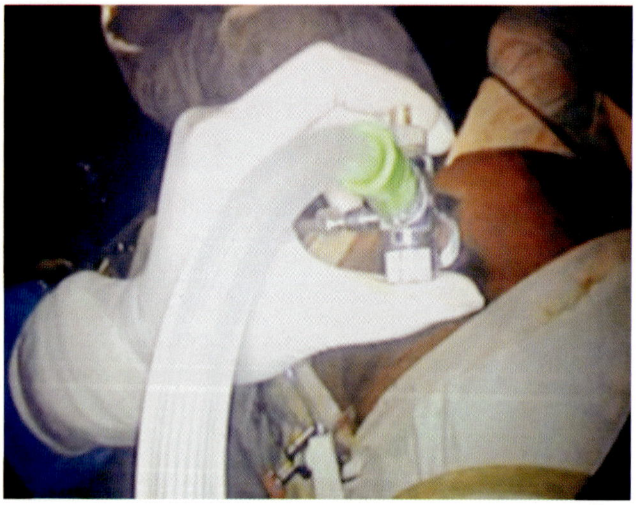

**Fig. 23.12:** Suction of the cyst fluid

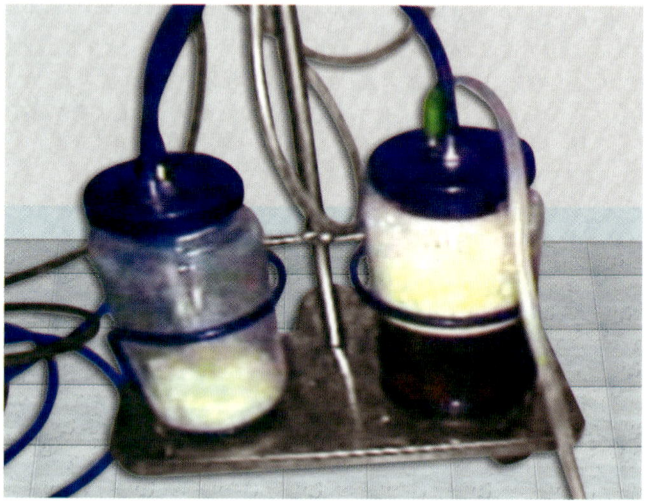

**Fig. 23.13:** Suction bottles showing collection of the cystic fluid in process

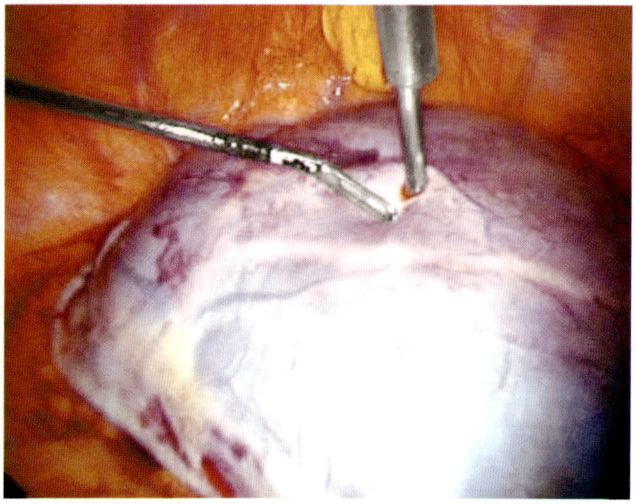

**Fig. 23.14:** Endoscopic view of cyst fluid being aspirated

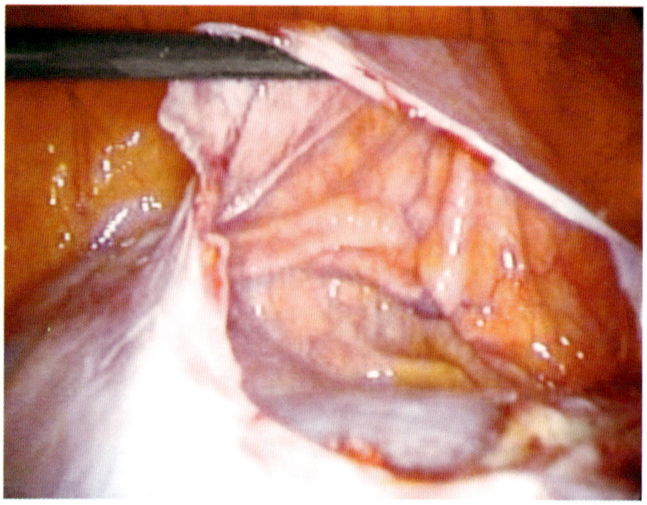

**Fig. 23.15:** Cystoscopy showing benign inner cyst wall

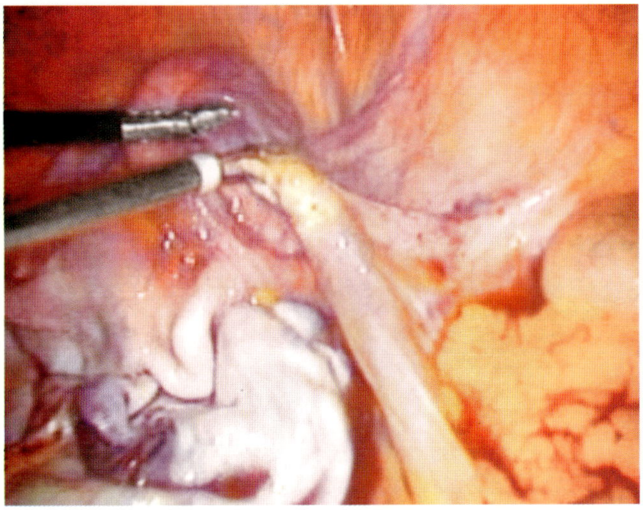

**Fig. 23.16:** Right adnexectomy being performed

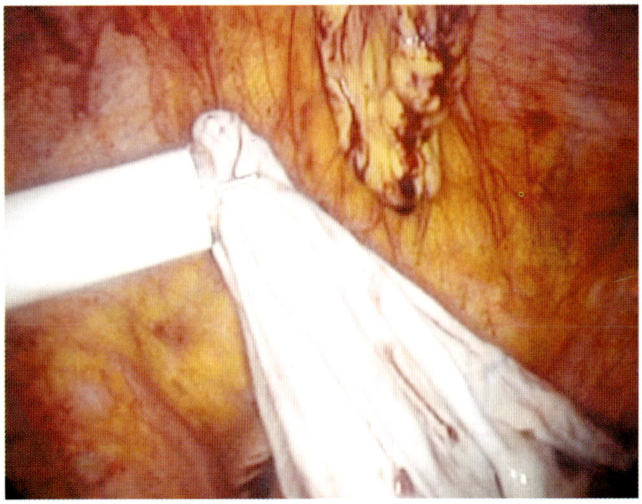

**Fig. 23.17:** Morcellation of adnexa with huge cyst wall

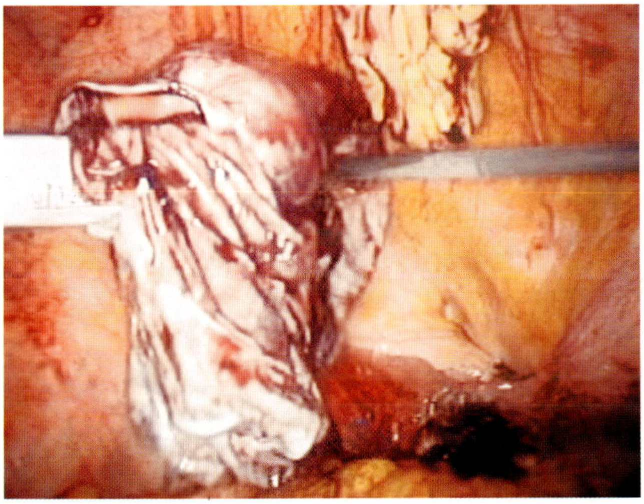

**Fig. 23.18:** Cyst morcellation in process

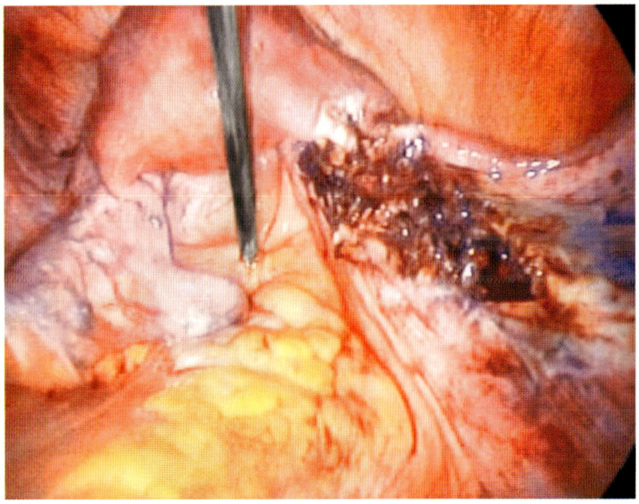

**Fig. 23.19:** Thorough lavage given. End result—clean pelvis

A 45-year-old female presented with acute pain in the lower abdomen. USG revealed a twisted huge left ovarian cyst. Tumor markers and sonography confirmed benign nature of the cyst.

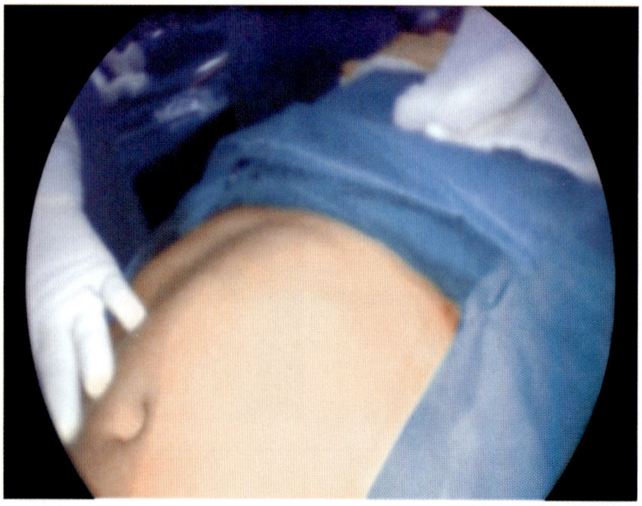

**Fig. 23.20:** Huge ovarian cyst—*note* the obvious abdominal distention

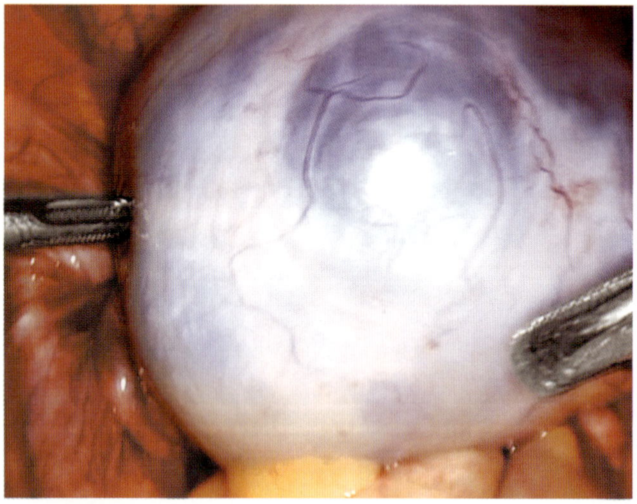

**Fig. 23.21:** Endo view of cyst

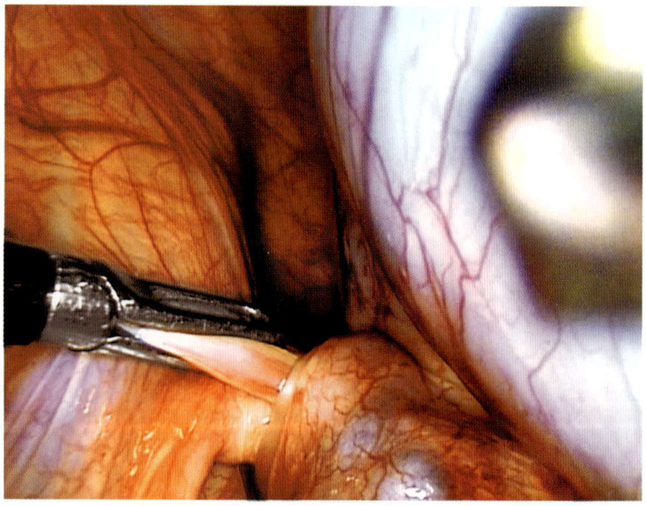

**Fig. 23.22:** Twist noted.

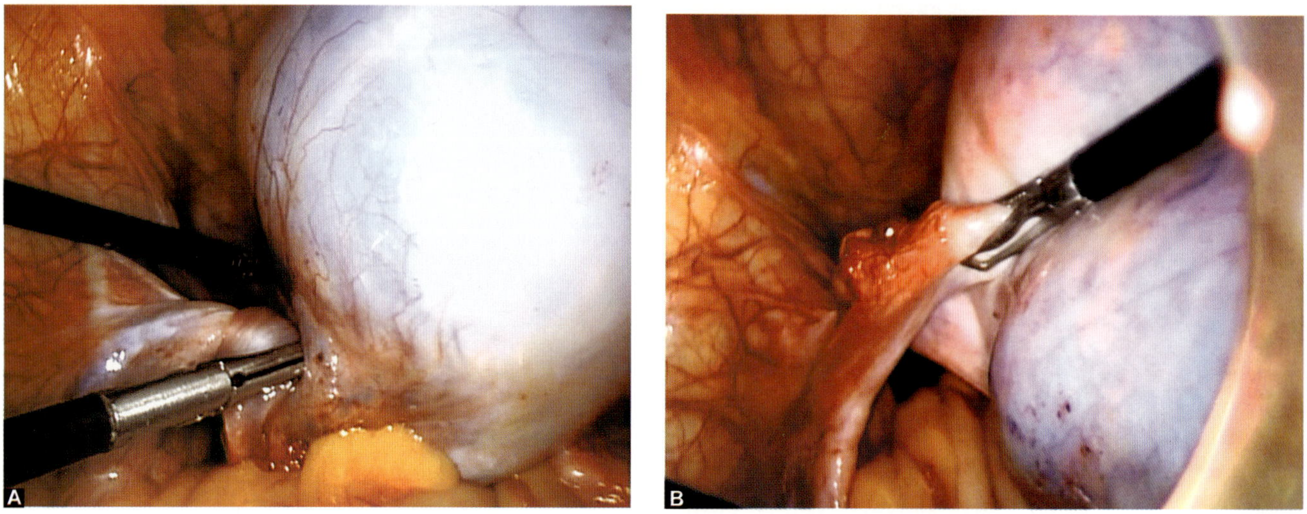


**Figs 23.23A and B:** Detorsion completed and adnexectomy performed

# Removal of Huge Ovarian Cyst

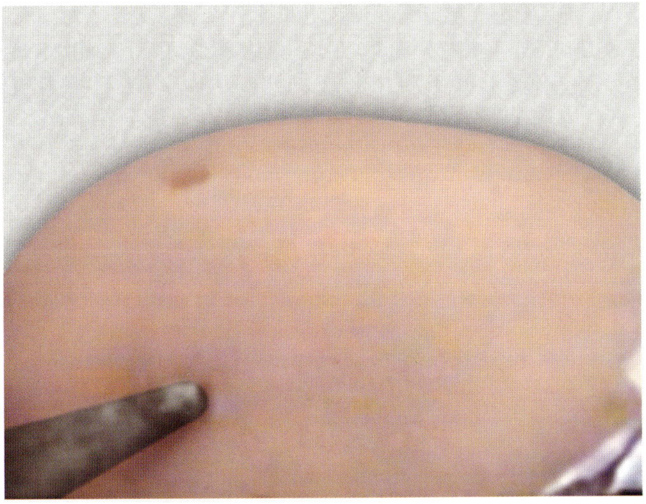

**Fig. 23.24:** Large benign ovarian cyst

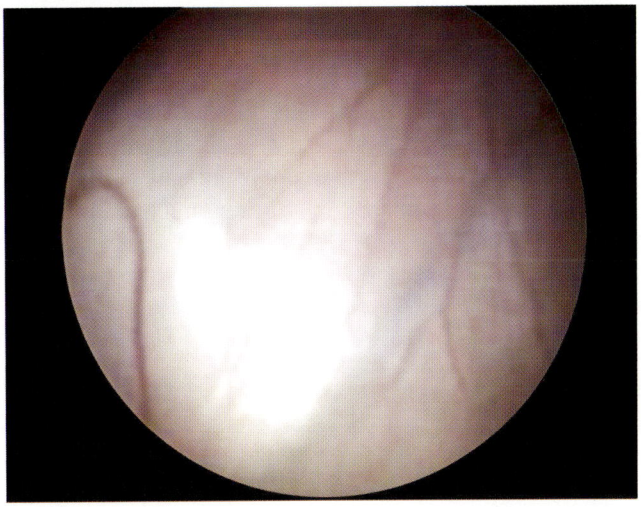

**Fig. 23.25:** Cyst from inside

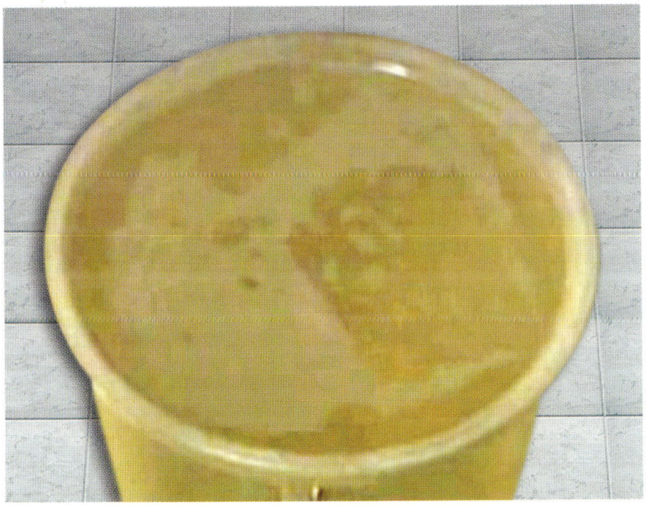

**Fig. 23.26:** Aspirated cyst fluid

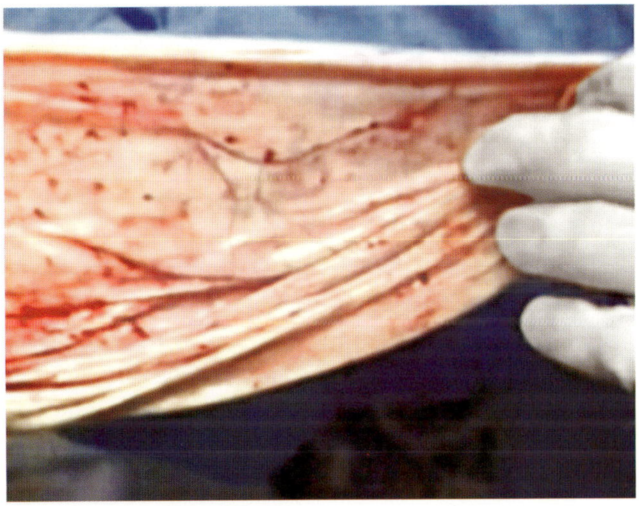

**Fig. 23.27:** Peeling of the cyst wall

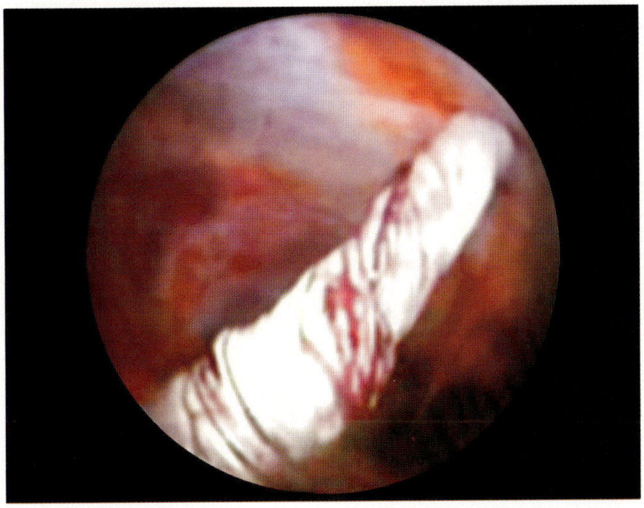

**Fig. 23.28:** Cyst wall removed from the side port

## BENIGN CYSTIC TERATOMAS

- Teratomas often can be excised intact.
- But if the cyst ruptures, the resulting contamination would be greater than if the cyst was opened and aspirated.
  Development of the plane is very important, sharp cut is taken on cortex and then plane is created either with hydrodissection or scissors, further enucleation of cyst is performed.
- After the cyst is excised, the base is coagulated with the help of bipolar forceps if bleeding is present.
- The edges of the ovary are left open to heal.
- Suturing is avoided since this causes unnecessary bleeding, collection of the blood in the ovarian cortex and postoperative adhesion.
- After laparoscopic removal, the tumor is retrieved through posterior colpotomy incision, if cyst is less than 6 cm and larger cyst is retrieved in a lapsac.
- In case, the cyst ruptures, the abdominal cavity should be cleaned off of sebaceous material and hair, which may be cumbersome.

**TIPS**

- In case of large defects, sutures can be taken inside the ovary with no. 2-0 delayed absorbable material.
- Incomplete removal of the material may cause peritonitis.

A 23-year-old unmarried girl, known case of dermoid had left-sided oophorectomy by laparotomy at the age of 18, came to us with right-sided 3 ovarian dermoid. It was very important to perserve ovarian tissue as much as possible.

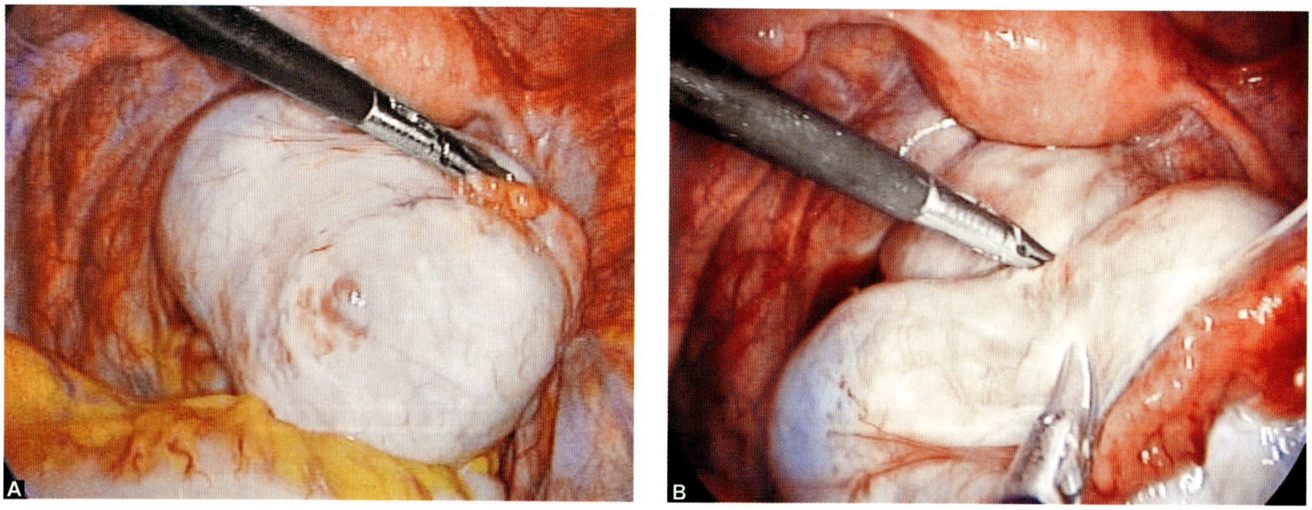


**Figs 23.29A and B:** Right ovarian dermoids. *Note* absence of left ovary

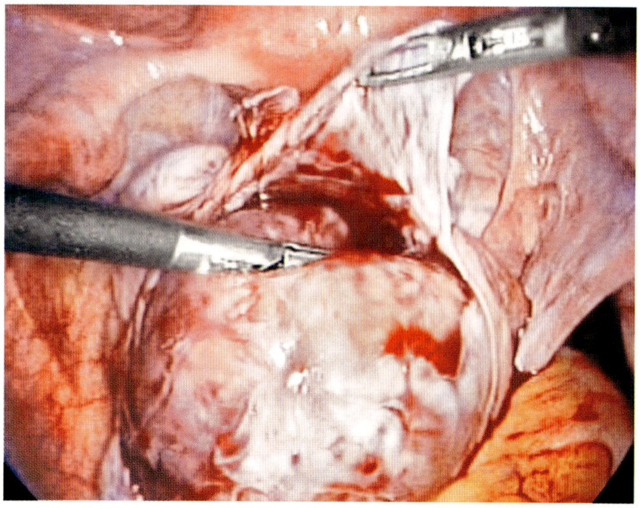

**Fig. 23.30:** Dermoid cysts excision in process

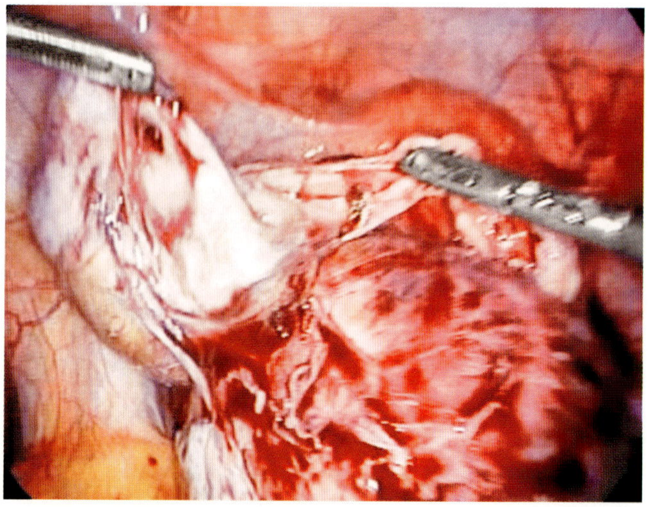

**Fig. 23.31:** Second dermoid cysts excision in process

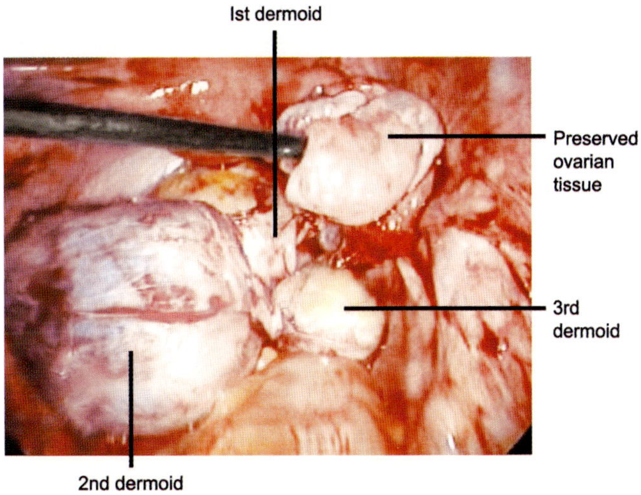


**Fig. 23.32:** All 3 dermoids removed and placed in the POD. Adequate amount of ovarian tissue preserved

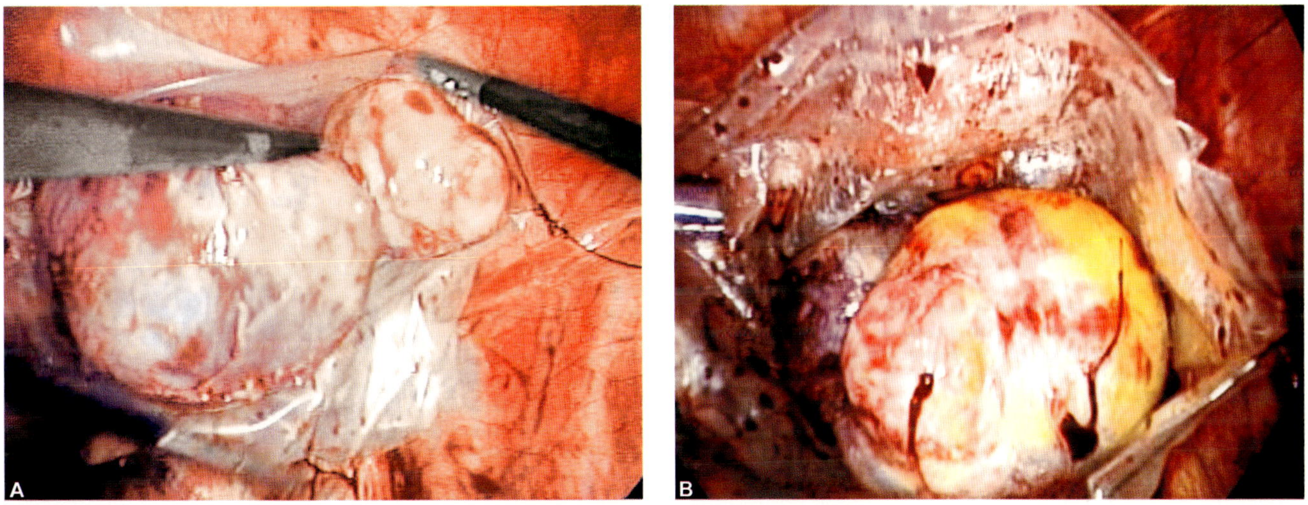


**Figs 23.33A and B:** Dermoid cysts placed in endobag

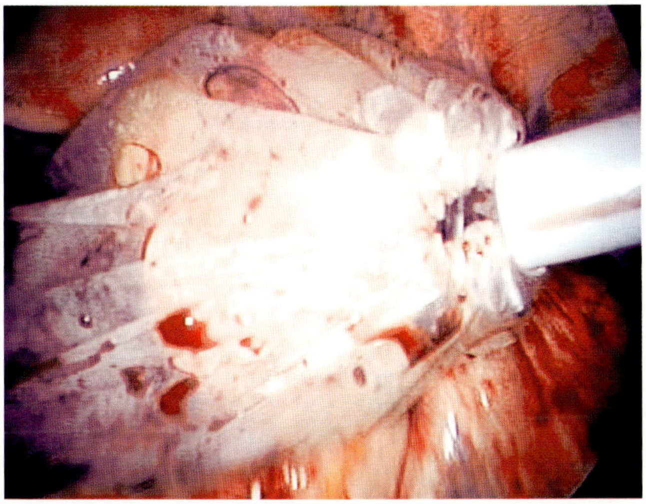

**Fig. 23.34:** Endobag being extracted through the secondary 10 mm port

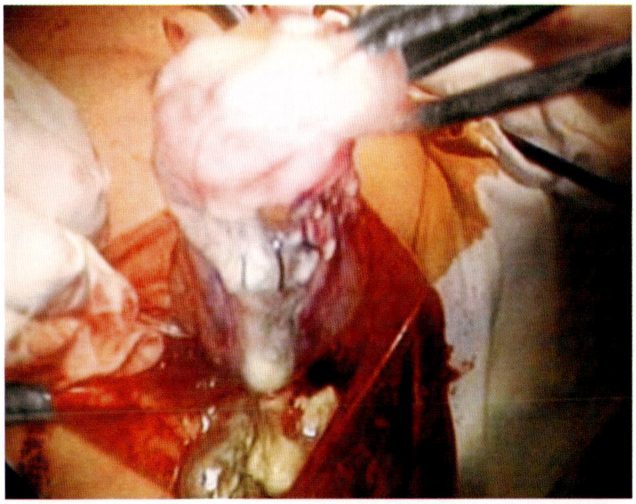

**Fig. 23.35:** External view of dermoid cyst getting removed. Precaution has to be taken to keep endobag intact to avoid spillage

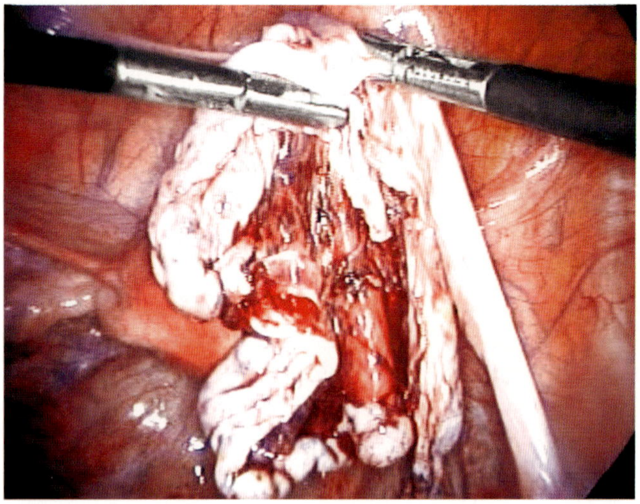

**Fig. 23.36:** Good amount of healthy ovarian tissue is preserved and the edges of the ovary are left open to heal

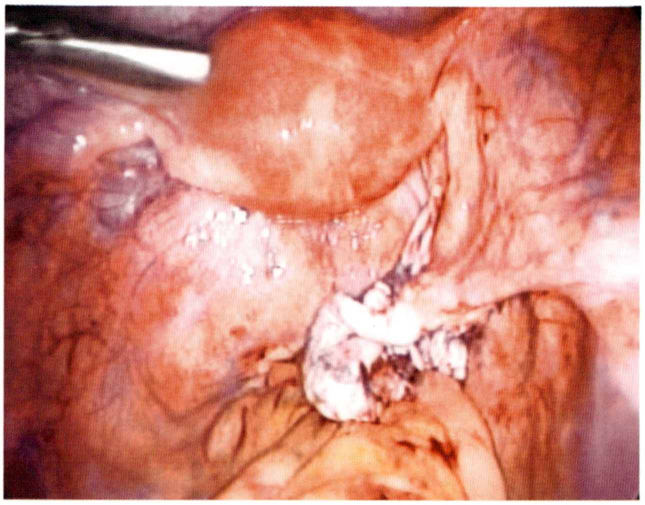

**Fig. 23.37:** End result

Chapter 24

# Laparoscopic Management of Tubal Ectopic

*Sunita R Tandulwadkar, Sejal Naik*

## UNRUPTURED ECTOPIC

### Preoperative Evaluation

- Diagnosis by thorough history and USG.
- No other preoperative preparation needed for unruptured ectopic.
- Ruptured ectopic can be tackled laparoscopically if the patient is hemodynamically stable.

### Preoperative Preparation

Blood needs to be organized as per patient's condition.

### Important Instruments

- One 10 mm and two/three 5 mm trocars.
- Two non-traumatic graspers.
- Bipolar forceps.
- Monopolar microneedle.
- Suction irrigation cannula.

## SALPINGOSTOMY

- A standard 10 mm laparoscope is introduced with three side ports, two on the left side and one on the right side.
- 5–10 cc of vasopressin in 1:100 dilution can be instilled in mesosalpinx with laparoscopic needle at the site of ectopic pregnancy (though this is not practiced by many endosurgeons).
- With a non-traumatic grasper, the tube is stabilized proximal to the ectopic mass.
- A linear cut is given with a monopolar microneedle on the antemesenteric border of the ectopic mass by using a cutting cautery current.
- Usually the ectopic mass will extrude out, otherwise it is squeezed out by holding fallopian tube with two nontraumatic graspers proximal and distal to the ectopic mass. It is then gently removed.
- Copious lavage is also given through the salpingostomy incision so that blood clots can be washed through the fimbrial end.
- If there is any bleeder at the incision site, it is seen under water flow and cauterized precisely with bipolar.
- The ectopic mass can be removed through the 5 mm port.

  * Milking of ectopic pregnancy in the ampullary region is not advised. But if the ectopic is at the fimbrial end, it can sometimes be milked out of the fimbrial end.

  * Linear salpingostomy is not successful in case of the isthmic ectopic pregnancy.

  In the era of ART, salpingostomy has limited rule.

**TIPS**

- The suture at the linear salpingotomy does not offer any advantage over the non-suture technique.
- If the ectopic has occurred due to the narrowing of the proximal part of fallopian tube, which is not corrected, there are chances of repeat ectopic in the same tube.

## Unruptured Ectopic

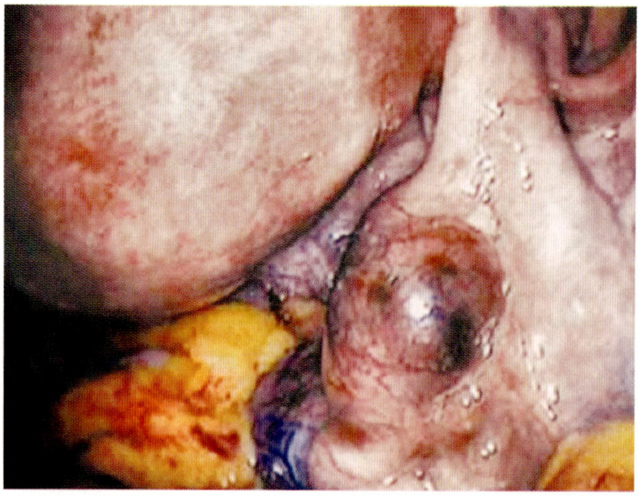

**Fig. 24.1:** Right tubal unruptured ectopic pregnancy

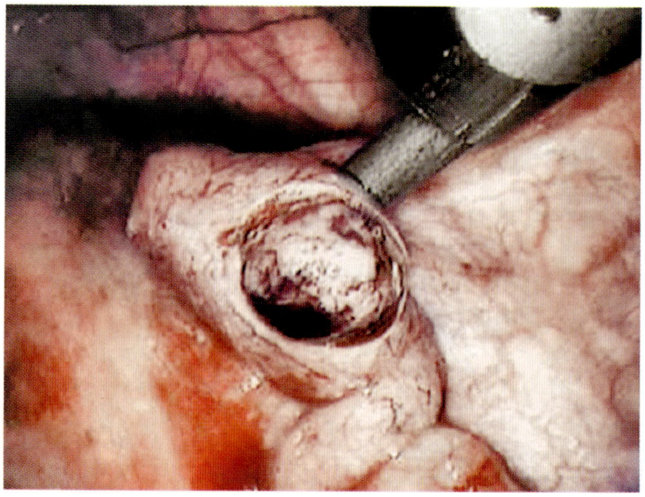

**Fig. 24.2:** Ectopic tissue seen protruding after linear incision with needle using monopolar cutting current

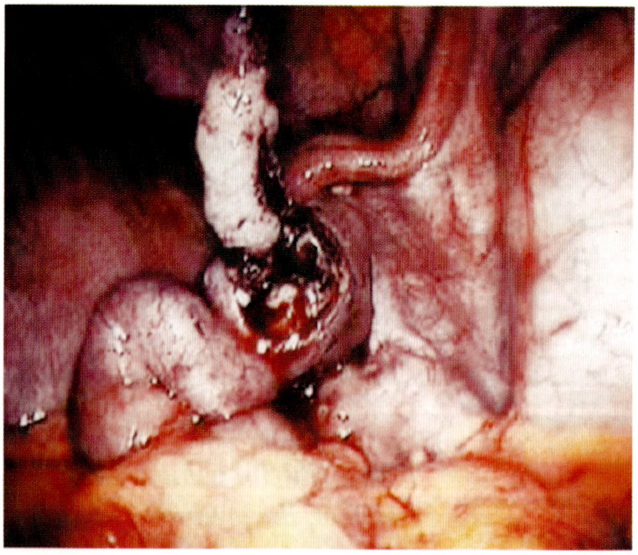

**Fig. 24.3:** Ectopic tissue removed with non-traumatic grasper

## SALPINGECTOMY

### Indications

- Isthmic pregnancy
- Ruptured ectopic
- Recurrent ectopic
- Associated hydrosalpinx
- Damaged tube.

### Procedure

1. Fallopian tube to be excised is held at the distal end and is lifted up to visualize mesosalpinx of the fimbrial end, which can be cauterized precisely without damaging the blood supply to the ovary.
2. Serial cauterization and cutting is done so as to remove the whole length of the tube.
3. Removal of specimen—5 mm telescope is passed through secondary port and 10 mm grasper is passed through the primary port and the specimen is removed always under vision.
3. Usually blood is squeezed on the bowel loops from the specimen while removing the specimen out through the primary port, which should be sucked.

## RUPTURED ECTOPIC

### Instruments

- Two 10 mm and two/three 5 mm trocars
- Two nontraumatic graspers
- Bipolar forceps
- Monopolar needle
- 10 mm suction irrigation cannula.

### Procedure

1. If patient is hemodynamically stable, one can proceed with laparoscopic salpinectomy.
2. If one is familiar with direct trocar insertion, it is preferred, as it will save time.
3. If a bleeding spurter is seen, it should be held with nontraumatic forceps and cauterized first.
4. Rest of the procedure—salpingectomy is performed as usual.
5. To hasten the speed of removal of blood clots from peritoneal cavity, 10 mm suction cannula is used.
6. Thorough lavage should be given to remove all blood and blood clots from the peritoneal cavity, which at times may be tedious. But this is an important step otherwise adhesions may be formed.
7. Drain can be kept from the side port for 12 hours.

## Ruptured Ectopic

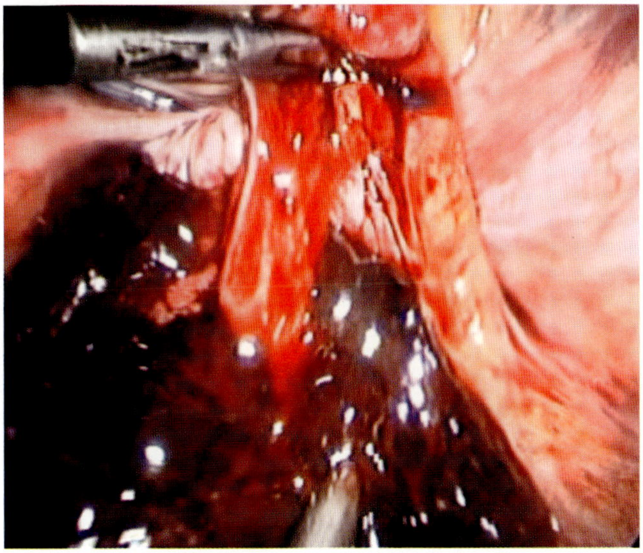

**Fig. 24.4**

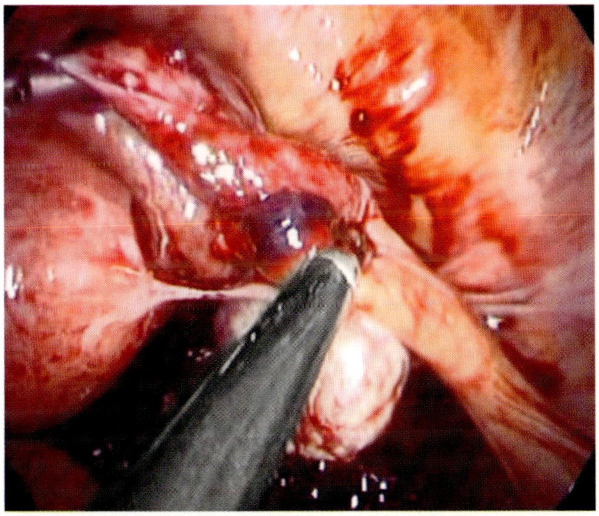

**Fig. 24.5:** Salpingectomy in progress

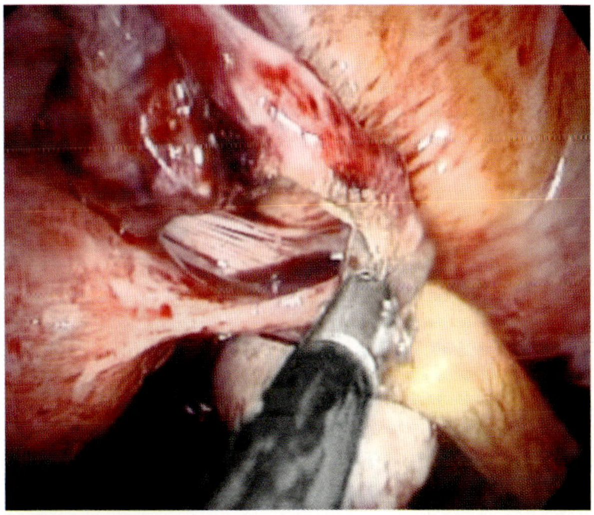

**Fig. 24.6:** Salpingectomy complete

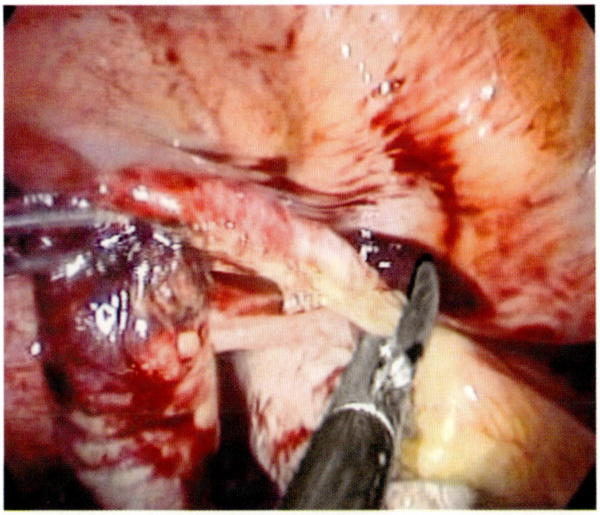

**Fig. 24.7**

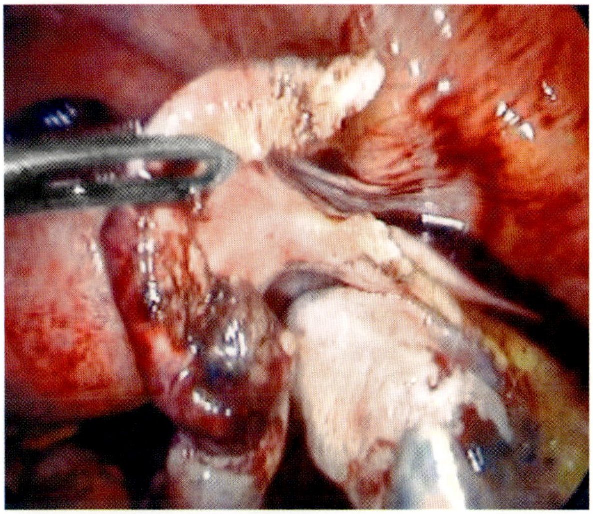

**Fig. 24.8**

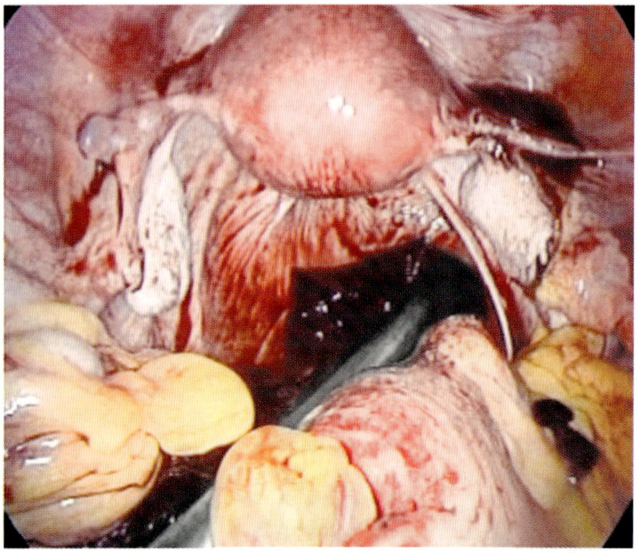

**Fig. 24.9:** Left side associated hematosalpinx so left cornu blocked as patient was for IVF

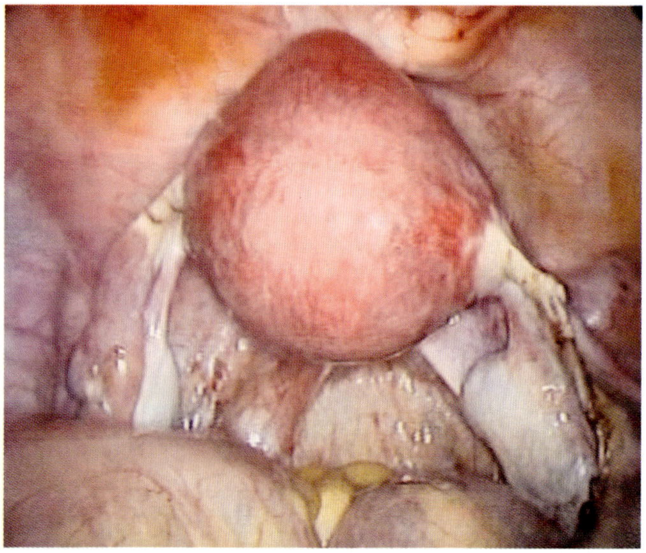

**Fig. 24.10:** End result

## Ectopic Pregnancies at Various Sites

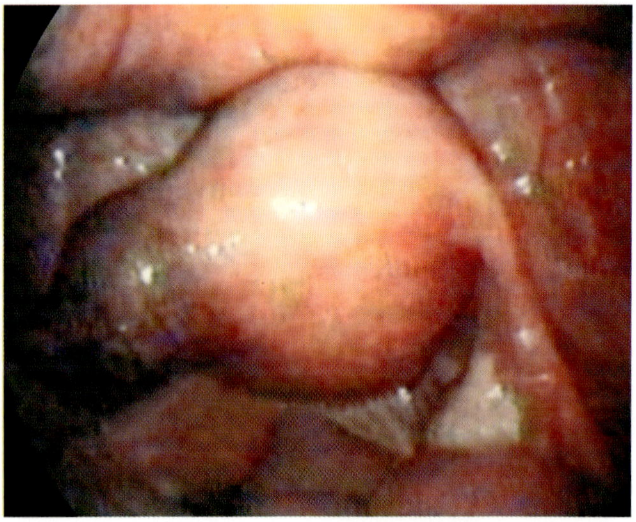

**Fig. 24.11:** Interstitial ectopic

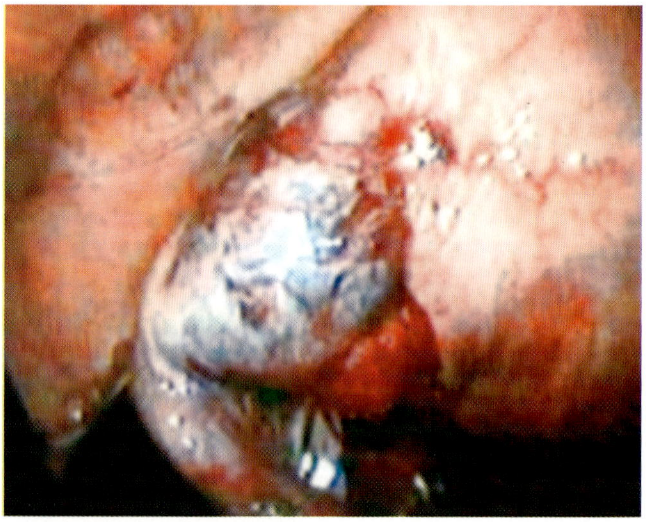

**Fig. 24.12:** Isthmic ectopic

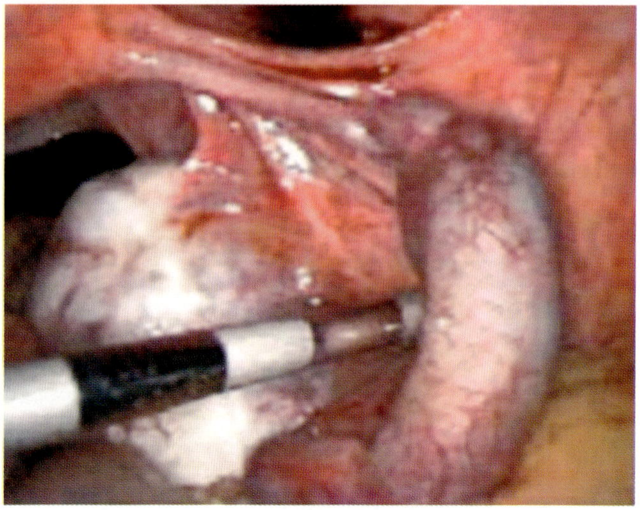

**Fig. 24.13:** Ampullary ectopic

## Ovarian Ectopic

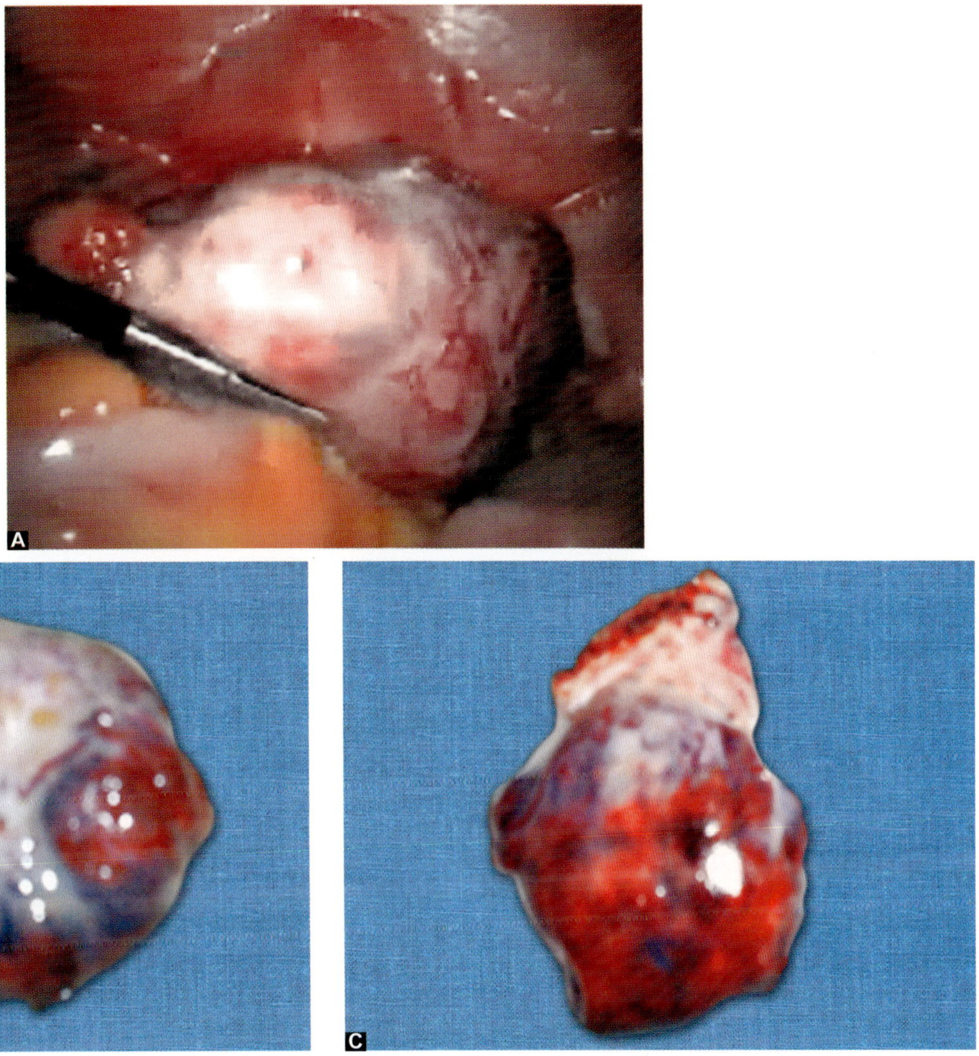

**Figs 24.14A to C:** Spontaneous ovarian ectopic pregnancy in a 43-year-old lady. Considering the high vascularily and age of the patient removed in toto

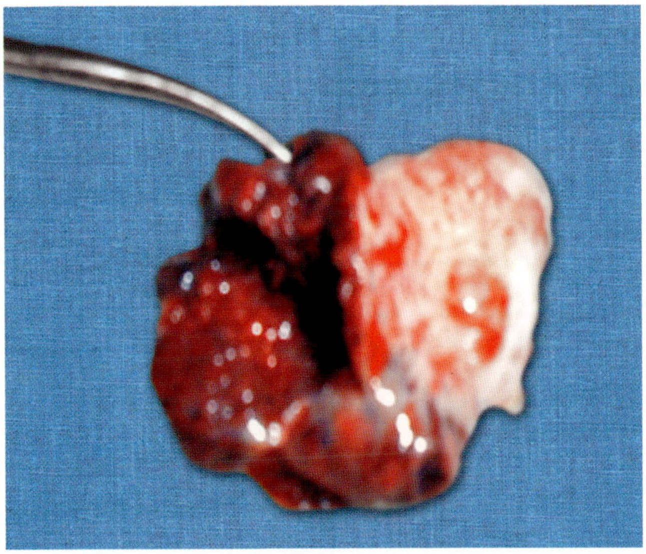

**Fig. 24.15:** Cut section

Chapter 25

# Laparoscopic Salpingectomy

*Sunita R Tandulwadkar*

## PREOPERATIVE EVALUATION

History and examination of patient.

## PREOPERATIVE PREPARATION

No specific preparation as such is needed.

## CRITERIA FOR SALPINGECTOMY IN AN INFERTILE PATIENT

- Written consent.
- Hydrosalpinx more than thumb size or easily seen on sonography.
- Hematosalpinx or pyosalpinx.

## INSTRUMENTS

- 5 mm zero degree laparoscope
- 10 mm zero degree laparoscope
- Single chip/three chip camera
- Bipolar forceps
- 10 mm tooth grasper
- Two nontraumatic graspers
- Suction irrigation system.

## PROCEDURE

1. 3 port laparoscopic entry.
2. The pathological tube is held with the nontraumatic grasper and the mesosalpinx is coagulated very near to the tube (so that ovarian blood supply is not compromised) with bipolar and cut with scissors. (If one has harmonic energy source, surgery becomes simplified as cauterization and cutting will happen simultaneously and also lateral thermal spread is minimal).
3. Removal of specimen—5 mm videoscope is passed through upper secondary port and 10 mm grasper with 10 mm reducer is passed through 10 mm primary port and the specimen is removed through it.
4. Thorough lavage is given at the end and hemostasis is confirmed.

**TIPS**

- Utmost care should be taken to avoid damage to the ovarian blood supply by staying close to the Fallopian tubes.

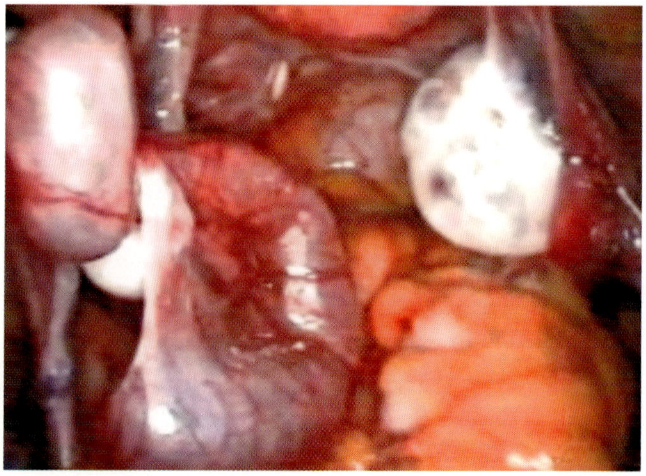

**Fig. 25.1:** Left hydrosalpinx

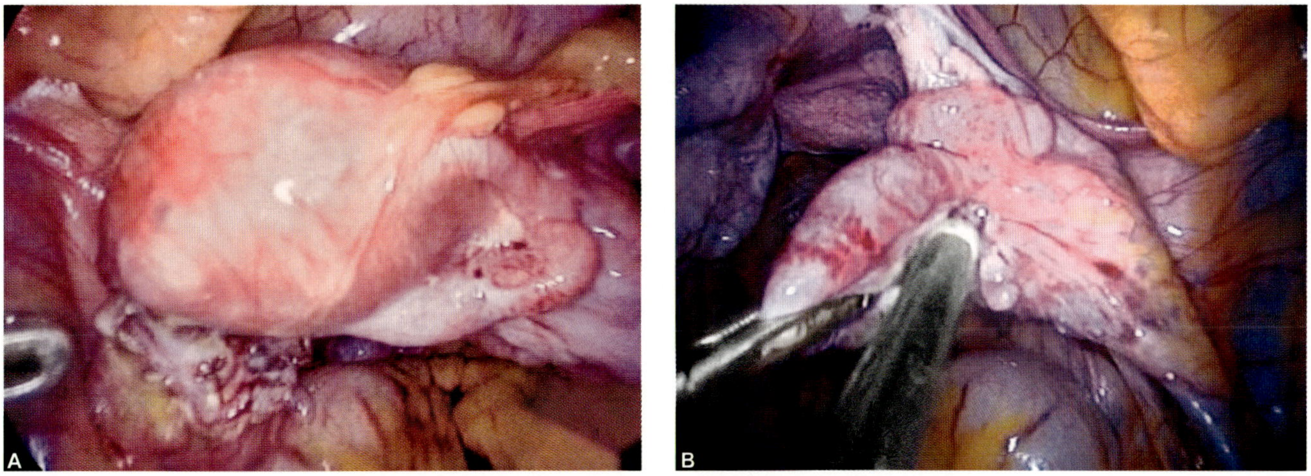

Fig. 25.2A and B: Right tuberculous salpingitis

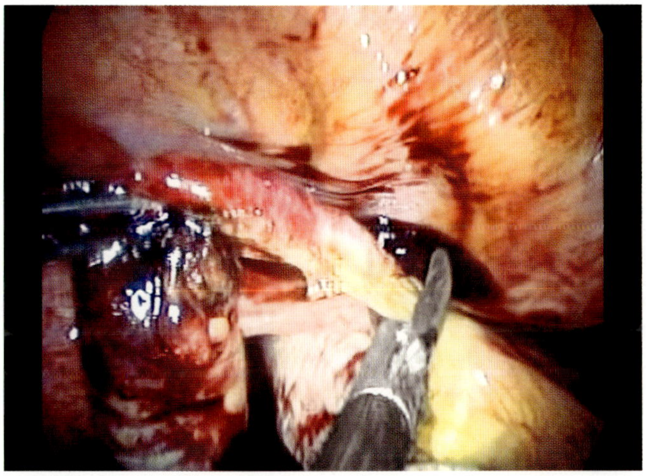

Fig. 25.3: Right salpingectomy for ectopic pregnancy with incision line next to mesosalpinx

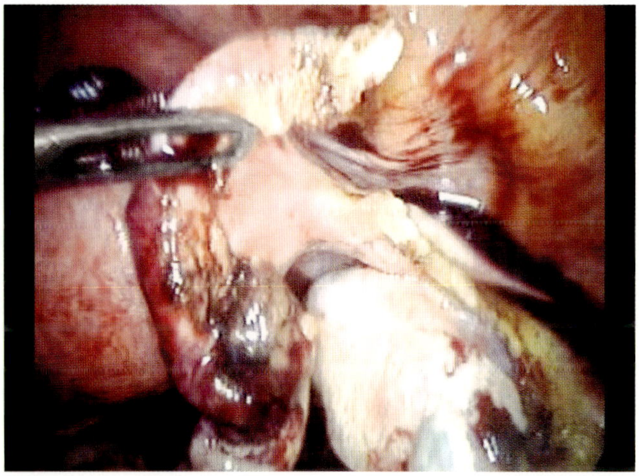

Fig. 25.4: Right salpingectomy completed

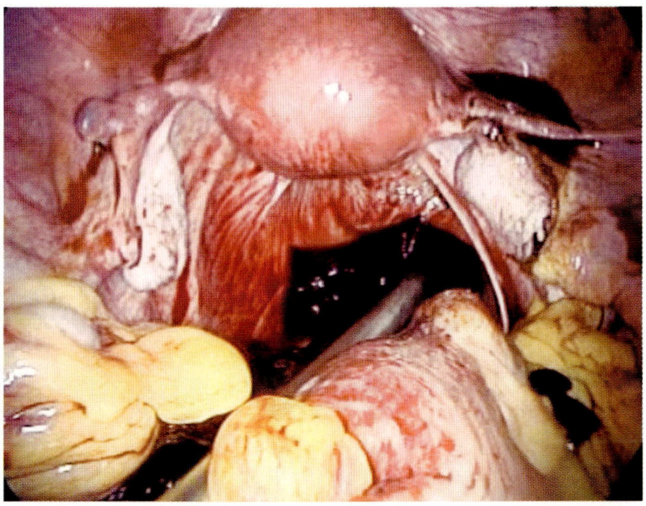

Fig. 25.5: Thorough suction and irrigation, left hematosalpinx also seen

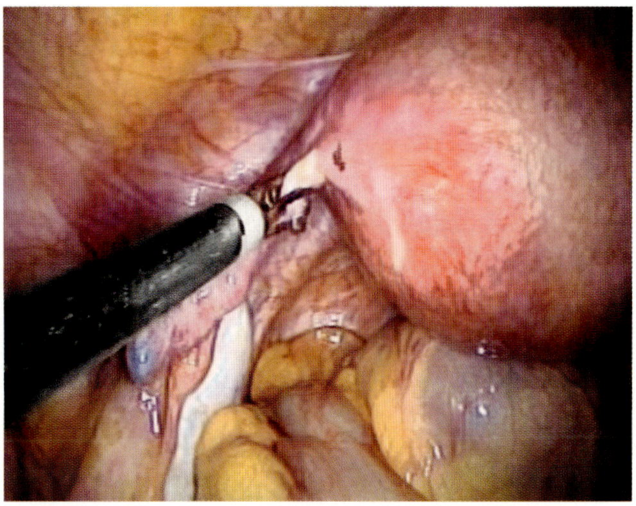

Fig. 25.6: Patient for IVF, left cornual end cauterized, as found to have hematosalpinx

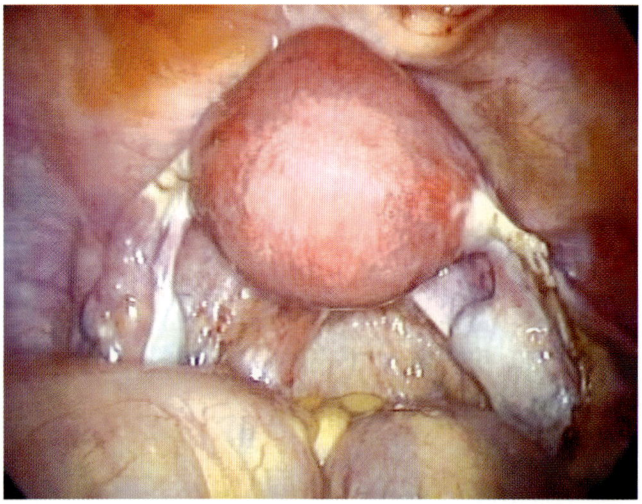

**Fig. 25.7:** End result—clean pelvis

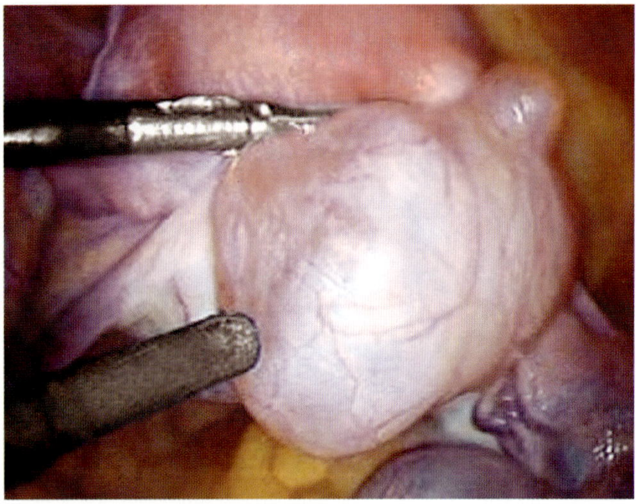

**Fig. 25.8:** Left hydrosalpinx

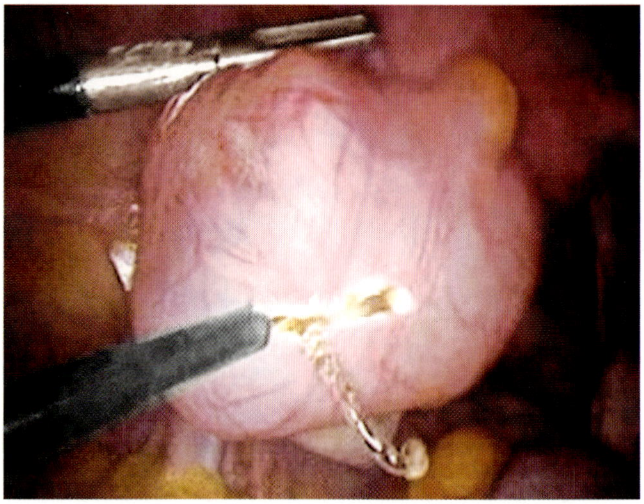

**Fig. 25.9:** Left hydrosalpinx drained

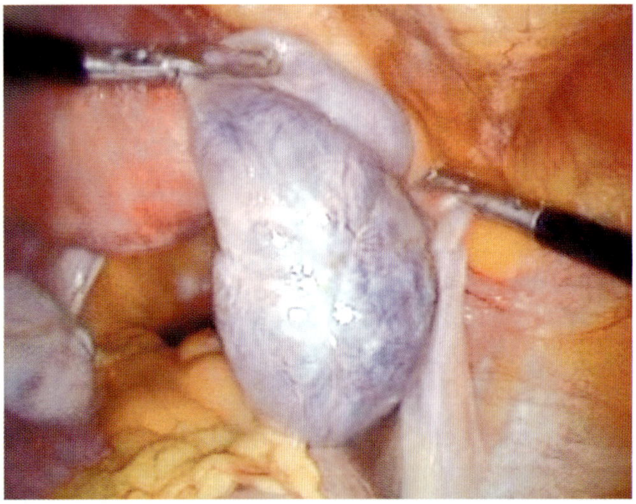

**Fig. 25.10:** Right hematosalpinx

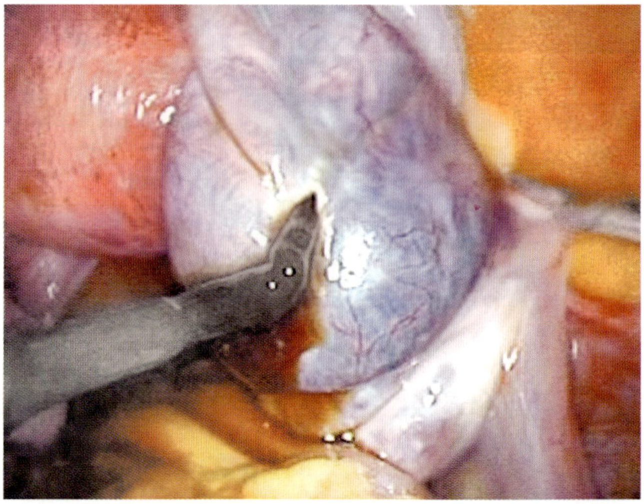

**Fig. 25.11:** Hematosalpinx drained

# Laparoscopic Sterilization

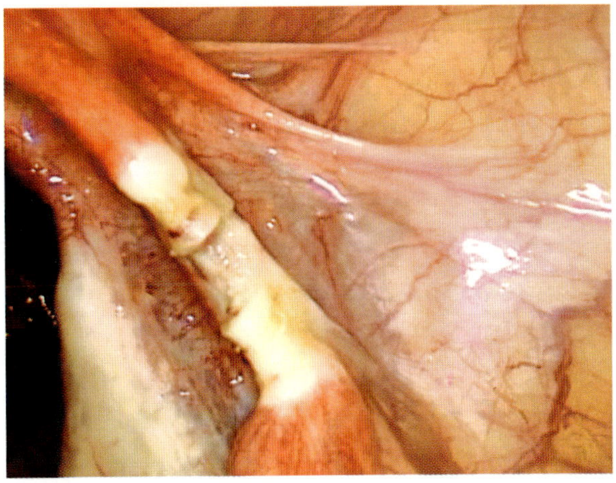

**Fig. 25.12:** Right Fallopian tube cauterized

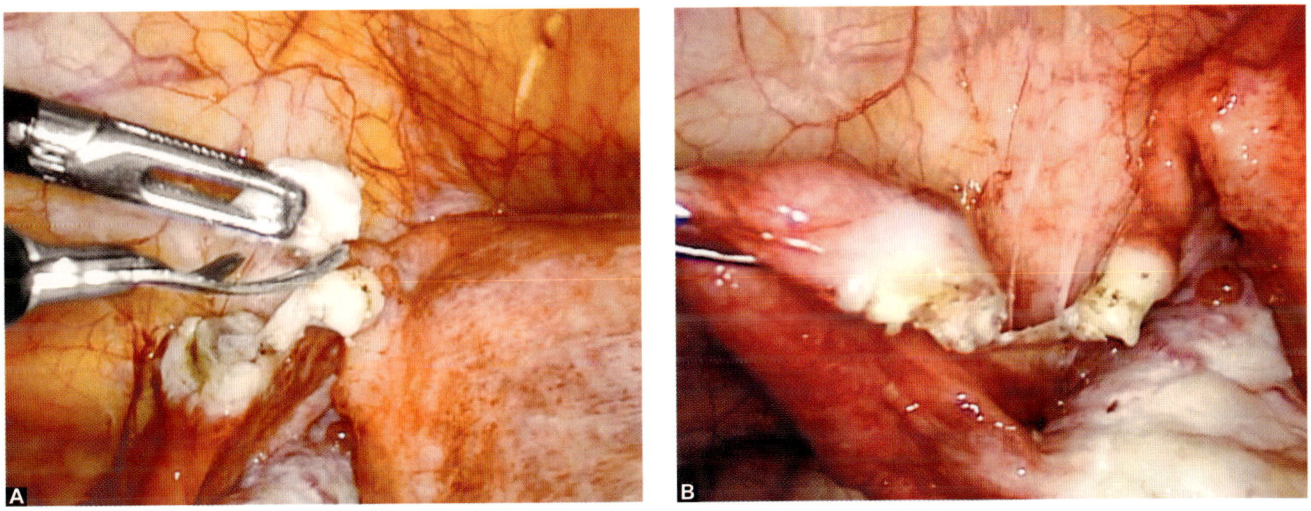

**Figs 25.13A and B:** Right Fallopian tube cauterized and cut

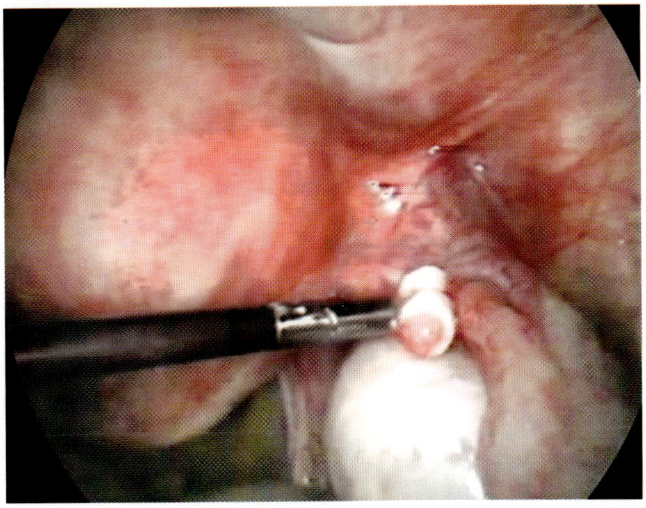

**Fig. 25.14:** Sterilization with sialistic bands

Chapter

26

# Conservation Laparoscopic Management of Hydrosalpinx

*Sunita R Tandulwadkar*

## PREOPERATIVE EVALUATION

- Diagnosis by thorough history and ultrasonography.
- Ultrasonography should reveal a normal uterine cavity with good ovarian volume.
- Normal male factor.
- Normal female hormonal assays and documentation of ovulation.
- Salpingoscopy§It should be performed at the time of laparoscopy. Major and minor mucosal folds are to be seen along with any intraluminal adhesions or strictures.

## PREOPERATIVE PREPARATION

- No other preoperative preparation needed for fimbrioplasty.

## IMPORTANT EQUIPMENT

- 10 mm zero degree laparoscope
- Single chip/three chip camera
- Monopolar needle
- Bipolar forceps
- Nontraumatic graspers
- Suction irrigation system.

## SURGICAL STEPS

1. Distended fimbrial end is stabilized with two nontraumatic graspers (Maryland's forceps are better) passed through the lower left and right contralateral ports.
2. A monopolar needle is passed through the left upper port.
3. Distended fimbrial end is punctured with monopolar needle with cutting current between 20 and 40 Watts, fluid is drained and cruciate incision is taken from the puncture site in all four directions (Figs 26.1 to 26.3).
4. The fimbrial ends are then everted and the ends are coagulated with the lowest possible power setting so as to coagulate only the serosa. This is done to avoid re-agglutination. (Some endoscopic surgeons do evert the fimbria by endosuturing) (Figs 26.4 and 26.5).
5. Methylene blue dye is injected and spillage is confirmed.
6. Thorough lavage is given and hemostasis achieved.
7. Under surface of diaphragm is checked for any adhesions.

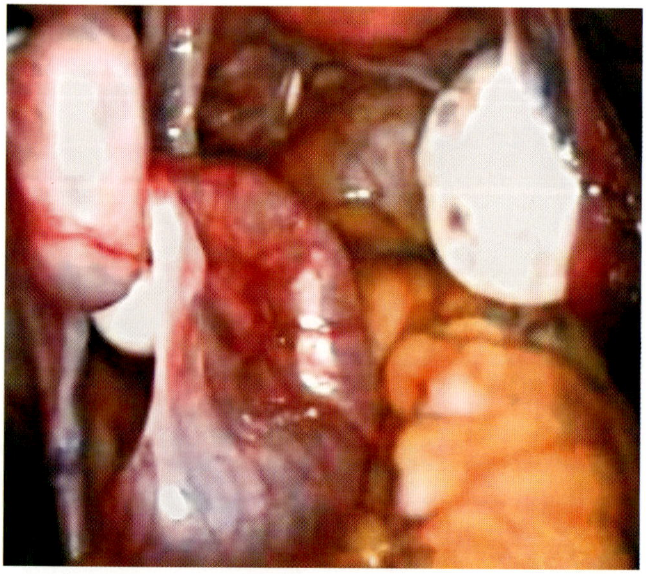

**Fig. 26.1:** Left hydrosalpinx

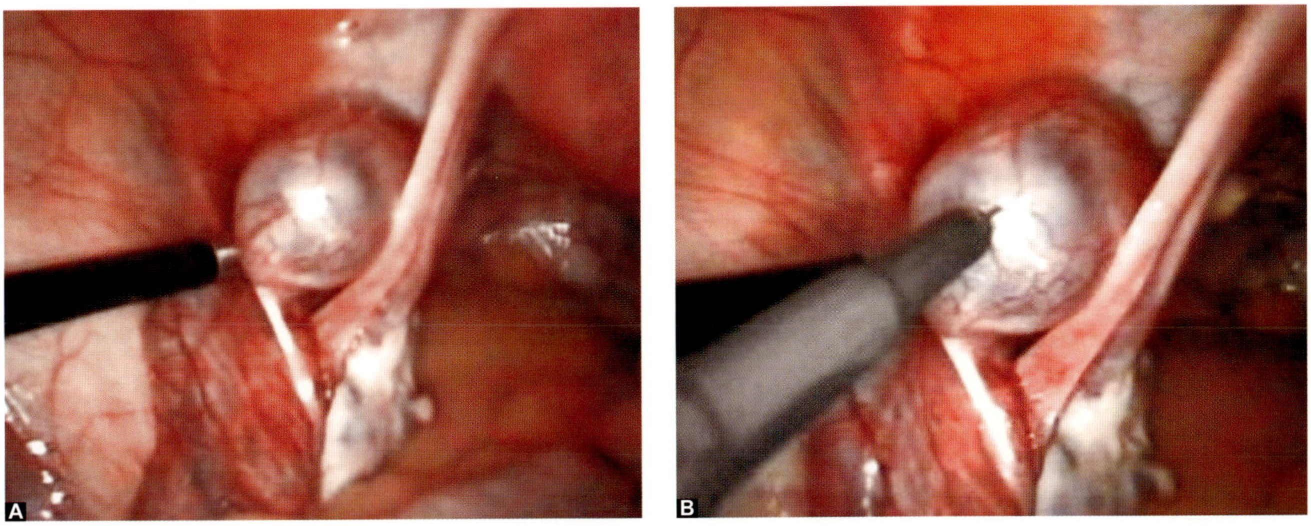

**Figs 26.2A and B:** Puncture with monopolar needle

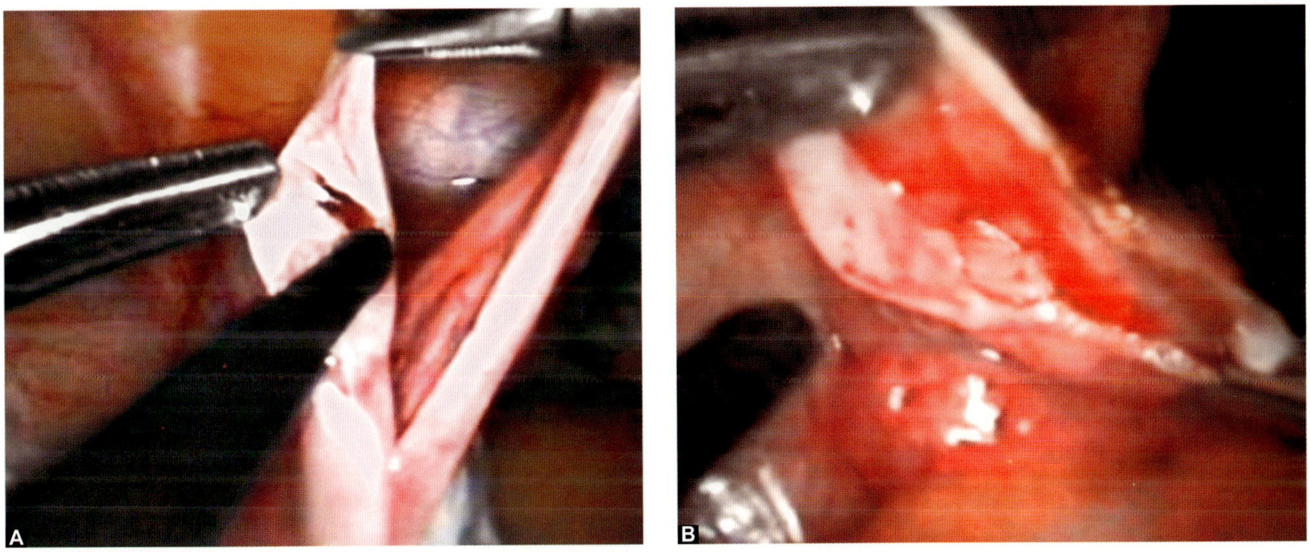

**Figs 26.3A and B:** Cruciate incision in progress

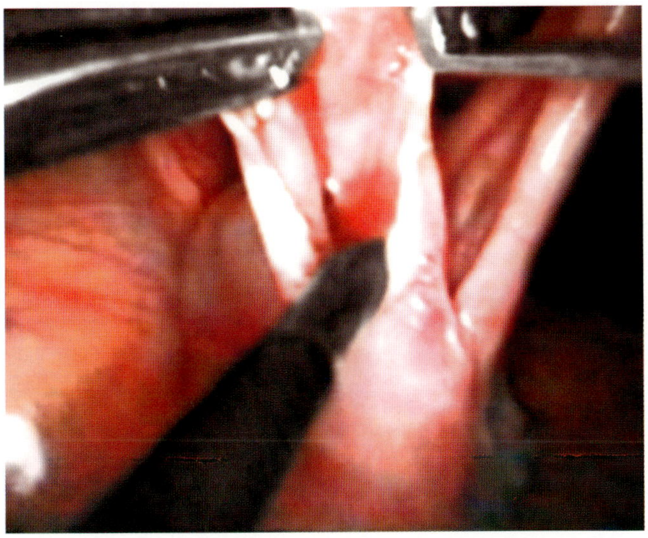

**Fig. 26.4:** Flattened fimbria seen inside the lumen

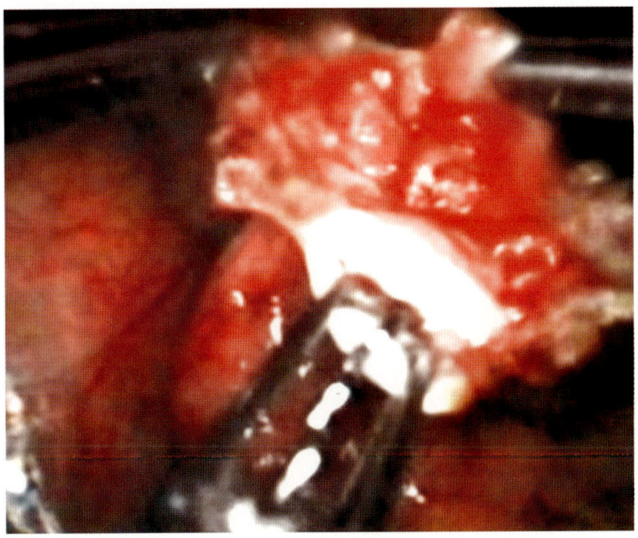

**Fig. 26.5:** Cauliflower fimbrial end—end result

## TIPS

- When the fimbria are encapsulated and hidden, the antimesentric border is incised to remove the fibrotic bands and expose the fimbria.
- After fimbrioplasty, a close watch should be kept on ectopic pregnancy.
- We recommend hysterosalpinoscintigraphy after 6 weeks to know functional patency of the Fallopian tubes (i.e. ciliary movements).
- In the era of ART, the role of this conservative management is questionable. But since IVF is expensive and not funded by Government or insurance companies in India, one might need to offer this to certain women.

Chapter

27

# Laparoscopic Tubotubal Anastomosis

*Sanjay Patel*

Laparoscopic microsurgery is a new discipline that synergizes the potential of classical microsurgery and laparoscopy. It can overcome the deficiencies in each of the techniques. Advent of microsurgical technique began by Swolin in 1967. First microsurgical reversal of the sterilization was done by Gomel and Winston in 1977.

## PREOPERATIVE EVALUATION

- Semen analysis: To rule out male factor.
- Day 3 serum FSH level to know the ovarian reserve.
- HSG to know the length and condition of the proximal tube.
- Saline infusion sonography and hysterosalpingography may be helpful.
- Details about the previous tubectomy.

## INDICATIONS

- Reversal of tubal sterilization procedure.
- Mid-tubal block secondary to various pathology.
- Tubal occlusion secondary to ectopic pregnancy treatment.
- Failed tubal cannulation for proximal tubal block.
- Failed previous macrosurgical sterilization reversal.

## CONTRAINDICATIONS

### Absolute Contraindications

- Aged 40 years or older.
- Decreased ovarian reserve or ovarian failure.
- Tubal infertility not amenable to tubal reconstruction.
- Extensive tubal damage.
- Hydrosalpinx with a diameter of more than 3 cm.
- Inadequate proximal or distal tubal segment for reanastomosis.
- Projected tubal length of less than 3 cm after the reconstruction procedure.
- Extensive pelvic/peritubal adhesions.
- Abnormal uterine cavity.
- Any contraindication to pregnancy or surgery.
- Severe male factor infertility or male sterility which otherwise needs ART treatment.

## EQUIPMENT AND INSTRUMENTS

### Magnification, Resolution and Digital Enhancement

- 25–40x magnification is essential to identify healthy mucosa of the Fallopian tube. 10–15x magnification is adequate for microsuturing.
- Use of endoscope, digital three chip camera with monitor has a 'multiplier effect' and the magnification can be achieved up to 27–25x.

### Microinstrumentation

- It is collectively known as 'KOH ultramicro series' (Fig. 27.1).
- Terminal serration of the jaw is especially treated so that microsuture material does not get crushed.
- Handle design should be such that least friction and maximum transmission of hand movement occur to the instrument tip. 130° angle between handle and shaft of the instruments provides better movements.

## SUTURES, NEEDLES AND ENERGY

- More rigid needles are better for micro-endosuturing.
- The suture material should be 6-0 to 8-0 polypropylene, depending upon the surgeon's experience of material handling and preference.

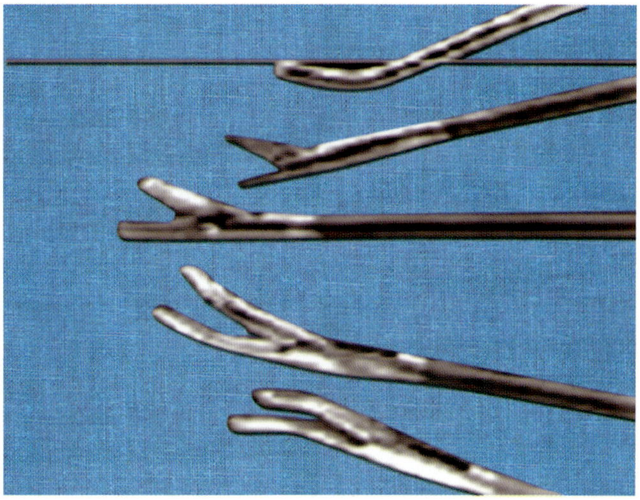

**Fig. 27.1:** KOH ultramicro series

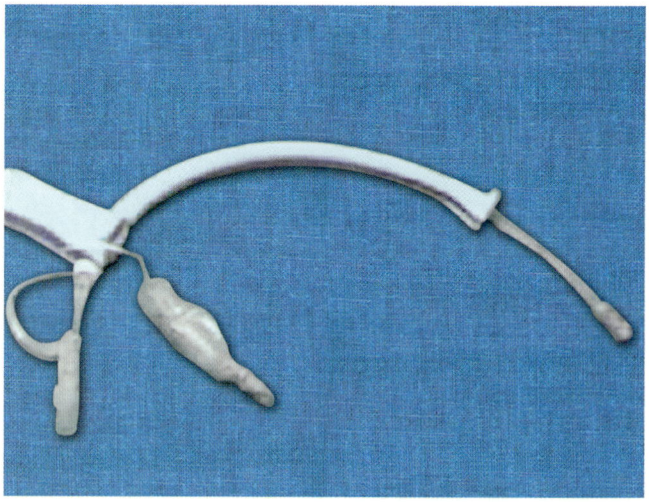

**Fig. 27.2:** Handlin's uterine manipulator

- Electrosurgery: 15-27 W for cutting and 15 W for fulguration, use minimum cautery to preserve sub-tubal vasculature (Fig. 27.12).
- *Handlin's Uterine Manipulator* is a fine disposable instrument (Fig. 27.2), which allows administration of the dye and manipulation of the uterus without causing any significant trauma.

## SELECTION OF CASES

### Length of Tubal Damage in Various Methods of Ligation

| *Type of TL* | *Length of Damage* | *Case Type* |
|---|---|---|
| Monopolar diathermy | 50 mm | Unfavorable |
| Filshie's clip (Fig. 27.3) | 4 mm | Most favorable |
| Bipolar diathermy (Fig. 27.4) | 30 mm | Intermediate |
| Falope Ring TL (Fig. 27.5) | 40 mm | Unfavorable |
| Pomeroy's method | 30 mm | Intermediate |
| Hulka clip | 7 mm | Favorable |

Other non-suitable cases are pathological tubes with PID, salpingitis isthmica nodosa and failed tubal cannulation.

## INTRA-OPERATIVE EVALUATION

Before proceeding for the tubal reconstruction, one must evaluate the inside of the tube, so as to be confirmed that the anastomosis is going to be fruitful or not at all worthwhile. This involves salpingoscopy and falloposcopy.

- Salpingoscopy allows direct inspection of tubal mucosa in the ampullary part.
- The degree of tubal mucosal damage is probably the major factor in establishing the prognosis for tubal surgery.
- Brosen's classification is useful for evaluation according to the degree of mucosal atrophy and mucosal adhesions.

**Salpingoscopy Grade 1: (Fig. 27.6)** Normal intraluminal findings with healthy major (primary) and minor (secondary) folds.

**Salpingoscopy Grade 2: (Fig. 27.7)** Mucosal nuclear staining with methylene blue dye.

**Salpingoscopy Grade 3: (Fig. 27.8)** Tubercles minimal flattening and minimal adhesion (↓) of endosalpinx.

**Salpingoscopy Grade 4: (Fig. 27.9)** Moderate flattening of endosalpinx with intraluminal adhesion.

**Salpingoscopy Grade 5: (Fig. 27.10)** Severe flattening of mucosa with severe interluminal adhesions.

## SURGICAL TECHNIQUE (FIGS 27.11 AND 27.12)

**Total 5 ports are used**

1. 10 mm laparoscope through the primary umbilical port.
2. Four ancillary ports, two 5 mm and two 3 mm.
3. The lower pelvic port of 5 mm is placed 4 cm medial and above the anterior superior iliac spine, i.e. ipsilateral Port.
4. Contralateral port of 3 mm size placed exactly opposite to ipsilateral port.
5. Another ipsilateral port of 3 mm is para-umbilical and laterally in the anterior axillary line.
6. One 5 mm central port, 2-3 cm above the pubic symphysis.

'The position of the ports is critical in enabling fluent two handed operating as well as suturing. The so-called 'fulcrum effect' is virtually eliminated by adopting specific port positions.'

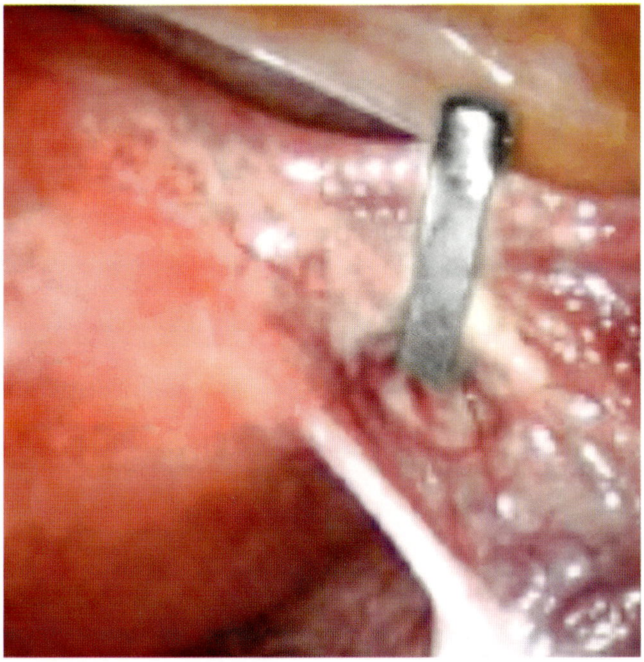

**Fig. 27.3:** Filshie's clip

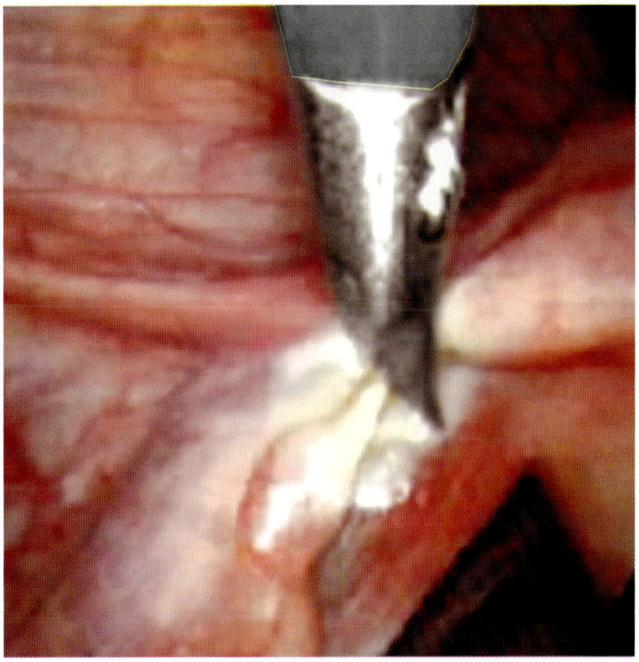

**Fig. 27.4:** Bipolar diathermy

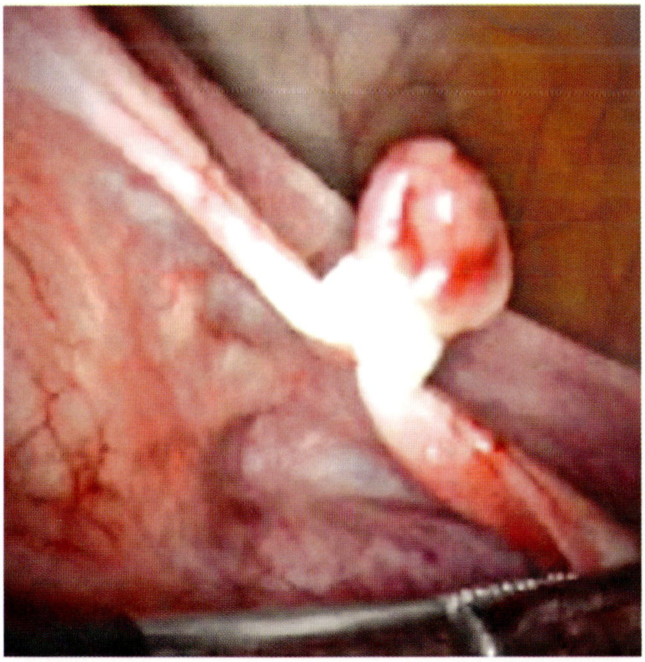

**Fig. 27.5:** Folope ring T2

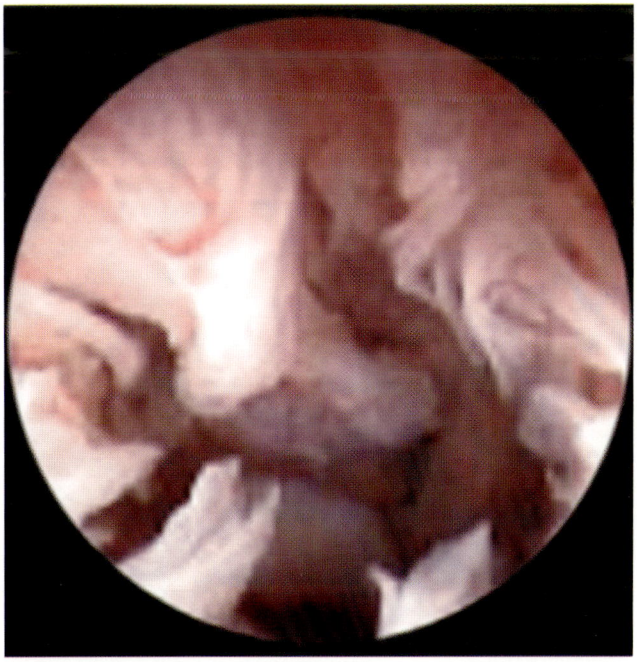

**Fig. 27.6:** Salpingoscopy Grade 1

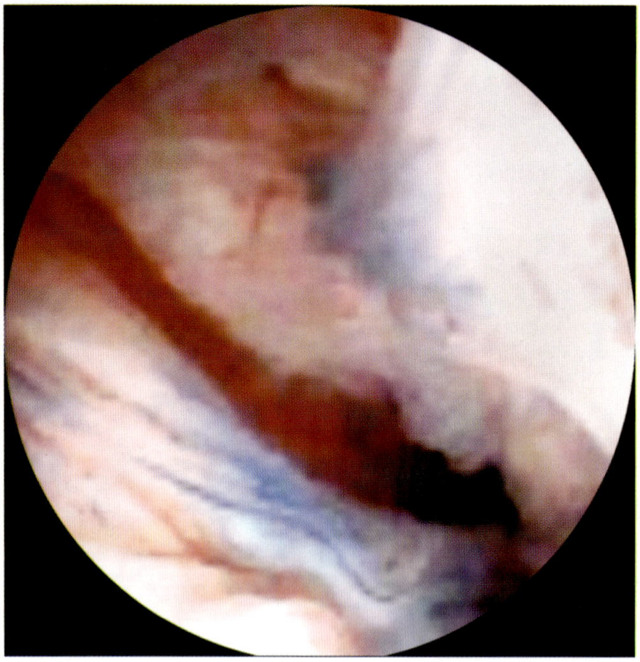

Fig. 27.7: Salpingoscopy Grade 2

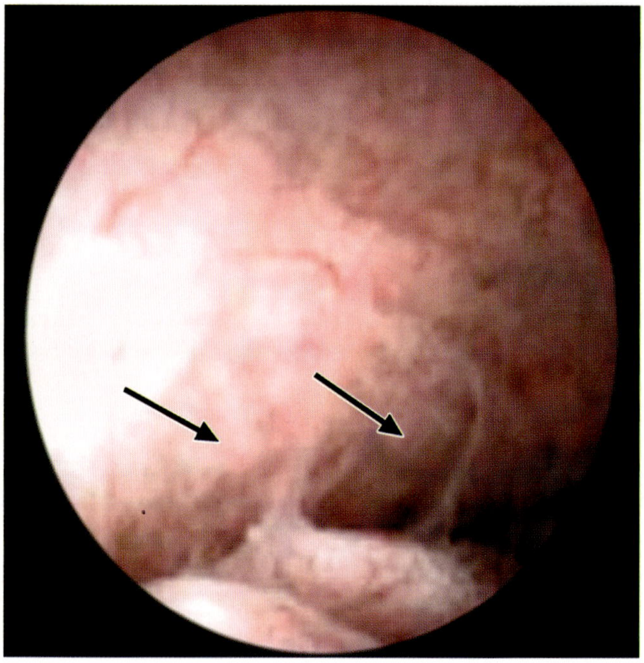

Fig. 27.8: Salpingoscopy Grade 3

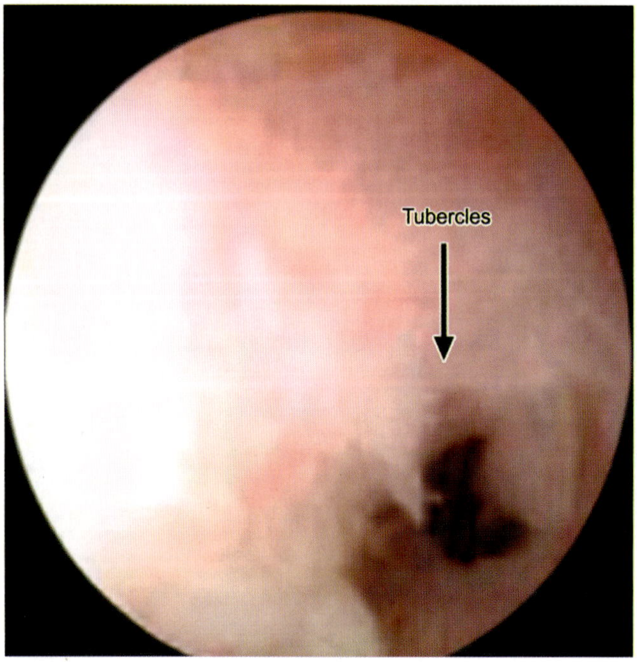


Fig. 27.9: Salpingoscopy Grade 4

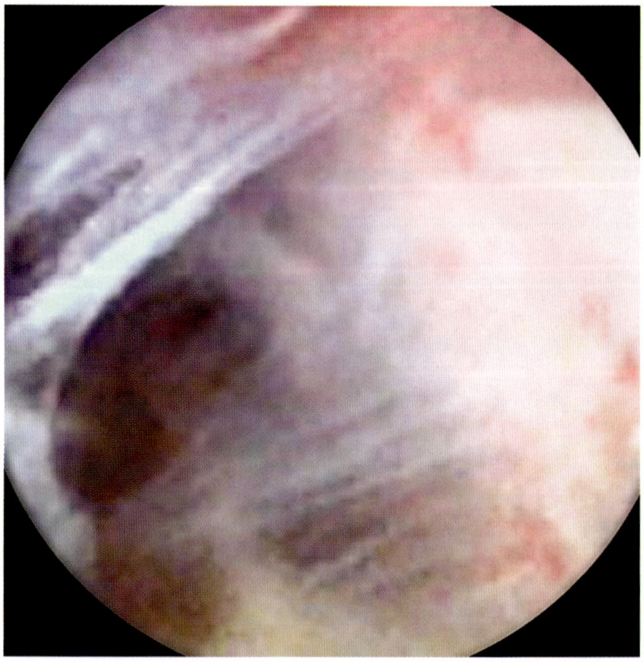

Fig. 27.10: Salpingoscopy Grade 5

### Port Positioning Sub-tubal Vessels

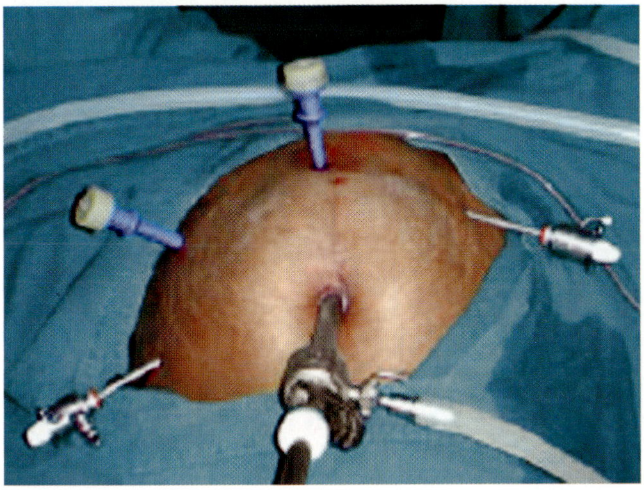

Fig. 27.11

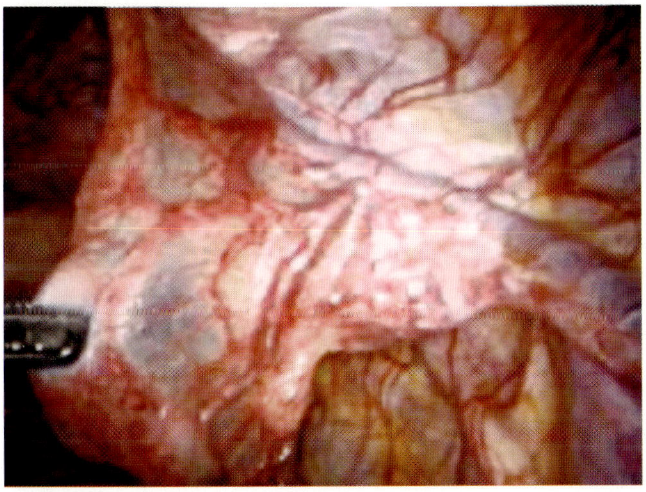

Fig. 27.12

### Important Surgical Steps

The surgical procedure involves transection of the tubal stumps and removal of scar tissue, approximation of the mesosalpinx, anastomosis of the muscle and mucosa, and approximation of the serosal layer.

## PROCEDURE

1. Dilute vasopressin is infiltrated into the mesosalpinx for hemostasis and hydrodissection.
2. It is very important to prepare the tube in two layers for a good anastomosis. Inclusion of any scarred portion in anastomosis can lead to poor healing.
3. The site of tubal obstruction is identified and held with a fine grasper. A circular incision is made on the serosa of the proximal stump about half a centimeter from the probable site of transection with a fine monopolar needle. Sharp scissors are used to excise the obstructed portion of Fallopian tube leaving a smooth edge to the patent lumen.
4. It is important that the dissection is halted at the level of the mesosalpinx to avoid injuring the blood vessels and compromising the vascularity of the tube (Fig. 27.12).
5. Chromopertubation is performed through the cervix to check the patency of the proximal stump.
6. The distal segment is also prepared in 2 layers in a similar manner. The patency of the segment is also checked by retrograde chromopertubation.
7. The mesosalpinx is approximated with a 6-0 polypropylene suture.

Tube is then approximated which is most difficult and important step.

**First Layer,** the mucosal-muscularis layer:
- Most important is 6 O'clock position stitch.
- To keep the knot outside the lumen, stitches are taken from outer to inner side on proximal end and vice versa on distal end.
- Rest of the stitches are taken at 12, 3, and 9 O' clock position in the similar manner.
- After approximation of the inner layer, chromopertubation should demonstrate tubal patency.
- The serosa is then approximated with two or three interrupted 7-0 sutures.

**Second layer,** the sero-muscularis layer:
- Sutured with 6-0 polypropylene.
- Thorough peritoneal irrigation with Ringer's lactate solution throughout the operation.
- Postoperative care is the same as for any other laparoscopic surgery. The patient is usually discharged on the evening of surgery or the first postoperative day.

## TYPES OF ANASTOMOSIS

### Isthmo-isthmic Anastomosis

- Lumen size is 500 μm–1 mm.
- Equal lumen size and thick muscularis allow technically easier and better anastomosis.

### Isthmo-ampullary Anastomosis

- Luminal disparity is the potential problem which can be adjusted by cutting the isthmic end.

### Ampullo-ampullary Anastomosis

Technically difficult anastomosis due to thin muscularis and tendency for mucosal folds prolapse.

### Tubo-cornual Anastomosis

Wedge excision in the cornual end mobilizes good length of interstitial tube.

### Pathological Tubes

Salpingoscopy plays a key role in decision making for reconstructive surgery of such tubes.

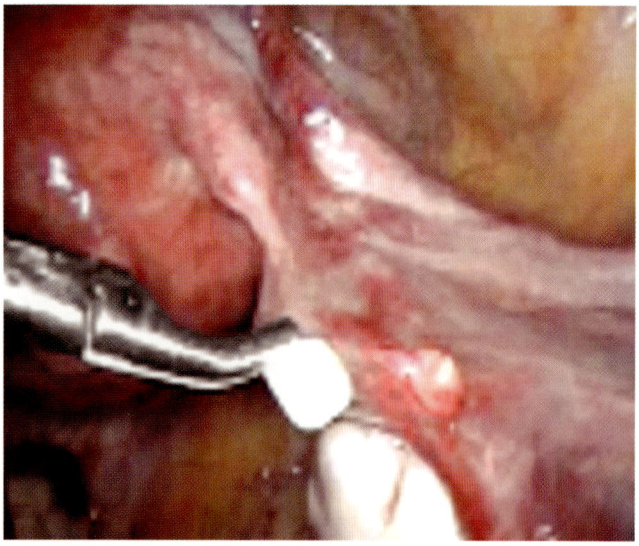

**Fig. 27.12:** Falope ring excision

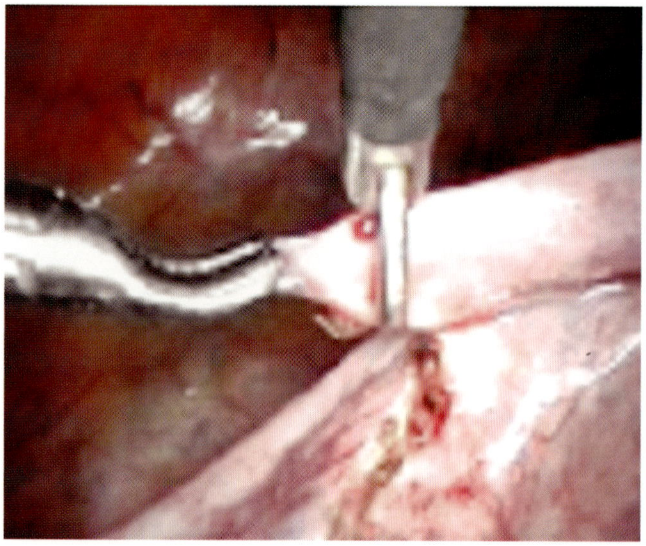

**Fig. 27.13:** Refreshening of edges

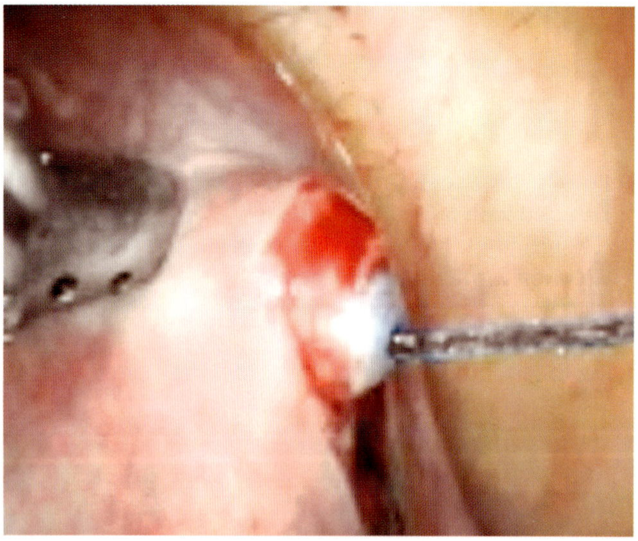

**Fig. 27.14:** Free dye flow

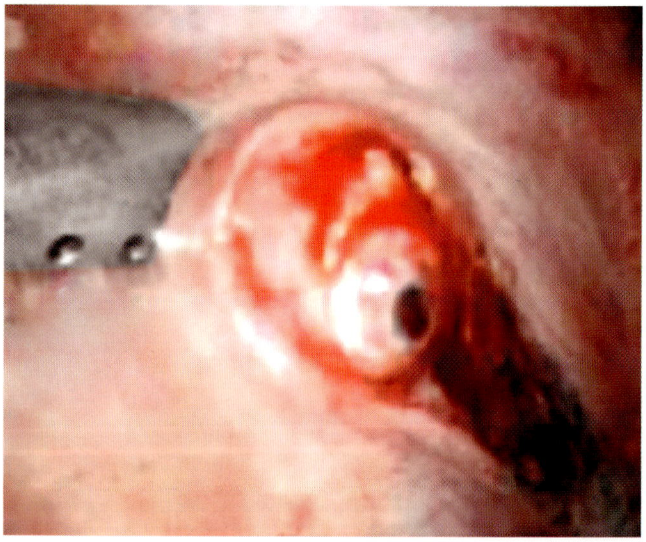

**Fig. 27.15:** Magnified view

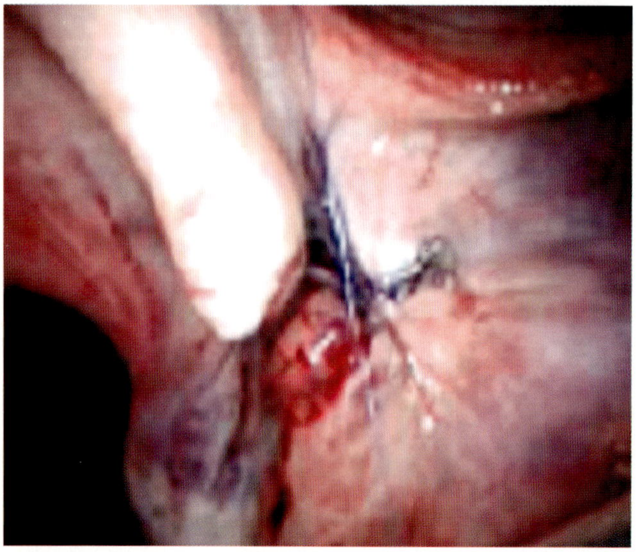

**Fig. 27.16:** Mesosalpinx stitch

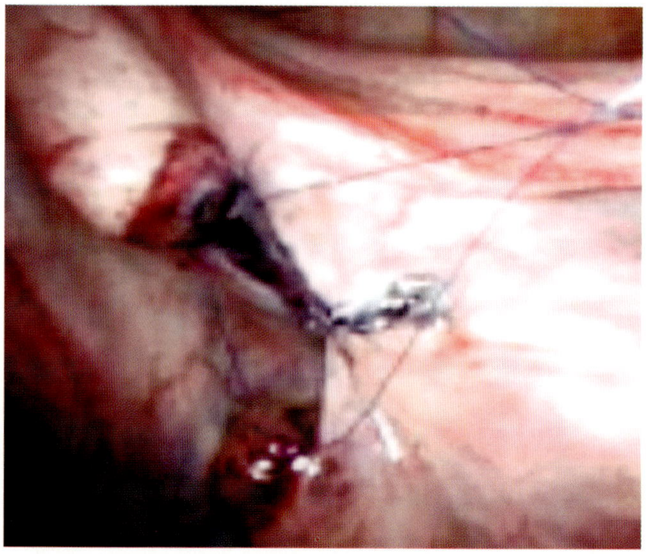

**Fig. 27.17:** 6 O'clock stitch

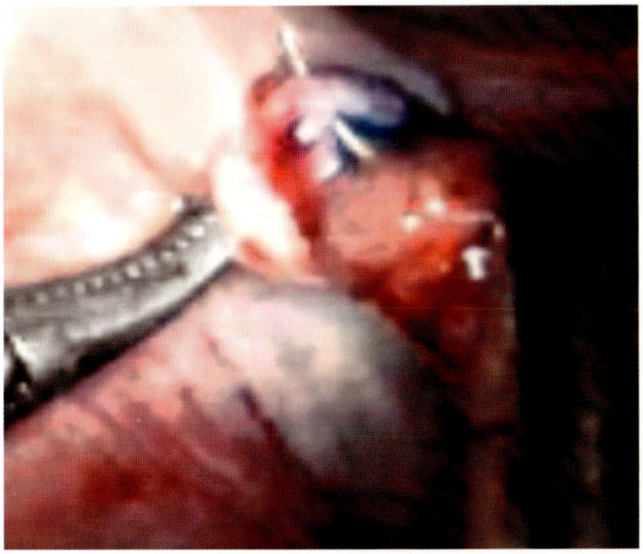

**Fig. 27.18:** 12 O'clock stitch

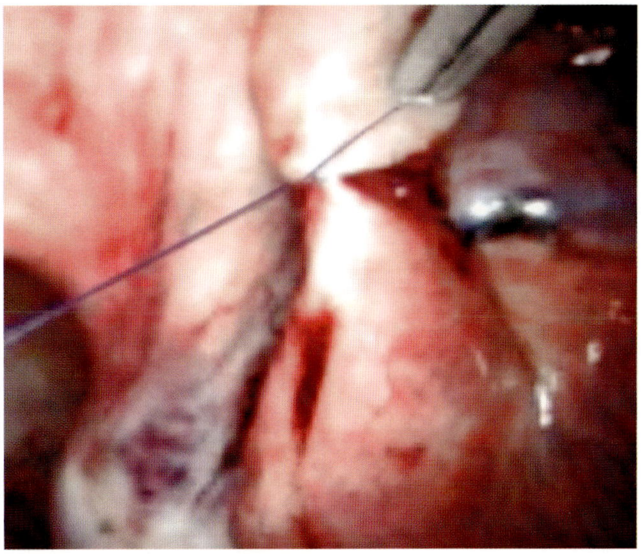

**Fig. 27.19:** Second layer

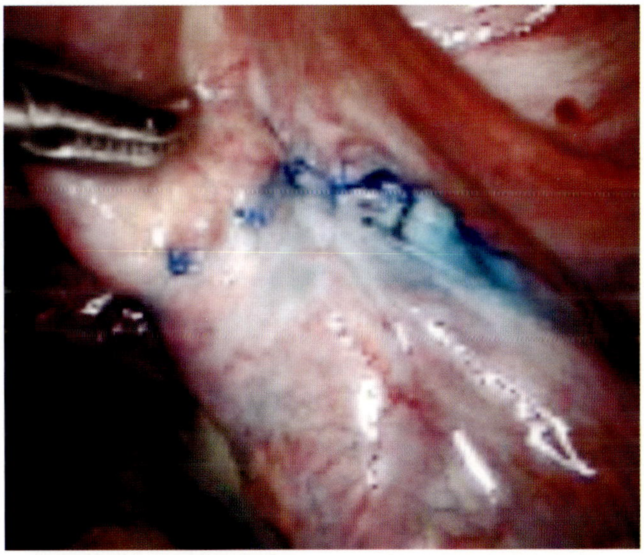

**Fig. 27.20:** No leak at the site of anastomosis

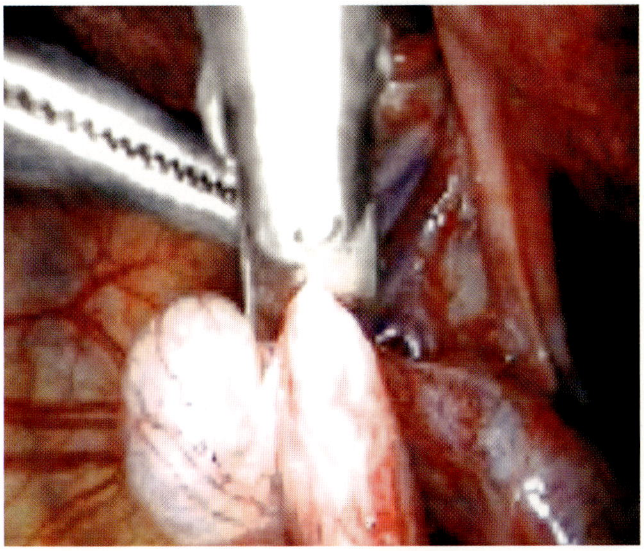

**Fig. 27.21:** Refreshening ends

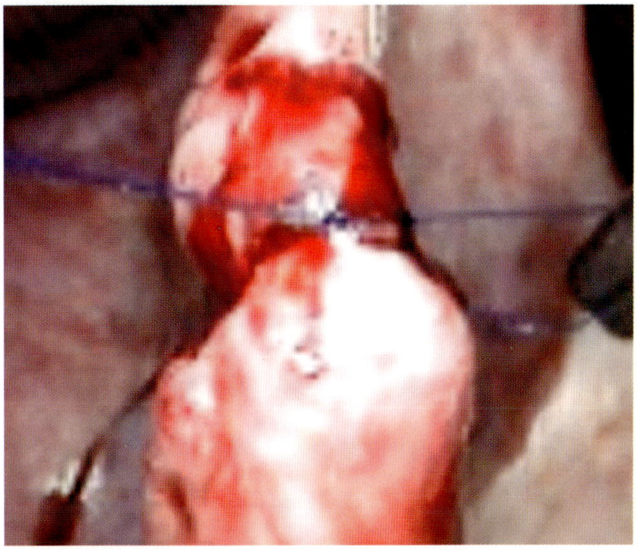

**Fig. 27.22:** First layer

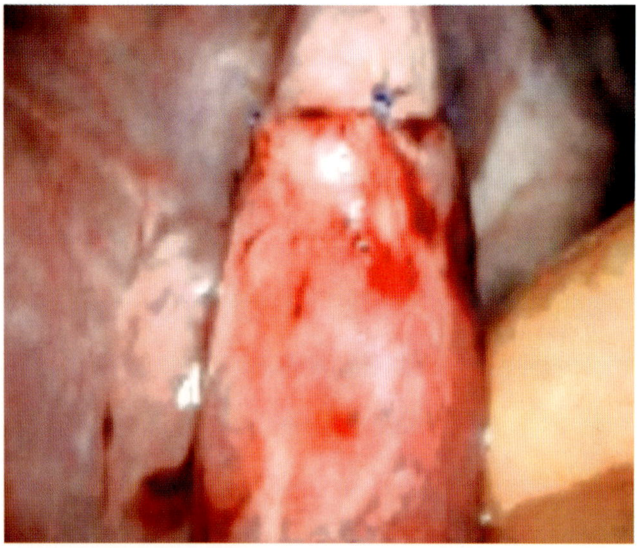

**Fig. 27.23:** Second layer

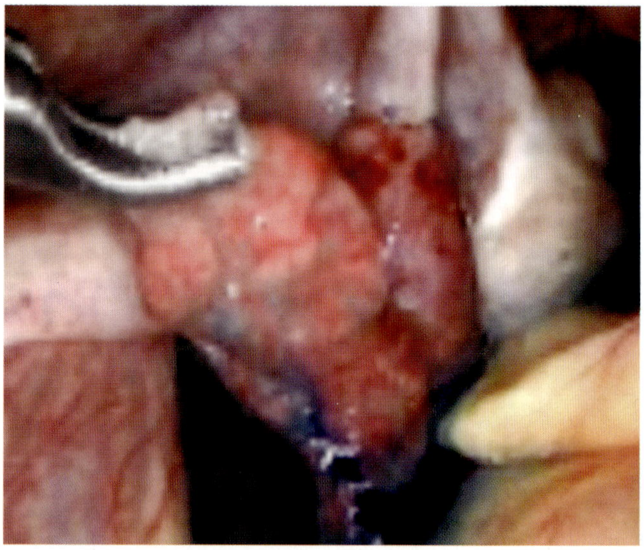

**Fig. 27.24:** Free spill

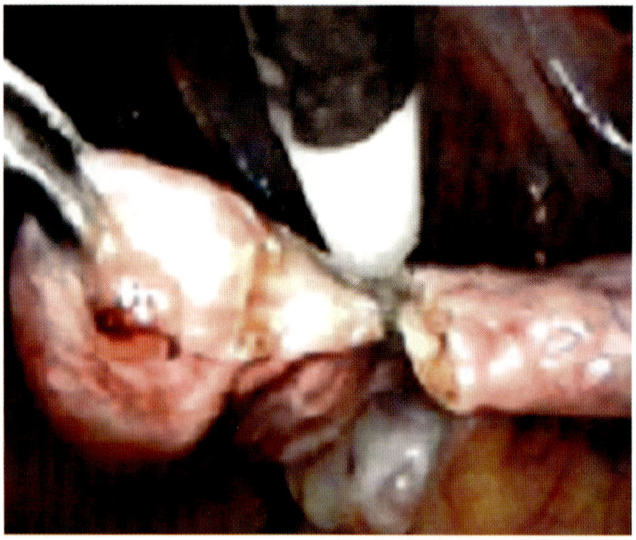

**Fig. 27.25:** Refreshening ends

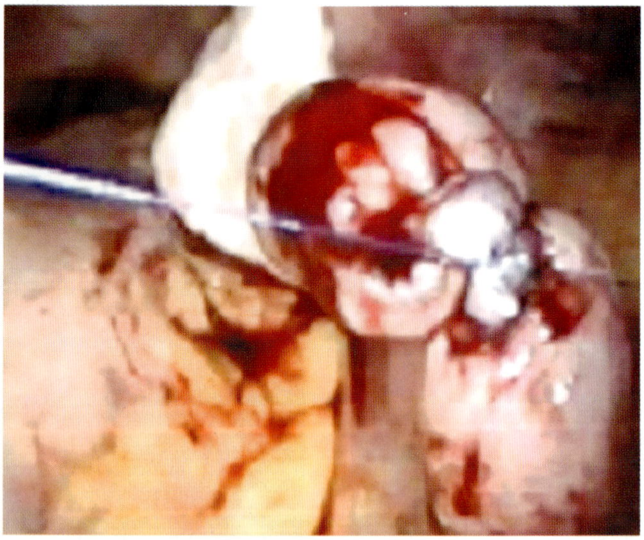

**Fig. 27.26:** First layer

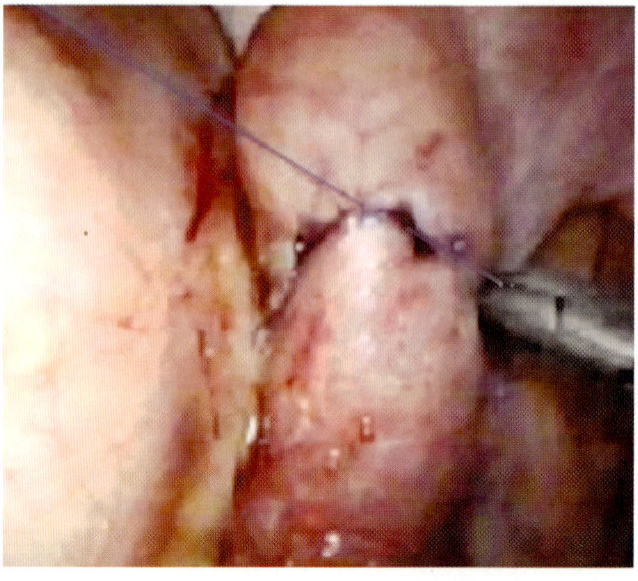

**Fig. 27.27:** Second layer

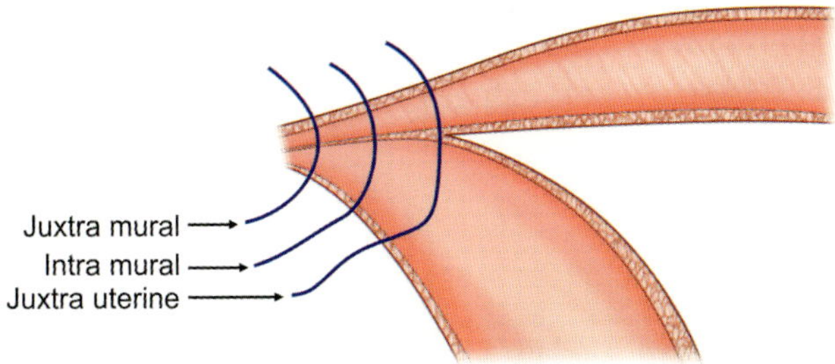


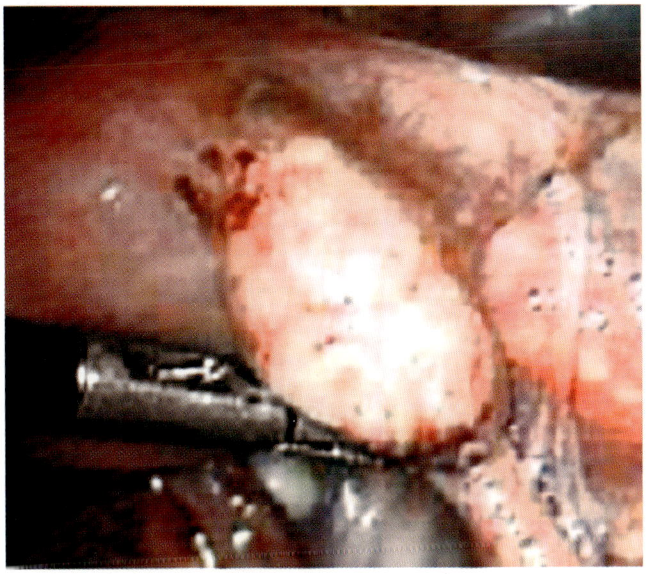

Fig. 27.28: Cornual pathology

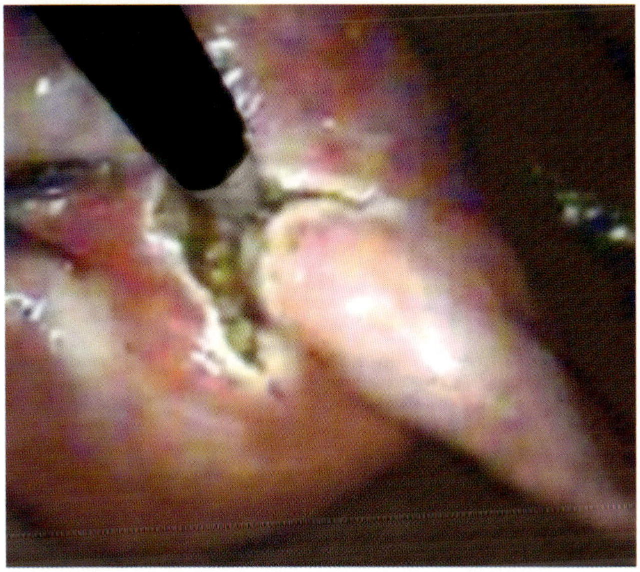

Fig. 27.29: Wedge incision

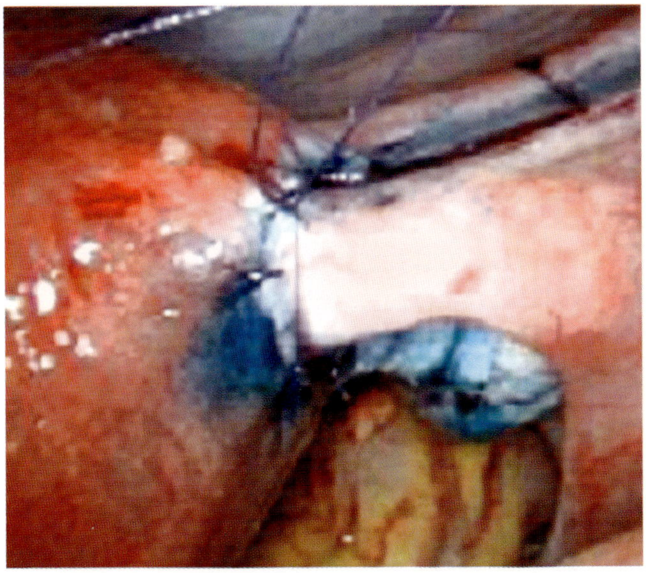

Fig. 27.30: Interstitial anastomosis

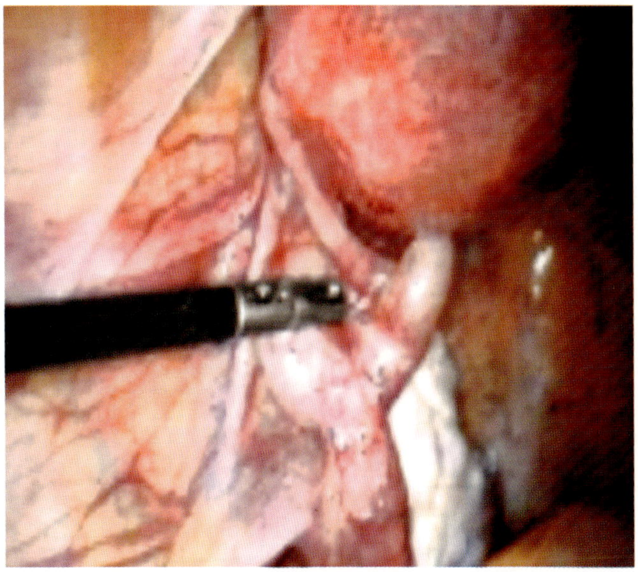

Fig. 27.31: Mild hydrosalpinx

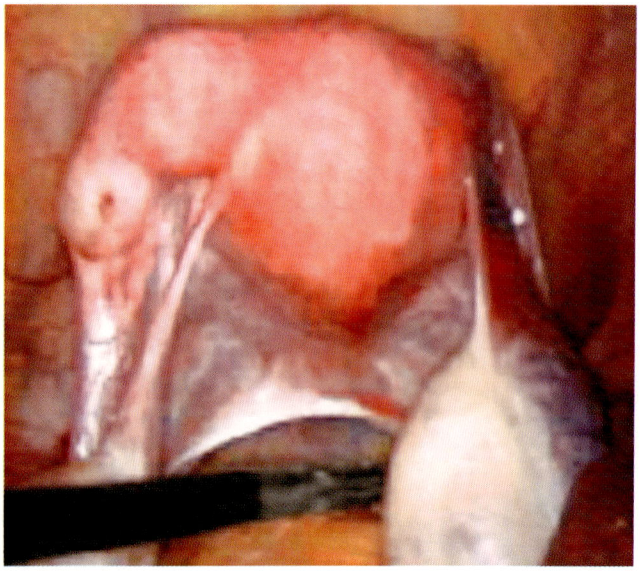

**Fig. 27.32:** Cornual pathology

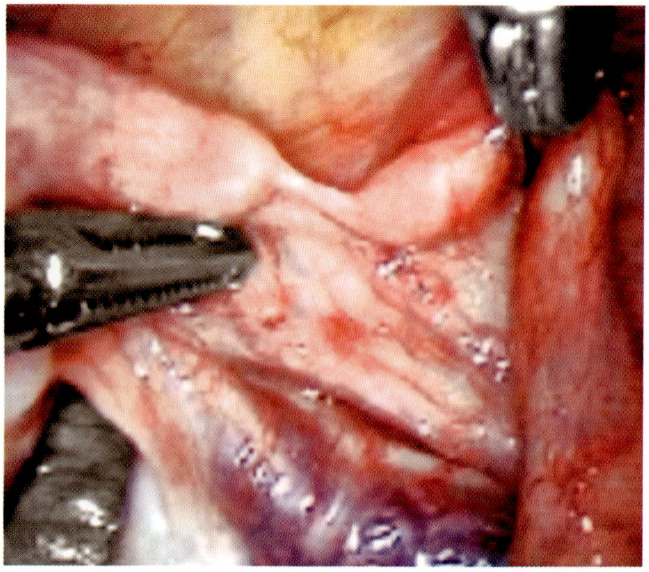

**Fig. 27.33:** Proximal tubal block

## TIPS

- Pregnancy rates are comparable with open tubal re-canalization.
- Salpingoscopy is very helpful in presence of pathological block.
- In cases of ectopic pregnancies, segmental excision is best option as compared to salpingostomy or total salpingectomy, if the ectopic sac is <2 cm of size.
- More cost-effective than IVF in the long run.
- Single step treatment as compare with IVF which may require multiple steps in each cycle.
- Make sure that the incision does not extend beyond the mesosalpinx.
- Ensure the right angled cut of the tubal ends for better alignment and approximation.

Chapter

# 28

# Laparoscopic Management of Endometrioma

*Sunita R Tandulwadkar*

## PREOPERATIVE EVALUATION

Thorough history with investigations like USG, Ca 125.

## PREOPERATIVE PREPARATION

### Bowel Preparation

- Diet: One day prior to surgery, soft diet till afternoon followed by liquid diet and then, nil by mouth for 8 hours prior to surgery.
- Peglec powder: Dissolve the pack in 2 liters of water to be given within 2–3 hours on previous evening.

OR

- Exelyte solution 90 mL to be added in 300 mL of limca/fruit juice to be given on previous evening.

## IMPORTANT EQUIPMENT

- 10 mm 0º laparoscope
- 5 mm laparoscope
- 5 mm atraumatic grasping forceps, toothed grasping forceps, microdissecting forceps and other standard operative endoscopy instruments
- Good suction irrigation cannula (5 mm)
- Monopolar needle
- Bipolar forceps
- Scissors
- 10 mm grasper (for extraction of specimen)
- Rectal and vaginal probe
- Lapsac bag
- Rumi/Hulka's uterine manipulator.

### Position of the Patient

Patient is placed in a low modified lithotomy position on the Allen's stirrups with adjustable and padded leg rest.

### Port Placement

Standard port placement (refer to chapter on port placement).

A 10 mm 0º laparoscope or occasionally 30º laparoscope is introduced through primary port. $CO_2$ is used for pneumoperitoneum at a rate of 3–9 liters/minutes with a pressure cut off at 15 mm Hg.

Trendelenberg's position is always given after primary port placement.

Whether endometrial cyst wall ablation or cystectomy depends upon:

- Size of the endometrioma
- Feasibility of excision
- History of previous surgeries for endometrioma
- Symptomatology—whether pelvic pain or infertility.

### *Usually*

- Endometrium <3 cm—Ablation of cyst wall
- Endometrium >3 cm—Cystectomy.

## ABLATION OF CYST WALL

1. After seeing the site of endometrioma, its relation with adjacent organs—ureters, bowel and lateral pelvic wall, and the point at which the endometrioma should be punctured is decided (Fig. 28.1).
2. Usually ovary is adherent and does not need stabilization, little lifting may be needed before puncturing.
3. Endometrioma is punctured with a needle with monopolar cautery current/harmonic scalpel/scissors (Fig. 28.2).
4. Chocolate material is completely drained. The incision is extended so as to visualize the inner cyst wall. Thorough inspection of inner cyst wall is an important step (Figs 28.3 and 28.4).

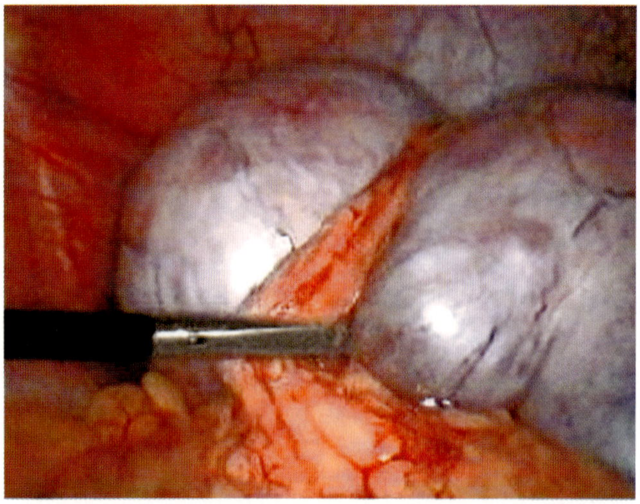

**Fig. 28.1:** Huge endometriomas

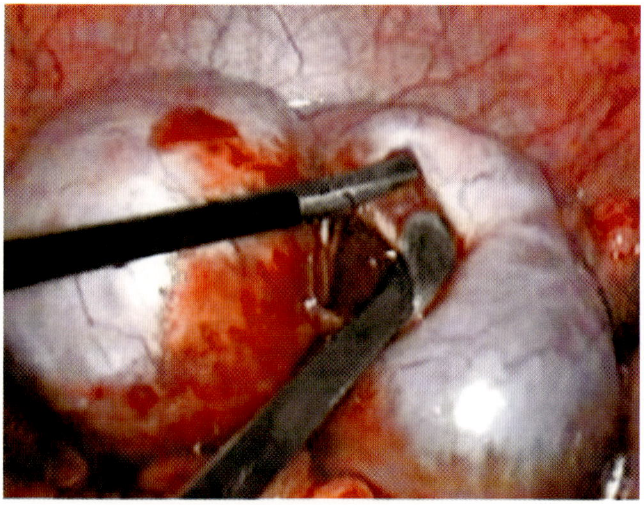

**Fig. 28.2:** Puncture and suction of chocolate fluid

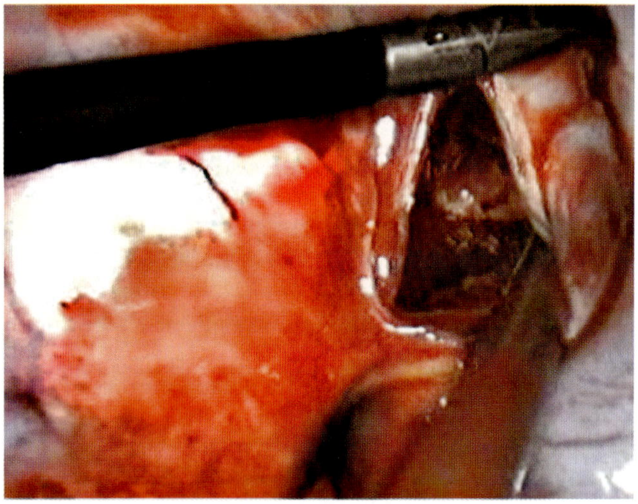

**Fig. 28.3:** Extending the incision

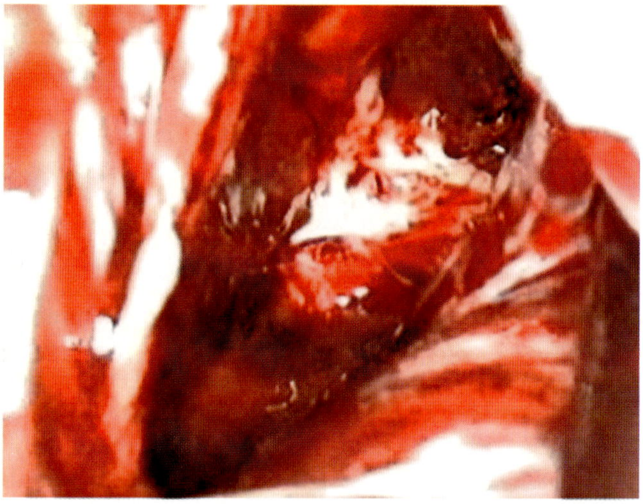

**Fig. 28.4:** Cystoscopy, i.e. inspection of the cyst wall

5. A small cyst wall piece is taken and sent for histopathological examination.
6. Rest of the cyst wall is ablated with bipolar cautery/laser.
7. Thorough lavage should be given.
8. Always aim at a clean pelvis as the end result.
9. Ovarian wound is left open to heal (and not sutured).

## CYSTECTOMY

1. Again the point of puncture is decided and the endometrioma is punctured with the monopolar needle/harmonic scalpel/scissors.
2. The incision is extended with scissor or the same monopolar needle so as to accommodate suction irrigation cannula.
3. Suction cannula is inserted into cyst and the chocolate material is completely drained out. This avoids excessive spillage of chocolate material in the lower abdomen especially in case of a large cyst.
4. The incision is further extended.
5. Inner cyst wall is inspected thoroughly (Fig. 28.4).
6. Cyst wall is identified and separated from ovarian tissue by applying two claw forceps on the cyst wall and the nontraumatic sturdy grasper with firm grip on ovarian wall, and pulled apart (Figs 28.5 and 28.6).
7. Forceps are advanced from time to time to stay closer to the cleavage line for proper traction and countertraction and hence dissection in a vascular plane.
8. Once the cyst wall is excised completely, the bed is observed for any active bleeder under water.
9. With simple grasper, the pressure is applied on the ovarian tissue to stop oozing.
10. During this time, through the other port, suction cannula is inserted and the pelvis is thoroughly lavaged.
11. Usually capillary oozing stops with pressure and only active bleeder seen under water flow can be cauterized with bipolar.
12. Avoid excessive cauterization of the bed as it will further reduce ovarian reserve.

13 Removal of cyst wall: 5 mm telescope is passed through secondary port and 10 mm grasper is passed

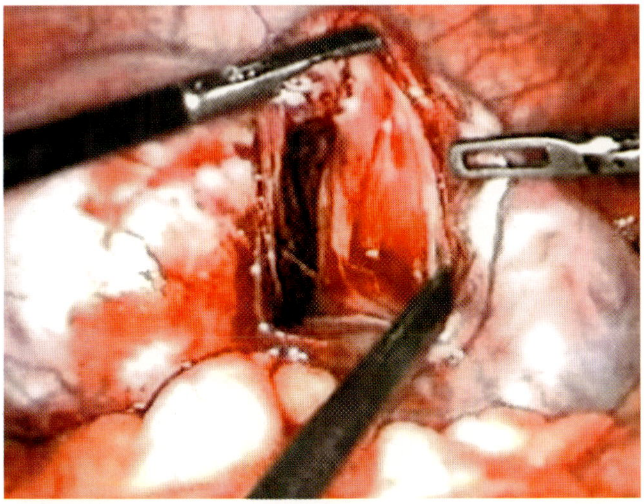

**Fig. 28.5:** Creating plane

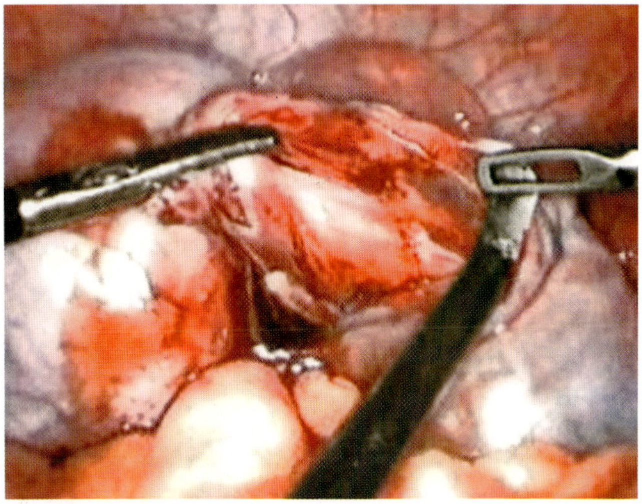

**Fig. 28.6:** Cystectomy in process

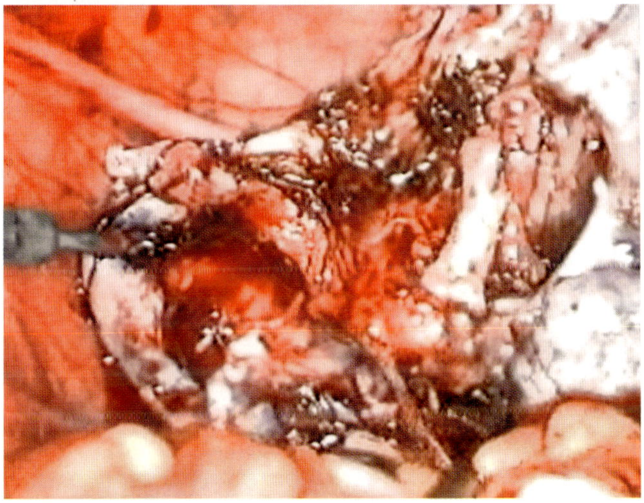

**Fig. 28.7:** Coagulation of bleeders to achieve hemostasis

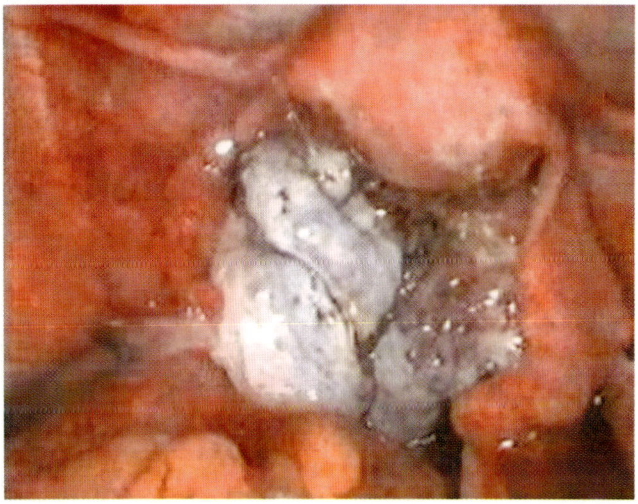

**Fig. 28.8:** End result

through the primary port and the specimen is removed always under vision. If specimen is small, it can be removed by withdrawing it in 10 mm reducer passed through primary port, but if it is bulky, either cut in 2 pieces and remove as above or remove in Lapsac.

14. Cauterization of any endometriosis spots if present in pelvis should be performed.
15. Thorough lavage should be given and a clean pelvis as an end result should be achieved (Figs 28.7 and 28.8).
16. Again, reconstruction of ovarian bed is not necessary but in cases of large endometrioma, simple 2 or 3 stitches to approximate the opposite walls can be taken to avoid adhesions.

## Postoperative Care

- All patients should be discharged by evening, as early mobilization is equally important in reducing postoperative adhesions.
- Immediately, after laparoscopic drainage, 3 injections of GnRH analogues (once every 4 weeks) or 3 months depot injection can be given. Second look laparoscopic surgery may be advocated.

### TIPS

- Good Trendlenberg position, adequate pneumoperitoneum and bowel preparation will keep bowel away from the field.
- Before proceeding for the surgery, if there are pelvic adhesions they should be removed either with sharp scissors or ultrasicion.
- During adhesiolysis in patients with extensive endometriosis, try to go from the lateral pelvic wall to the medial, and proceed from identifiable tissue organs to unidentified ones.
- Always aim at conserving ovarian tissue and minimizing postoperative adhesions.

## Laparoscopic Management of Endometrioma with Extensive Adhesions

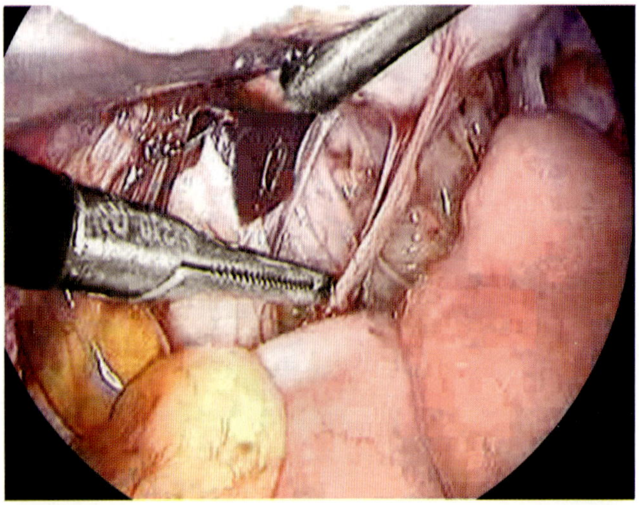

**Fig. 28.9:** Endometrioma opened

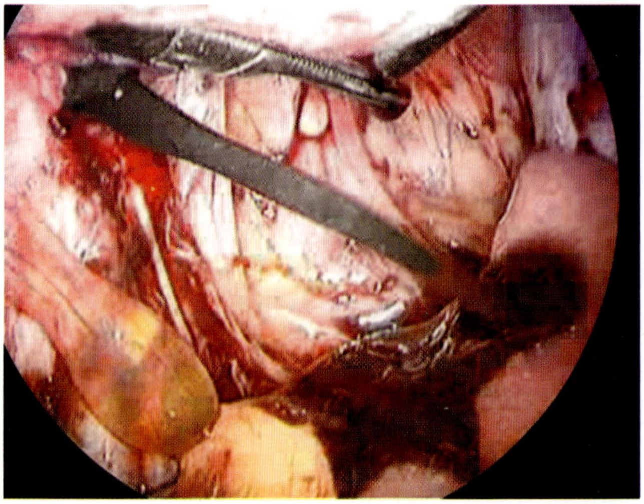

**Fig. 28.10:** Chocolate material is drained

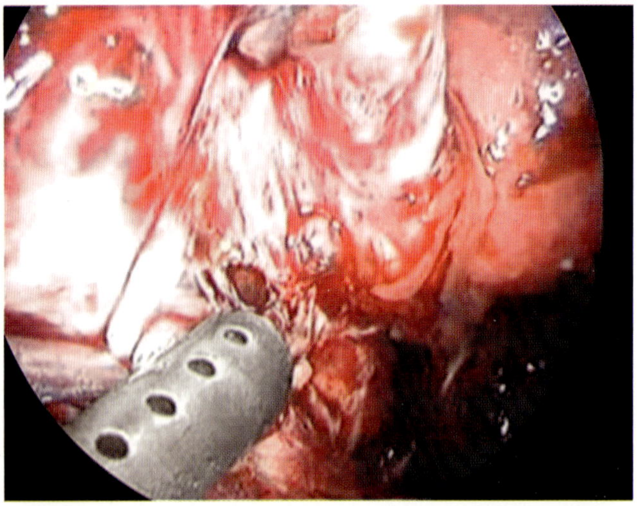

**Fig. 28.11:** Opening of the endometrioma

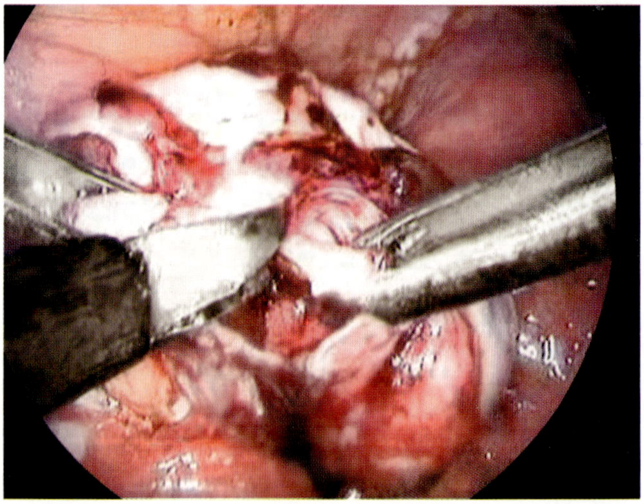

**Fig. 28.12:** Relaxing incision

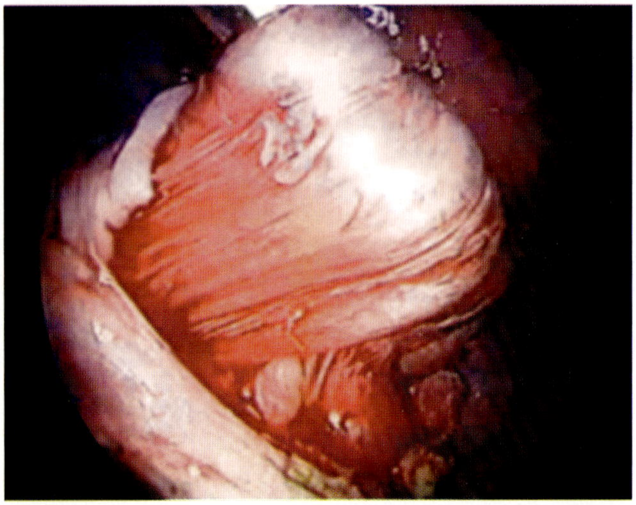

**Fig. 28.13:** Peeling of cyst wall

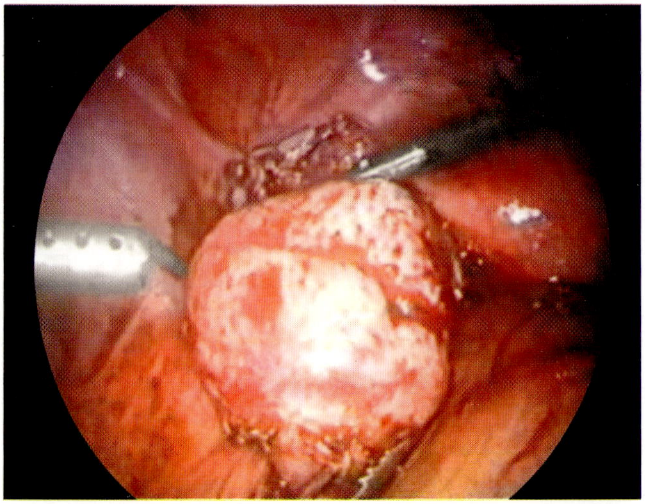

**Fig. 28.14:** Evertion to expose cortex

## Laparoscopic Excision of a Large Endometrioma in an 18 year-old Girl

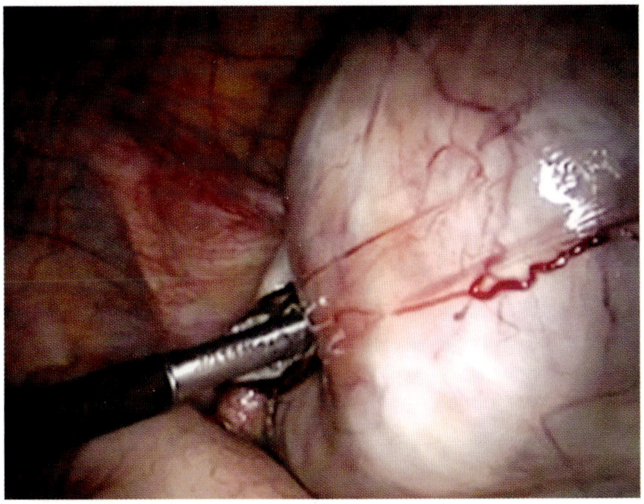

**Fig. 28.15:** Examination

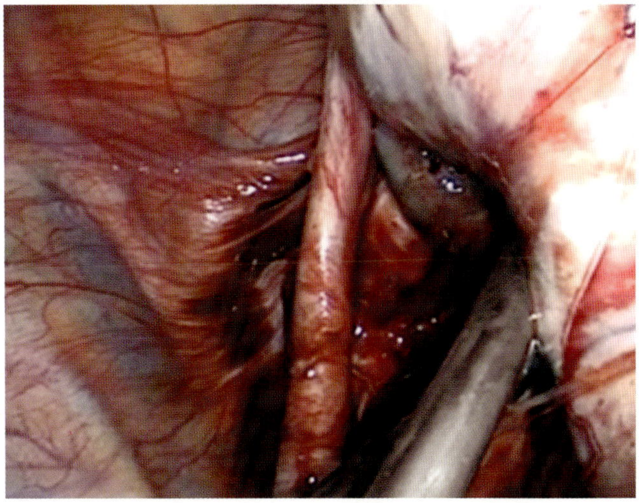

**Fig. 28.16:** Adhesions present and separated

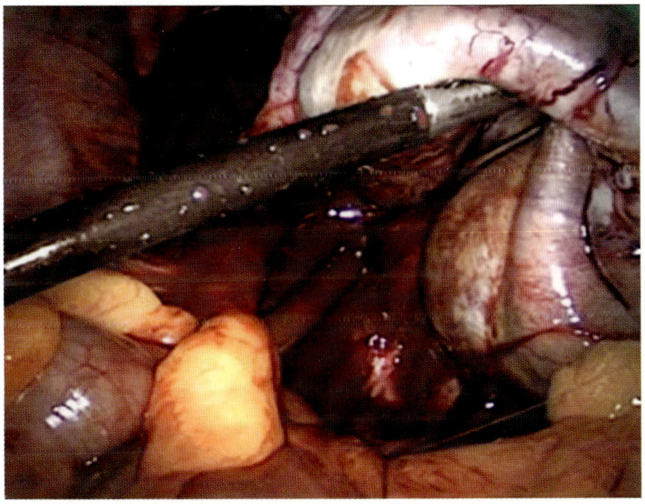

**Fig. 28.17:** 'Chocolate' fluid drained

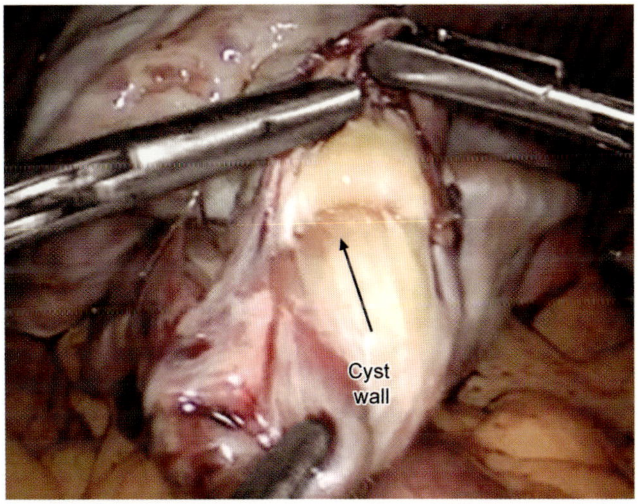


**Fig. 28.18:** Cyst wall excised from normal ovary

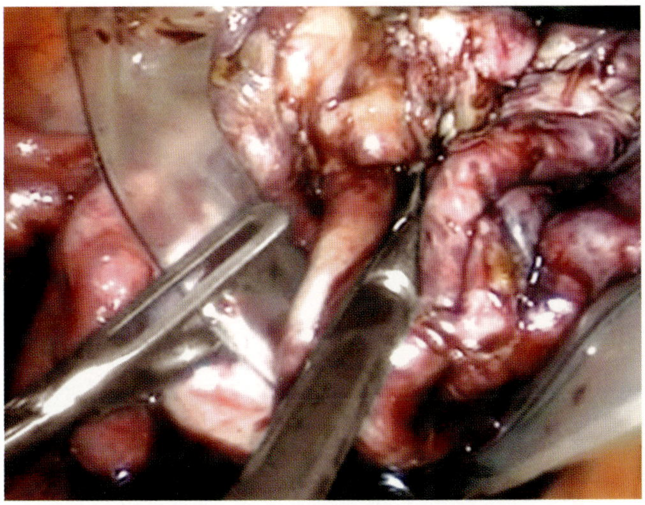

**Fig. 28.19:** Cyst wall removed in endobag

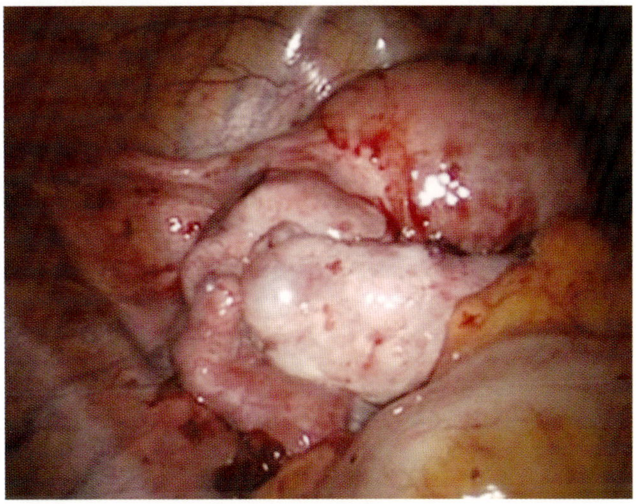

**Fig. 28.20:** End result: Clean cavity

Chapter 29

# Salpingoscopy

*Sanjay Patel*

It is the endoscopic examination of the mucosal folds of the distal segment (ampullary portion) of the Fallopian tube which has an important role in the investigation of infertility.

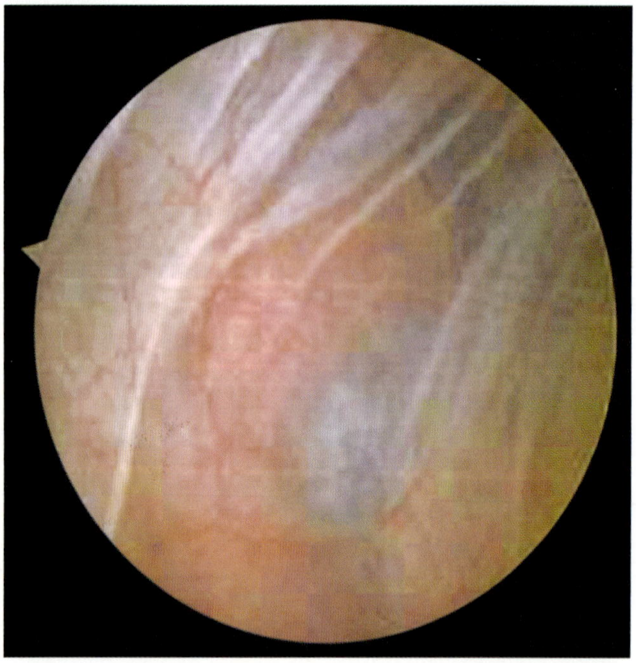

## INSTRUMENTS AND PROCEDURE OF SALPINGOSCOPY

Salpingoscopy is performed under laparoscopic guidance. Two separate laparoscopic cameras (Karl Storz, Tuttlingen, Germany) each with separate monitors should be used.

Salpingoscopy is performed using 2.9 mm diameter telescope with 12° angle (Figs 29.1 and 29.2). 2.9 mm telescope with diagnostic sheath of 4 mm in diameter.

- Normal saline is used for distension of the Fallopian tubes without any positive pressure.
- Occasionally dilatation of the fimbrial end is performed using a retrograde dye tester instrument (Figs 29.3A and B) or a 5 mm Maryland grasper (Figs 29.4 and B).
- Retrograde dye tester is a hollow, light and smooth conical tip instrument. It was actually designed to be used at laparoscopic tubal recanalization for retrograde dye test.

Extreme caution and gentleness is required in handling fimbriae as they play the most important role of ovum pick up and are indeed very delicate structures (Figs 29.5A and B).

It is preferred to introduce the salpingoscope through the 5 mm midline secondary port, under vision from the primary telescope.

Fluid gently distends the ampullary portion of the tube and allows detailed assessment of the tubal endothelium.

There are usually 4–6 larger folds of endothelium which are described as major or primary folds.

In between two major folds, there are 3–4 smaller thin folds, which are minor or secondary folds.

Prof. Brosen has classified salpingoscopy into 5 grades depending upon the visual impression of the tubal endothelial folds which are modified slightly as following:

### Grade I (Fig. 29.6)

It is the normal, pink healthy looking major and minor mucosal folds. Major folds can be seen floating freely as the fluid passes through the tubal lumen.

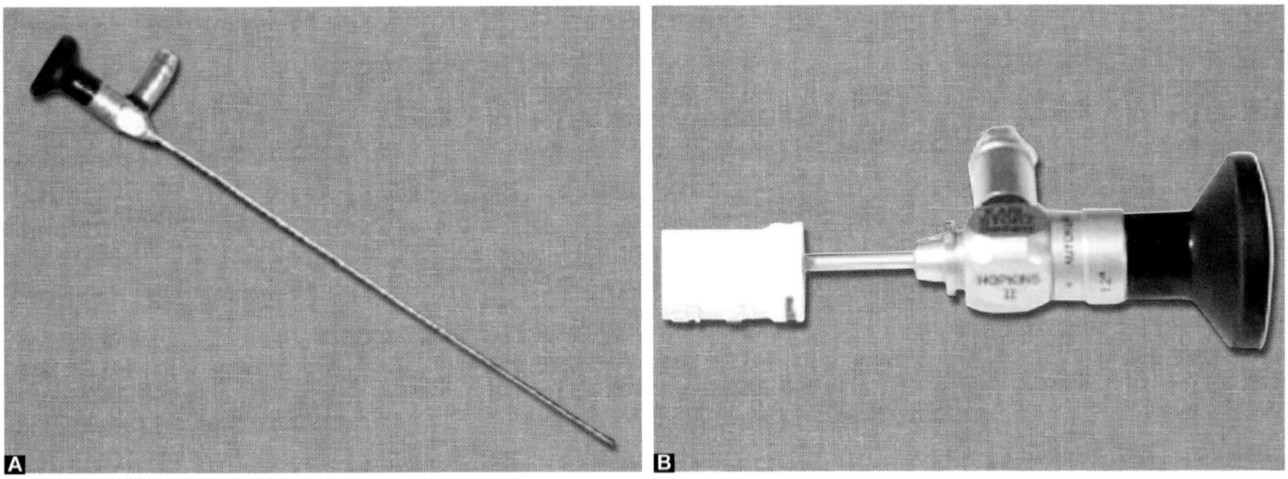

**Figs 29.1A and B:** Telescope 2.9 mm

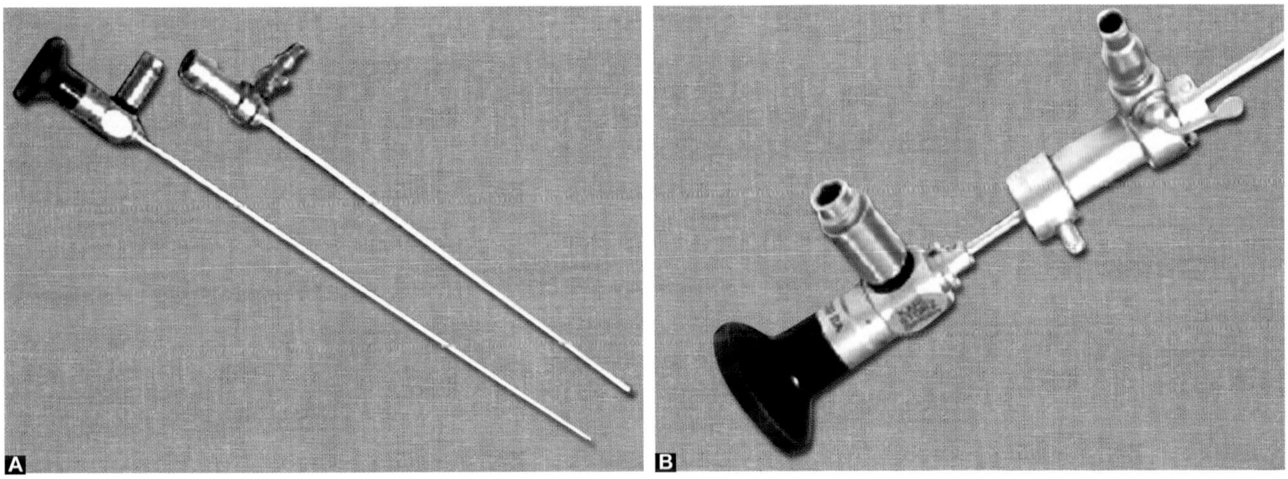

**Figs 29.2A and B:** Telescope with diagnostic sheath (4 mm)

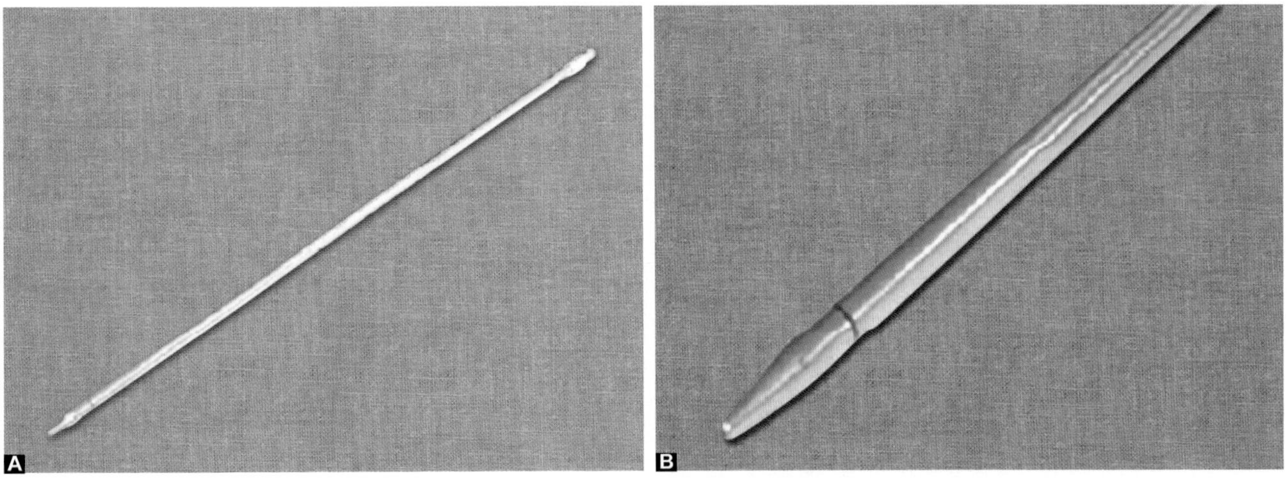

**Figs 29.3A and B:** Retrograde dye tester

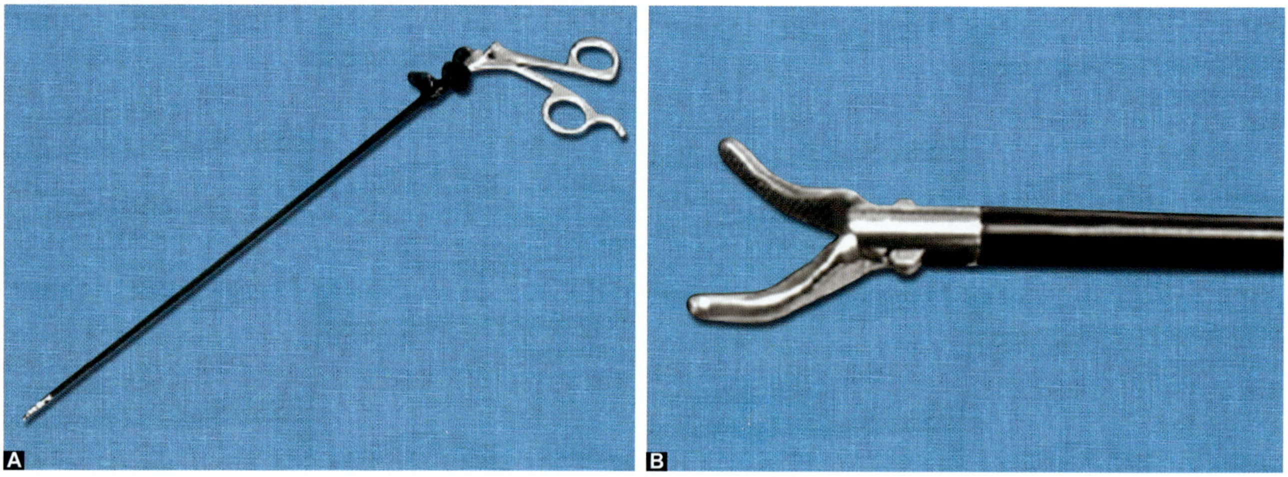

**Figs 29.4A and B:** Maryland grasper

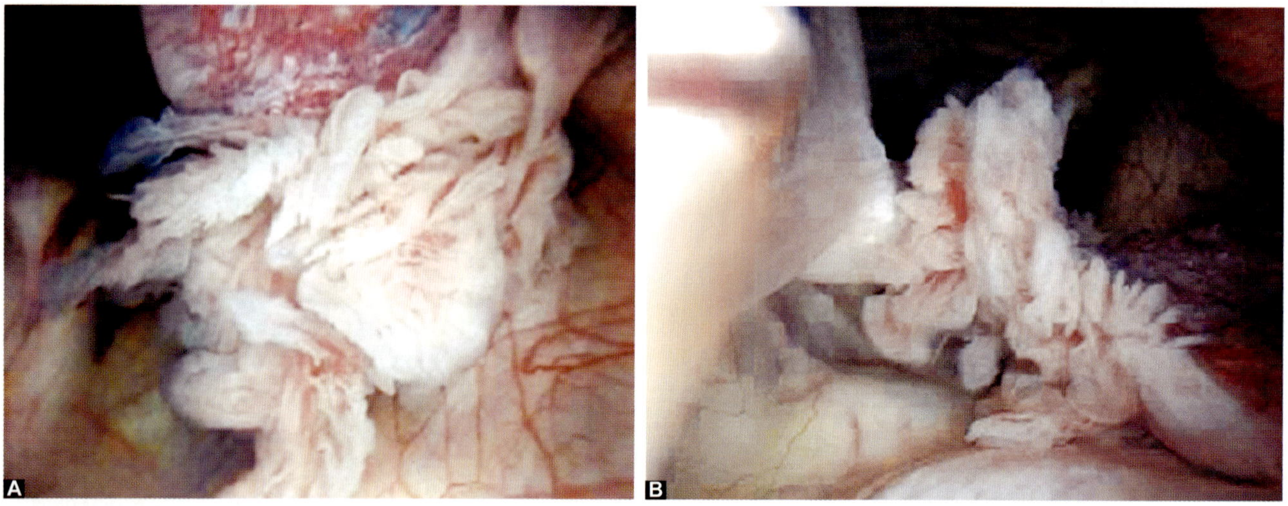

**Figs 29.5A and B:** Healthy fimbriae

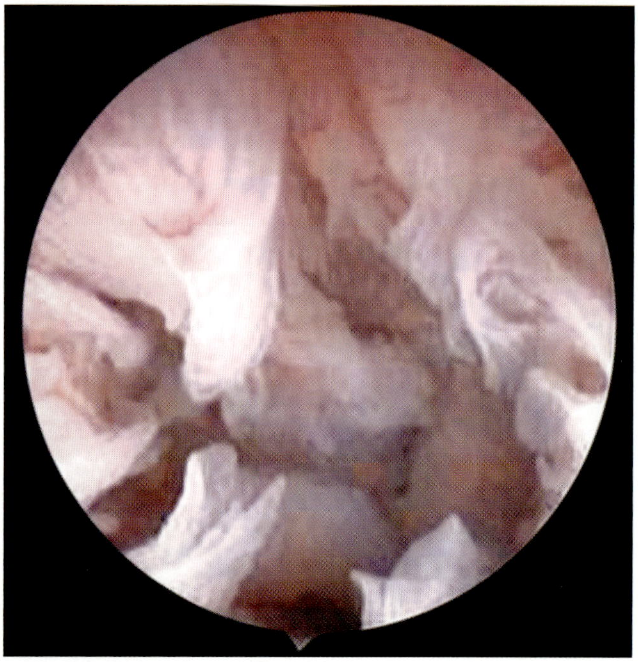

**Fig. 29.6:** Grade I Salpingoscopy

## Grade II (Figs 29.7 and 29.8)

Methylene blue is passed before salpingoscopy to confirm tubal patency.

Patchy staining of endothelial folds with methylene blue dye is seen and/or there is minimal flattening of major folds with separation of major and minor folds.

It indicates the inflammatory reaction within the endothelium.

This can be further divided in:

Grade IIA: Only staining of the endosalpinx (Fig. 29.7).

Grade IIB: Staining along with mild flattening of major folds with single band of adhesion (Fig. 29.8).

On contact micro-salpingoscopy with upto 150x magnification, inflammatory cells are seen as blue dots very clearly. They are nothing but the inflammatory cell nucleus which stain on methylene blue dye test (Fig. 29.9).

Rest of the mucosa appears healthy.

## Grade III (Fig. 29.10)

Variable degree of flattening of the endothelial folds with moderate adhesions between them. Flattening of

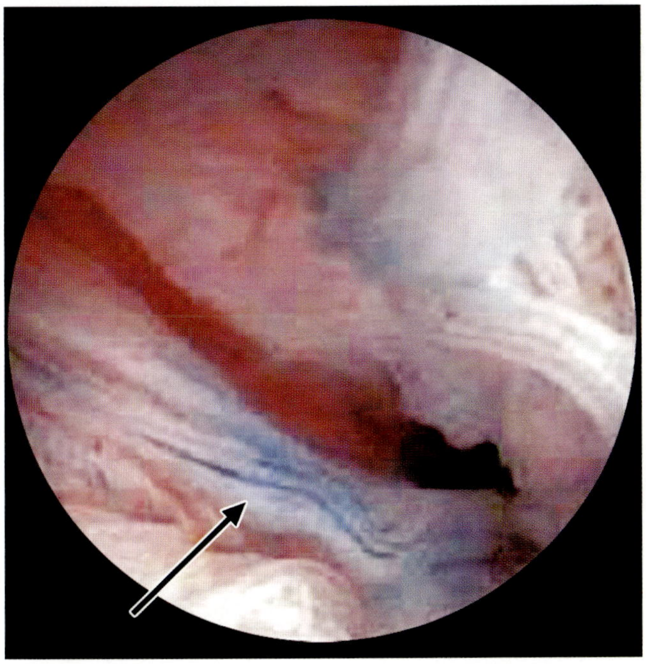

**Fig. 29.7:** Staining of the endosalpinx (Grade IIA)

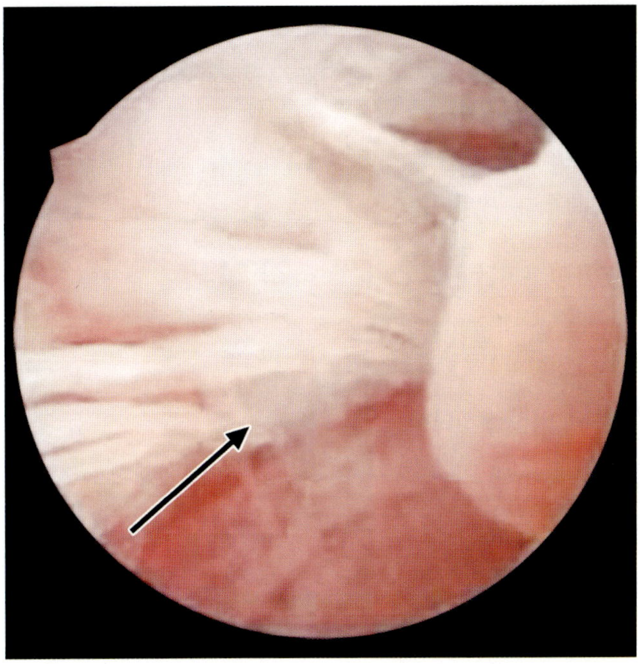

**Fig. 29.8:** Grade IIB salpingoscopy

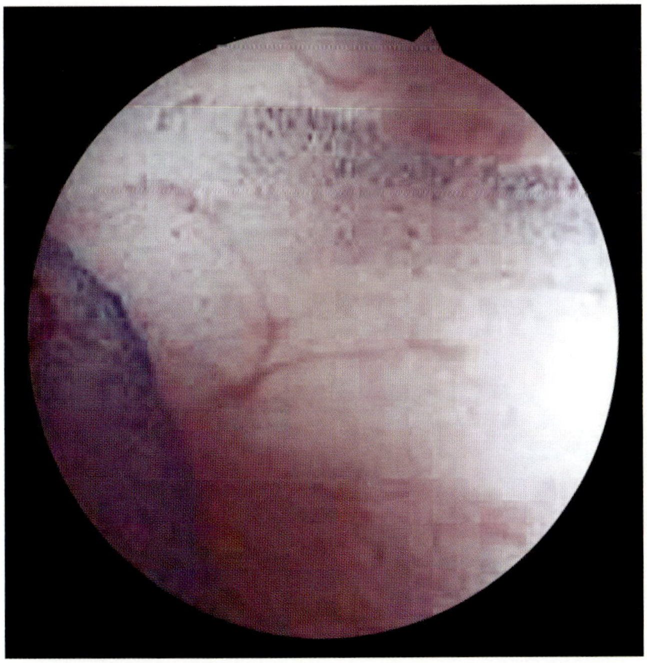

**Fig. 29.9:** Methylene blue stained imflammatory cell nucleus

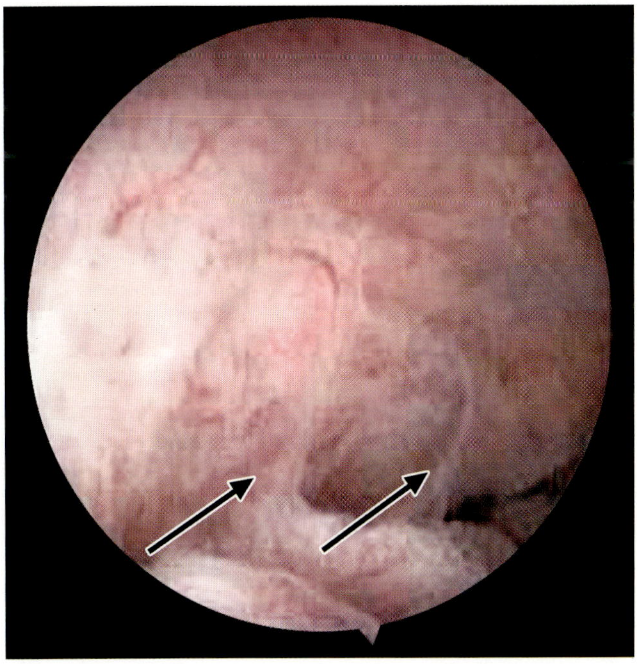

**Fig. 29.10:** Grade III salpingoscopy

endothelial folds give wide bore appearance of the lumen, and adhesions may cause restriction of free movements of major folds.

## Grade IV (Fig. 29.11)

Severe degree of flattening with severe adhesions of the mucosa. Tube appears wide, rigid and bald from inside. It may be patent or even blocked.

## Grade V (Fig. 29.12)

Lumen appears obliterated due to severe intraluminal cob-web type of adhesions. There is total destruction of endothelium leading to loss of the normal architecture and blockage of lumen at various sites.

These are totally dysfunctional Fallopian tubes and they should be excised rather than conserved. Spontaneous intrauterine pregnancy is highly unlikely in these cases and if she conceives the risk of ectopic is significantly high.

## Genital Tuberculosis (Fig. 29.13)

It often results in tubal damage. The external appearance of the tube may be normal. Often, tubes appear less supple, rigid and fibrotic. It may be patent or even blocked. It often shows the presence of small tubercles on the endothelium.

## Endosalpingeal Polyp (Fig. 29.14)

Rarely small endosalpingeal polyps are seen, however, they don't seem to be of any significance.

## Difficulties and Pitfalls

It is not always possible to perform salpingoscopy easily. The learning curve is steep and long. Fimbrial stenosis and accessory ostia can cause difficulty in performing the salpingoscopy.

## Accessory Fimbrial Ostiae (Fig. 29.15)

Gentle fimbrial dilatation is recommended using Maryland grasper or retrograde dye pusher.

Occasionally a false passage (Fig. 29.16) may occur in the muscularis wall of the tube and it can appear like grade 5 salpingoscopy findings. However, it can be differentiated by identifying pulsatile vessels in between myofibrils.

It is recommended to use gravity-fall system to pass the fluid for distension. If it is allowed to flow under pressure, one can experience 2 problems:

1. It can result in tubal wall edema and
2. It causes temporary flattening of the folds, therefore giving false positive salpingoscopy findings.

## Tubal Edema (Fig. 29.17)

**Generalized Endothelial Staining (Fig. 29.18)**

However, a pathological tube shows focal staining of endothelium.

## Tubal Diverticulum (Fig. 29.19)

The fimbrial diverticulum is a normal anatomical variant and it may cause difficult introduction of the telescope.

If the telescope enters the diverticulum, it is a thin part of the tube and it may appear as severely flattened tube and may give false positive findings.

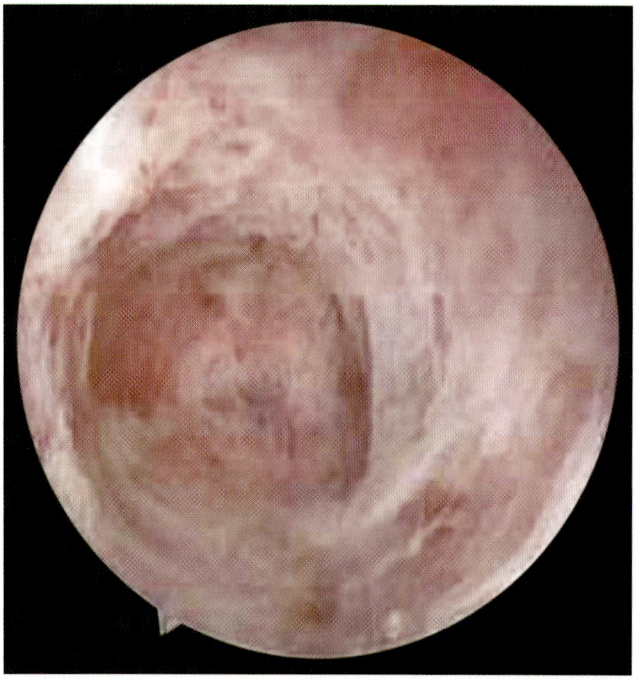

**Fig. 29.11:** Grade IV salpingoscopy

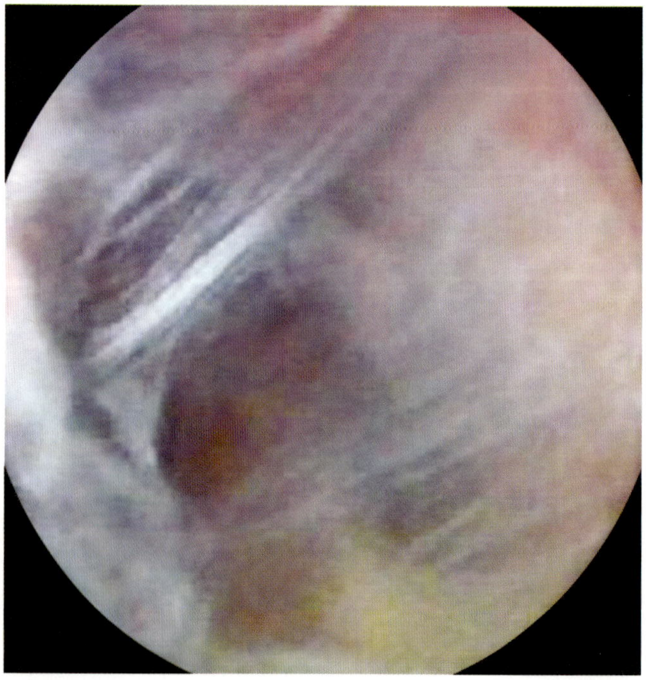

**Fig. 29.12:** Grade V salpingoscopy

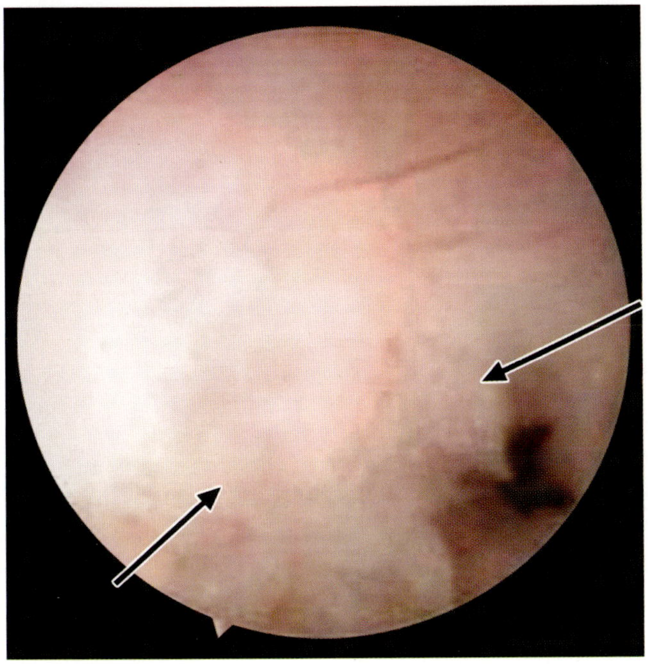

**Fig. 29.13:** Genital tuberculosis

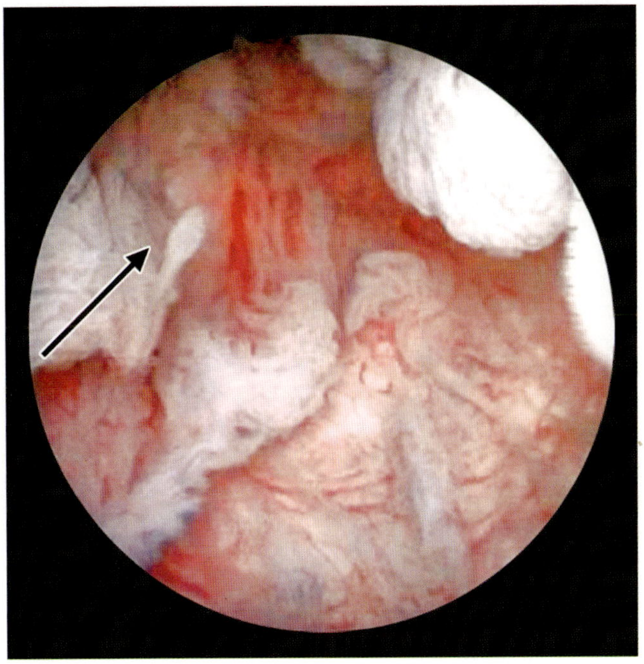

**Fig. 29.14:** Endosalpingeal polyp

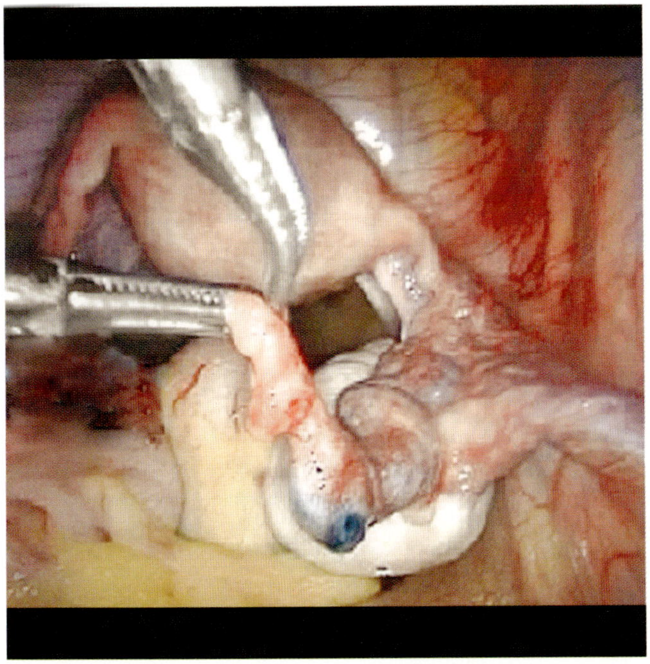

**Fig. 29.15:** Accessory fimbriae ostiae

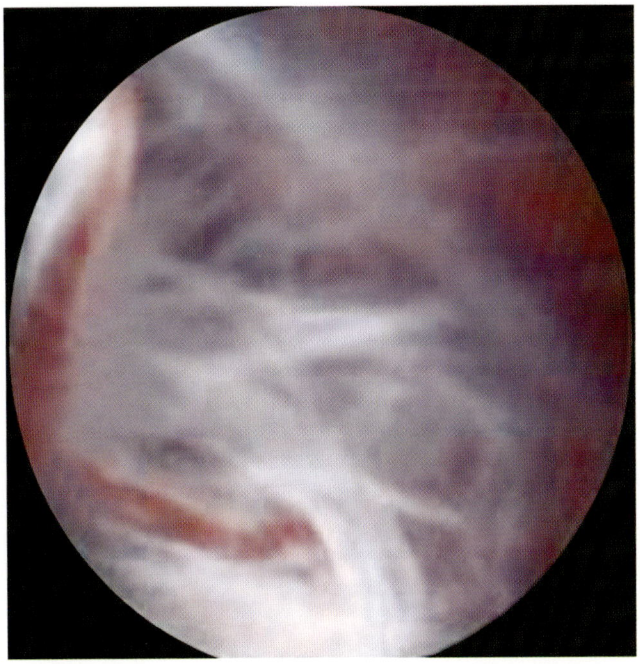

**Fig. 29.16:** False passage in muscularis wall of the tube

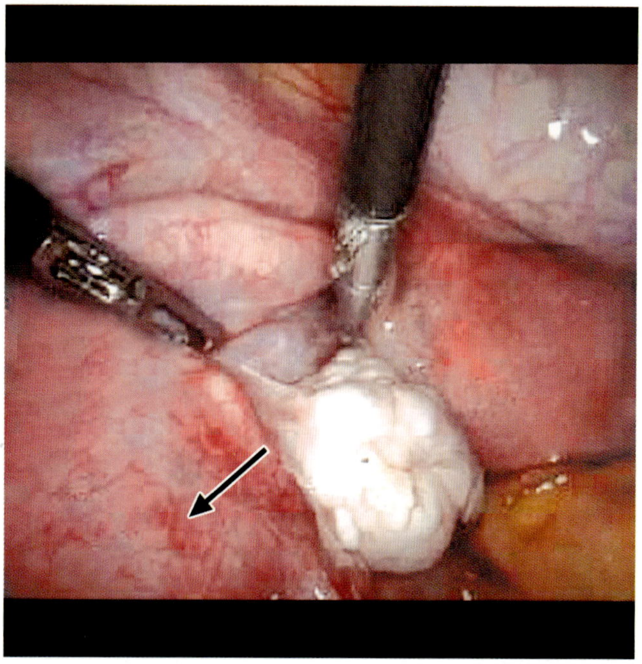

**Fig. 29.17:** Tubal edema

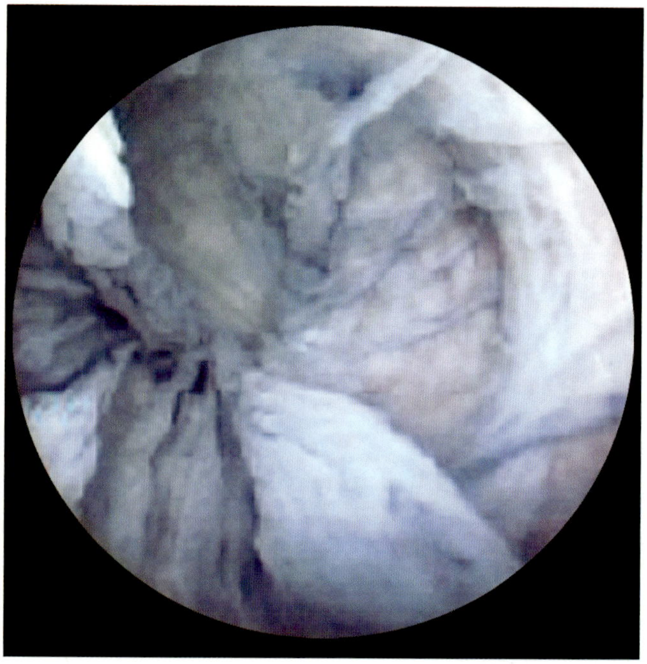

**Fig. 29.18:** Generalized endothelial staining

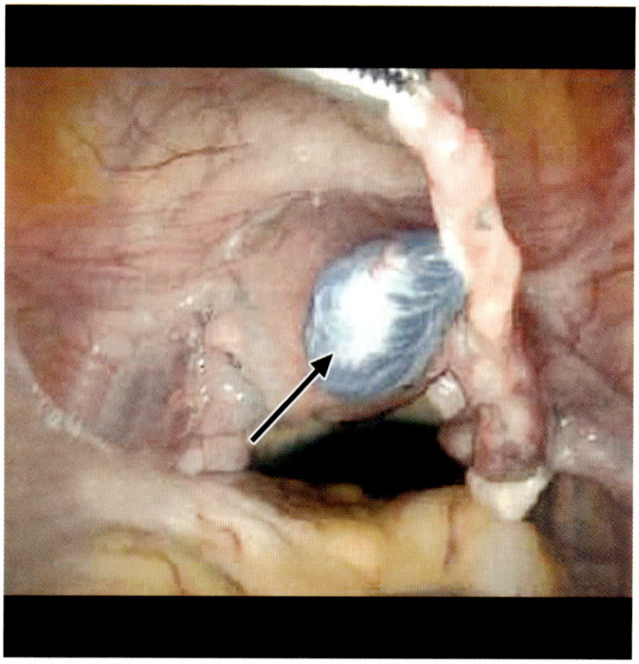

**Fig. 29.19:** Tubal diverticulum

## TIPS

- Dilute 3 drops of methylene blue dye into 100 mL of normal saline. If more concentrated methylene blue dye is used, it may cause uniform staining of the endothelium giving false positive findings.
- In cases with Grade III and more, IVF-ET is the preferable option rather than IUI. Spontaneous pregnancy or IUI would involve significantly higher ectopic pregnancy rate.

Chapter

# 30

# Laparoscopic Management of Adenomyoma

*Sanjay Patel, Yogendra Jhala*

## DEFINITION

The heterotypic presence of the functioning endometrium glands and stroma within the myometrium at least 2.5 mm deeper to the basal layer is termed as adenomyosis.

Common in patients with previous history of MTP, dilatation and curettage or any previous surgery on the uterus.

## CLASSIFICATION

As per its morphological occurrence:

- If localized adenomyoma.
- Diffused adenomyosis.

## TRANSVAGINAL ULTRASONOGRAPHY

- Adenoma is usually diagnosed on ultrasound. It appears uncapsulated, heterogenous, anechoic areas. All these

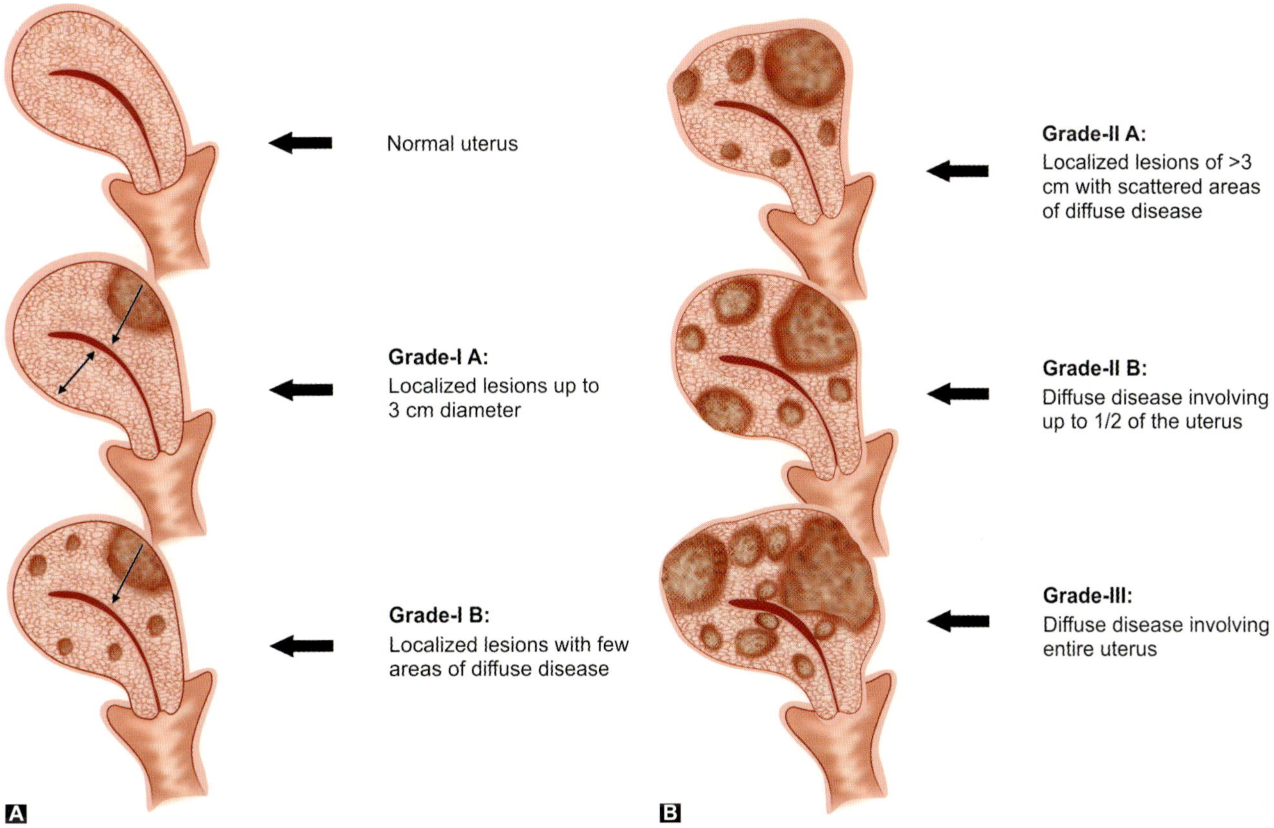


**Figs 30.1A and B:** Dr Sanjay Patel's Classification of adenomyoma

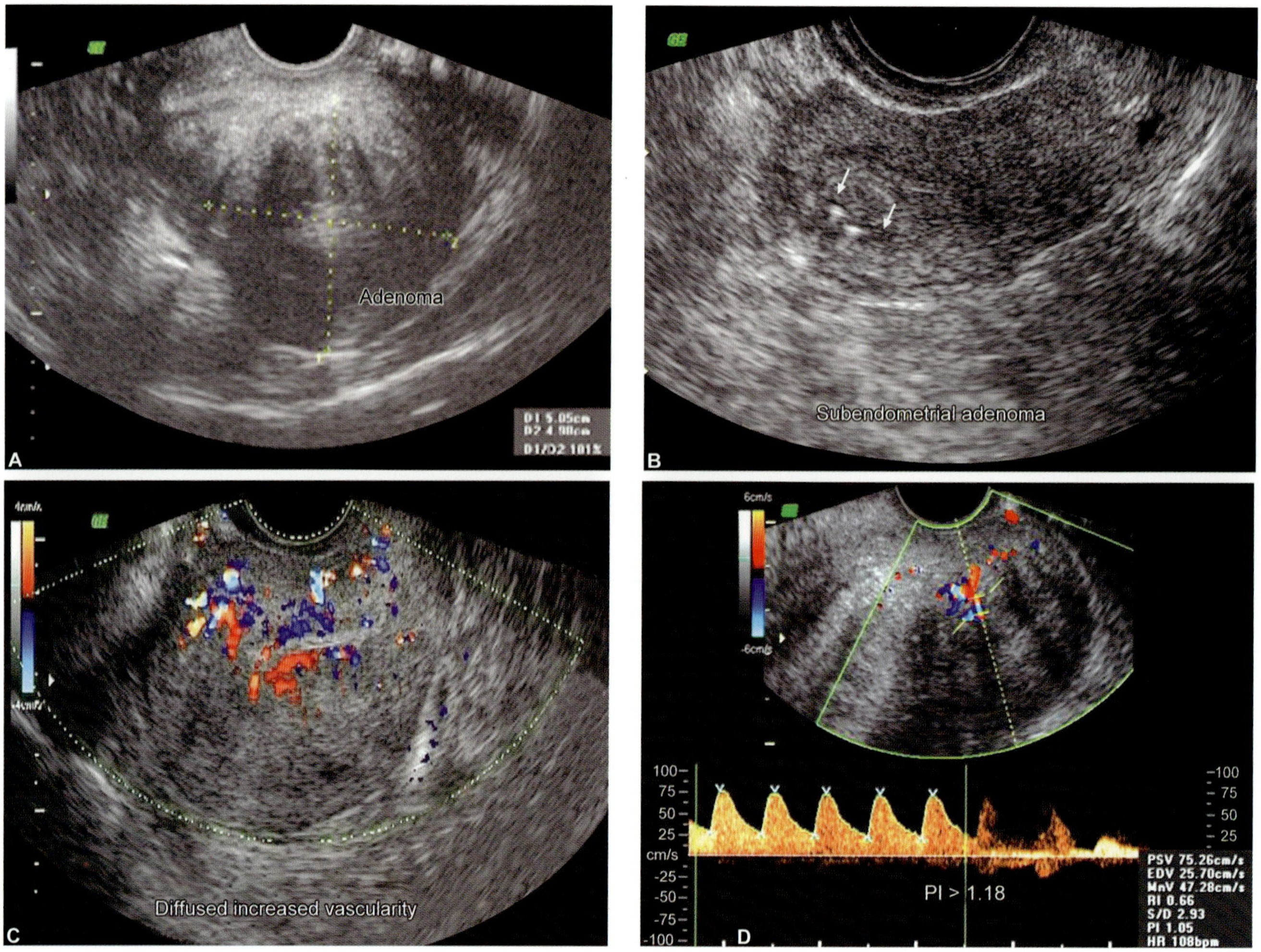


**Figs 30.2A to D**

changes will be more pronounced if you do it during menstruation.

- On color Doppler it may appear as diffuse, increased over all vascularity (PI >1.18 cm/s).

## ADENOMA ON LAPAROSCOPY

Adenoma may be misdiagnosed as fibroid on ultrasound. If during surgery, one finds difficult to find the plane of cleavage, then it is more likely to be adenoma.

There may be chocolate-colored fluid collection in the myometrium (intramyometrial cyst).

## ADENOMA ON HYSTEROSCOPY

- Hysteroscopy shows increased endometrial vascularity.
- Subendometrial adnenoma on hysteroscopy.
- Endometrial puckering (looking like adhesions) due to adenomyosis.

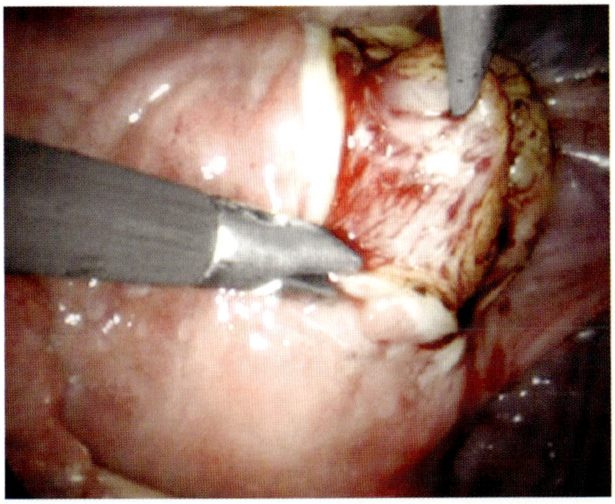

Fig. 30.3

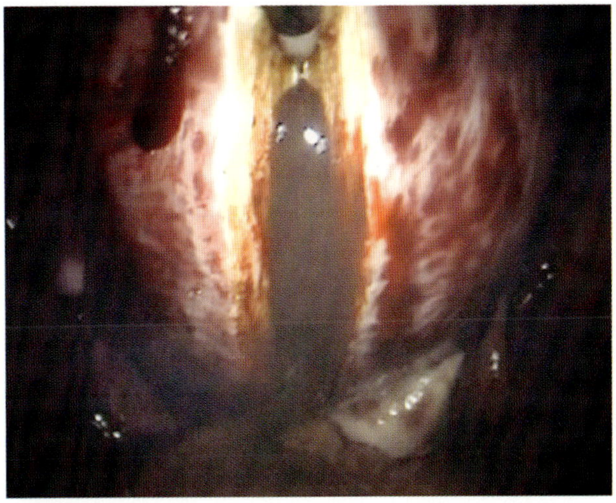

Fig. 30.4

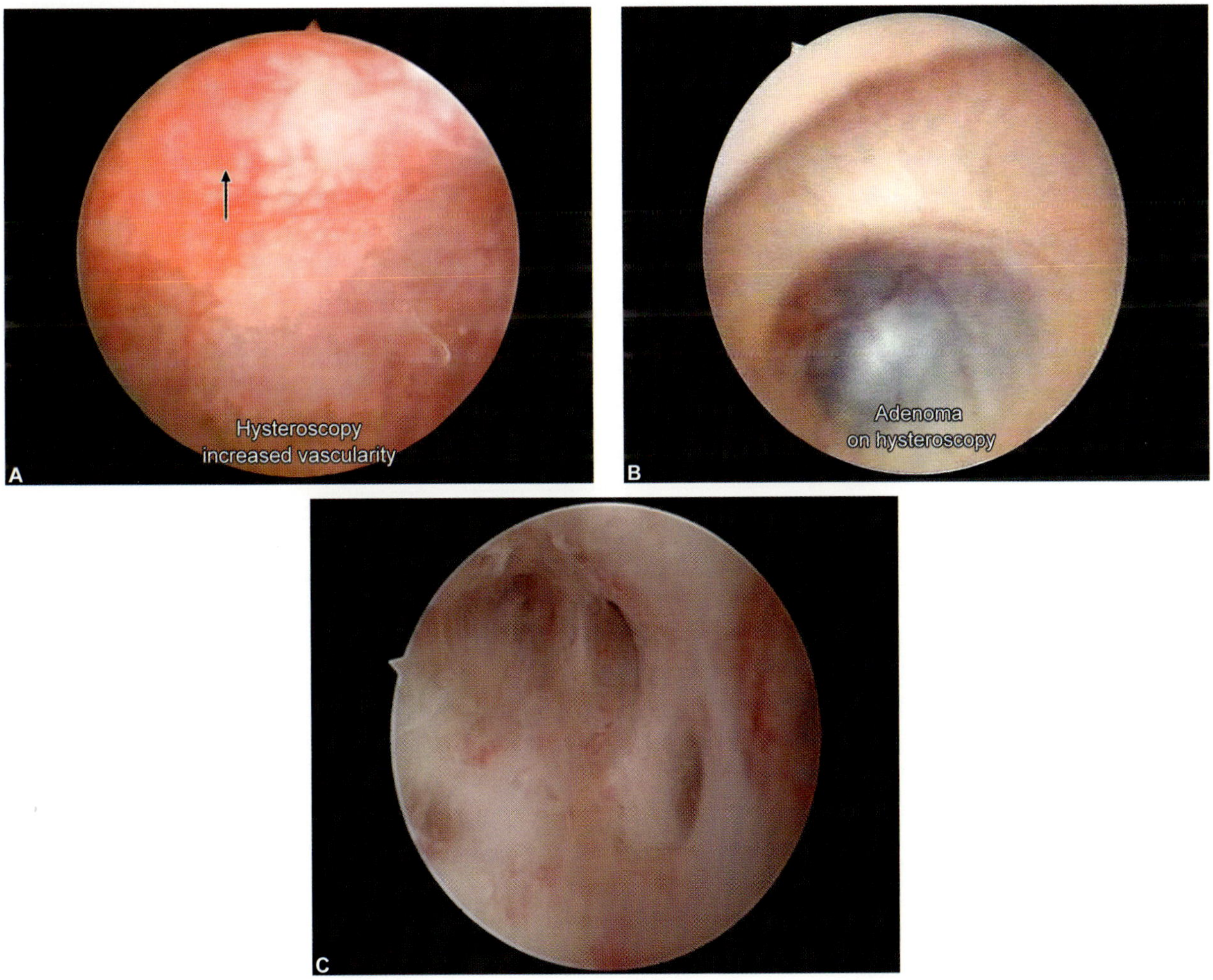


Figs 30.5A to C

## COEXISTING PATHOLOGIES

Adenomyosis/adenoma may coexist with endometriosis, fibroid, endometrial polyp/hyperplasia, Uterine adhesions.

## PREOPERATIVE ADENOMA MAPPING

We routinely make a map depicting size, location of adenoma before starting the surgery.

Intraoperative transvaginal sonography is also done when needed

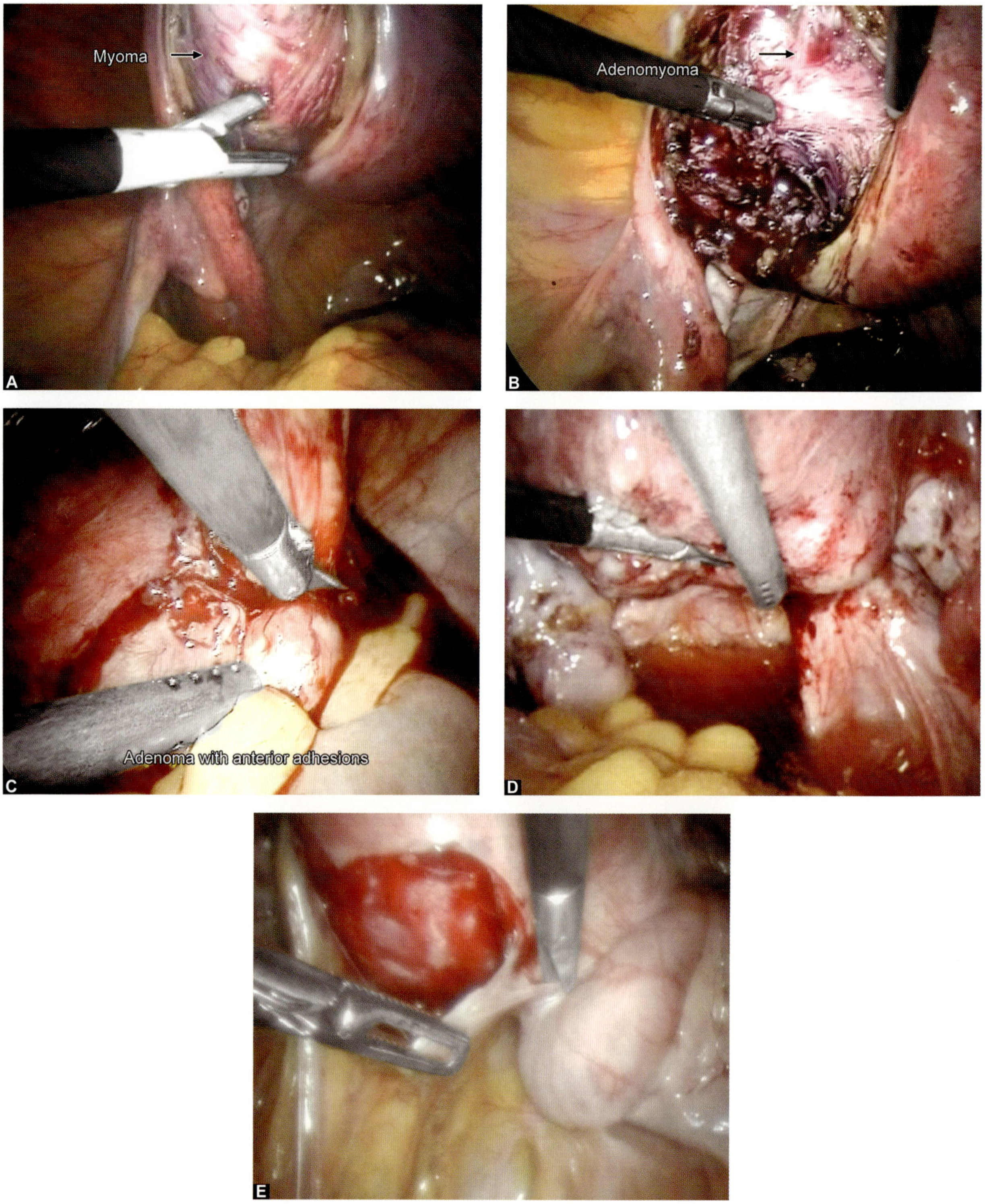


**Figs 30.6A to E:** Adenoma with posterior adhesions

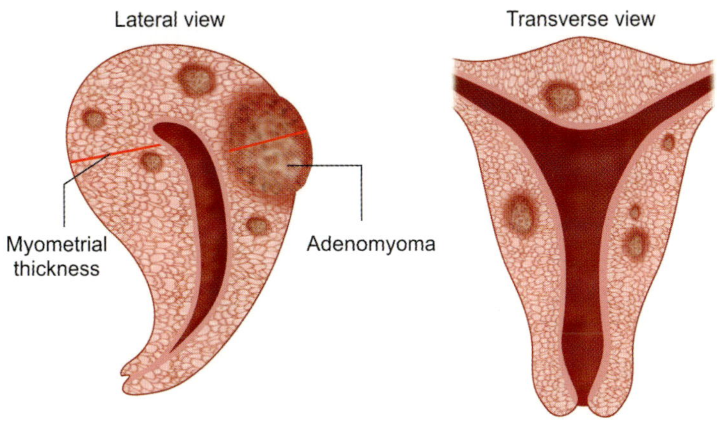


Fig. 30.7: Endoscpy OT2

## AIM OF THE ADENOMA RESECTION

Resection helps in improving the symptoms by reducing the uterine vascularity, thus improving pain, menorrhagia and fertility. As adenoma/adenomyotic tissue is tough, it is better to use monopolar pure cutting current than scissor. Too much smoke generated during use of monopolar current should be evacuated periodically.

## TECHNIQUE OF ADENOMYOMA RESECTION

Three techniques of adenoma resection:

1. Elliptical strip excision technique for Grade I adenoma: Elliptical strip excision would be better for adenoma resection rather than attempting enucleation as in fibroid.

   It may be difficult to locate adenoma intraoperatively, for which intraoperative transvaginal sonography is useful.

   Adenoma bleeds minimal. So if surgeon encounters more bleeding while resecting then he may have entered the healthy myometrium. The aim of resection is to reduce tension in myometrium (similar to debulking surgery of benign SOL of brain without injuring vital areas of brain) which can be achieved by debulking the affected myometrium which is sometimes upto 50% leading to hemi-hysterectomy.
2. Hood technique for Grade II without involvement of serosal layer of uterus by disease.
3. Slice technique for Grade II with involvement of serosal layer of uterus by disease.

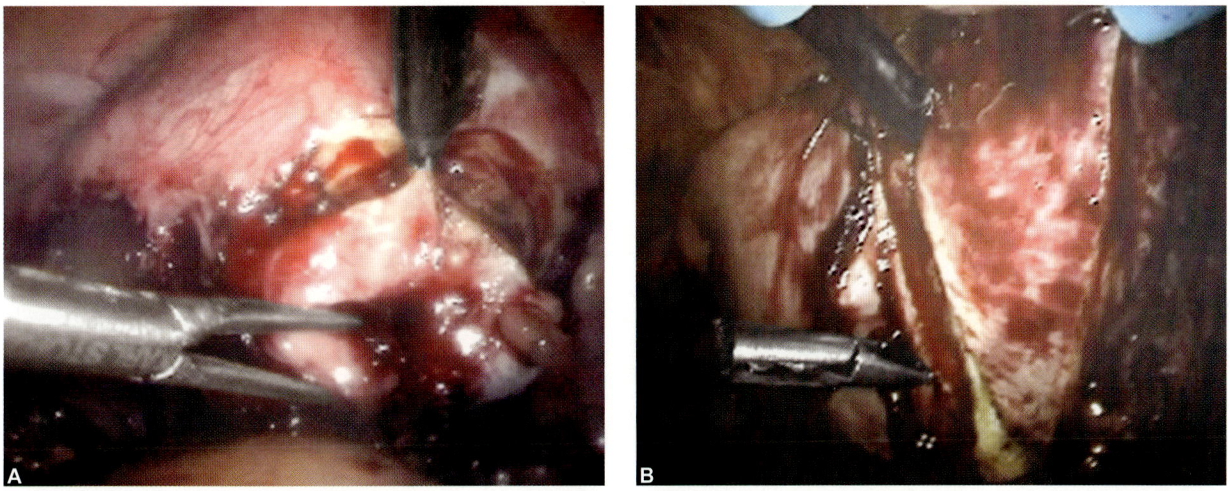


Figs 30.8A and B

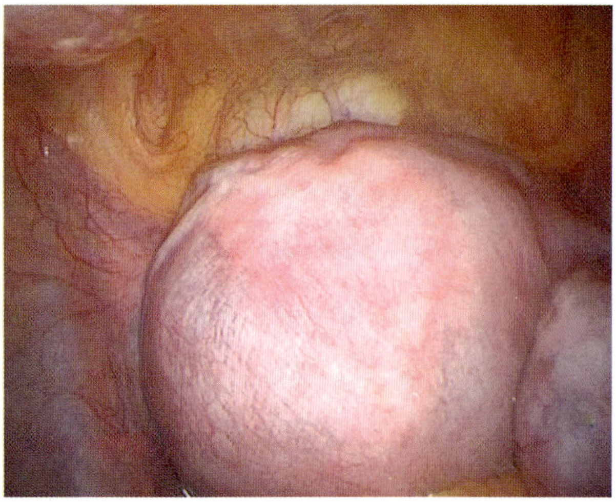

**Fig. 30.9:** Posterior wall adenoma with normal serosa

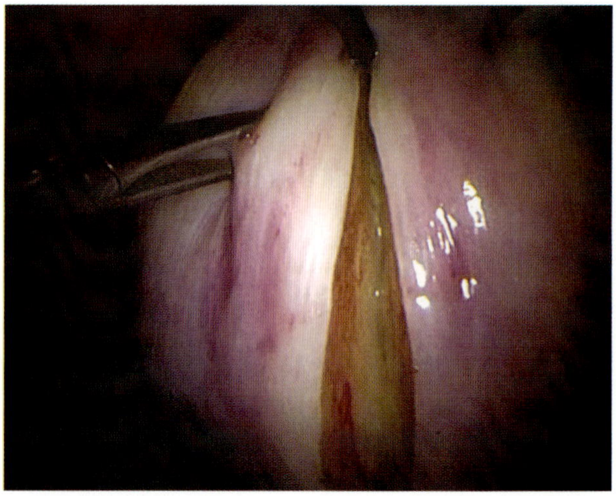

**Fig. 30.10:** Incision made using monopolar needle

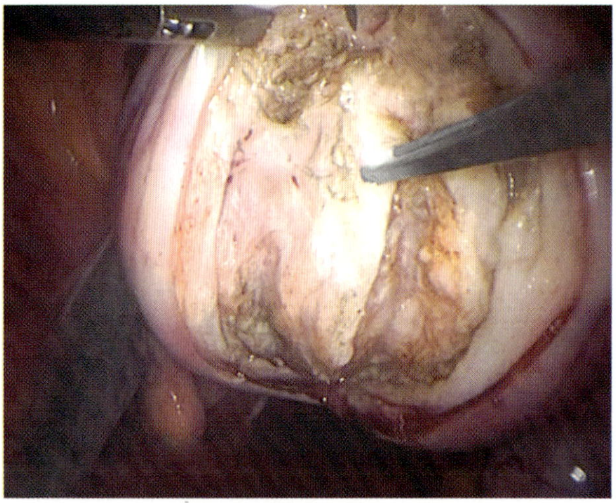

**Fig. 30.11:** Hood made by coring below the normal uterine serosa

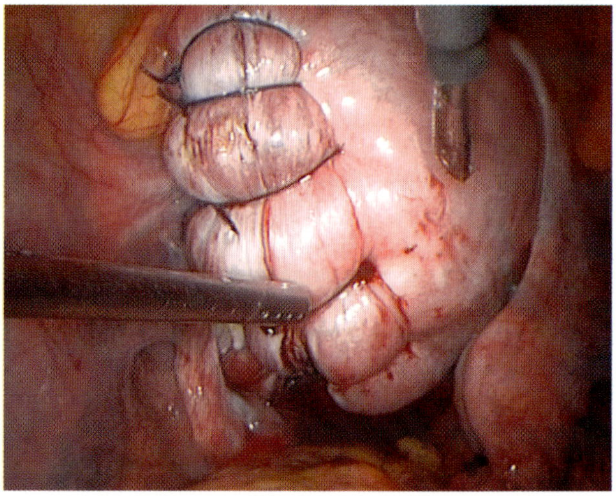

**Fig. 30.12:** Suturing done by slip knot technique

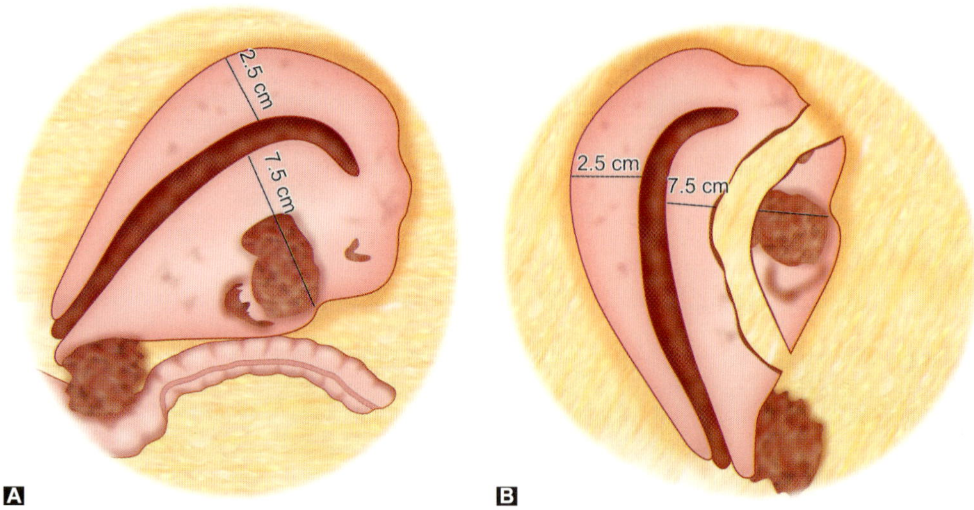


**Figs 30.13A and B:** Posterior wall adenoma with serosal involvement by the disease

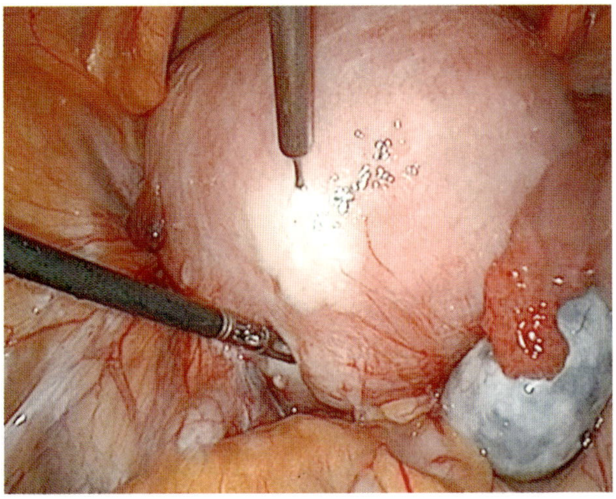

**Fig. 30.14:** Inj. Pitressin (1:200 mL dilution) injected in adenoma

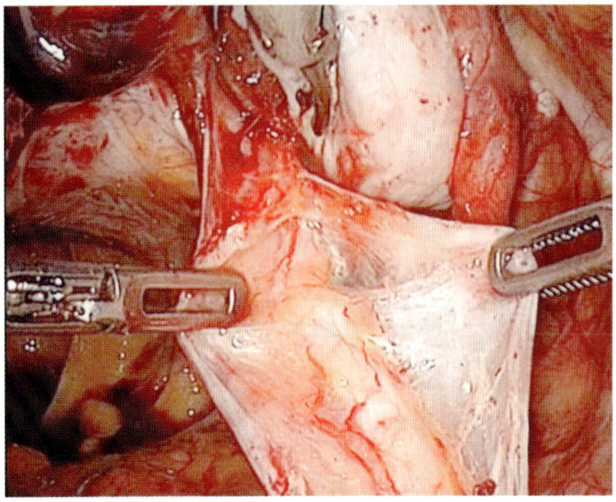

**Fig. 30.15:** Lateral mobilization of the ureter

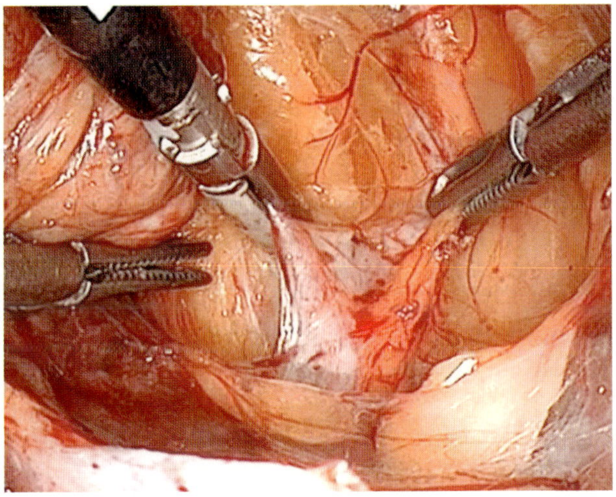

**Fig. 30.16:** Uterine artery ligated at the origin

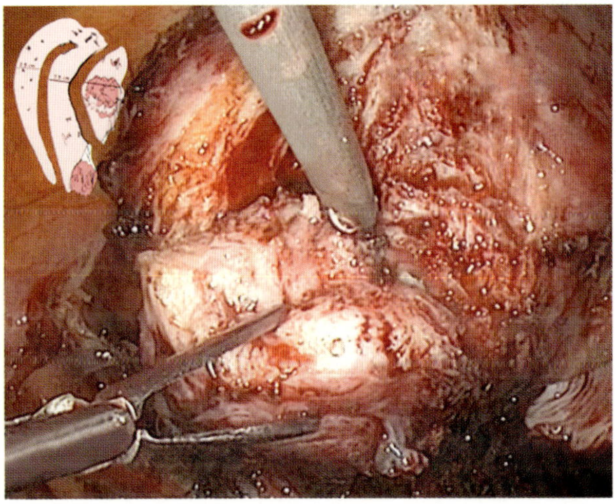

**Fig. 30.17:** Slice of adenoma excised

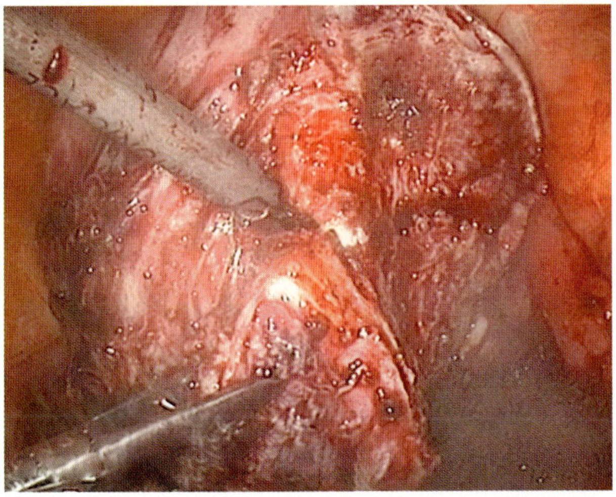

**Fig. 30.18:** Slice of adenoma excised

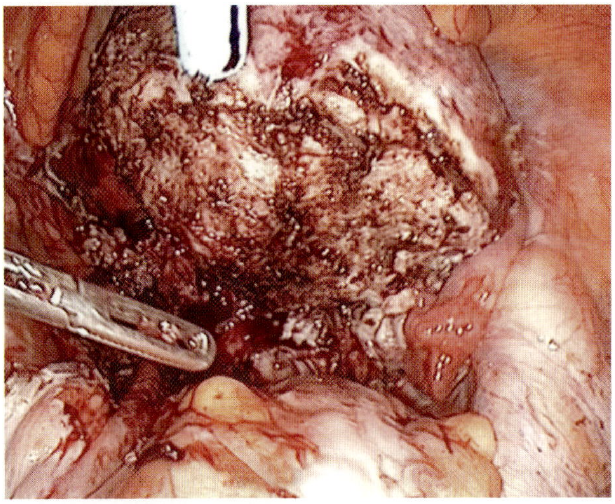

**Fig. 30.19:** Half of the adenomyotic posterior wall removed

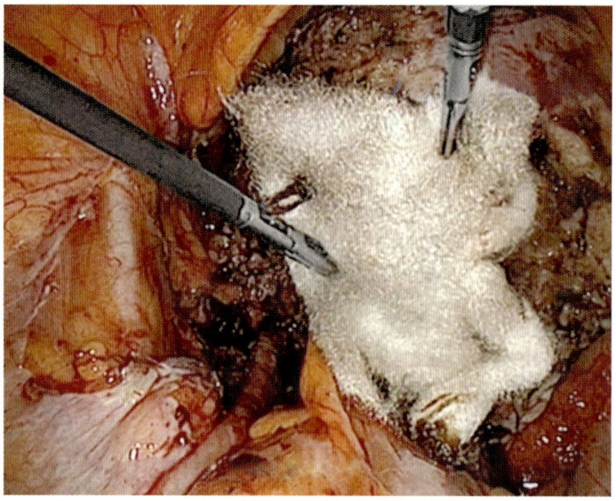

Fig. 30.20: Surgicel (J&J) placed over the raw area for hemostasis

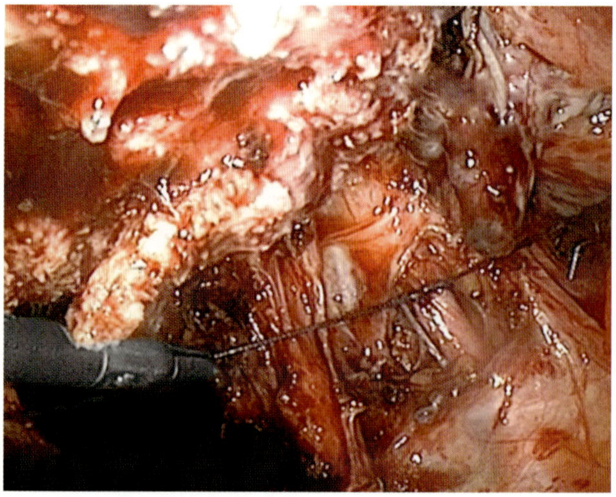

Fig. 30.21: Internal iliac artery ligated for hemostasis

## TECHNIQUE OF ENDOSUTURING: INTRA-CORPOREAL SLIP KNOT TECHNIQUE

Proper approximation should be done after resection. It can be achieved by intracorporeal slip knot technique.

First we take full thickness bite on right edge and then on left edge. Then we place first half hitch and over we place a second half hitch. This makes it a square surgical knot. This loose knot is then slipped as far as down as it goes. This knot is not tightened and is not complete and secured as yet. It is left half way through. First stitch acts as an assistant holding the edges together for us.

Then we go for second stitch 1 cm lower down in same manner as first stich.

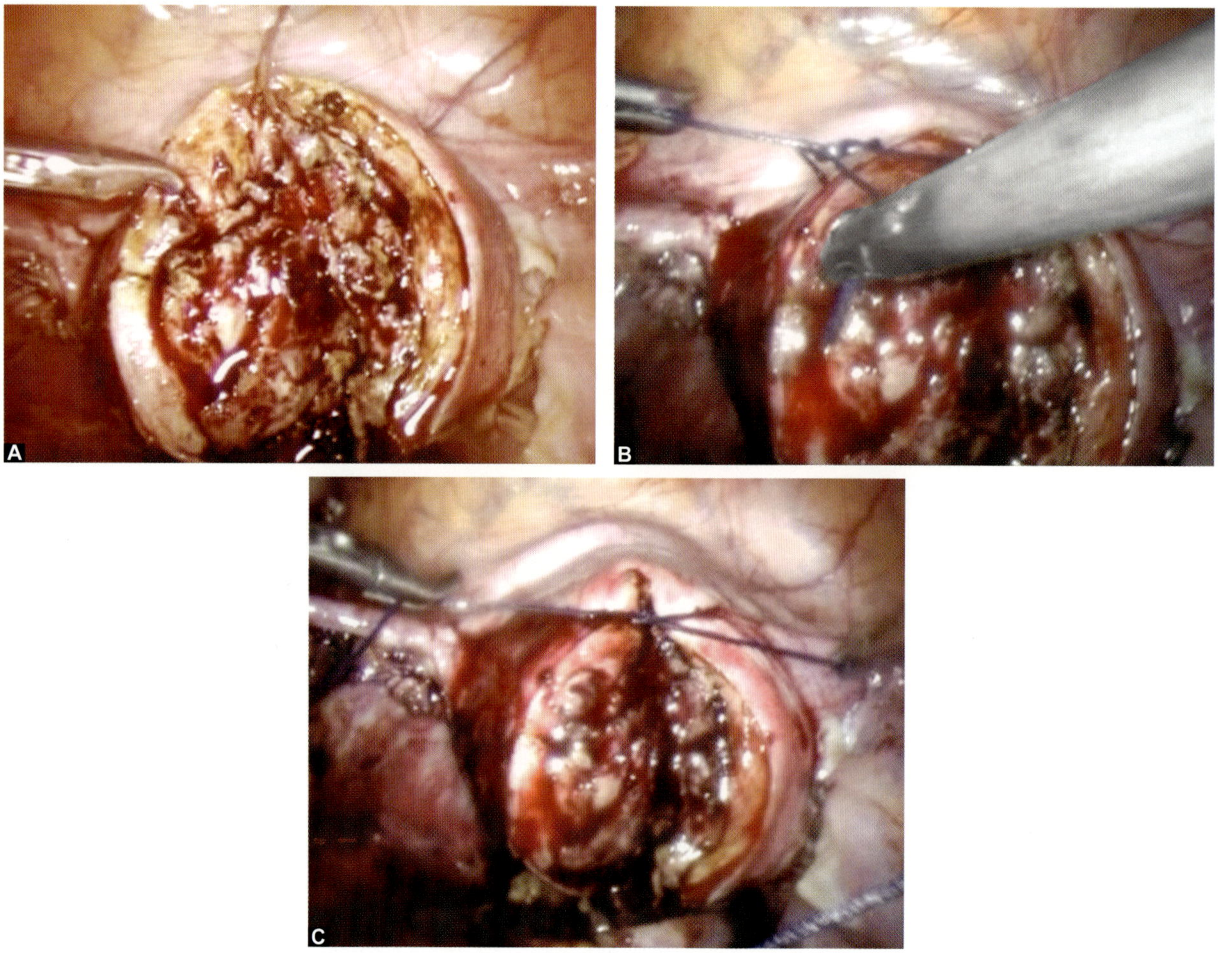

Figs 30.22A to C

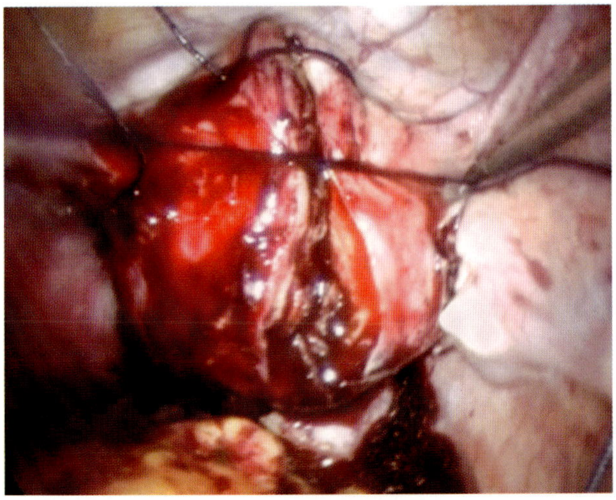

Fig. 30.23

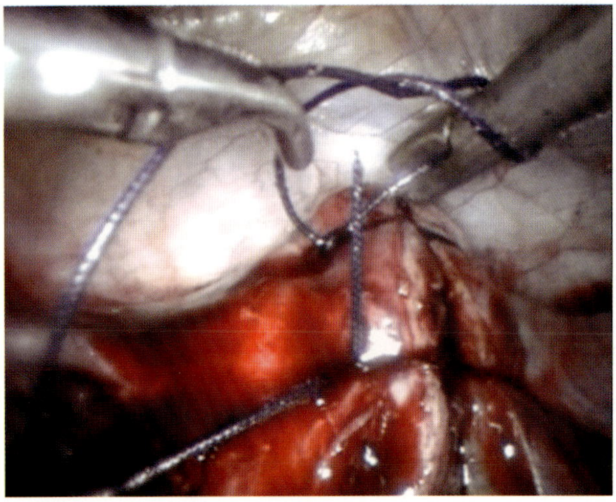

Fig. 30.24

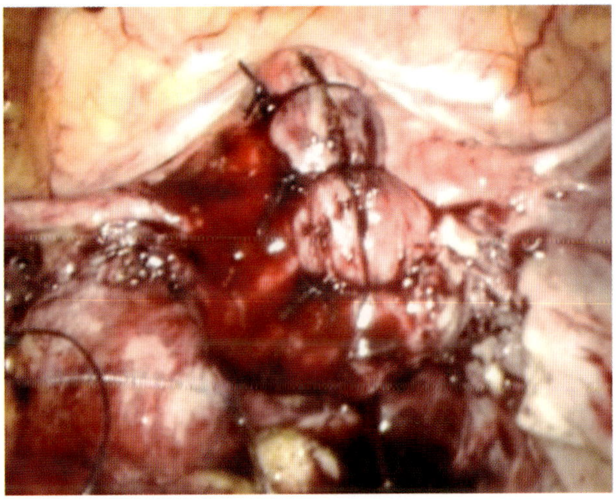

Fig. 30.25

Then we go back to first stitch which is further tightened completely to secure it further approximating the myometrium.

This is how entire length of myometrium is approximated without leaving any residual dead space.

## OUR EXPERIENCE

| ***Our series*** | ***Year 1996–2005*** |
|---|---|
| Localized adenoma | 210 cases |
| Diffuse disease | 46 cases |
| Total | 256 cases |

### Symptomatic Improvements

| | | |
|---|---|---|
| Dysmenorrhea | 92% | 236 cases |
| Menstrual loss | 84% | 215 cases |
| Recurrence rate after 3 years | 38% | 97 cases |

*Note:* Recurrence rate is higher in Grade II and Grade III.

### Pregnancy Rates

| *Group* | *No. of cases* |
|---|---|
| Localized Adenoma | 87 cases (37%) |
| Diffuse adenomyosis | 20 cases (8%) |

## CONCLUSION

Adenoma resection is technically more difficult but quite a rewarding surgery in early stage of the disease in terms of fertility and improvement in symptomatology in whom hysterectomy cannot be advised.

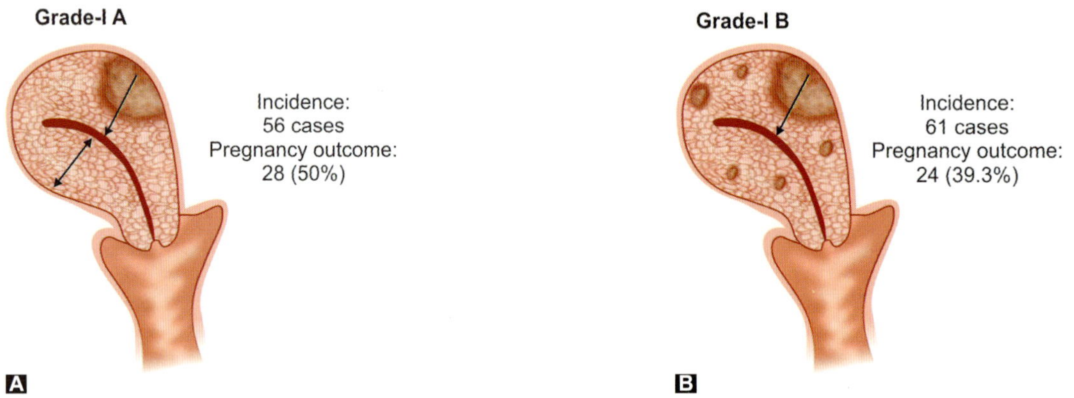


**Figs 30.26A and B**

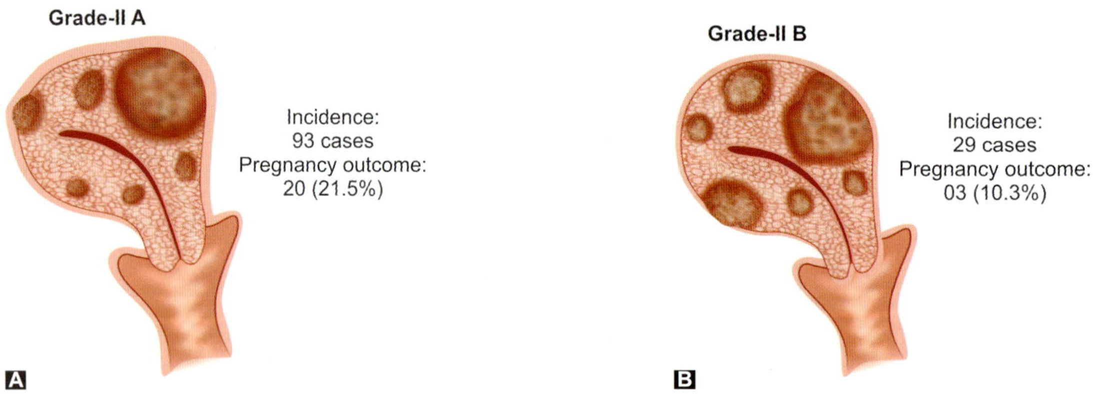


**Figs 30.27A and B**

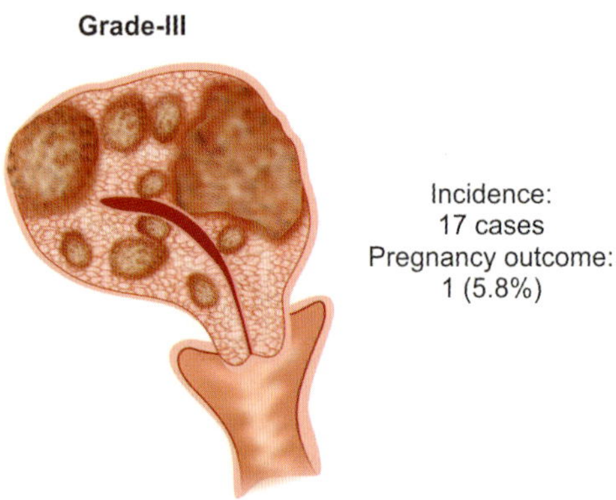


**Fig. 30.28**

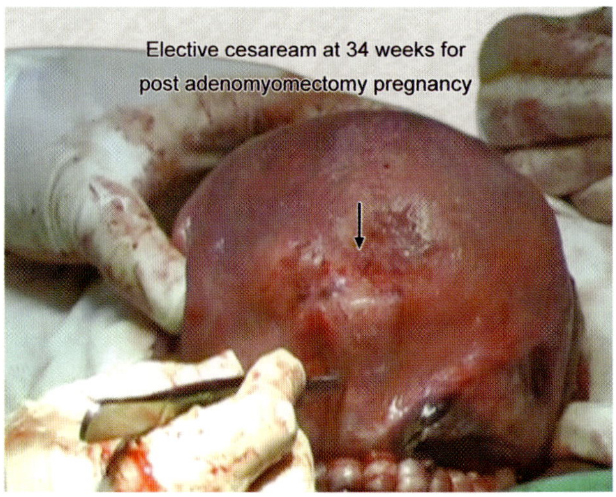


**Fig. 30.29**

Chapter

31

# Anatomy of Pelvic Floor and Laparoscopic Prolapse Repair

*Revaz Botchorishvili, Sara Campos*

## PREOPERATIVE EVALUATION

- Transvaginal ultrasound for uterine/endometrial evaluation
- PAP test if last evaluation > 1 year ago
- Urodynamics evaluation in case of doubtful clinical presentation concerning stress urinary incontinence

## PREOPERATIVE PREPARATION

The patient is installed as for any operative laparoscopy:

- General anesthesia.
- Lies on her back.
- Legs semi-flexed at 45°.
- Indwelling bladder catheter.
- Uterine cannulation to allow mobilization of the uterus—this cannulation is achieved using Tintara uterus manipulator (*Karl Storz GmbH & Co.KG, Tuttlingen, Germany)* identical to that used for tubal sterility work-up (no cervical dilatation) rather than the device used for total hysterectomy (requiring cervical dilatation), with the aim of avoiding cervical dilatation in order to decrease trauma and potential prosthesis contamination to a minimum (Fig. 31.1).
- Bowel preparation is not routinely required but a fiber-free diet is recommended for 3–5 days prior to surgery.
- Antibiotic prophylaxis: cephazolin IV 2 g, single dose, 30 minutes before induction of anesthesia.

## SPECIFIC INSTRUMENTS AND EQUIPMENT

Most of the instruments used are same as for any operative laparoscopy.

- RoBi™ dissecting rotating bipolar forceps (*Karl Storz GmbH & Co.KG, Tuttlingen, Germany*) - The surgery of prolapse requires long and precise dissection and the use of an adequate dissecting bipolar forceps is particularly helpful (Fig. 31.2).
- Disposable scissors (*Vectec, Hauterive, France*).
- T'Lift™ tissue retraction system (*Vectec, Hauterive, France*).

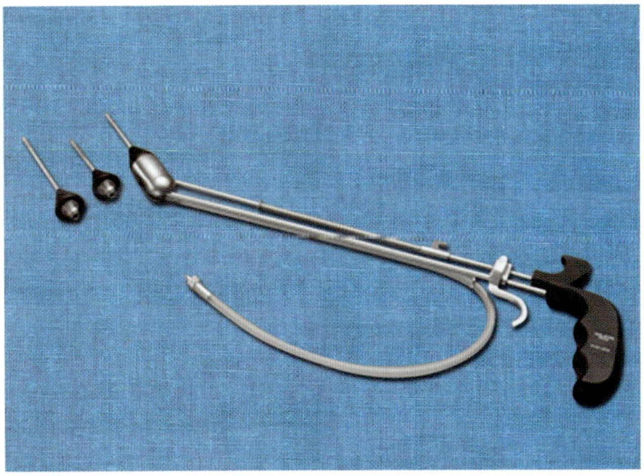

**Fig. 31.1:** Tintara™ uterine mobilizer (Karl Storz GmbH & Co.KG, Tuttlingen, Germany)

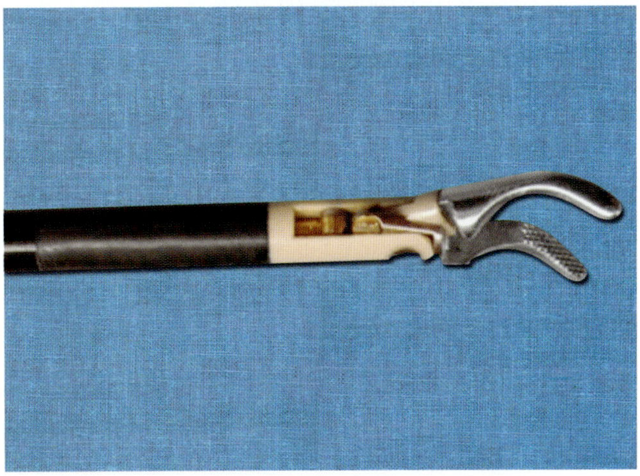

**Fig. 31.2:** RoBi™ dissecting rotating bipolar forceps - tip detail (Karl Storz GmbH & Co.KG, Tuttlingen, Germany)

- Berci Fascial Closure Instrument (*Karl Storz GmbH & Co.KG Tuttlingen, Germany*).
- Chardonnens morcellation knife (*Karl Storz GmbH & Co.KG, Tuttlingen, Germany*) or Brucker/Messroghli Supraloop™ monopolar cutting device (*Karl Storz GmbH & Co.KG, Tuttlingen, Germany*).
- Polypropylene meshes (Surgimesh™ XLight Prolapse, *Aspide Medical, La Talaudière, France*).
- Laparoscopic extraction bag (*ExBag™, Matrics Medical, Berlin, Germany*).
- Rotocut G1 Morcellator (*Karl Storz GmbH & Co.KG, Tuttlingen, Germany*).
- Tintara uterus manipulator (*Karl Storz GmbH & Co.KG, Tuttlingen, Germany*).
- Sutures (*Ethicon, Issy-les-Moulineaux, France*) or similar:
  - 3 Monocryl™ 1 (poliglecaprone 25: Monofilament synthetic absorbable suture with a curved 36 mm needle, in 70 cm strands).
  - 2 Monocryl™ 0 (poliglecaprone 25: Monofilament synthetic absorbable suture with a curved 36 mm needle, in 70 cm strands).
  - 3 PDS™ II 2-0 (polydioxanone: Monofilament synthetic absorbable suture with a curved 26 mm needle, in 70 cm strands).
  - 6 Ethibond Excel™ 0 (polyester: Coated braided synthetic non-absorbable suture with a curved 26 mm needle, in 90 cm strands).
  - 1 Ethibond Excel™ 1 (polyester: Coated braided synthetic non-absorbable suture with a curved 30 mm needle, in 75 cm strands).

## PREREQUISITES

- Mastering on intra and extracorporeal suturing.

## PORT PLACEMENTS (FIGS 31.3 AND 31.4)

- 1 × 10 mm umbilical port for the optics
- 3 ancillary ports for the instruments:
  - 2 × 5 mm trocars, which are inserted in the iliac fossa outside the outer edge of the *rectus abdominis* muscle level with or above the anterior superior iliac spine
  - 5 mm trocar inserted on the midline (at least 8 to 10 cm below the umbilical trocar). After dissection has finished this trocar is replaced by a 10 mm trocar to allow easy insertion of the needles and prosthesis.

## ANATOMICAL LANDMARKS IN PORT PLACEMENT

- Inferior epigastric vessels
- *Rectus abdominis* muscle (lateral margin)

## KEY STEPS OF THE PROCEDURE

### 1st Phase: Exposing the Promontory

- Peritoneal dissection enough to allow one or two sutures to be placed in the anterior common vertebral ligament without any risk for the surrounding structures.

It may be necessary to briefly accentuate the Trendelenburg position so that this procedure can be carried out under good conditions.

To help promontory and pouch of Douglas exposition, it is helpful to fasten the sigmoid to the left flank, for what we use T'Lift™ passing through epiploic appendices (Fig. 31.5).

In obese patients and patients with a low aortic bifurcation particular care must be taken respecting the left iliac vein which is often flattened by the pneumoperitoneum pressure.

#### *Promontory Anatomical Landmarks (Fig. 31.6)*

- L5-S1
- Aorta bifurcation

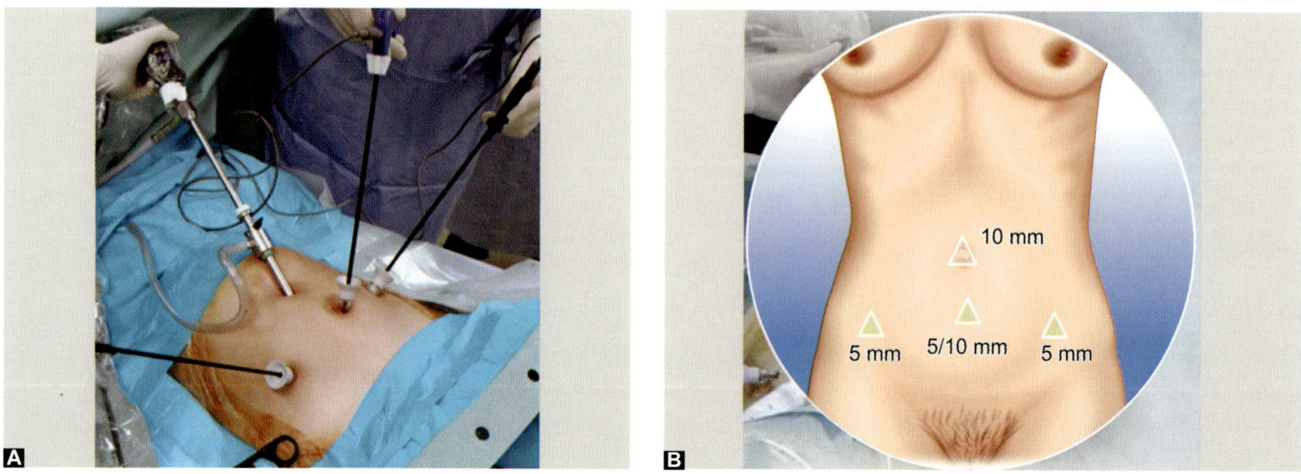


**Fig. 31.3:** Trocars placement—external view

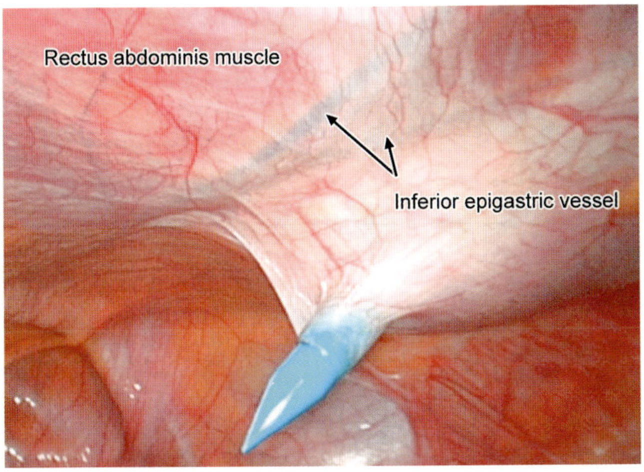


**Fig. 31.4:** Trocars placement—internal view, right lateral wall

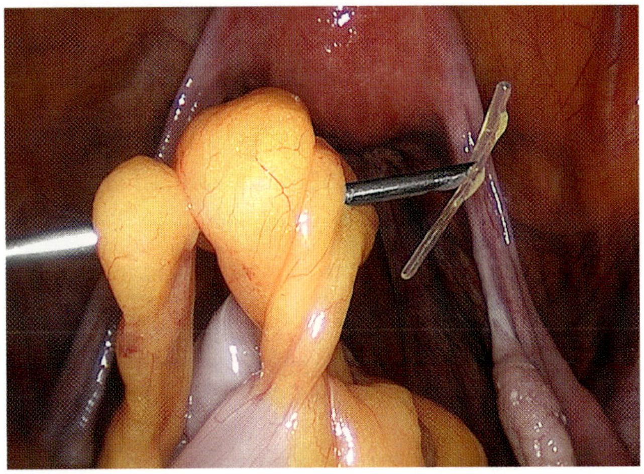

**Fig. 31.5:** Transparietal sigmoid suspension for promontory and Douglas exposition using T'Lift™ tissue retraction system

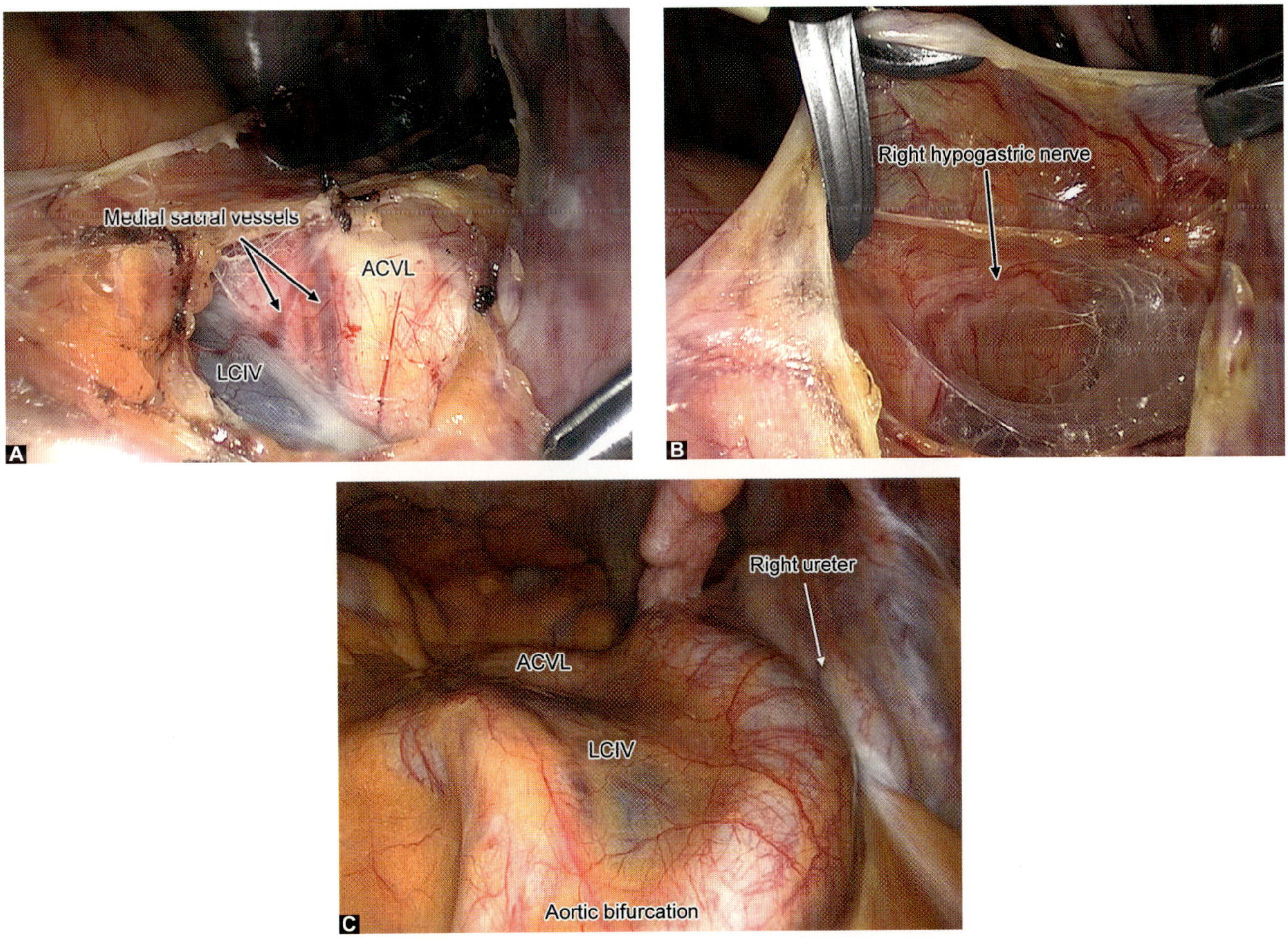


**Figs 31.6A to C:** Promontory anatomical landmarks. LCIV: left common iliac vein; ACVL: anterior common vertebral ligament

- Right ureter
- Lower edge of the left common iliac vein
- Medial sacral vessels
- Right hypogastric nerve.

## 2nd Phase: Pararectal and Rectovaginal Dissection

- Extension of the peritoneal incision started at the promontory forwards and caudally towards the pouch of Douglas, running lateral to the rectosigmoid and medially at an adequate distance from right ureter. This incision will allow the prosthesis to be peritonized at the end of surgery. It is prolonged until the pouch of Douglas, medially to the right uterosacral ligament. During the dissection, integrity of right hypogastric nerve should be preserved in order to decrease post-operative obstructive defecation syndrome.
- Rectovaginal dissection starts after drawing the rectum backwards and pushing the uterus forwards. The rectum is grasped by the assistant using bowel forceps then strong traction is applied downwards and backwards. The peritoneum opposite the *torus uterinus* is stretched in an arc; it is coagulated then sectioned two centimeters below its uterine insertion. The cleavage plane is identified as close as possible to the vaginal wall and is then guided by the relief of the posterior vaginal wall (Fig. 31.7).
  Dissection of this plane is simple, if exposure has been properly achieved. It is made easier by the phenomenon of pneumodissection, creating the "bubbles" in the low density connective tissue, the traction applied to the rectum and the thrust applied to the uterus.
- Lower limit of dissection lies at the anorectal angle. Dissection continues laterally to the anorectal angle and inwards to reveal the *levator ani* muscles to which the prosthesis will be attached.
  At this point dissection must go far enough to allow easy access for the sutures in this space directly in contact with the pelvic floor.

### *Rectovaginal Dissection Anatomical Landmarks (Fig. 31.8)*

- Anorectal angle (medially)
- Middle rectal vessels, *levator ani* muscles and pelvic sidewall (laterally)
- Vagina (anteriorly)
- Rectum (posteriorly).

## 3rd Phase: Start of Supracervical Hysterectomy

Hysterectomy is preferred as it facilitates the procedure, namely the prosthesis fixation. We perform supracervical hysterectomy once it avoids vaginal opening and the consequent risks of infection involving the prosthesis. The hysterectomy technique is standard and has already been described.

### *Advantages of Supracervical Hysterectomy*

- The cervix is conserved thus providing a sturdy point to which the prosthesis can be attached firmly
- There is no opening created in the vagina thus reducing the risk of sepsis due to contact with the prosthesis; an uterine morcellator can be used (with appropriate concomitant endoscopic bag usage) so that the morcellated uterus can be easily extracted without any colpotomy.

## 4th Phase: Vesicovaginal Dissection

- Dissection of the vesicovaginal space is achieved by drawing the prevesical peritoneum upwards, incising the peritoneum then opening the vesicovaginal space along the midline, taking the incision downwards while

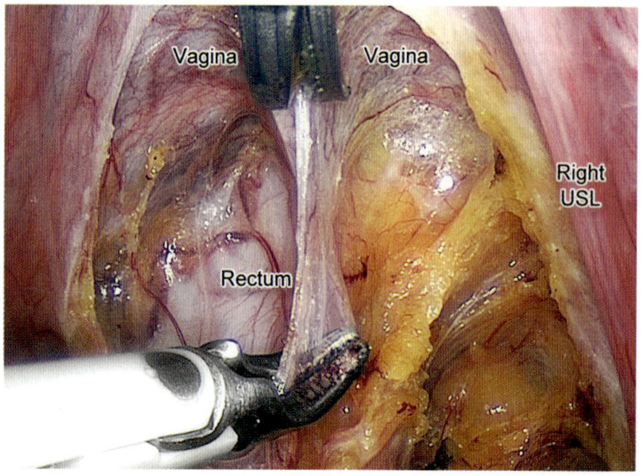


**Fig. 31.7:** Recto-vaginal dissection. USL: Uterosacral ligament

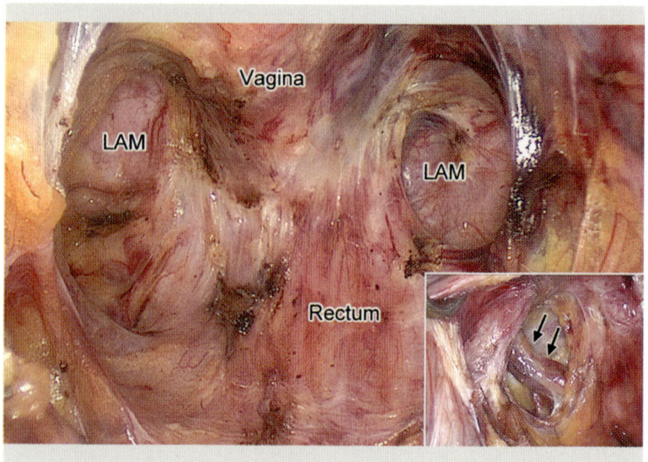


**Fig. 31.8:** Recto-vaginal dissection—final view. (A: anatomical landmarks. B: middle rectal vessels—detail on left side.) LAM: levatori ani muscles

pushing the bladder in between the internal bladder pillars.

Dissection must continue as low as possible, in close proximity to the bladder neck identified by the outline of the urinary catheter balloon, and over a surface wide enough to allow the anterior part of the prosthesis to be spread out completely.

The space in which the prosthesis will be installed is triangular and variable in size, with the lower point close to the bladder neck.

Suspension of the prevesical peritoneum with a T'Lift™ device will help subsequent steps.

### *Vesicovaginal Dissection Anatomical Landmarks (Fig.31.9)*

- Bladder neck (inferiorly)
- Bladder (anteriorly)
- Internal bladder pillars (laterally)
- Vagina (posteriorly).

## 5th Phase: End of Supracervical Hysterectomy

- After hemostasis of the uterine pedicles, the cervix is sectioned as high as possible after removing the manipulator. Various means can be used for this section. We ourselves prefer to use a cold knife in an endoscopic holder (*Chardonnens morcellation knife)* or monopolar cutting device Supraloop™.
- Irrigation of cervical stump with povidone-iodine.
- The cervical stump is carefully sutured using two or three stitches of poliglecaprone 25 (Monocryl™1) (Fig. 31.10).
  Suturing the cervical stump is important because it protects the prosthesis against any vaginal contamination.
  Once the hysterectomy has been completed, it is convenient to suspend temporarily the cervical stump from the anterior pelvic sidewall in order to leave the assistant's instrument free to help with suturing. We use a Berci Fascial Closure Instrument to pass the threads of the last stitch through the abdominal wall at suprapubic level.
- The uterus is left waiting to be sectioned inside an endoscopic bag at the end of the procedure.

*When there has been a previous hysterectomy*

- The vaginal vault is exposed with the help of a compress held in long-handled forceps inserted in the vagina in order to make dissection easier (Fig. 31.11).
  Vesicouterine dissection is, however, more difficult. In these cases there is a greater risk of vaginal or bladder perforation.

*If the uterus is conserved*

- A passage must be prepared through the broad ligament for the two arms of the prosthesis.
- Dissection is thus continued laterally by opening the two (anterior and posterior) peritoneal layers of the broad ligament, remaining level with the isthmus but at a distance from the uterine pedicle, which is easy to identify.
  Care must also be taken not to go too deep into the broad ligament in order to avoid the ureters and uterine vessels, specially uterine veins.

## 6th Phase: Installing the Prosthesis

- The prosthesis is inserted via the 10 mm trocar, which replaced the 5 mm midline trocar.
- Two polypropylene meshes may be used. The anterior prosthesis consists of a rectangle with a triangular anterior extremity, and the posterior part presenting a

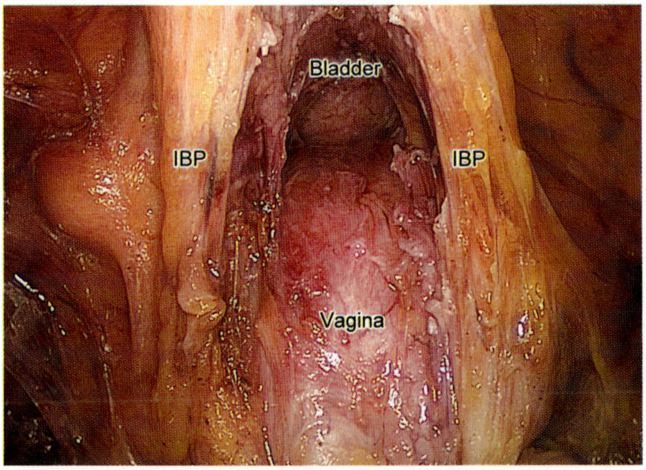


**Fig. 31.9:** Vesico-vaginal dissection—final view (IBP: internal bladder pillars)

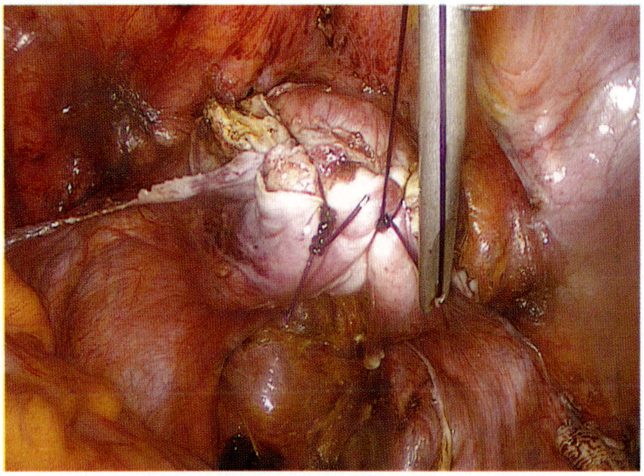

**Fig. 31.10:** Cervical stump suturing

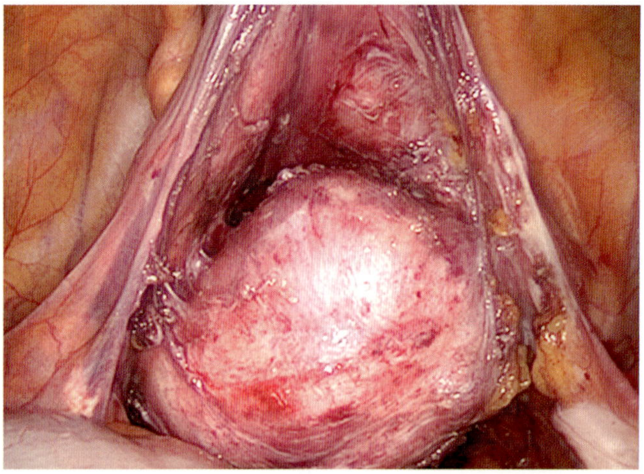

**Fig. 31.11:** Vaginal vault dissection after hysterectomy (exposition achieved thanks to a vaginal swab held in long-handled forceps)

curve downwards and to the rear to allow the rectum to pass between the two arms, which are attached to the *levator ani*.

- The rear part of the tape is fixed first. The posterior prosthesis is attached to the *levator ani* muscles each side using one stitch, and one more stitch to the posterior vaginal wall, medially. The sutures consist of polydioxanone (PDS II™ 2-0) (Figs 31.12 and 31.13). The prosthesis is then fixed to cervical stump with two or three polyester stitches (Ethibon Excel™ 0), to achieve a sturdy anchorage (Fig. 31.14). The sutures are closed with extra-corporeal knots of the half-hitch type using knot pusher.
  It is easier to take the needle through the *levator ani* muscles using the right hand, from outside inwards (Fig. 31.12).
  When the prosthesis is to be fixed to the vaginal vault particular care must be taken not to transfix the latter.
- The anterior prosthesis is placed beneath the bladder and fixed with one non-transfixing stitch to the anterior vaginal wall, then with one stitch level with the extremity of the cervix, using polyester (Ethibond Excel™ 0) (Fig. 31.15).
- The anterior and posterior prosthesis are then attached to each other laterally and medially by stitches which also takes up the cervix, using the same suture (Fig. 31.16).
  It is essential not to have any stitches that transfix the vagina in order to avoid any risk of prosthetic contamination.

*If the uterus is conserved*

- The two arms of tape are taken through the openings made in the posterior layer of the broad ligament.
- Then knotted behind the isthmus using a flat knot in the area deperitonized where the rectovaginal detachment was started.

## 7th Phase: Peritonization

Must be meticulous, aiming at complete extraperitonization of the prosthesis.

- There are 2 steps, before and after the prosthesis is fixed to the promontory, respectively:
  - Vesicouterine and rectovaginal peritonization. This step is achieved by taking up the anterior and posterior peritoneum using a "back and forth" running suture (Fig. 31.17A).
  - Running suture closes the line of the incision going from the promontory to the pouch of Douglas (Fig. 31.17B).
- The suture material used is a poliglecaprone 25 (Monocryl™ 0).
  Peritonisation will prevent incarceration of a loop of bowel, which otherwise is always possible. The tape is thus routed exclusively behind the peritoneum.

## 8th Phase: Fixing to the Promontory

- Fixation with one or two stitches of polyester (Ethibond™ 1) (Fig. 31.18).
  The suture is made using the left hand, from the inside towards the outside and from bottom to top.
  The needle must only take up the fibrous layer of the ligament, meaning it remains visible by transparency, to ensure that the disc is not perforated in any way. Staples are not recommended in this location, for the same reason.
  Avoid to route the needle to medially at the promontory, in order to avoid middle sacral pedicle and right hypogastric nerve.
- Apply sustained traction to check that they are firmly attached.
- Place the mesh on the promontory in tension-free fashion, then fixe it in position. We make a peroperative clinical examination to check that a normal anatomical situation is restored by this promontofixation.
- The final peritonization stitches are made after the mesh has been fixed to the promontory (Fig. 31.19).

## 9th Phase: Paravaginal Repair and Burch Colposuspension

In case of paravaginal defect, its repair is mandatory. Urinary incontinence can easily be treated with Burch colposuspension after retropubic space dissection.

- Retropubic space (space of Retzius) is opened by an incision in the peritoneum above the bladder running from one umbilical artery to the other, after pulling the peritoneum downwards (Fig. 31.20).
- The urachus is coagulated then sectioned and dissection must then continue along a vertical plane towards the pelvic sidewall. The umbilicovesical fascia needs to be crossed in order to achieve the retropubic space. Pneumodissection helps open the space.

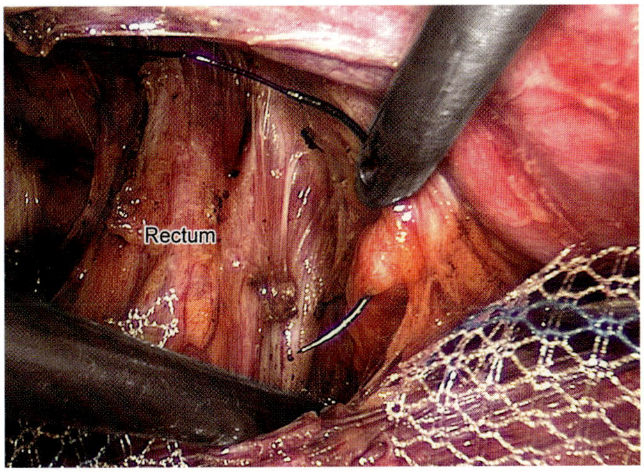


Fig 31.12: Suture placement for posterior mesh fixation to right levator ani muscle

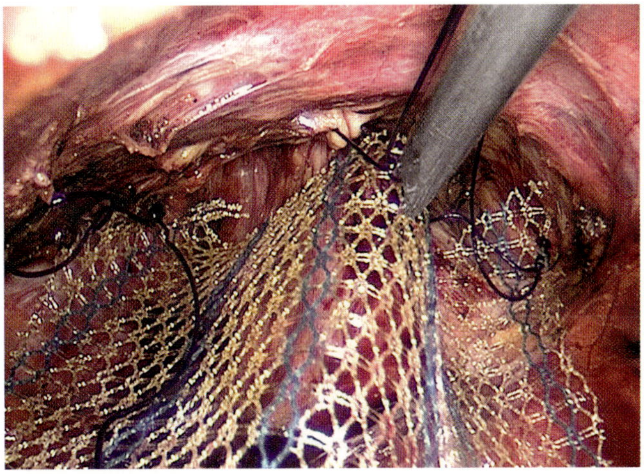

Fig. 31.13: Fixation of posterior mesh to levator ani muscles and posterior vaginal wall—final view

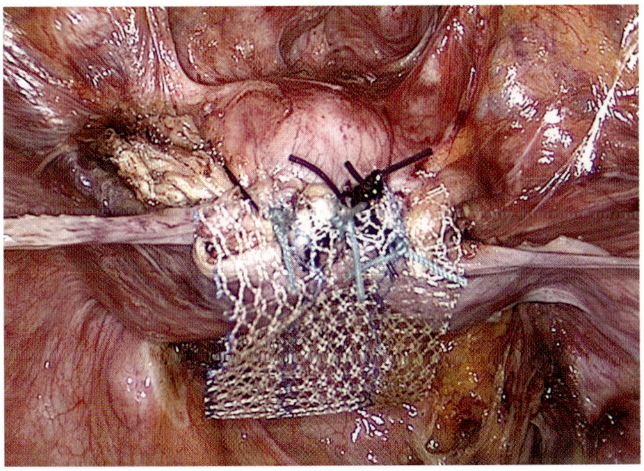

Fig. 31.14: Posterior mesh fixation to cervical stump. Note that the posterior mesh placement should be completely tension-free

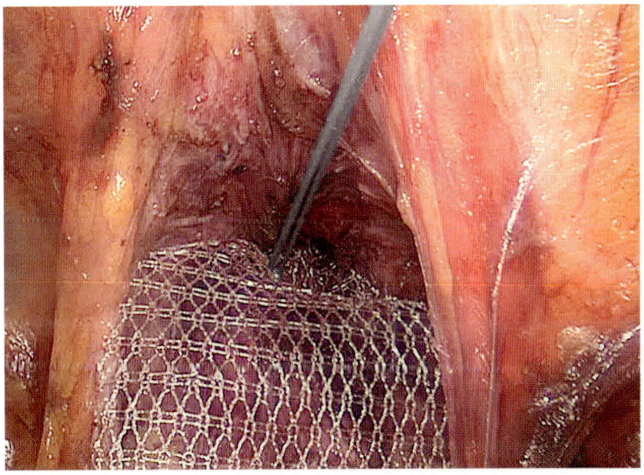

Fig. 31.15: Anterior prosthesis fixation to anterior vaginal wall

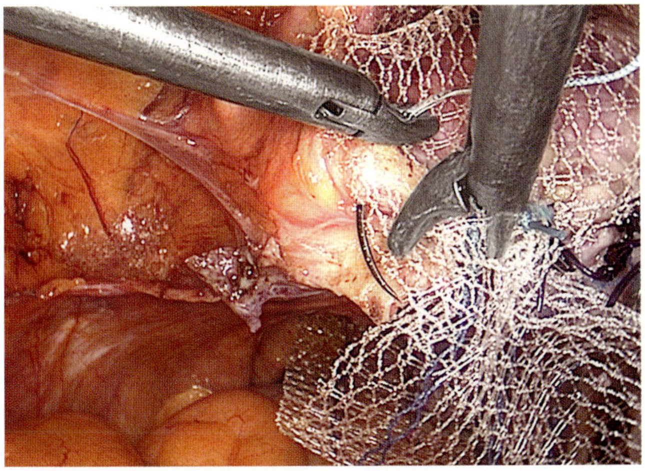

Fig. 31.16: The anterior and posterior meshes are attached to each other and to cervical stump with lateral and medial stitches

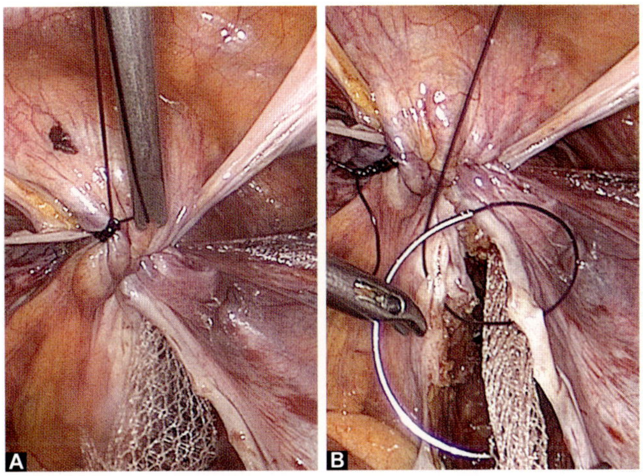


Figs 31.17A and B: First and second steps of peritonization

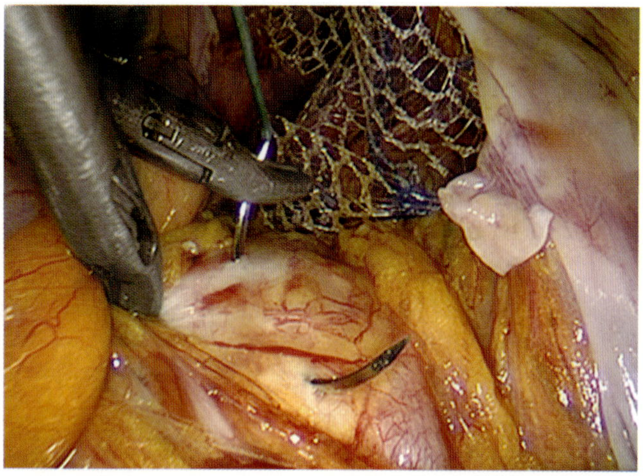

**Fig. 31.18:** Needle passing through anterior vertebral ligament, from left to right, bottom to top

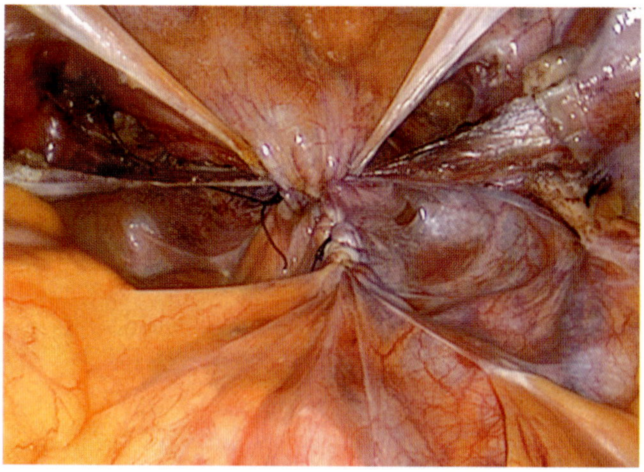

**Fig. 31.19:** Peritonization—final view

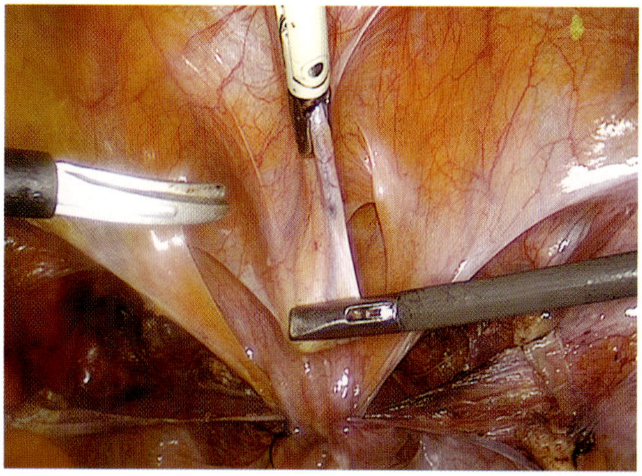

**Fig. 31.20:** Approaching retropubic space—beginning of dissection

- The right and left pectineal (Cooper) ligaments revealed on each side mark the upper limit of the space of Retzius.
- The space is opened up completely by simply breaking down the fat tissue until the internal obturator muscle revealing tendineus arch of pelvic fascia (TAPF) and paravaginal defect. Dissection continues backwards until just below the obturator foramen.

### Retropubic Dissection Anatomical Landmarks (Fig. 31.21)

- Pubic symphysis (superoanteriorly)
- Ischiopubic *ramus* with pectineal ligaments (superolaterally)
- Bladder (posteriorly)
- Bladder neck and vagina (inferiorly)
- TAPF and internal obturator muscles (laterally).

### Colposuspension

- The suture is first taken from top to bottom through the pectineal ligament, then through the vagina, from the inside outwards, without transfixion. Two to four sutures are placed each side. Traction must be moderate. The surgeon's experience is extremely important in this respect.
- The suture material used is polyester (Ethibond Excel™ 0) with extracorporeal knotting technique (Fig. 31.22). Before carrying out colposuspension, the positive pressure of the pneumoperitoneum allows inspection of the lateral defects that are almost always present in cases of complex prolapse. They show up as hernias running from the TAPF to the vagina itself. If there is a paravaginal hernia like this, it must be repaired (Fig. 31.23).

### Paravaginal Repair

- We repair this defect by carrying out a colposuspension to pectineal ligament, catching the TAPF, using at least three anchorage points with polyester (Ethibond Excel™ 0), which thus brings the vagina up level with the TAPF, closing the defect (Fig. 31.23). In order to close the defect completely and encourage fibrosis, a floating prosthetic reinforcement is positioned paravaginally (Fig. 31.24). In fact this is a modification of the prosthetic Retzius plasty technique proposed by H. Manhes.
- The colposuspension and paravaginal repair phase is completed by peritonization using a running suture of poliglecaprone 25 (Monocryl™ 0).
- Uterine morcellation using a cold knife in an endoscopic holder inside an endoscopic bag.
- Closure of the aponeurosis at the location of the infraumbilical 10 mm trocar.

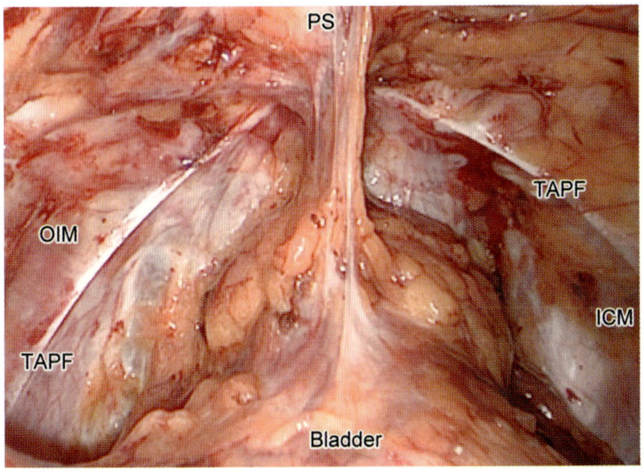


**Fig. 31.21:** Retropubic space dissection—final view. (PS: pubic symphysis; TAPF: tendinous arch of pelvic fascia; OIM: obturator internus muscle; ICM: iliococcygeus muscle)

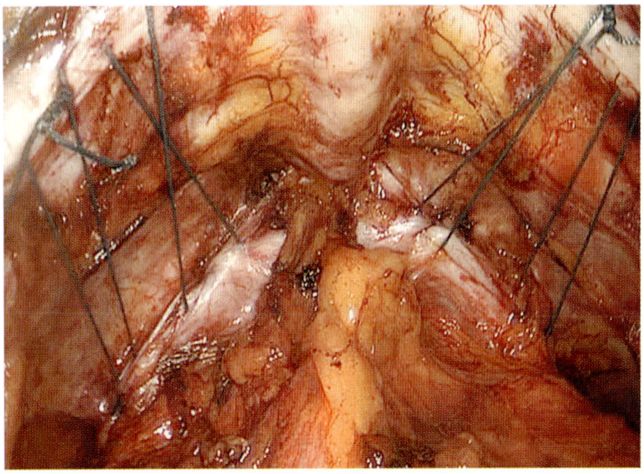

**Fig. 31.22:** Burch colpossupension

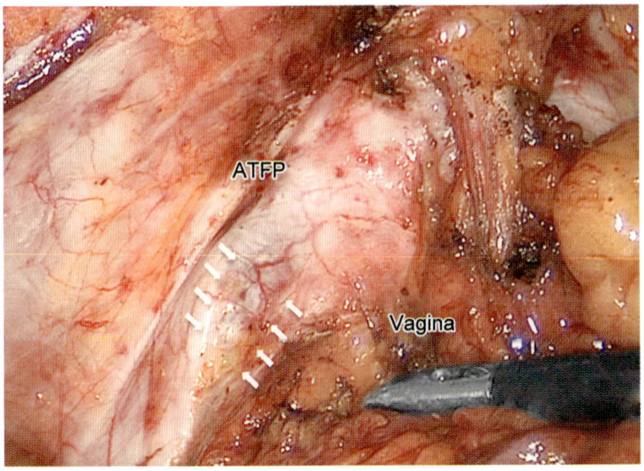


**Fig. 31.23:** Paravaginal defect. ATFP: tendinous arch of pelvic fascia

## Postoperative Management

- Thromboprophylaxis: Enoxaparin 40 mg SC qDay, for 3 weeks.
- Avoid physical efforts for 3 weeks
- Constipation prevention: Osmotic laxative Movicol™ (Macrogol, sodium bicarbonate, sodium chloride, potassium chloride) qDay to q12 hours, enough for daily dejection
- Discharge in 48 hours
- First consultation 1 month after the surgery.

**The technique described can be adapted to all types of pelvic organ prolapse if some rules are followed:**

- Avoid vaginal opening
- Avoid over-traction
- Use polypropylene mesh
- Avoid thread transfixion
- Complete prolapse treatment.

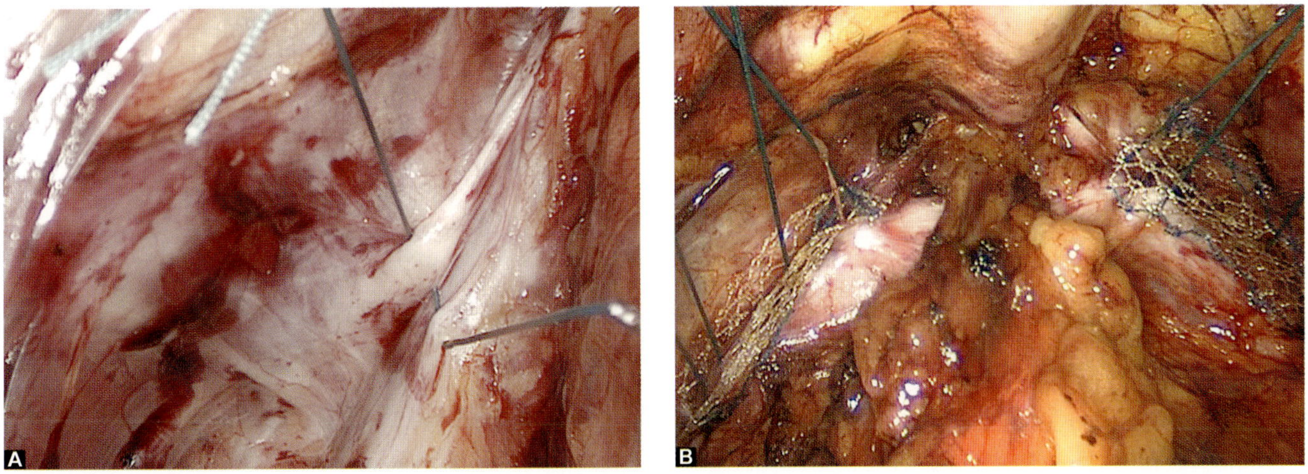


**Figs 31.24A and B:** (A) Paravaginal defect repair in case of tendinous arch detachment; (B) Retzius plasty with free prosthesis placed around sutures

Chapter

32

# Laparoscopic Sling Surgery

*Sunita R Tandulwadkar, Nirzari Mangeshikar*

## LAPAROSCOPIC SACRO-SPINOUS FIXATION FOR UTERINE PROLAPSE

This procedure can be performed for a young woman with uterovaginal prolapse, who desires preservation of uterus.

A sacrospinous fixation will benefit such a patient. It can be done unilaterally or bilaterally. When one does bilaterally, they have to take psoas loop on the left side. So most of the gynecologists prefer unilateral right-sided sling (Soonawala sling).

### Preoperative Evaluation

- History and examination of the patient.
- Ensure that it is utero-vaginal prolapse and not cervical elongation, in which case this procedure will not be suitable.
- Baseline tests as required prior to administration of general anesthesia.

### Preoperative Preparation

- Thorough bowel preparation by laxatives administered evening prior to surgery, especially in obese patients.

### Instruments and Materials

- 10 mm zero degree laparoscope
- Camera system
- Bipolar forceps
- 10 mm tooth grasper
- Two non-traumatic graspers
- Suction irrigation system
- Scissor
- Harmonic scalpel (if available helps in dissection at L5)
- Allis forceps (for vaginal part)
- Long artery forceps
- Prolene mesh 6"x 2"
- Tackers for fixation.

### Procedure

1. Apply Allis forceps posterior lip of cervix and give upward traction.
2. A horizontal incision is given on the posterior vaginal wall and dissection is done to create space. Care is taken not to open the Pouch of Douglas.
3. Laparoscopically, the L5 region is identified and its overlying peritoneum is dissected. All loose areolar tissue on the anterior aspect of ligament are dissected taking care of the vessels. (otherwise mesh will not be anchored well). Harmonic definitely helps in doing the bloodless dissection.
4. Through this retroperitoneal incision, the space in the lateral pelvic wall medial to the ureter is created. This helps the assistant who is passing the long artery forceps, retroperitoneally along the pelvic wall from the vaginal end.
5. Through primary 10 mm port, polypropylene mesh of 6" x 2" is introduced.
6. One end of the mesh is held tight by the assistant, while the other end is kept free for the artery forceps which is coming from the vaginal end to pick up.
7. Under laparoscopic vision, a long artery forceps is introduced through the vaginal incision and

negotiated upwards along the lateral pelvic wall, medial to the ureter, all length till reaches the peritoneal incision at L5 level.

8. During this passage, artery forceps can be negotiated more easily by doing small opening and closing of the jaws in the loose areolar tissue along the lateral pelvic wall.
9. Once it reached the L5 incision level, the jaw is opened and the other end of the mesh is held tightly and is pulled down till the vaginal end.
10. Assistant holding the other end of the mesh allows the easy pull down without losing the grip on the other end of the mesh.
11. The mesh is fixed at the isthmic area at three points with Gortex/Prolene sutures.
12. Vaginal incision is closed with Vicryl No. 1-0.
13. Now the cervix is pushed up and the other end of the mesh held with the strong forceps is pulled up. The mesh is then anchored to the ligament of L5 vertebra either with tucker or with 3 to 4 stitches with Gortex.
14. The mesh is pulled up sufficiently so that the tip of the cervix is above the ischial spine level, but at the same time taking care that the colon is not completely compressed.
15. Excessive length of the mesh is cut and peritoneum is closed with Vicryl 1-0.

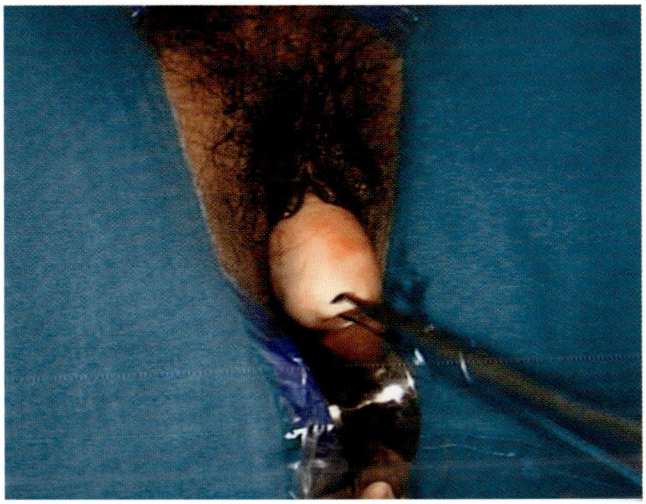

**Fig. 32.1:** 3rd degree uterocervical prolapse

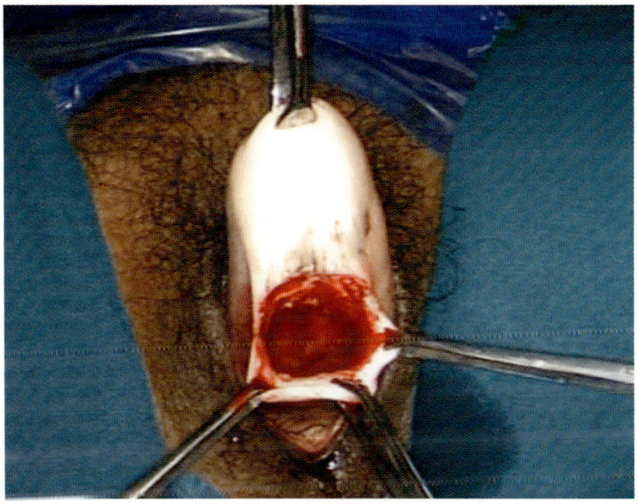

**Fig. 32.2:** Horizontal incision on posterior vaginal wall at the level of isthmus and dissection in the rectovaginal pouch without opening POD

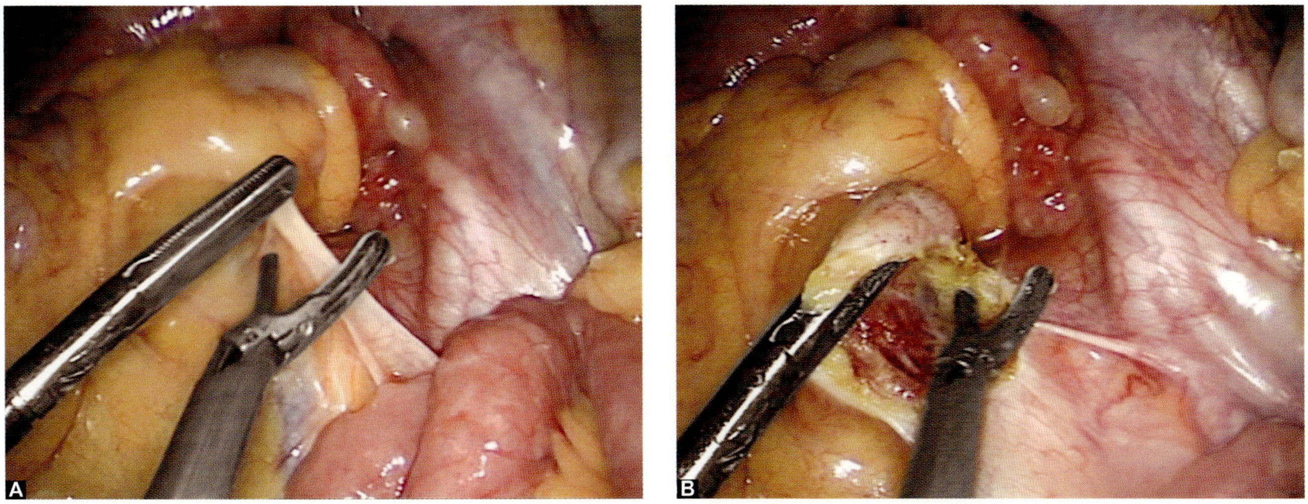

**Figs 32.3A and B:** Peritoneum over L5 vertebra identified and dissected

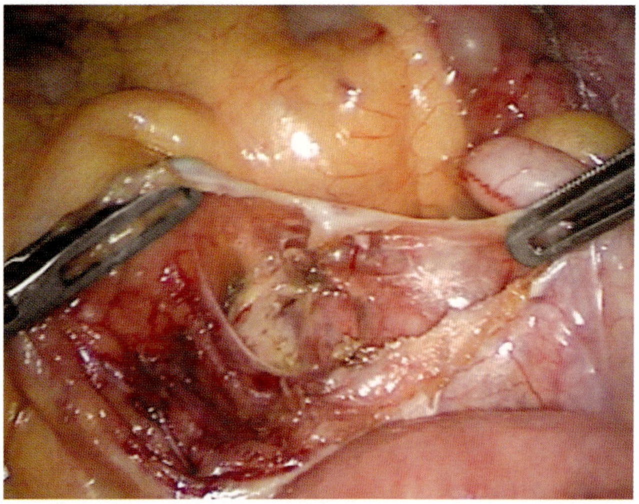

**Fig. 32.4:** Loose areolar tissue is completely removed

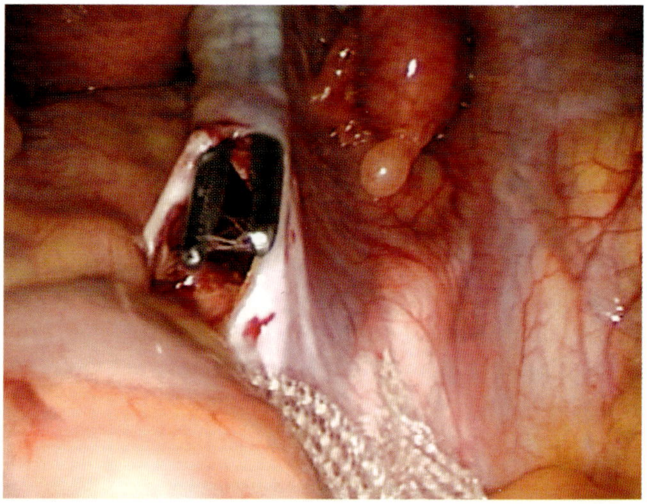

**Fig. 32.5:** Artery forceps introduced through vaginal incision along the lateral pelvic wall medial to the ureter

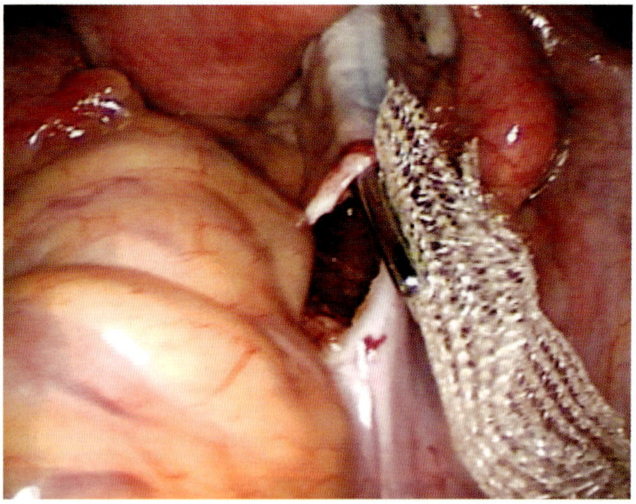

**Fig. 32.6:** Prolene mesh grasped with artery forceps and pulled towards the vaginal end

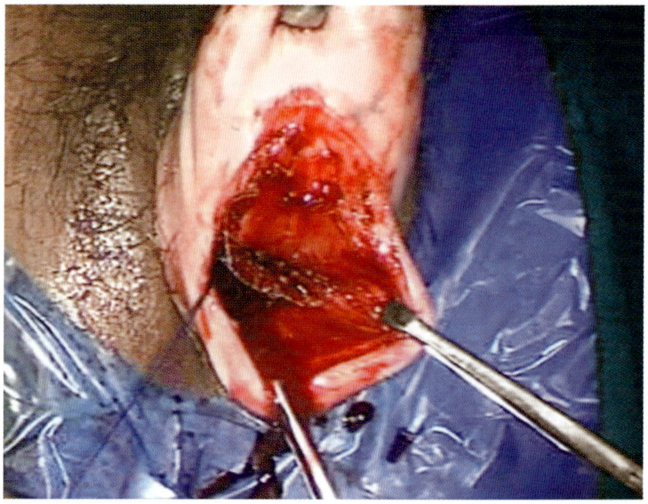

**Fig. 32.7:** Mesh sutured at vaginal end with no.1 prolene suture

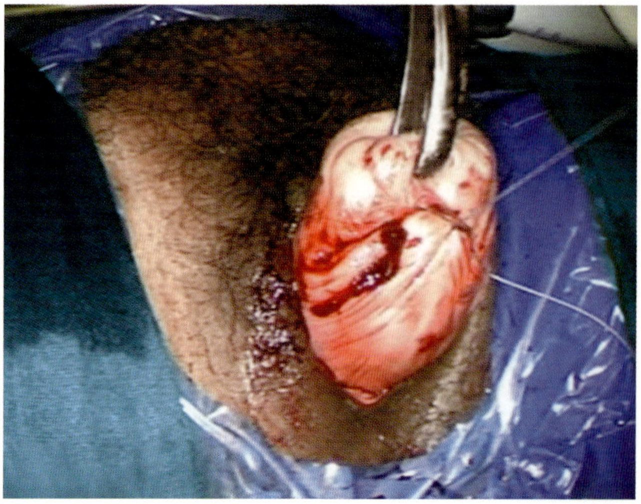

**Fig. 32.8:** Vaginal incision closed with no.1-0 Vicryl in continuous fashion at this stage only

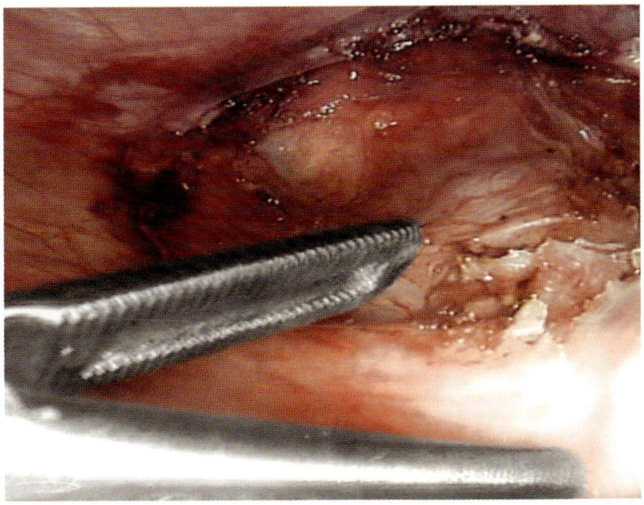

Fig. 33.1: UV fold of peritoneum dissected and bladder separation is done and paracervical loose areolar tissue also dissected so as to loosen up descending cervical artery

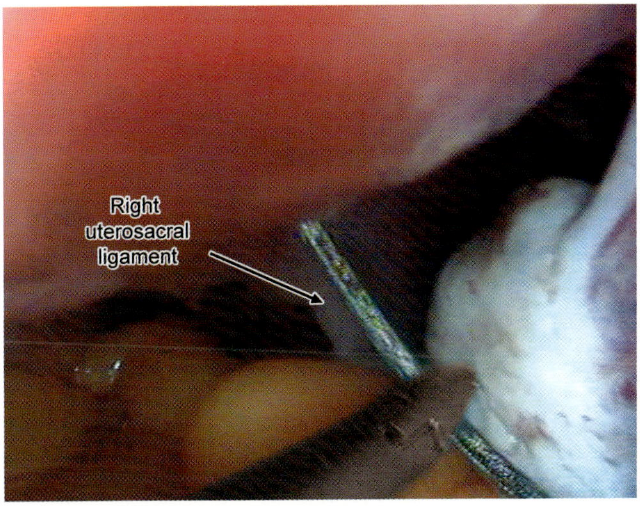


Fig. 33.2: Stitch taken posteriorly above the level of uterosacral ligament

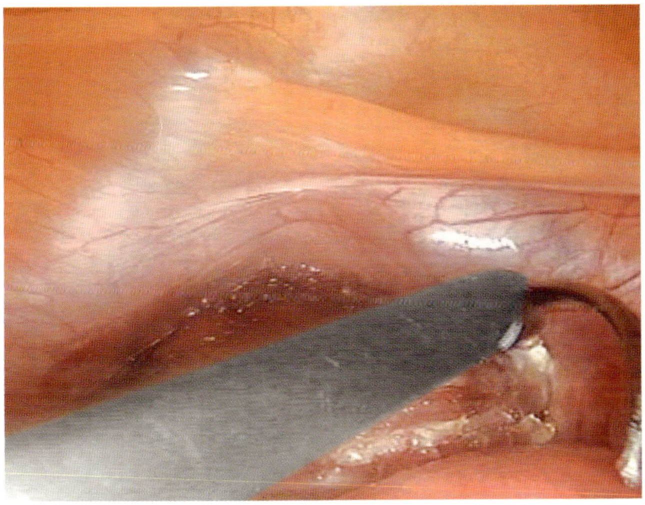

Fig. 33.3: Needle brought out anteriorly on right side

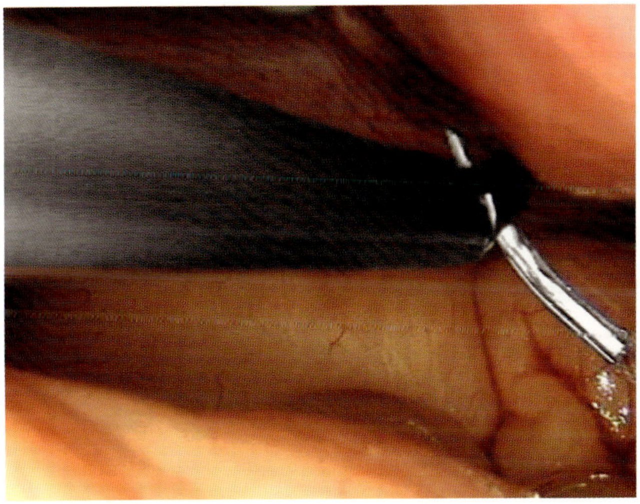

Fig. 33.4: Needle then inserted above the left uterosacral ligament

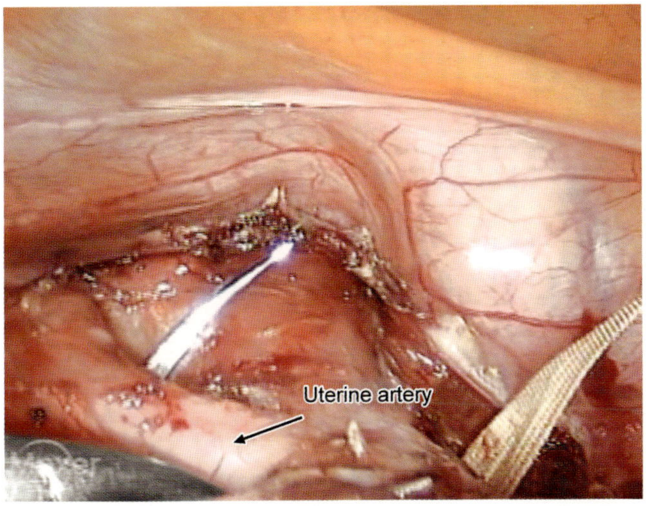


Fig. 33.5: Needle taken out anteriorly, medial to the descending part of uterine artery

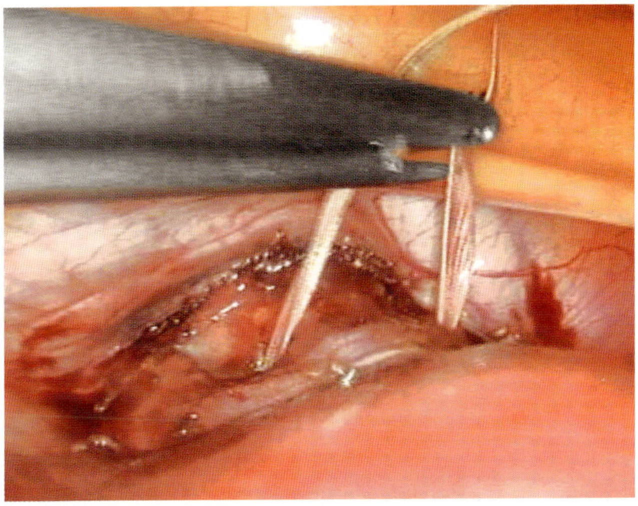

Fig. 33.6: Tape tightened by pulling up both ends of the tape

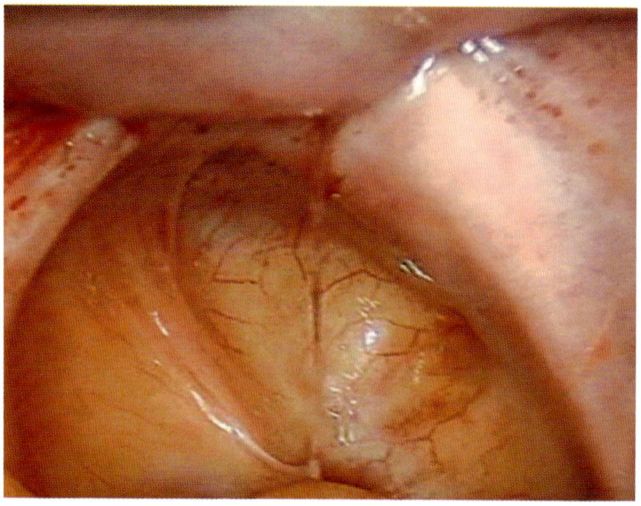

**Fig. 33.7:** Position of tape is confirmed on posterior aspect

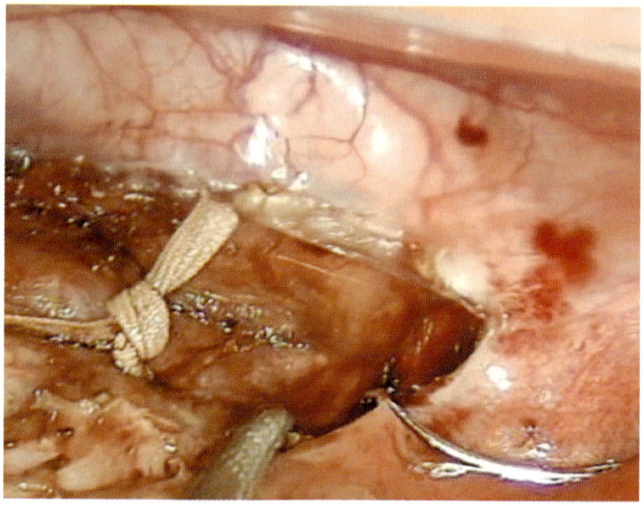

**Fig. 33.8:** After tightening satisfactorily, knot is tied anteriorly

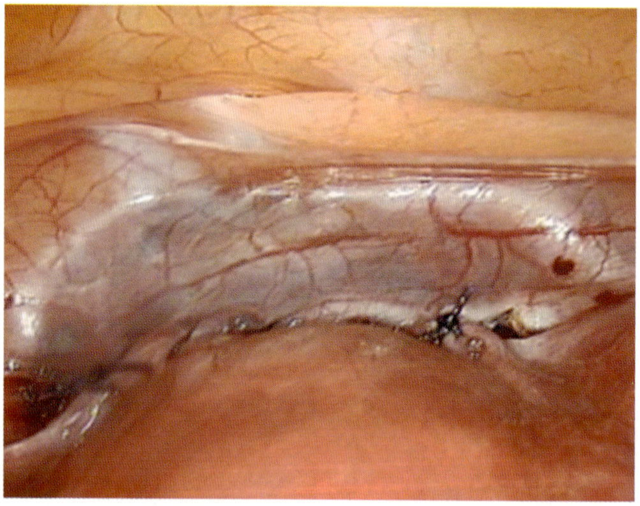

**Fig. 33.9:** Peritoneum closed with NO. 1-0 Vicryl® suture

## TIPS

- Tape has to be placed medial to the descending cervical vessels.
- To avoid the injury to the descending cervical vessel, dissection of the paracervical loose areolar tissue should be done after the bladder dissection. This loosens up the vessel from the cervix.
- Harmonic scalpel helps in making the dissection bloodless.
- During pregnancy uterine manipulation cannot be done and may need the help of an assistant for gentle uterine manipulation by putting right sided port. Considering bulky uterus of pregnancy, 30 degree telescope enhances the vision.

Chapter 34

# Single Incision Laparoscopic Surgery Using Common Laparoscopic Instruments

*Sevellaraja Supermaniam*

## PREOPERATIVE EVALUATION

Proper case selection is necessary. When starting to perform this technique, it is best to select simple cases first. A good case to start is a small uterus with no previous surgery.

## PREOPERATIVE PREPARATION

### Bowel Preparation

No special diet is necessary.

The patient is asked to dissolve 2 bottles of fleet phosphosoda and drink it about 8 hours before surgery.

### Position of Patient

Patient is placed in a low modified lithotomy position on stirrups. Yellofin stirrups are good because the position of the leg can be adjusted during surgery. In single incision surgery, the surgeon (right handed) will be standing on the left of the patient holding 2 instruments close to the laparoscope at the umbilicus (see Figure 13). This may be tiring. So tilting the patient slightly to the left (toward the surgeon) can reduce stress on the back of the surgeon.

## IMPORTANT EQUIPMENT

- One 10 mm trocar (choose a trocar that does not have a large "head")
- Two 5 mm trocars
- Two rubber bands
- One 30 degrees 10 mm laparoscope
- One right angle connector (Fig. 34.1)
- One vessel sealer which can coagulate and cut (e.g. ligasure, enseal, bicision, harmonics)
- One bipolar forceps (choose a bipolar which has the cable parallel to the shaft)
- Monopolar hook
- Uterine manipulator
- Needle holders
- Graspers (1 Maryland grasper for suturing)
- Myoma screw.

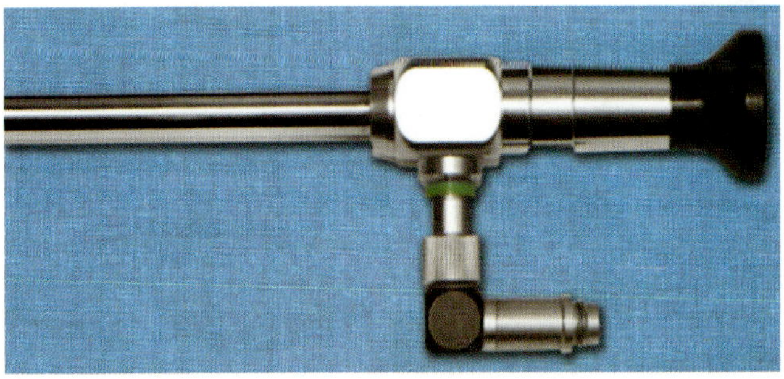

**Fig. 34.1:** Right angle light connector

## TECHNIQUE

### Manipulator

Uterine manipulator used will depend on the surgery performed. For single incision total laparoscopic hysterectomy, a RUMI with a KOH cup and occluder is ideal.

## Skin Preparation and Port Placement

1. Make a mark using a sterile ruler, 2.5 mm across the umbilicus (Fig. 34.2).
2. Make a midline incision connecting these 2 marks (Do not go beyond these marks) (Fig. 34.3).
3. Detach the skin of the umbilicus from its attachment in the midline. Be careful not to enter into the peritoneal cavity (Fig. 34.4).
4. Create a space of about 1.5 cm under the skin and above the rectus sheath all around the incision (Fig. 34.5).
5. Use a veress needle to insufflate the abdomen in the center of the incision (Fig. 34.6).
6. Take a 10 mm trocar and tie 2 rubber bands about 1.5 cm from the tip. This is to prevent it from slipping into the abdomen during surgery.
7. Insert the trocar into the abdomen in the usual way. (Fig. 34.7)
8. If you have accidentally made a large opening in the rectus sheath, enter the 10 mm trocar directly into the abdomen and place a purse string around it to prevent leakage of gas (Fig. 34.8).
9. Place the laparoscope with the right angle light connector attached and visualize the abdomen and pelvis for adhesions.
10. Place the 5 mm trocar on the right side as laterally as possible stretching the skin. Choose a 5 mm trocar with an extension for gas input (Fig. 34.9)
11. Place a grasper to see that the trocar is well-placed in the abdomen.
12. Remove the grasper.
13. Place the second 5 mm trocar on the left side as laterally as possible stretching the skin and then place a grasper to ensure that it is properly placed (Fig. 34.10).
14. You are now ready to perform the surgery. Figure 34.11 showing positions of trocars and instruments.

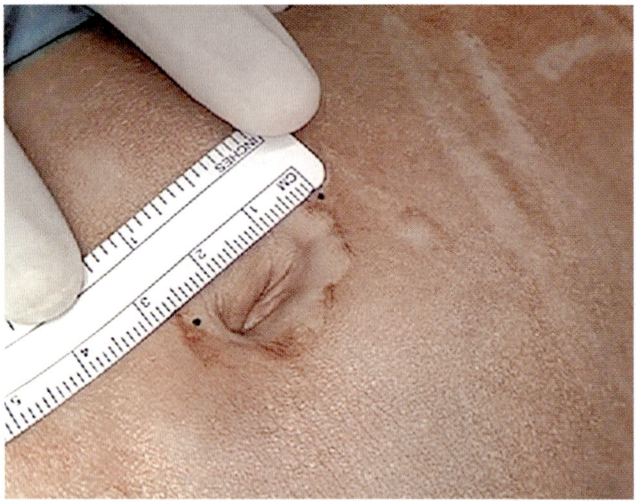

**Fig. 34.2:** Make a mark across the umbilicus 2.5 mm apart

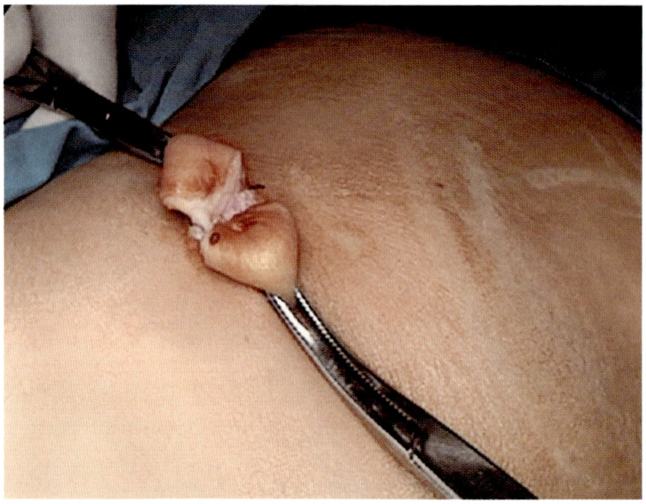

**Fig. 34.3:** Make a midline incision connecting the 2 marks

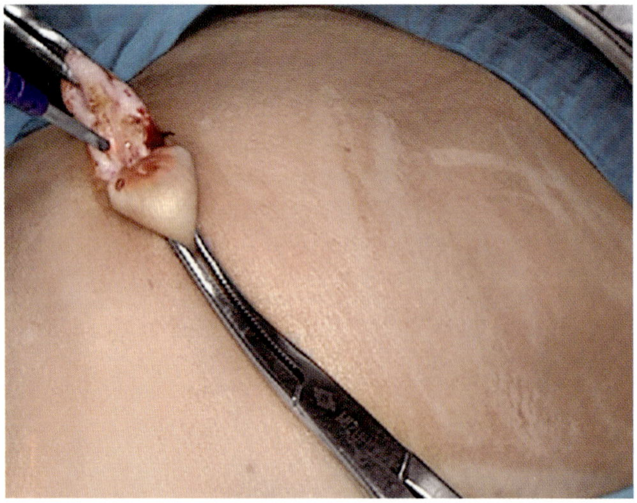

**Fig. 34.4:** Separate the skin from the rectus sheath

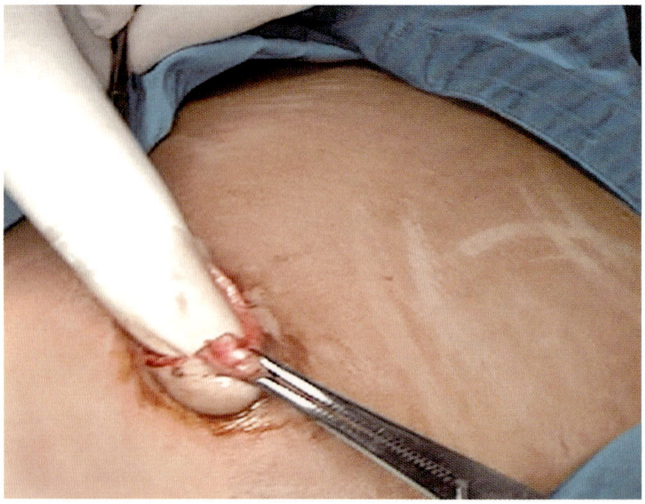

**Fig. 34.5:** Create a space of about 1.5 cm all around the skin above the rectus sheath

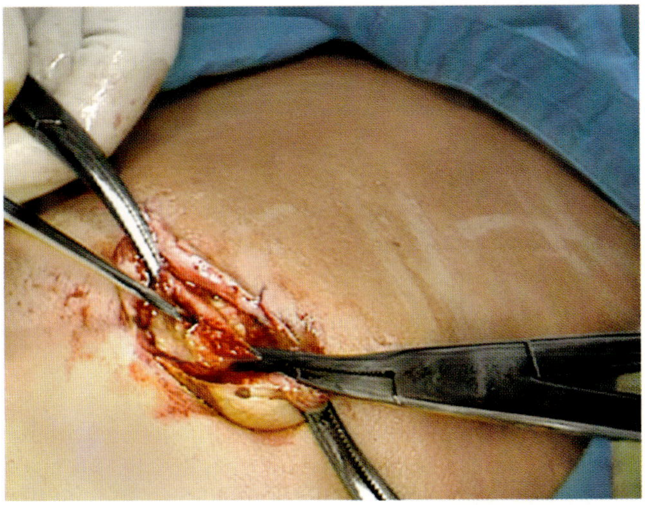

**Fig. 34.6:** Use the veress needle to insufflate the abdomen

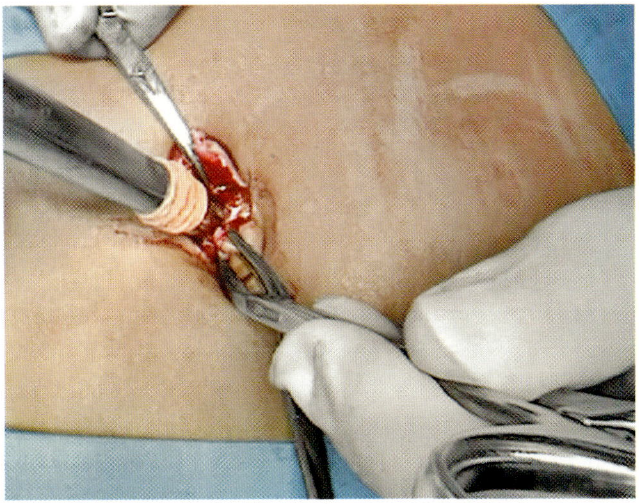

**Fig. 34.7:** Introduce the 10 mm trocar

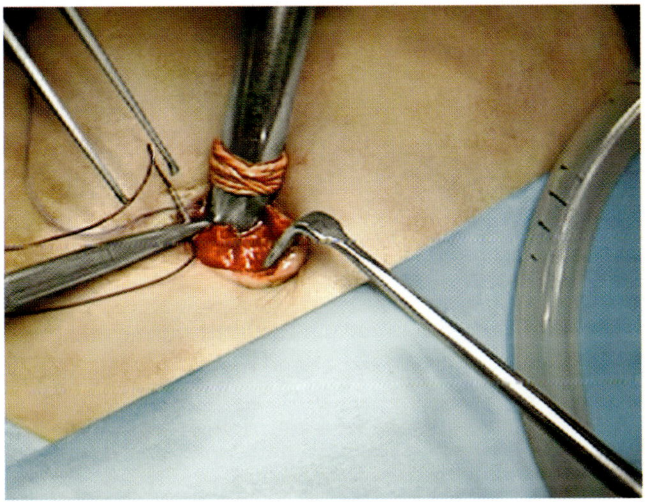

**Fig. 34.8:** Place a purse string if a large hole has been accidentally made in the rectus sheath

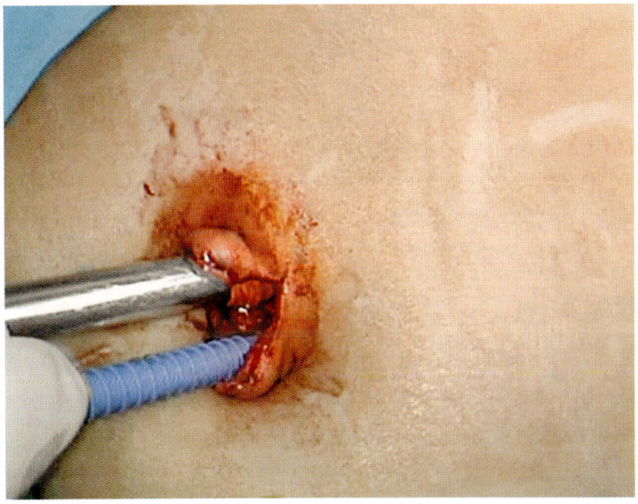

**Fig. 34.9:** Place the 5 mm trocar as laterally as possible on the right

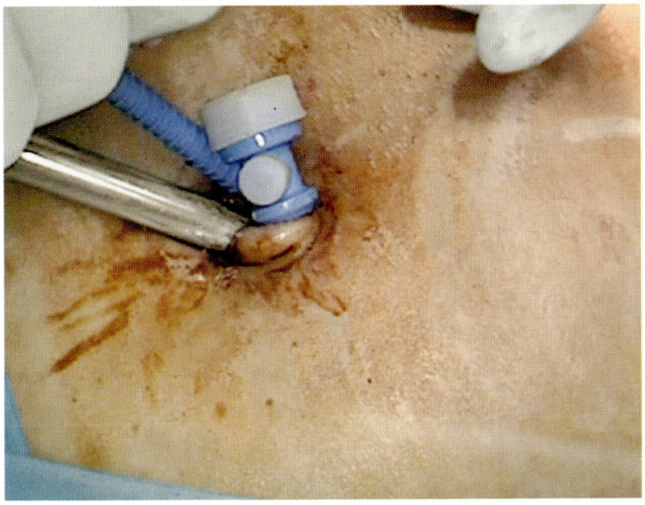

**Fig. 34.10:** Place the second 5 mm trocar as laterally as possible on the left

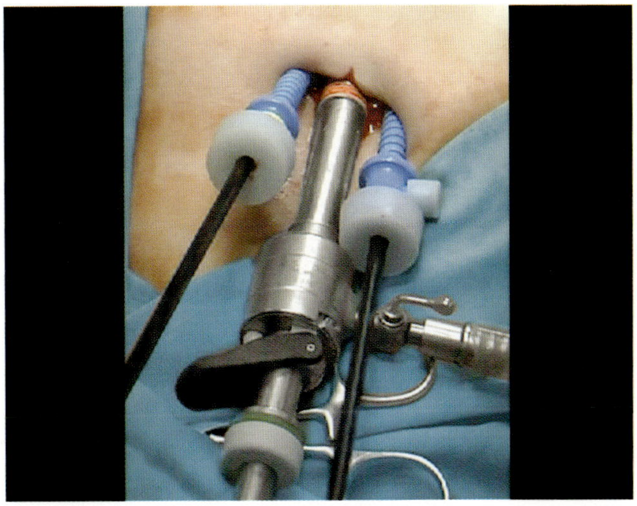

**Fig. 34.11:** Position of trocars and instruments during single incision laparoscopic surgery

## STEPS FOR PERFORMING SINGLE INCISION LAPAROSCOPIC HYSTERECTOMY

1. Inspect the pelvis for suitability to perform the hysterectomy by single incision.
2. Place a vessel sealing instrument in the right port and a grasper in the left port.
3. Begin by coagulating and cutting the right tube and right ovarian ligament (even when you plan to do a salpingo-oorphorectomy, leave the ovaries and tubes in the pelvis first and come back and remove them after the hysterectomy. In this way, the presence of the tubes and ovaries attached to the uterus will not obstruct your view when dealing with the ascending branches of the uterine arteries) (Figs 34.13 to 34.15).
4. Coagulate and cut the broad ligament until the uterine vessels are reached.
5. Release the peritoneum overlying the bladder and cut it and separate the bladder from the cervix (Figs 34.16 and 34.17).
6. Coagulate and cut the left ovarian ligament and tube. Usually it is possible to do it with the vessel sealant in your right hand. This will involve crossing your instruments. If this is awkward, change so that the vessel sealant is in your left hand and the grasper is in your right hand (Figs 34.18 and 34.19).
7. Once both uterine vessels are seen, bring a needle into the abdomen through the skin (Use a large needle so that it is easy to pass through the skin) (Fig. 34.20).
8. With the needle holder in the right hand, suture the left uterine artery first. Then use the Maryland grasper in your right hand which will make tying the knot easier. Use the clinch knot (Figs 34.21 and 34.22).
9. Suture the right uterine artery next. It is preferable to suture both the uterine arteries from top to the bottom. So for the left uterine artery, hold the needle holder with your left hand in the left port.
10. After suturing both the uterine arteries, the needle can be hooked on the anterior abdominal wall and removed from the vagina later or brought out through the skin (Fig. 34.23).
11. Coagulate and cut the uterine arteries and the cardinal ligaments. One can use the vessel sealant or just a normal bipolar followed by the scissors (Figs 34.24 and 34.25).
12. Use a monopolar hook to cut on the KOH cup and make a circumferential incision to detach the uterus from the vagina. Use the 30 degrees lens to look at the various angles when performing this. To do the posterior part one, can rotate the laparoscope 180 degrees (Figs 34.26 and 34.27).
13. Remove the uterus from the vagina.
14. Remove the tubes or the ovaries at this juncture (Fig. 34.28).
15. Bring a needle through the vagina using a vaginal tube.
16. If the bladder is obstructing the view of the vault, bring in non-absorbable suture on the straight needle through the skin, then hitch up the peritoneum of the bladder.
17. Suture the angles of the vaginal vault (Figs 34.29 and 34.30).
18. Place two more interrupted sutures in the middle to close the vault (Figs 34.31 and 34.34).
19. Inspect the vault for bleeding and attain hemostasis.
20. Remove the 2–5 mm trocars, then release the carbon dioxide and remove the 10 mm trocar.

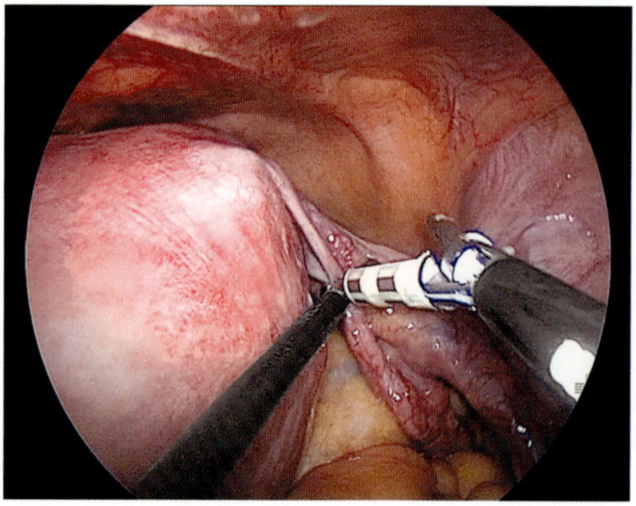

**Fig. 34.12:** Right adnexa held with a grasper and a vessel sealant used to coagulate the pedicle

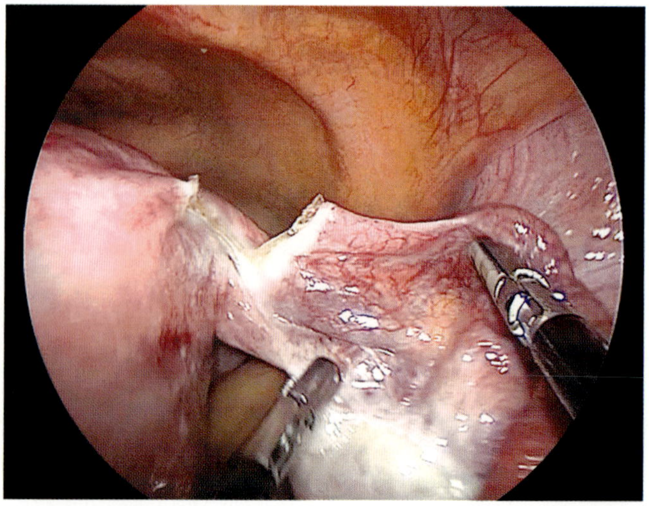

**Fig. 34.13:** Right tube is coagulated and cut

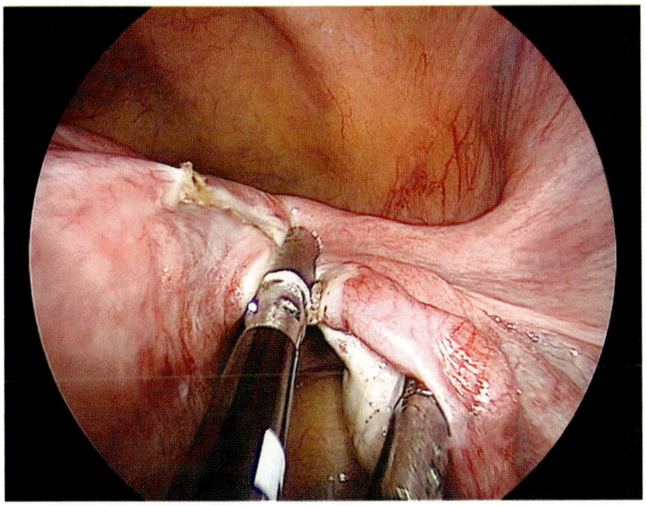

**Fig. 34.14:** Right ovarian ligament is coagulated and cut

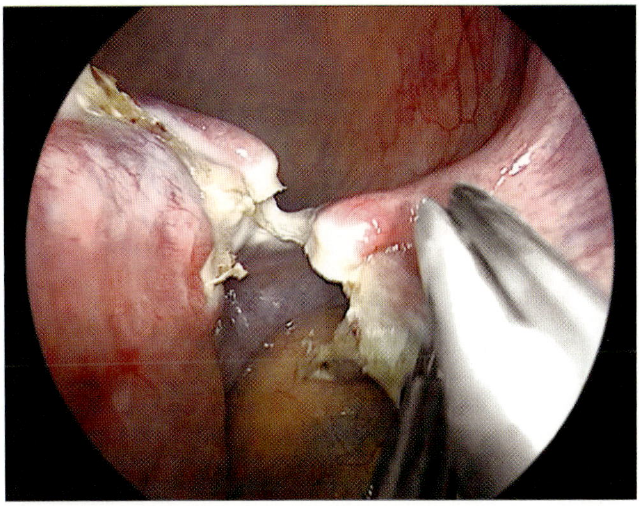

**Fig. 34.15:** Right round ligament is coagulated and cut

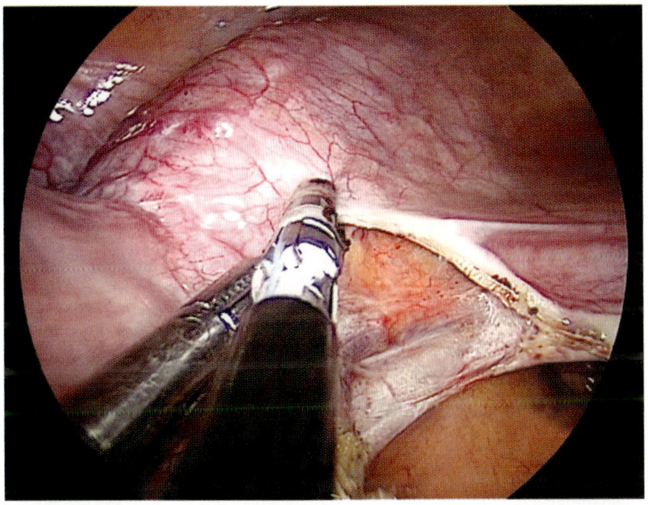

**Fig. 34.16:** Peritoneum overlying the bladder is separated

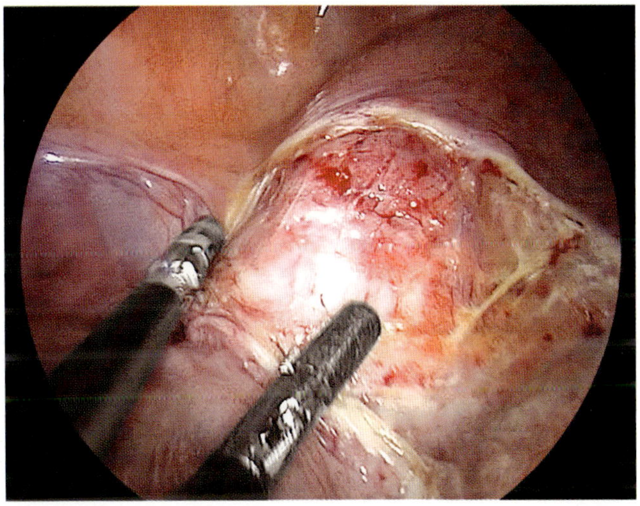

**Fig. 34.17:** Bladder is push down

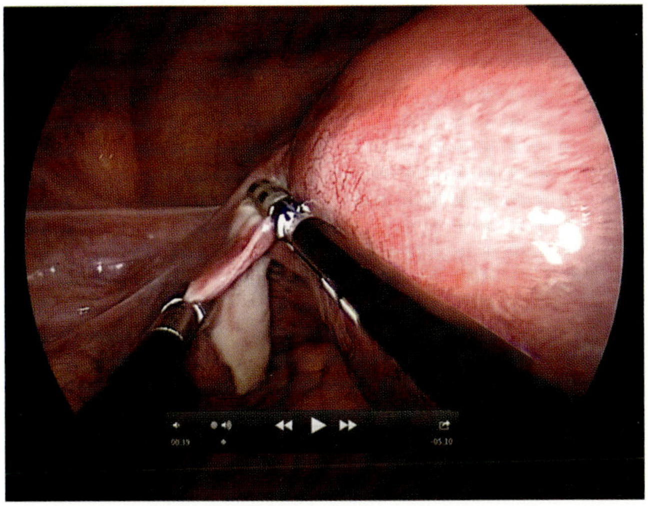

**Fig. 34.18:** Left adnexa is separated

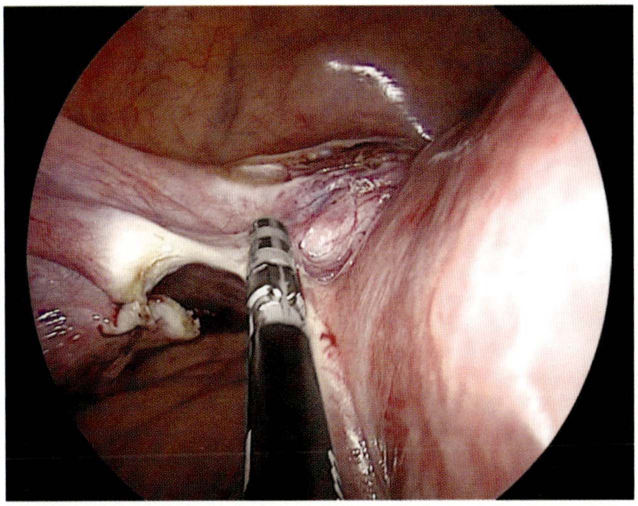

**Fig. 34.19:** Left broad ligament is incised

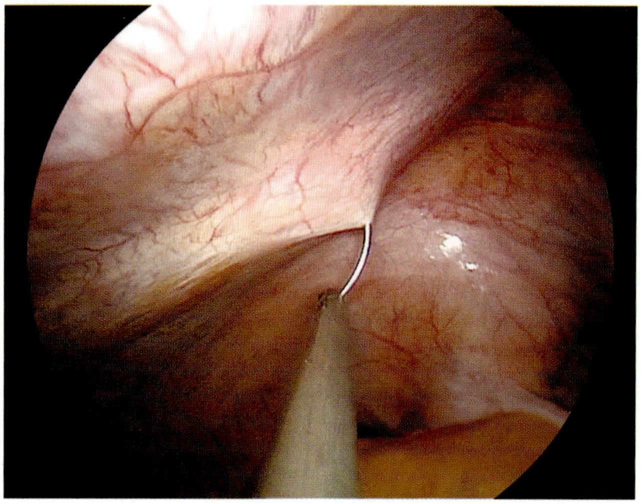

Fig. 34.20: Needle is brought out through the skin

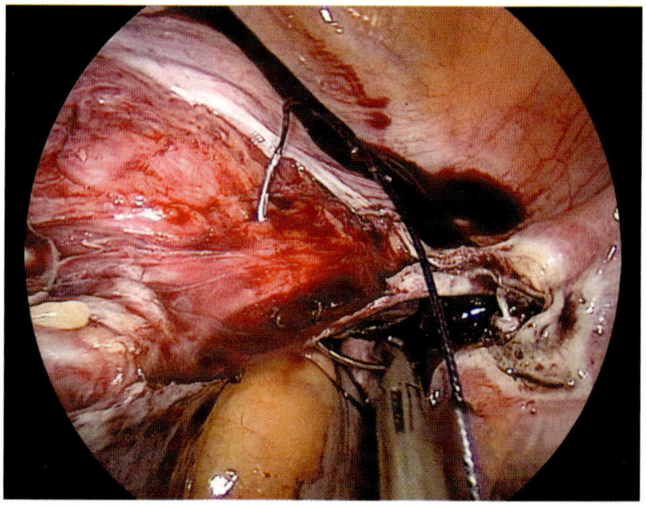

Fig. 34.21: Right ascending branch of uterine artery sutured

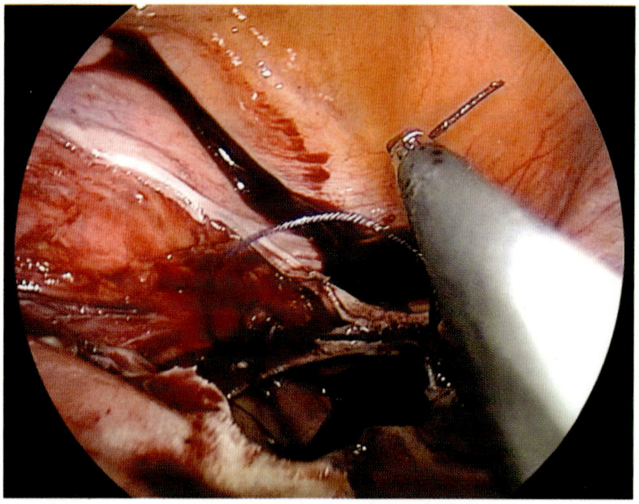

Fig. 34.22: Clinch knot

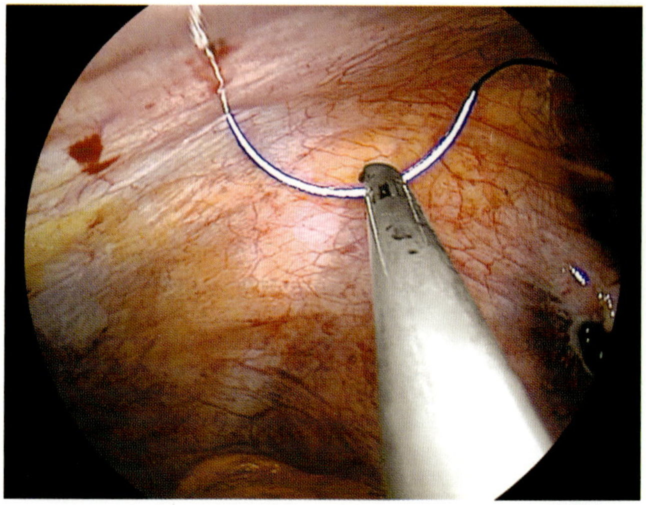

Fig. 34.23: Needle brought out of the skin

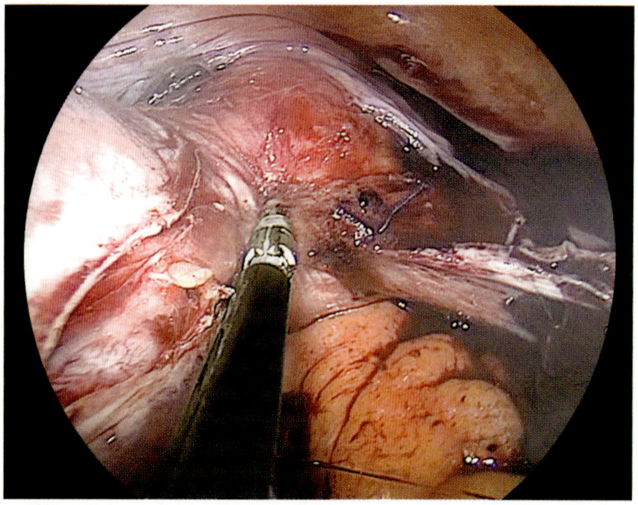

Fig. 34.24: Right uterine artery is coagulated and cut

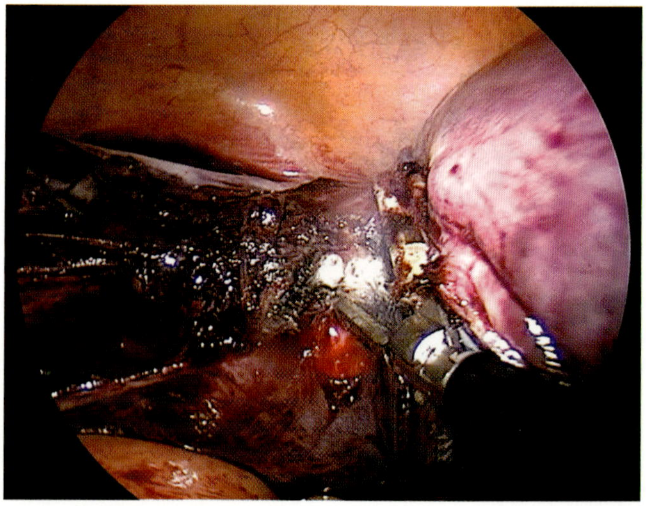

Fig. 34.25: Left uterine is coagulated and cut

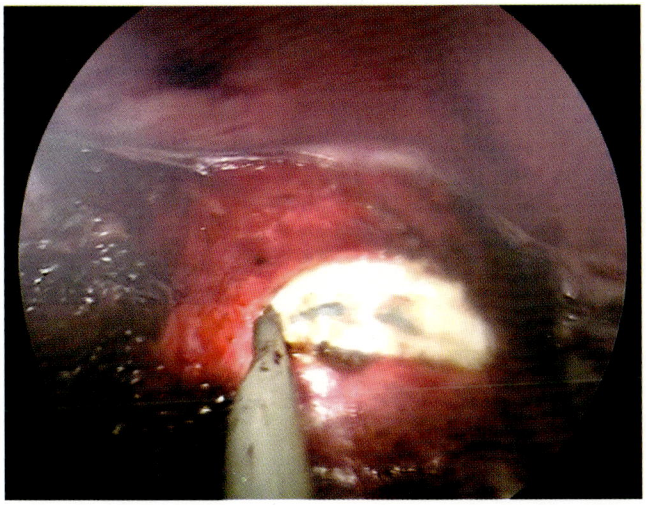

**Fig. 34.26:** Anterior colpotomy is performed

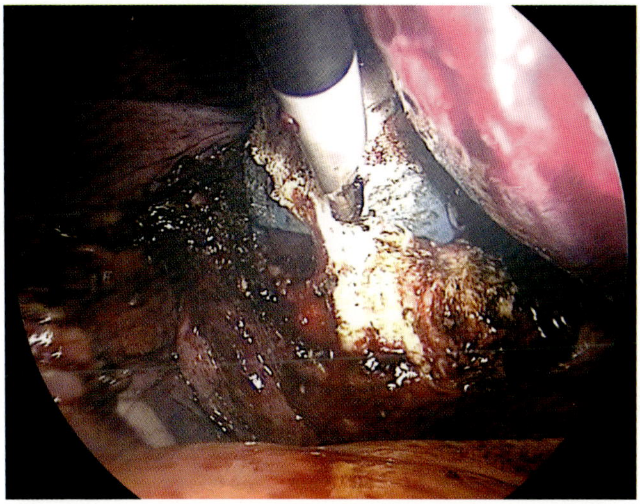

**Fig. 34.27:** Cervix is detached

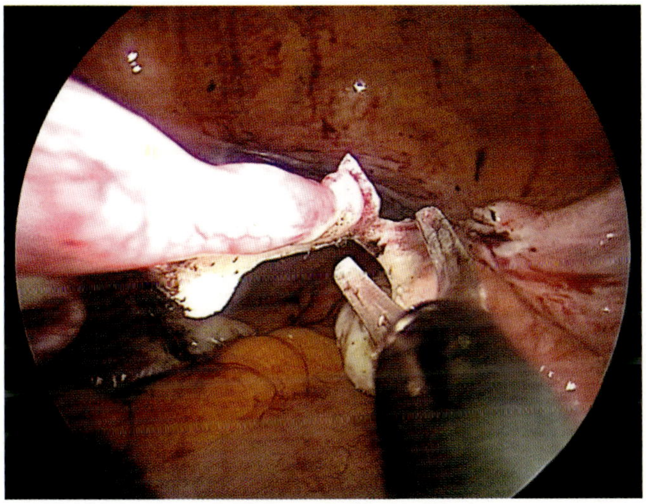

**Fig. 34.28:** The tubes are removed

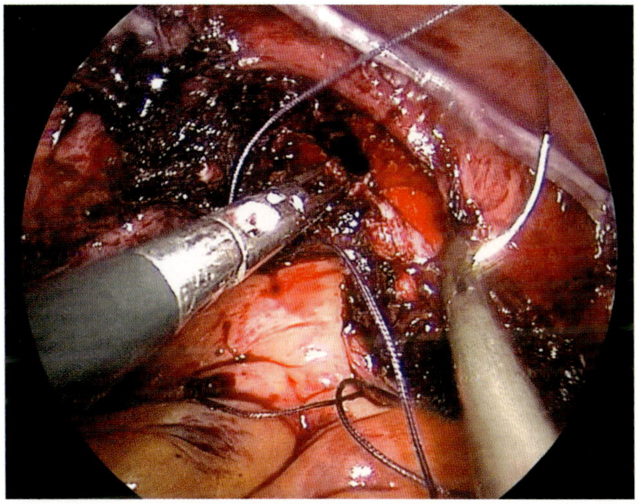

**Fig. 34.29:** Right angle is sutured

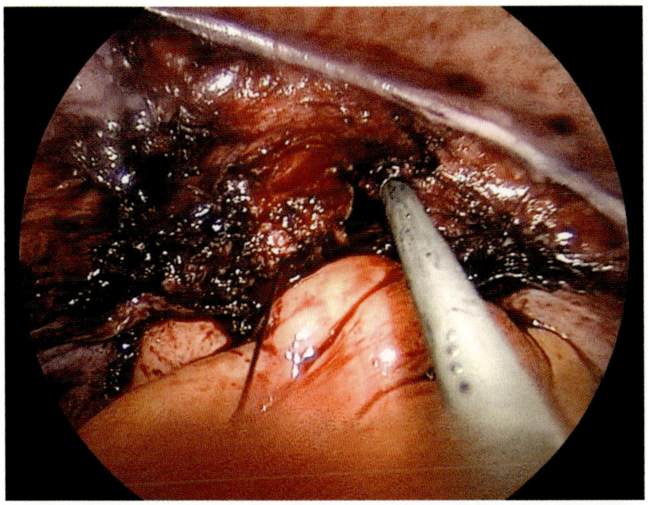

**Fig. 34.30:** Left vault angle is sutured

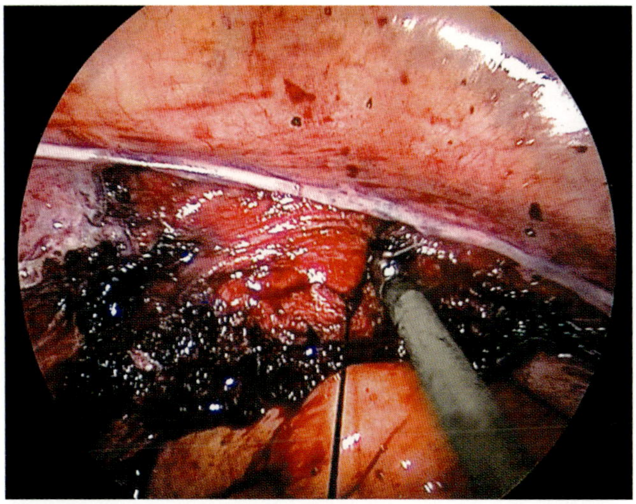

**Fig. 34.31:** Closing the middle part of the vault with interrupted sutures

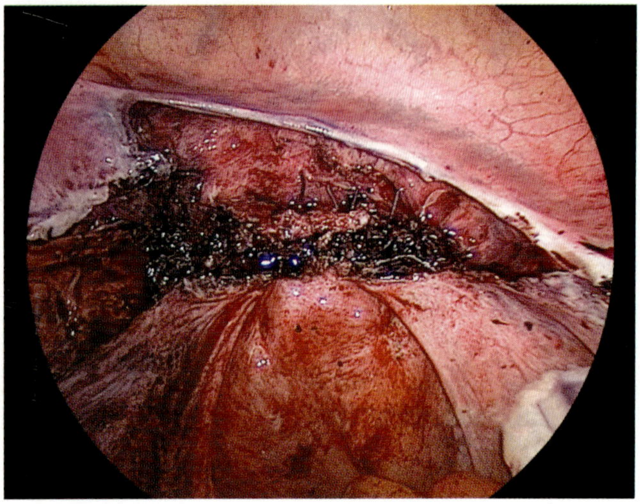

Fig. 34.32: Vault after completion of vault closure

### Reconstruction of the Umbilicus

1. Suture the 10 mm port opening carefully using a 1 PDS suture (Fig. 34.33).
2. Using a 3-0 PDS suture, reattach the skin to the rectus sheath in the midline. This is crucial for a good cosmetic result (Figs 34.34 and 34.35).
3. Close the midline incision using interrupted suture. 5-0 quick absorbing sutures (e.g. RapidVicryl or SafilQuick) should be used (Figs 34.36 and 34.37).
4. Close the wound with a small gauze and a waterproof dressing (Figs 34.38 and 34.39).
5. Use a syringe to create a vacuum in the dressing so that pressure is applied to the wound (Fig. 34.40).

## POSTOPERATIVE MANAGEMENT

There is no need for Foley's catheter post operation unless there is excessive bladder dissection.

Clear fluids an be given after 6 hours and nourishing fluid and soft diet can be commenced after the patient has passed flatus. She could be discharged 24 hours to 48 hours later.

## OTHER PROCEDURES THAT CAN BE PERFORMED BY THIS TECHNIQUE

### Laparoscopic Myomectomy

Choose cases with a single anterior subserous fibroid, for suturing of the wound is easier. Use a midline incision on the fibroid for due to the location of the needle holder at the umbilicus, suturing will be easier. The fibroid can be removed via a colpotomy or by converting to a 5 mm laparoscope and morcellating from the umbilicus.

### Laparoscopic Salpingoophorectomy or Salpingectomy

This can easily be performed using this technique. The difficulty will be placing the cyst in a bag. A bag can be passed into the abdomen from the 10 mm port and 2 graspers can be used to open up the bag to place the cyst/tube in the bag. This can sometimes be technically difficult. One can use fluid to open up the bag and then place the cyst in the bag.

Tips and tricks in performing single incision laparoscopic surgery in gynecology using common laparoscopic instruments

1. If you are unsure whether you can perform SILS surgery, make a small incision in the umbilicus, insufflate with Veress needle and use a 5 mm scope to look into the abdomen first and then decide whether the case is suitable for single incision surgery.
2. If there is a worry of umbilical adhesions, Veress needle can be placed at the palmar point and a needle scope

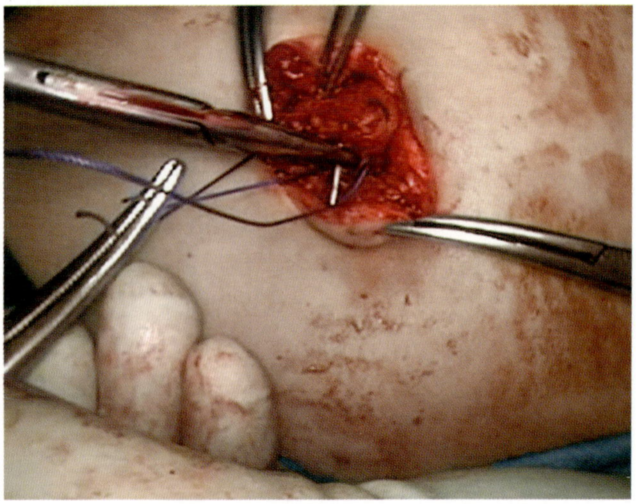

Fig. 34.33: Rectus sheath is closed with PDS 1 suture

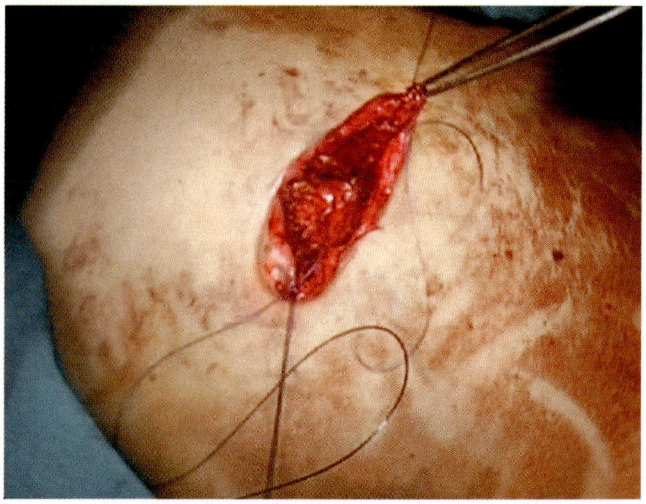

Fig. 34.34: Everted skin is reattached to the rectus sheath using PDS 3-0 suture

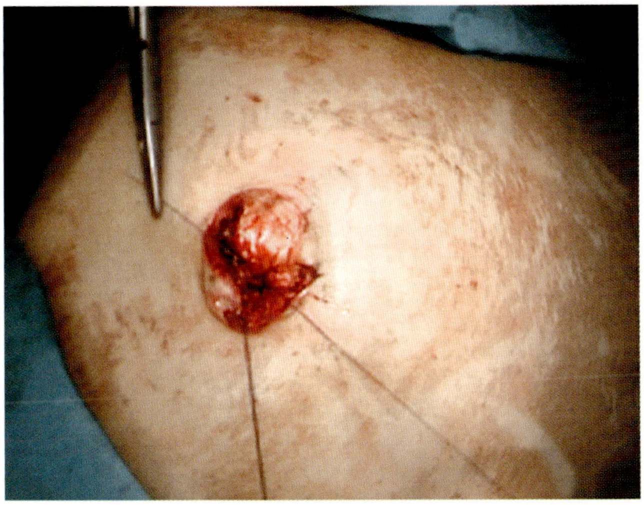

**Fig. 34.35:** Skin is reattached to the rectus sheath

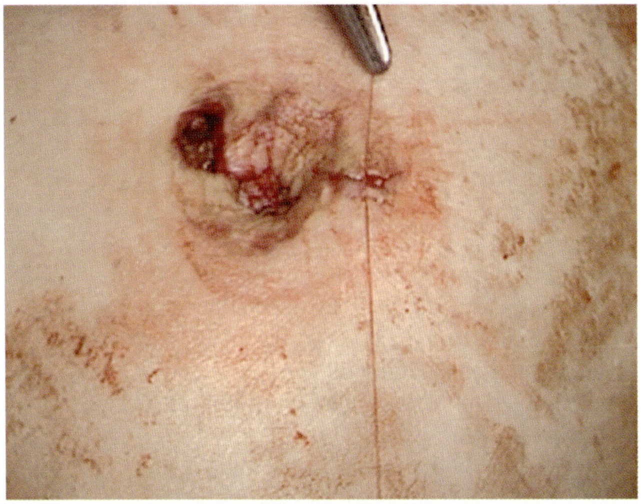

**Fig. 34.36:** Skin is closed using interrupted rapid absortiong 5-0 sutures

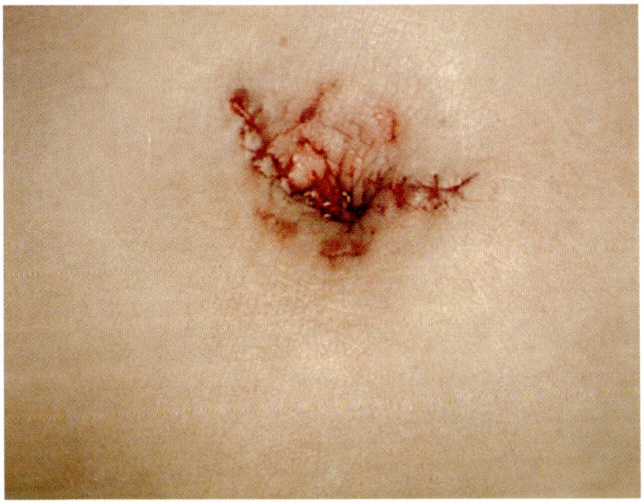

**Fig. 34.37:** Reconstruction completed

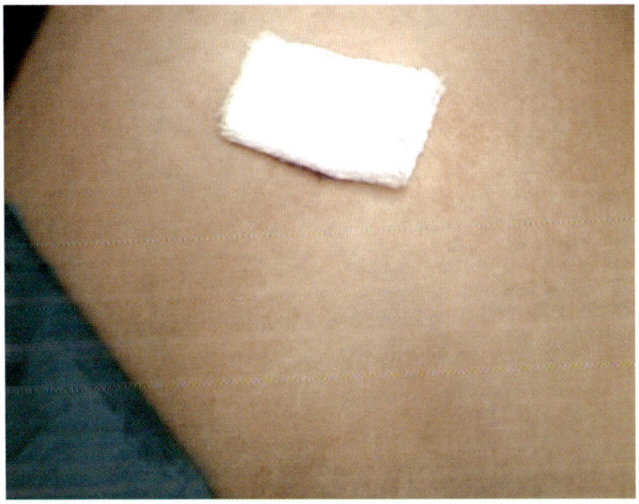

**Fig. 34.38:** Small piece of gauze is placed on the wound

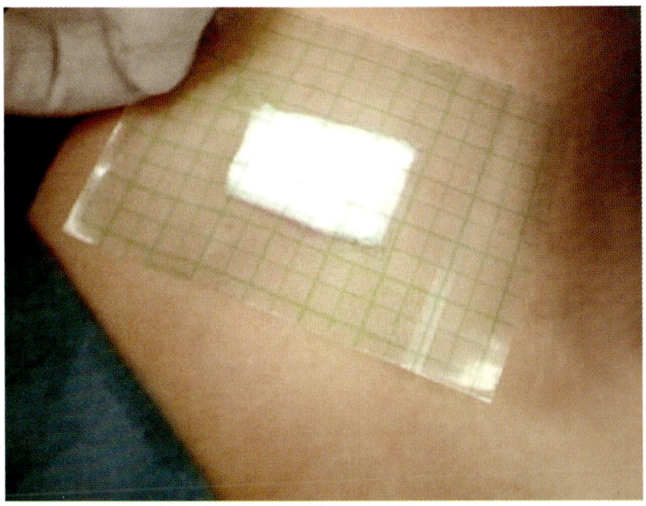

**Fig. 34.39:** Sterile waterproof dressing placed

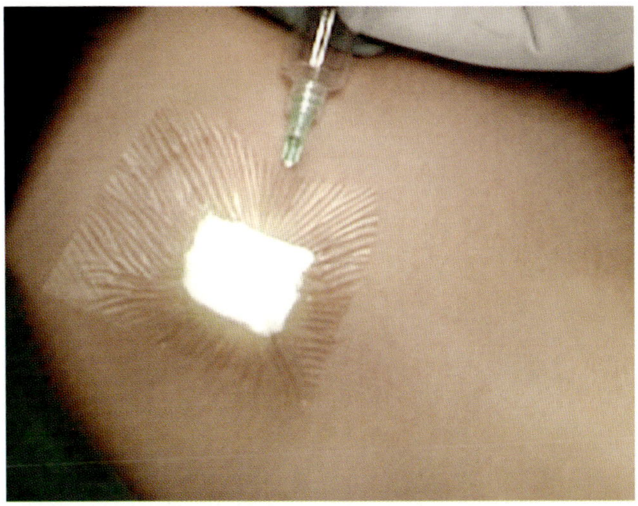

**Fig. 34.40:** Vacuum created with a syringe

can be inserted from here to view the umbilicus before deciding on single incision surgery.

3. Choose 10 mm and 5 mm trocars with a small "head." Choose hand instruments with no side projections (e.g. diathermy attachments). Cable should come parallel to the hand instruments.
4. Use instruments with multifunction to reduce operating time.
5. Long bariatric instruments, especially needle holder, can bring the handle of the needle holder far away from the head of the 10 mm trocar so that there will not be clashing of instruments.
6. When instruments are clashing at the site of the camera head, zoom-in.
7. Sutures can be used as retractors. Bring the sutures through he skin and use them as retractors.
8. Rescue a difficult surgery with an accessory 5 mm or 3 mm trocar.
9. Fogging of the laparoscope may occur. This can be reduced by changing the carbon dioxide input to the right 5 mm trocar.

**MESSAGE BOX**

Single incision laparoscopic surgery can be performed using common laparoscopic instruments available in most operating theaters. The only accessory required is a right angle light connector. Choose simple cases to start of with. A small uterus will be ideal of SIL TLH. Choose a 10 mm trocar and 2, 5 mm trocars with small "head" to prevent clashing of instruments. Choose instruments with multifunction and with no side or perpendicular projections. Pay particular attention to skin preparation because leakage of gas will cause difficulty during surgery. Tilt the patient to your side if you suffer from back pain.

Chapter 35

# Robotic Surgery in Gynecology

*Charles Miller, Kirsten Sasaki*

## INTRODUCTION

Robotic-assisted laparoscopic surgery using the da Vinci® Surgical System (Intuitive Surgical®, Sunnyvale, California) has been approved by the Food and Drug Administration (FDA) for use in gynecology since April 2005. It provides an additional tool for performing minimally invasive gynecologic procedures, and has been widely adapted by new and established surgeons. This chapter will review the clinical basics of applying robotic-assisted surgery to the gynecologist's surgical practice.

## SELECTION OF CASES

- General gynecology:
  - Total or supracervical hysterectomy
  - Myomectomy
  - Excision of endometriosis, including stage IV
  - Presacral neurectomy
  - Ovarian cystectomy.
- Urogynecology:
  - Sacrocolpopexy
  - Uterosacral ligament suspension
  - Retropubic colposuspension (Burch).
- Reproductive endocrinology and infertility
  - Tubal reanastomosis.
- Gynecology oncology:
  - Radical hysterectomy
  - Pelvic and para-aortic lymph node dissection.

## PREPARATION FOR SURGERY

- Preoperative testing/imaging
  - Laboratory and cardiac evaluation per hospital guidelines
  - Urodynamics when indicated
  - Pelvic Imaging
    - Transvaginal ultrasound
    - Saline infusion sonohysterogram
    - Magnetic resonance imaging (MRI).
- Bowel preparation
  - Clear liquids day prior to surgery
  - Magnesium citrate preparation at evening prior to surgery.
- Patient and bed positioning
  - Dorsal lithotomy with sacrum at edge of operating room bed
  - Arms tucked and padded with thumbs turned upward in order to avoid nerve compression and injury.

### Robotic Components

*Robotic Cart*

- Consists of three or four arms that dock onto the camera and robotic trocars.
- Instruments are placed through these trocars and are manipulated by the surgeon seated at the console.
- Docked to the patient cart is the camera trocar, through which the da Vinci® vision system is placed.

### Da Vinci® Vision System

- Two cameras, each with a separate light source.
- Provides 3-dimensional, high-definition images to the surgeon console.
- Available in 8.5 mm and 12 mm.

### Surgeon Console

- Adjustable binocular viewer
- Camera control that enables up to 15 × magnification.
- Instrument controls through the use of pedals and hand controls.
- Dual console available for the da Vinci® Si(T) system
  - This enables two surgeons to operate at the console together for complex procedures or training of new robotic surgeons.

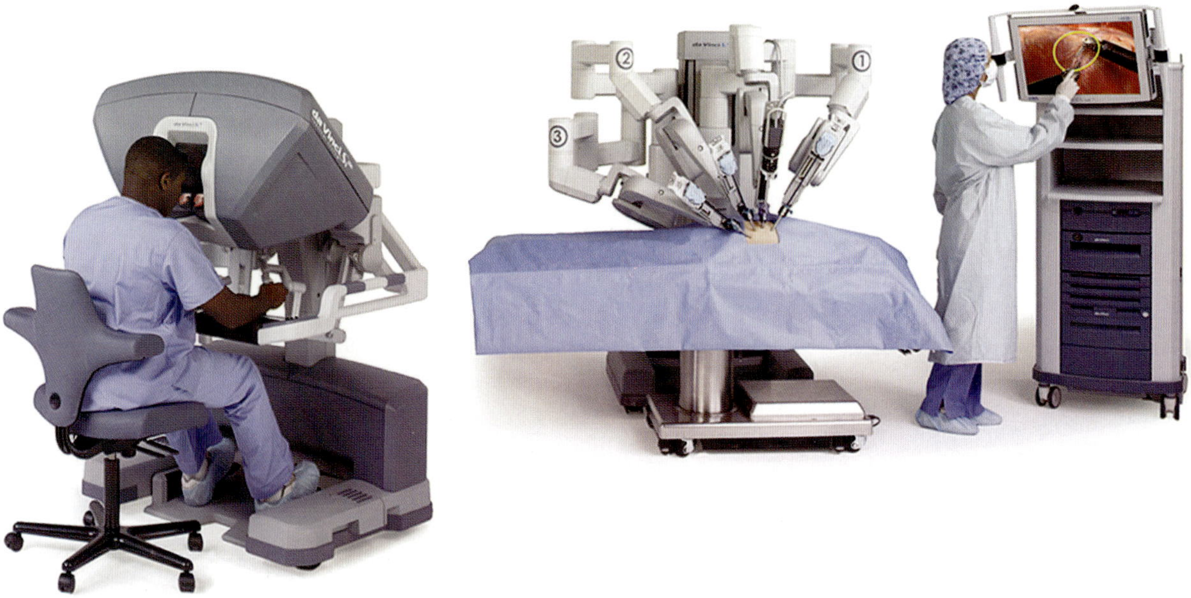

**Fig. 35.1:** da Vinci® robotic components: Surgeon console, patient cart and da Vinci® vision system

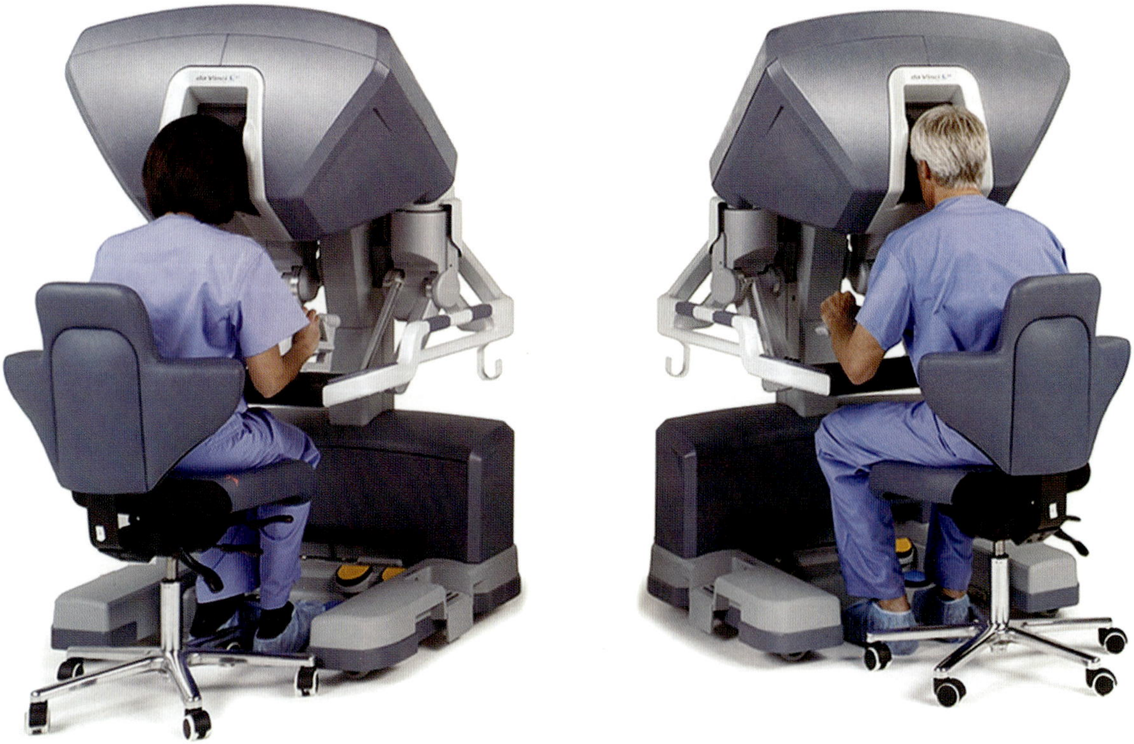

**Fig. 35.2:** da Vinci® dual console

## Technique

- *Trocar placement*
- *Camera trocar*
  - Placement of camera trocar approximately 8-10 cm cephalad from the fundus of the uterus.
  - Survey of abdomen and pelvis to determine use of 3 or 4 robotic trocars as well as assistant trocar.

### *Robotic Trocars*

- 8 mm robotic trocars generally used for gynecologic procedures.
- 5 mm robotic trocars available, but surgical workspace and instrument availability may be limited given current technology, used primarily in pediatric surgery
- Place robotic trocars approximately 8 cm apart to avoid collision of the robotic arms.
- Often placed at or below the level of the camera trocar (Fig. 35.3).
- If 4 robotic arms used, place third arm opposite of the assistant trocar (Figs 35.4 and 35.5).

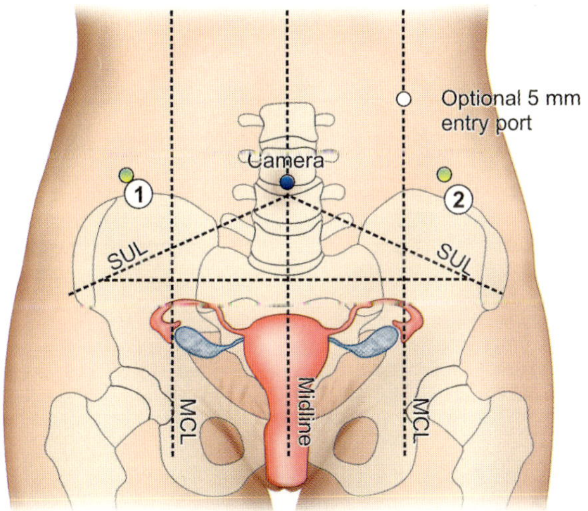


**Fig. 35.3:** Trocar configuration with three robotic arms and an optional assistant port

### *Assistant Trocar*

- Placed at the same level on the opposite side of the 3rd robotic arm.

### *Docking*

- Lower bed to floor.
- Place patient in adequate amount of Trendelenburg in order to complete procedure as well as tolerated by patient.
  - This may require decreasing the pressure of the pneumoperitoneum in order to limit rise in peak airway pressures
- Determine whether "straight" or "side" docking
- If "straight" docking, robotic cart center column and camera port are aligned. The robotic cart should be brought in until the camera arm is nearly touching the camera port, and all arms should be in the blue "sweet spot".
- If "side"docking, the operating bed can be rotated, or if the room configuration allows, the cart can be angled so that it is brought in at a 30-45° angle to the bed. Robotic arms do not have to be within the "sweet spot" bands.
  - Provides more room for the person manipulating the uterus
  - May not be feasible in all operating rooms.
- Once docked, the operating bed cannot be moved. Movement can affect the placement and depth of the trocars and instruments, with potential for abdominal or pelvic injury.

## Equipment for Surgery

- 8.5 mm or 12 mm trocar for robotic camera.
- 2 or 3 robotic trocars with sealing cap (5 mm or 8 mm). If only two robotic trocars are used without an assistant trocar, each trocar should have a port to allow insufflation and smoke evacuation via the robotic trocars and away from the camera trocar.

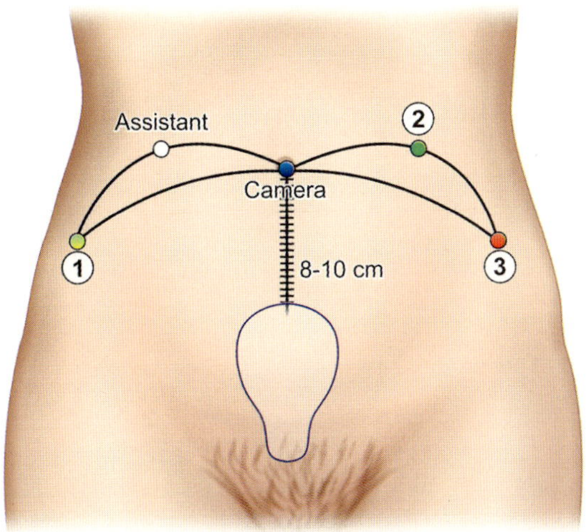


**Fig. 35.4:** Trocar configuration for 4 robotic arms and assistant port

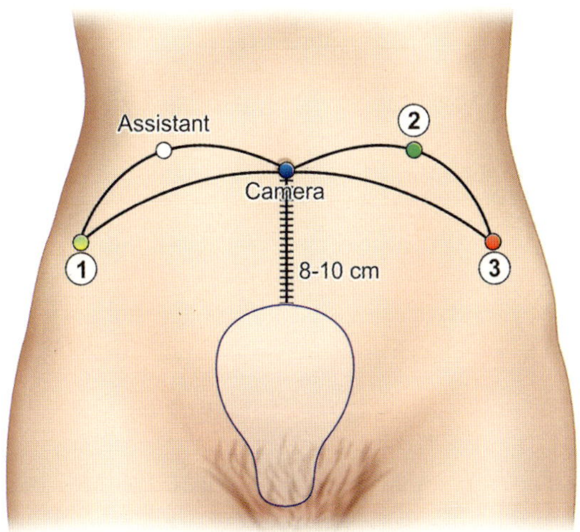


**Fig. 35.5:** Port placement with 4 robotic arms and an assistant trocar for larger pathology

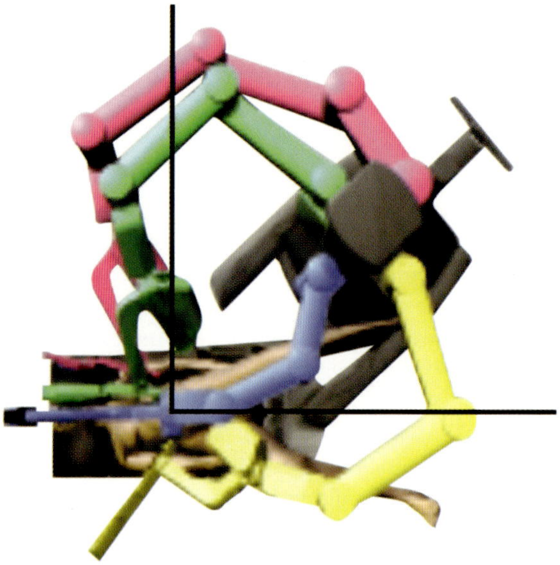

Fig. 35.6: Side-docking with 4 robotic arms. Patient cart is brought in at approximately a 45 degree angle to operating bed, and straddles the corner of the bed

- 5 mm or 12 mm assistant trocar (if desired).
- 8.5 mm or 12 mm robotic camera.
  - Robotic camera available in 0 and 30° (which can be placed up or down).
- Laparoscopic needle driver.
- Suction-Irrigation device (Robotic or Laparoscopic).

## Instruments for Hysterectomy

- Bipolar Instruments: Maryland forceps, PK™ dissecting forceps (Olympus, Southboro, MA), fenestrated forceps, or Endowrist® One™ Vessel Sealer for da Vinci® Si™ which provides both dessication and cutting.
- Monopolar instruments: Hot shears™, hook, or spatula
- Atraumatic grasping instruments: Prograsp™, Cadiere, or long-tip forcep.
- Needle driver: Mega™ and large needle driver both available with or without suture cutting ability.
- Additional instruments: Harmonic Ace® (Ethicon, Cincinnati, OH) may be used in place of a monopolar instrument.

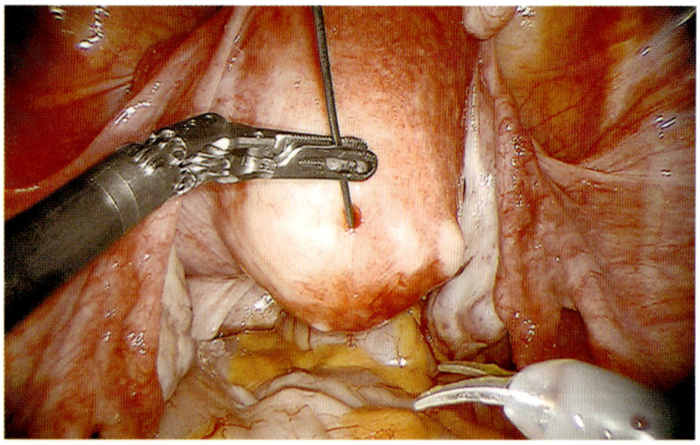

Fig. 35.7: Injection of dilute vasopressin with guidance of needle transabdominally by Prograsp™

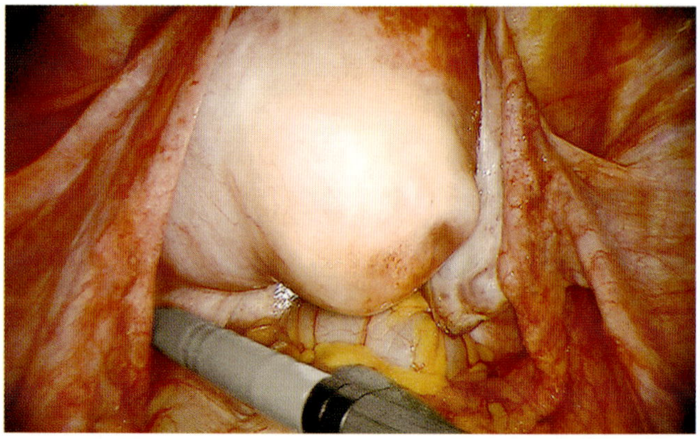

Fig. 35.8: Blanching of uterus after injection of dilute vasopressin

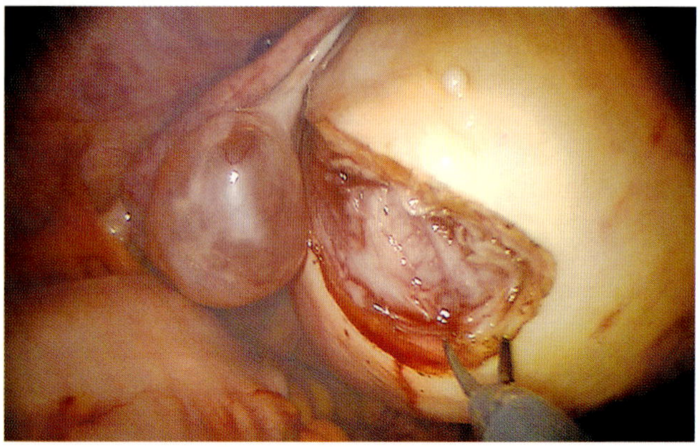

Fig. 35.9: Creation of hysterotomy with Hot Shears™

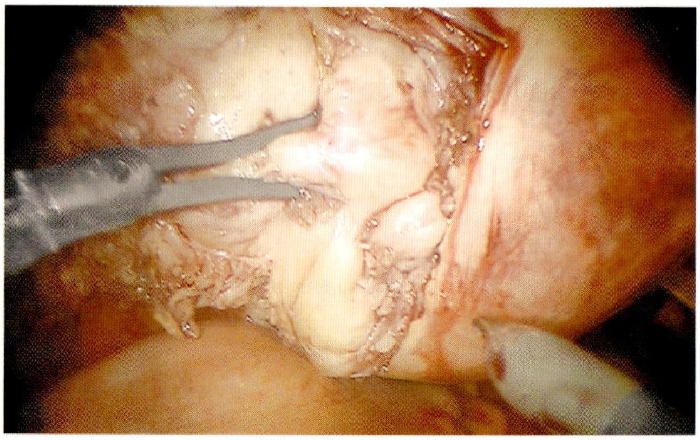

Fig. 35.10: Traction applied with tenaculum forcep to remove myoma

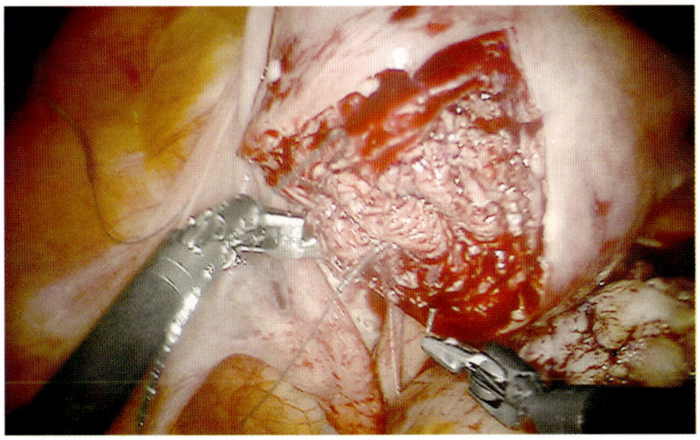

**Fig. 35.11:** Suturing with Prograsp™ and Mega™ needle driver

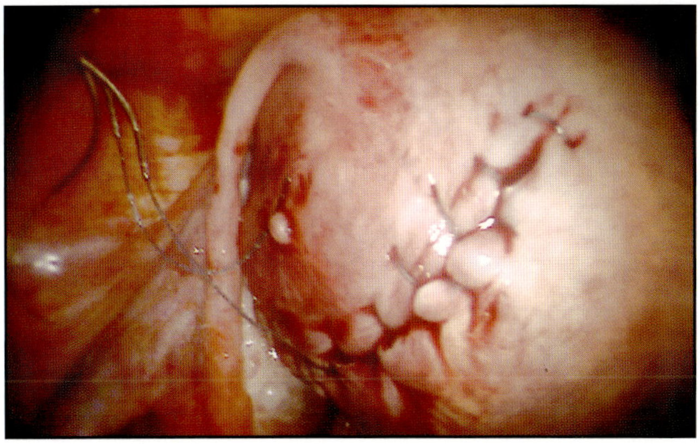

**Fig. 35.12:** Completion of myomectomy

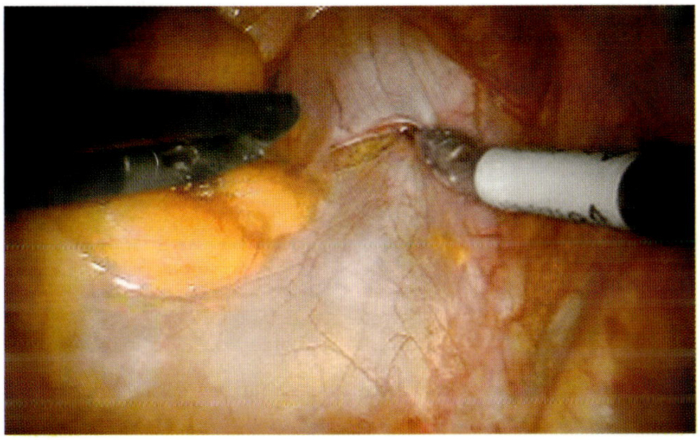

**Fig. 35.13:** Incising peritoneum over sacral promontory with Hot Shears™

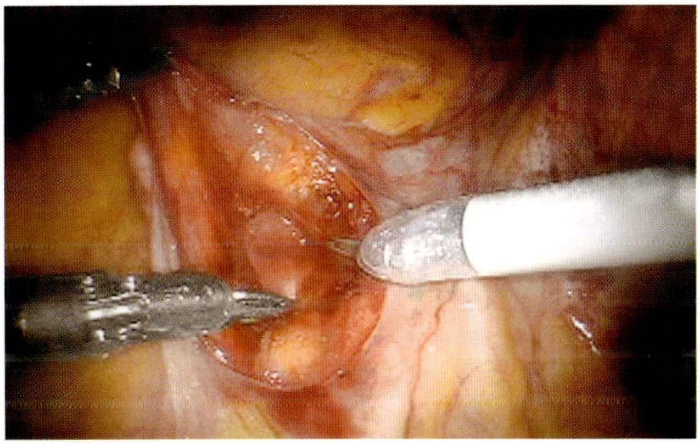

**Fig. 35.14:** Opening presacral space with Maryland Bipolar and Hot Shears™

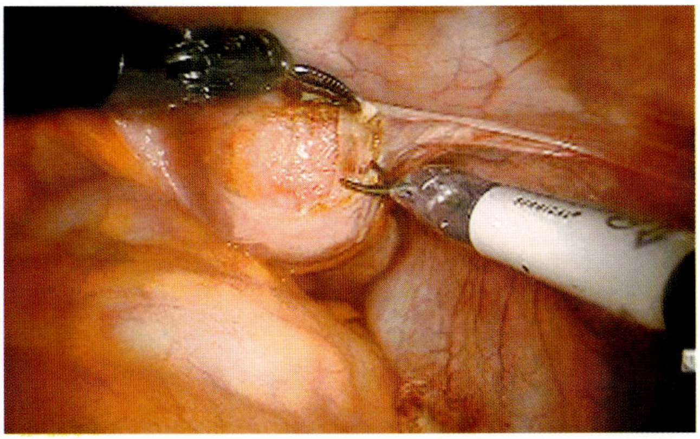

**Fig. 35.15:** Opening peritoneum over anterior vaginal wall with Hot Shears™

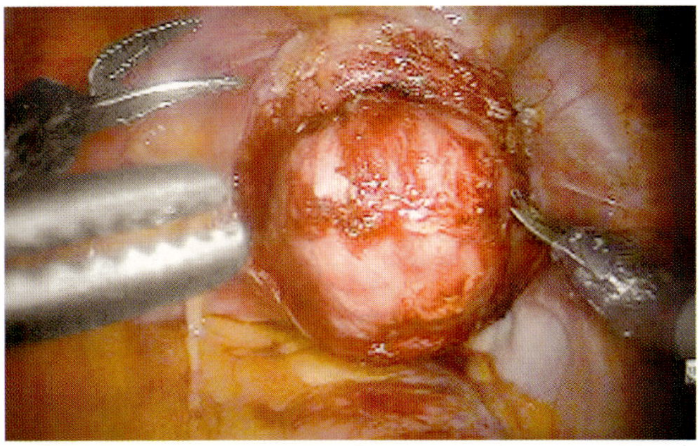

**Fig. 35.16:** Peritoneum dissected off of the anterior and posterior vaginal walls

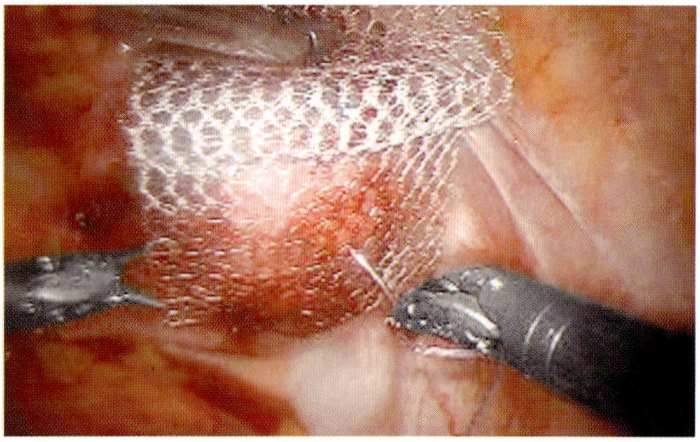

**Fig. 35.17:** Suturing mesh to vaginal apex with two large needle drivers

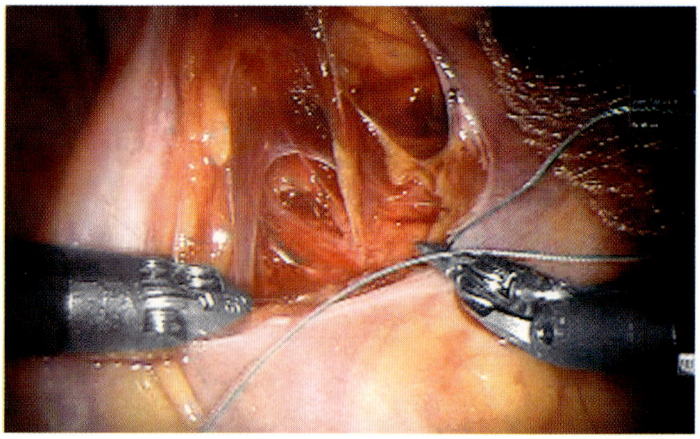

**Fig. 35.18:** Suturing anterior longitudinal ligament with two large needle drivers

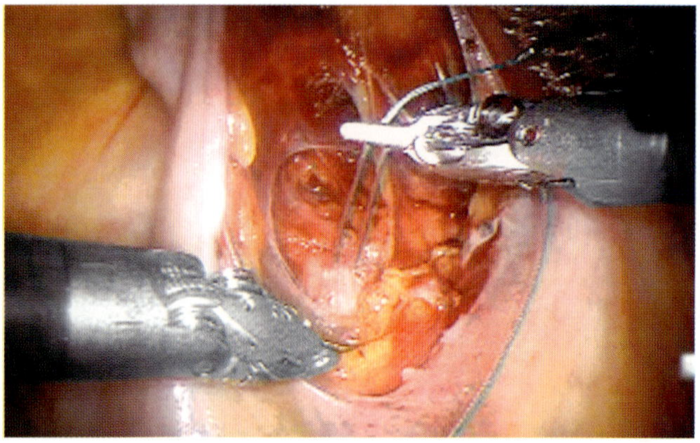

**Fig. 35.19:** Suture placed through anterior longitudinal ligament

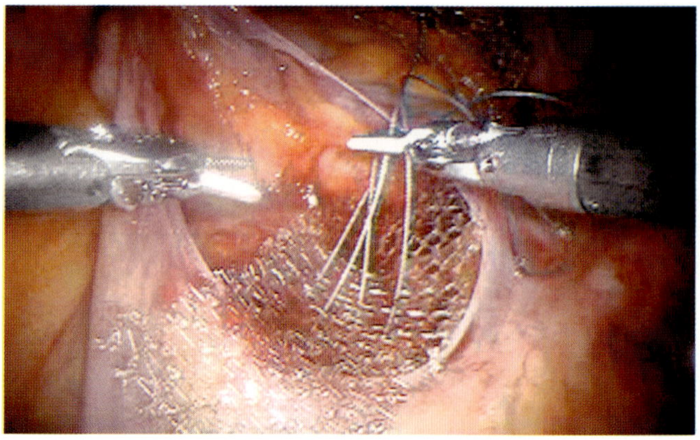

**Fig. 35.20:** Both sutures through anterior longitudinal ligament and mesh

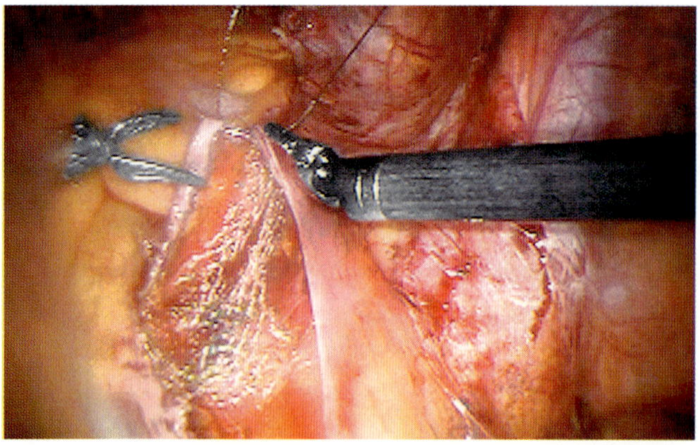

**Fig. 35.21:** Suturing peritoneum over mesh with large needle driver

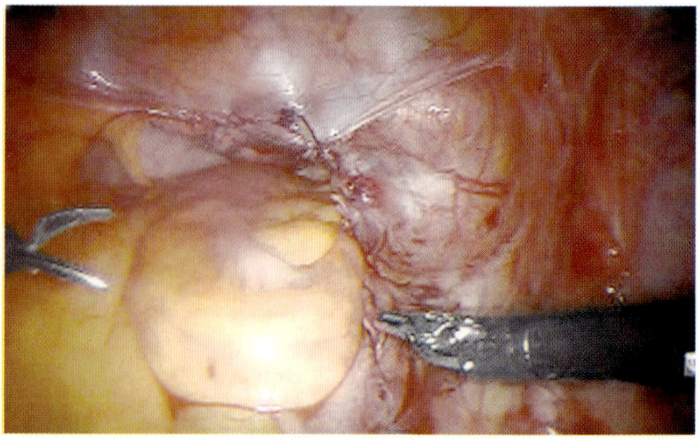

**Fig. 35.22:** Completed image

## Instruments for Myomectomy

- Atraumatic grasping instrument: Prograsp™, Cadiere, or long-tip forcep.
- Traumatic grasping instrument: Tenaculum forcep (Preferred) or Cobra grasper.
- Hot Shears™.
- Needle Driver.

## Instruments for Sacrocolpopexy

- Prograsp™.
- Mega™ suture cut needle driver or large needle driver
- Hot Shears™.
- PK™ dissecting forceps or Maryland bipolar.

## Advantages and Disadvantages of Robotic Surgery

*Advantages*

- 7 Degrees of movement versus 4 degree in traditional laparoscopic surgery
  - Allows surgeon to move his/her hand as in open surgery
  - Robotic suturing is significantly easier to perform compared to traditional laparoscopic suturing.
- Three-dimensional visualization
  - Overcome lack of depth perception experienced in traditional laparoscopic surgery.
- 15 times magnification with scaled down motion
  - Assists with performance of delicate dissections in a controlled fashion such as lymph node dissections and ureterolysis.
- Elimination of fulcrum effect experienced with traditional laparoscopic surgery
  - Instrument moves in same direction as hand and arm.
- Tremor filtration which facilitates fine dissection.
- Additional technology including Tile Pro™, Da Vinci® Firefly™ Fluorescence and Single Site® surgery.

### *Tile Pro™*

- Available for the S™ and Si™ systems.
- Allows surgeons to view radiologic images at the surgeon console. May be helpful for fibroid mapping.

### *da Vinci® Firefly™ Fluorescence*

- Assist in identifying blood vessels during surgical dissection. Indocyanine green (ICG) dye is injected intravenously through a peripheral line and binds to albumin.
- Can facilitate gonadal vein transections, dissection of the pre-sacral space and has been used to identify tumor margin for resection.

### *Single-Site®*

- Used currently for benign hysterectomies and salpingo-oophorectomies.
- Eliminates cross body confusion and maintains the three dimensional visualization and magnification of the traditional robotic platform.

*Disadvantages*

- Fixed positioning of the patient and trocar configuration.
  - Once the robotic trocars are placed, and the robot is docked, the patient cannot be repositioned without first removing all of the instruments and undocking the trocars.
- Lack of haptics or tactile feedback. Some of this may be overcome with the improved visualization.
- *Cost:* Not all hospitals can afford the acquisition and maintenance cost of the robot.

Section

4

# Vaginal Surgery

Chapter 36

# Vaginal Surgery: Surgical Principles

*Andri Nieuwoudt*

## INTRODUCTION

The art of vaginal surgery is special for those who practice it. To be able to guard against the eroding of this art, it is up to the vaginal surgeons to see to it that those who come after us, will be able to take this forward. Due to the "flirting" with synthetic, and other materials, in vaginal reconstructive surgery, the surgeon had been "banned" from the vaginal surgery must be based on surgical skills again and not on the quality or quantity of these materials!

Basic surgical principles must apply:

- Knowledge of anatomy of the pelvic contents is the most essential element of these principles.
- The dissection planes available for the surgeon, especially in the vaginal wall, and from here to the sidewalls of the pelvis are the pathways of surgery to be done. Breaks in the walls of these pathways must be looked for and repaired; normal anatomy is the template of surgery.
- Perivaginal organization not only to simplify surgery, but also to improve results must be practiced.
- Reconstructive surgery must be done in a structured manner—a staged approach must be possible if additional surgery is indicated at a later date.
- The right instruments form an essential part of any surgical procedure, and it must be used right.
- The same applies to suture materials and needles.

These will form the basis of this essay.

## ANATOMICAL CONSIDERATIONS

Detailed pelvic floor and cavity anatomy is discussed elsewhere. The vaginal surgeon must know his/her way around the pelvic cavity—a three dimensional mindset is the best to describe the orientation needed for this type of minimal invasive surgery. It is not always possible to directly visualize the landmarks and tissues to be utilized in the procedures. The eye is sometimes on the index finger!

## PERIVAGINAL ORGANIZATION

A few basic rules apply in vaginal surgery:

1. The different pelvic organs come from different embryologic sources—each brings its own blood supply. The embryologic planes between these organs allow the vaginal surgeon to follow dissection planes with minimal risk of injury to blood vessels (Fig. 36.1). Spaces between these organs allow independent movement of the organs and must not be breeched.
2. There is different areas of "safe" pathways where injury to adjacent organs is kept to a minimum.

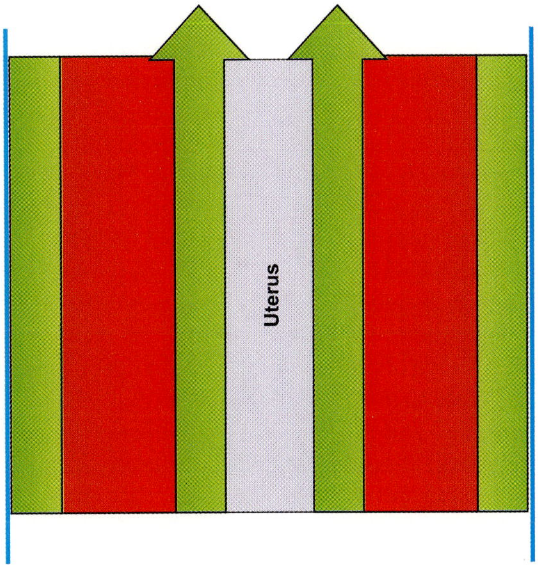


**Fig. 36.1:** The green zones will be the surgical "safe" zones, the red zones, the"danger" zones

If the vaginal surgeon uses any curved clamp in the pelvis it is always advised that the curve must be towards the blue areas, away from the red zones.

3. Suction must be kept to a minimum—if a bleeder is a nuisance then the bleeder must be identified and cauterized or tied. The suctioning of especially venous bleeders can result in excessive blood loss. Suction must be limited to improving visualization to enable the identification of a bleeding point.
4. The tying of bleeders in the pelvis is a special art: The bleeders can be associated with underlying structures (e.g. ureter) that can easily be injured with the tying of bleeders. It is advisable to do a "figure of 12" with Vycril 000: the needle is taken superficially through the bleeder point, lifting it by pulling on the two strands of Vycril, take a superficial "bite" adjacent to the bleeder on one side, and repeat it on the other side. If the suture is now tied, the bleeding point will be bundled up without compromising underlying structures.
5. When small calibre veins are seen in the operating field (e.g. on the inside surface of the vaginal skin) it is advisable to use the cautery as a "flame thrower" rather than taking a surgical forceps and cauterize it. If the cautery is set high, the spark will cauterize the vein without rupturing it or burning deep into the underlying tissues. This obviously will only be the case in small caliber veins. Arterial bleeders must either be tied or cauterized with direct contact, preferably via a small surgical forceps.
6. Suture material choice is preferably monofilament. If a nonabsorbable material is used it must be buried from contact with the vaginal skin. The absorbable delayed absorbable monofilament suture material is best for fascial surgery and nonabsorbable for ligaments. Vaginal skin can be closed with Vycril 000 (preferably Vycril Rapide, but not if there is underlying synthetic materials, then Vycril will do).
7. The needles used must be robust and strong, taper pointed and preferably with a 5/8 circle. The HGU-46 needle of Covedien fits the description. If prolene is used, the UR-6 needle is preferred. The CT-2 needle on Vycril plus suture 2-0 is good when Vycril is needed. Tying of pedicles (e.g. with vaginal hysterectomy) is best with Vycril 0 on a CT needle. To attempt vaginal surgery, especially prolapse surgery without these needles are not advised.
8. The placing of the needle in vaginal surgery needs extra care: Due to the laxity of the tissue, the needle cannot be placed and retaken with the same needle holder—the needle tends to swing away from the surgeon and sometimes out of view. To counter that, one needs to master the two needle holder technique: the suture is placed with one needle holder which is not removed but stabilizes the needle to enable one to grab the tip of the needle with needle holder number 2. Number 1 is now removed and the needle pulled through with number 2. This maneuver requires the use of needles that is robust and has a five-eighths circle (e.g. HGU-46 and UR-6). Skin closure and tying of pedicles can be done with the three-eighths circle needles.
9. Vaginal reconstruction surgery without a Lone Star (Cooper Surgical) or TLC self-retaining retractor system (Applied Medical Technology, Inc) is like driving without seatbelts! It is impossible to do vaginal surgery without the organizational help of these. It is impossible to do dissection plane surgery in the pelvis without the tension-countertension help these retractors provide with their hooks (Fig. 36.2). The nonsharp hook of the prepacked (8 per pack) of the TLC system suits this type of surgery best.
   There are disposable retractors from Lone Star and TLC systems available—the TLC system retractor is superior. The author prefers the metal reusable Lone Star ring, with the more superior and cheaper hooks from TLC. The Lone Star hooks do not fit in the TLC ring. A Lone Star APS disposable retractor (Cooper Surgical) can also be helpful especially when a vaginal hysterectomy is done (Figs 36.3A to C).
10. Positioning of the patient:
    There is a variety of leg support systems available for the patient in lithotomy. A KISS ("Keep It Simple and Stupid") method for these is probably best: Main requirement is that the buttocks of the patient must rest at the end of the table with good support for the sacrum and enough room for an Ovard speculum to swing freely over the edge. Care must be taken not to have too much strain on the flexed hips. The author prefers the candy cane type of leg supports—it gives more room for seated assistants (Fig. 36.4).
11. Positioning of the surgeon and assistants:
    A vaginal surgeon who stands is a vaginal surgeon who is uncertain: the vaginal surgeon must always be seated (at all times!) on a preferable hydraulic stool without a backrest. Vaginal surgery with a surgical table at the end of the bed support perivaginal

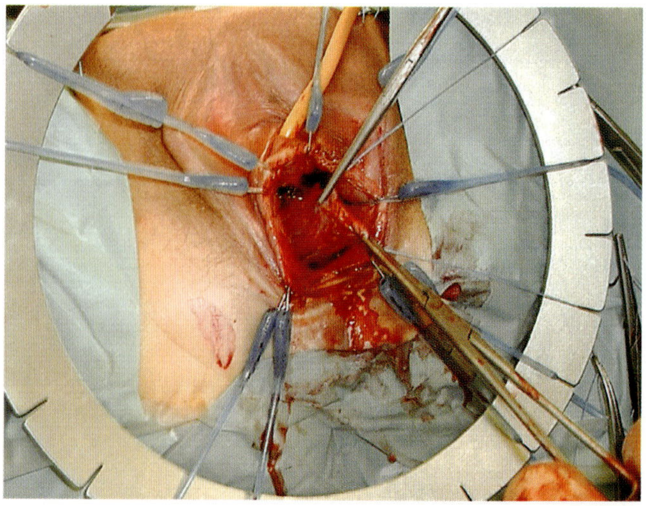

Fig. 36.2: The retractors are also utilized as supports for the suture pedicles

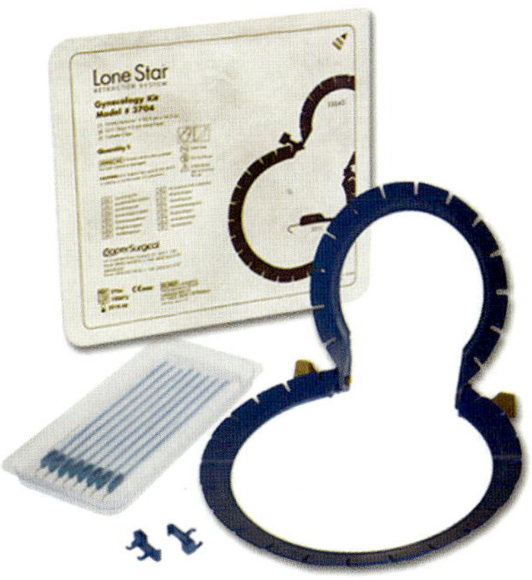


A

Disposable Lone Star

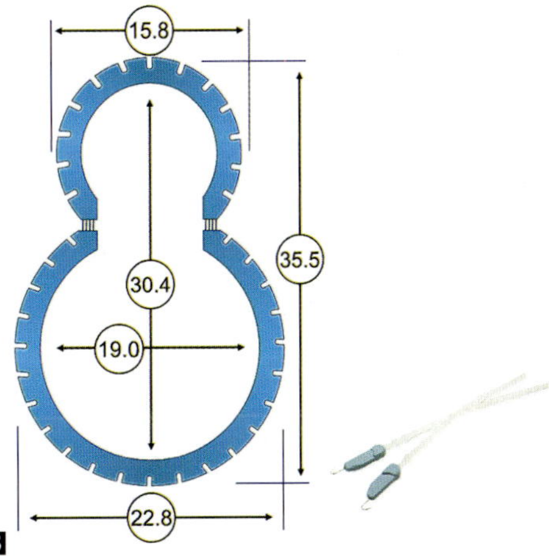


B

Disposable TLC Retractor

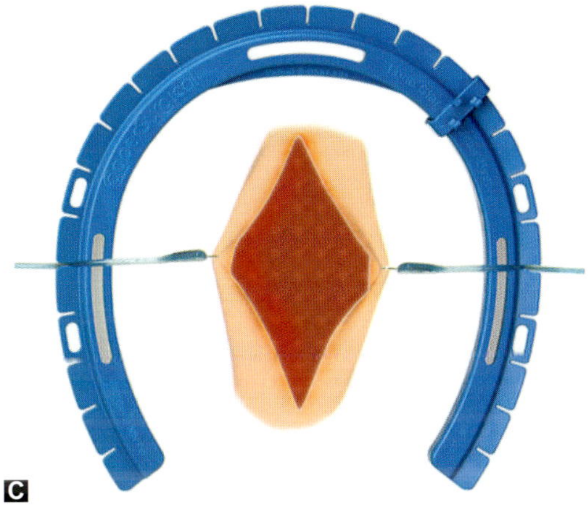

C

Disposable Lone Star APS retractor

**Figs 36.3A to C:** Disposable retractors

organization. The headrest of the theater table can easily be customized to fit at the end of the table. The assistants must be seated next to the surgeon—this involves them in the surgery (Fig. 36.5). A camera with direct video taping of the procedures is a helpful accessory; the screens must be visible to the patient and the operators. Usually, a magnified operating field can be utilized.

12. Instruments for vaginal reconstructive surgery:
    i. Needle holders: 2 × Sklar Baumgartner needle holders
    ii. Rochester-Pean straight forceps × 5.

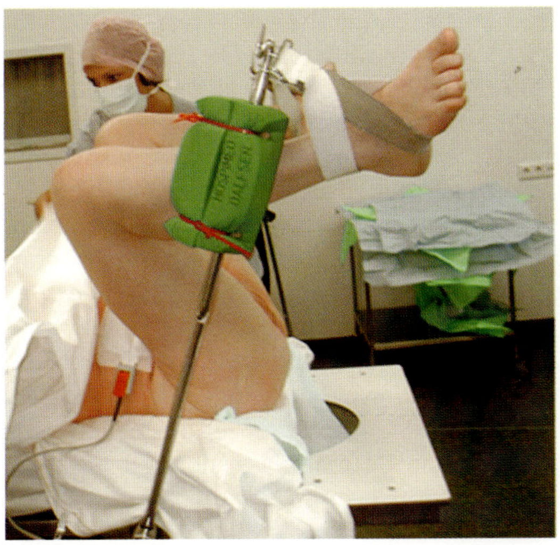

**Fig. 36.4:** Candy cane stirrups with customized surgeons' table

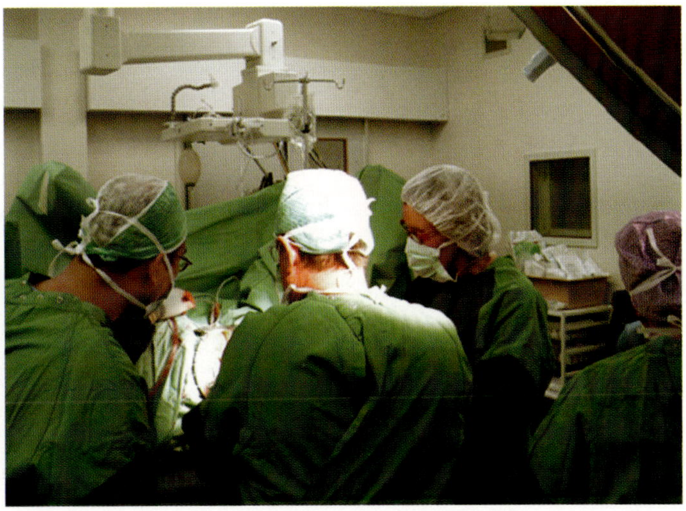

**Fig. 36.5:** Positioning of assistants

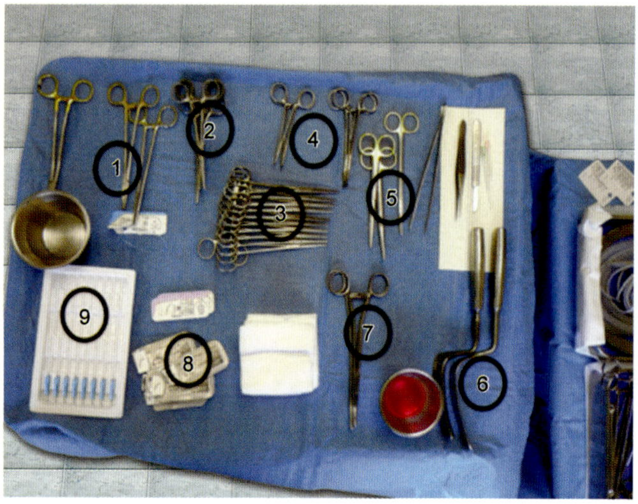


**Fig. 36.6:** Instruments required for vaginal reconstruction surgery

3. Small straight Kochers × 5.
4. Curved criles × 2 and curved mosquito clamps × 2.
5. Surgical scissors, including a Metzenbaum-Fino scissors.
6. Breisky-Navratil Vaginal Retractors × 2.
7. Artery forceps.
8. Suture materials.
9. TLC vaginal retractor hooks.

Extras: Surgical knives (not 10 or 20 blades!), fine toothed forceps for cauterizing, Thomson Walker needle holder.

It is non-negotiable to attempt vaginal surgery without the following:

- Vaginal retractors (Lone Star or TLC retractor systems) with hooks
- Breisky vaginal retractors
- Correct suture materials and needles
- Two needle holders
- Number 10 blade surgical knife and Metzenbaum-Fino scissors.

One can have the perfect organization around the surgery, but still lacks the skills and enthusiasm to make one a great vaginal surgeon. These can only be cultivated with the necessary experience and guiding. Operating through the vagina is the prerogative of the gynecologist: the gynecologist must guard this.

Teachers of this art in science can keep the vaginal approach to surgery alive.

## THE ROLE OF SURGICAL AUDITING IN DEFECT SPECIFIC SURGERY

> The reason for failure seems to be that the normal support of the bladder has not been sought for and restored, but instead an irrational removal of part of the anterior wall has been resorted to, which could only result in disappointment and failure.
>
> *George White (1866-1926)*

Surgical techniques develop continually in the experienced surgeon. Surgical shortcuts and non-repetitive maneuvers are the biggest dangers in experienced surgery. The only safeguard against this is to follow strict protocols with the application of surgical auditing—this especially applies if one leaves the comfort zone given by your teachers. In the following, a new avenue of pelvic reconstruction surgery the author had to follow this route. In this assay, the route taken as guided by a strict protocol with surgical auditing will be described. Only one experienced vaginal surgeon was involved in all procedures, as was all assessments. A strict adherence was given to the principle of "primum non nocere", with transparency of practice and patient safety as the primary end goals. The first step in transparency was to introduce colleagues and nursing personnel to the paradigm shift in thinking. From here the stepwise introduction of new techniques involved patience and time. The auditing protocol was to videotape all procedures enabling revision of the exact technique used in patients with both suboptimal and optimal results, as assessed after 6 months and 12 months. It was focus to have especially as near as possible to 100% follow-up at 6 months postoperatively as that is felt that future outcome predictions is most reliable at this time frame.

The main outcome measure was "need to treat" with functional and anatomical outcomes assessments during each visit. The quality of live questionnaires in use was the PISQ 12 and PFDI-20. All complications that can be related to the surgery were noted in the databank. In all patients, consent were obtained.

Peer review consists of regular communication with like thinking surgeons and regular invites to colleagues to attend round table discussions and theater sessions. Since 2008, regular organized meetings (5 per year) was held in the local hospital (Ziekenhuis Zorgsaam, Terneuzen) with invited colleagues, nationally and internationally. Groups of up to 10 attended a day seminar followed by a full day theater hands-on session. During these "master classes", the theory and the technical details of procedures in use were discussed. International guest surgeons were invited to participate during some of these sessions. The Dutch Society of Gynecology and Obstetrics (NVOG) accredited these meetings. Twenth eight of these meetings were done between 2008 and December 2012 with participation of 239 gynecologists from diverse countries.

The surgical starting point was conventional anterior colphorrhapy with 5 days hospital stay with a suprapubic catheter in place. The operation technique was changed—the hospital stay and indwelling catheter initially not.

Introduction of the Prolift TVM technique took the dissection laterally beyond the pubic rami to the sidewall. This anterior Prolift technique, although successful in treating the prolapsed anterior wall, lead to unwanted complications of which shrinkage and pain were the main concerns—this was discussed with the manufacturers

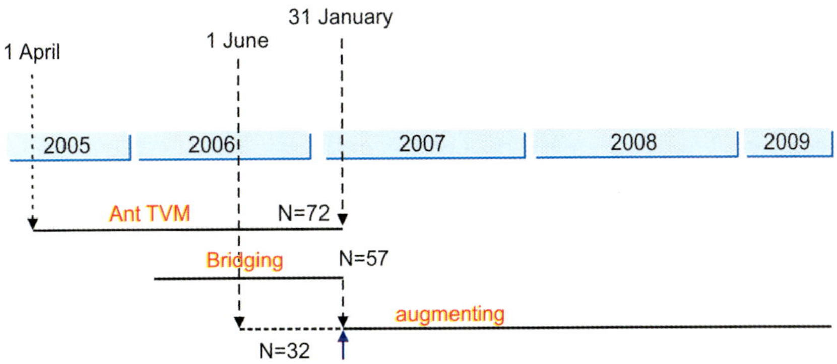


**Fig. 36.7:** Surgical auditing

and one of the main investigators (Dr Cosson from Lille University). Answers were unsatisfactory and the technique was abandoned on the 30th of January, 2007.

From 2006 Paravaginal repairs were introduced in Terneuzen by dr Richard Reid from Australia with a bridging technique using noncrosslinked xenograft (SurgiSIS-Cook Medical). The basis of the technique change was to take the dissection of the anterior wall to the pelvic sidewall, utilizing the anatomical dissection planes. The vesicovaginal space was not opened and Lone Star retractors (Cooper Surgical) were used in all cases. The defects that lead to vaginal wall prolapse could adequately be visualized.

Paravaginal repairs proved to be a safe procedure with minimal complications.

The initial repair technique was to place 4 Ti-Cron 0 (braided polyester-Covidien) sutures (numbered A, B, C and D) on the arcus tendineous fascia pelvis (ATFP) or Whiteline as shown in the Figure 36.8.

A prepared 4-layered sheet of SurgiSIS (Cook Medical) anchored to these points was placed as a bridge supporting the bladder base. It was sutured to the cervix with Vycril 000 sutures.

The initial advantage was a better understanding of what anatomical defects lead to the prolapsed vaginal wall. Bladder atonia and urinary retention were not seen; with the result that both hospital stay and removal of the urinary catheter were on the mean 24 hours postoperative-no need for suprapubic catheters was a direct result. This lead to change of protocols.

On the downside were important problems directly linked with the repair technique:

1. The braided polyester (Ti-Cron Covidien), although fantastic to work with, proved to be a bad choice in the vaginal wall: it was expelled through the vaginal skin in 10% of cases, with two who developed sinus tracts to the deeper knots. The needle (HGU-46 5/8 taper point Covidien) used was a good choice with the correct strength and curvature for vaginal surgery. The suture material was changed to monofilament polyglyconate (Maxon 0, Covidien). Suture length of 45 cm was adequate for the use intended.

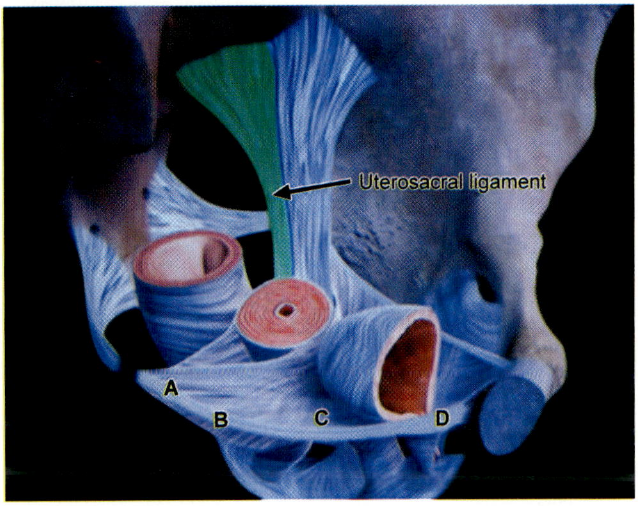


**Fig. 36.8:** Ti-Crona 0 sutures placed on arcus tendineous fascia pelvis

2. Bridging the pelvic cavity with a non-cross linked xenograft (SurgiSIS, Cook Medical) to support the bladder proved to be initially effective, but this support broke down after 6–12 months when the xenograft was replaced by native tissue.

| | *Prim >12 m* | *Sub-optimal* | *Time (months)* | *Anterior* | *Middle* | *Posterior* |
|---|---|---|---|---|---|---|
| Bridging | 59 | 31 | 7.3 m | 20 | 14 | 1 |
| | | 54% | | 35% | 24.6% | 1.7% |
| Ant tvm | 73 | 26 | 13 m | 16 | 12 | 6 |
| | | 35.6% | | 22% | 16.4% | 8.2% |

In the patients in which this happened secondary surgery proved to be add-on rather than undo-redo type of surgery with low morbidity—in itself an improvement to the conventional method of colphorrhapy. Utilization of native tissue countered this tendency for early breakdown of the repair.

Layer by layer suturing (first native tissue to ATFP followed by bolstering the native tissue with a non-crosslinked xenograft) proved to put too much tension on the native tissue: especially in previous colphorrhaphies and in the elderly, resulting in poor wound healing and suboptimal results.

When this was changed (plus changing the suture materials—*see* 4 and 5 below) to rather approximating the native tissue layers with the xenograft being suturing to the ATFP over the native tissue (layered suturing and nonlayered suturing—*see* later) putting all the strain on the xenograft, the results improved markedly to 9–70% need to treat.

| | **2010** | **2011** |
|---|---|---|
| **6 months** | 11 | 6 |
| | 19% | 40% |
| **12 months** | 35 | 9 |
| | 61% | 60% |
| **24 months** | 11 | |
| | 19% | |
| **Total(n):** | 57/136 | 15/143 |
| | 39% | 9,70% |

In an ongoing random control trail-layered suturing and nonlayered suturing are being compared. If the results proved to be the same, nonlayered suturing would be the safer option.

Reverting to a transverse incision and dissecting the skin only for 1 cm loose from the septum abolished the need for a large sheet of xenograft support. This also gives less scarring of the vaginal skin.

To improve wound healing with a lasting effect (e.g. in the elderly) a band of tension free synthetic mesh was approximated to the supracervical suture line and tension-free placed on both sides between the bladder and pelvic sidewall: this proved to give superior wound healing and resulted in fewer need to treat cases. Erosions of the synthetic are a problem in 10% of cases—this is attributed to too much skin tension applied by the tamponade sutures (see later). With care taken here this can be avoided. The erosion is easily being treated on an outpatient's basis due to the small amount of mesh being used: Central cutting and removal of the offending piece did not result in recurrences of the prolapse.

*In the 50 to 60, and 60 to 70 years age groups an ongoing random control trail is being conducted with and without synthetic mesh lining the suture line.*

3. The Xenograft in use (Biodesign, Cook Medical) if enclosed in a confined space seems to give rise to the formation of a seroma or fluid collection. These absorbed spontaneously, but in two cases, drainage was indicated. This stopped from happening when suture C and later suture D was abolished, allowing a drainage channel to the bladder sidewall and hence, the peritoneal surface. The seroma formation did not compromise sidewall attachment to the ATFP.
4. The utilization of three Maxon sutures to tie the severed septum back to the cervix proved in the elderly especially to last only until the Maxon dissolves after 3 months. Replacing two of the Maxon sutures with Prolene 00 proved to solve this. This was later applied to

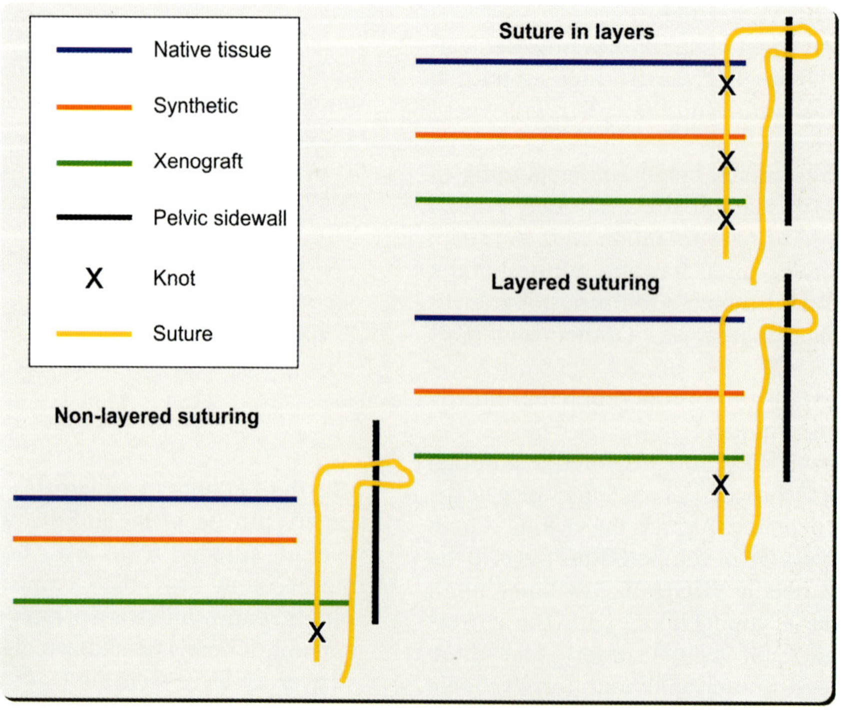


**Fig. 36.9:** Suturing techniques

all age groups. Special care is taken to bury the knot of the Prolene behind the fascia away from the vaginal skin to counter erosion of the Prolene through the vaginal skin.

5. The most frequent area of recurrence was on the anterior cervical ring with a HTD (High Transverse Defect, or defective anterior cervical ring). With focus on the suture material as outlined in 4, plus utilizing the non-crosslinked xenograft as a splint running from sidewall to sidewall at the level of the ischial spines supporting the suture line on the cervix adequately for 3 months till wound healing kicks in gave improved results. The splinting of the suture line is now advocated in 100% of patient.

*Primary defect specific surgery: Need to treat: 2010 compared to 2011*

| | 2010 (n = 136) | 2011 (n = 143) |
|---|---|---|
| **6 months** | 11/136<br>8% | 6/143<br>4,40% |
| **12 months** | 35/136<br>25,70% | 9/143<br>6,20% |
| **24 months** | 11/136<br>8% | |
| **Total:** | 57/136<br>39% | 15/143<br>9,70% |

The phase in which Defect Specific Surgery now enters can best be described as a "fine tuning" phase. The dissection technique whereby the defects can be diagnosed, the suture materials needed to close the defects and the materials needed to augment the primary tissue defect repairs are well-defined and described. To fine-tune these, one need to define in which age group of patients what materials to use need to be tested. Clustering patients into comparable groups depending on age, type of defect found, type of repair needed and type of associated other compartment defects will enable one to compare on a like-for-like basis. Attention to these is being given in ongoing random control studies.

All the answers are not in yet, but the results do show that without putting the patient at risk prolapse surgery can be taken to a new level with the focus on restoring normal anatomy. With native tissue as the primary building block and normal anatomy as the template, grafts and meshes can be utilized as augmenting rather than primary tools.

With the help of surgical auditing the present technique with a focus on the repair of defects present with a secondary improvement of the prolapsed vaginal wall proved to be free from serious complications, with an improvement of quality of life in all ages of women with prolapse.

This is paving the way for vaginal wall prolapse repair in the very young woman—a too long neglected patient in pelvic organ prolapse. The young sexually active woman with symptomatic prolapse is not too uncommon. Surgery on her had been with circumspection: she is the one in whom potential harm is the highest, she is the one that have high failure rates, and she is the one whose life can be destroyed by zealous treatment. If the reconstruction surgeon can do right with her, he can do right with all patients with vaginal wall prolapse!

Chapter

# 37

# Nondescent Vaginal Hysterectomy

*Sunita R Tandulwadkar*

## PREOPERATIVE EVALUATION

- Relevant indication.
- Routine investigation.
- TVS to know the exact size of uterus and the adnexal pathology.
- To assess mobility of the uterus and vaginal laxity.
- Decision to remove adenexa as per indication.

## PREOPERATIVE PREPARATION

- Vaginal disinfection.
- Preoperative antibiotics.
- Bowel cleansing.

## ANESTHESIA

- Spinal.
- Epidural.
- General.

## POSITION

- Lithotomy.
- Modified lithotomy (refer to chapter laparoscopic hysterectomy).

## TECHNIQUE

- Careful evaluation of descent of uterus and associated vaginal wall prolapse.
- Hold the cervix with two (preferably) long Allis' forceps.
- Saline adrenaline injection 50–150 mL as per the size of uterus and the comfort of the surgeon (Optional).
- Foley's catheterization.
- Transverse incision on the anterior lip.
- Pushing of bladder with wet gauze piece, perhaps in a single sweep upto bladder reflection.
- Posterior vaginal reflection over the cervix, identified and a bold transverse cut taken 1 cm below the reflection often opening the peritoneum in the same cut. Sim's speculum should compress the posterior vaginal wall so as to keep the bowel away from the incision line.
- Laterally, vaginal mucosa is not cut; in fact it is taken in the first clamp along with the uterosacrals.
- Uterosacral and Mackenrodts' are clamped, cut and transfixed and stumps kept long.
- Those trained in clampless surgery may directly ligate and cut.
- The bladder peritoneum if not opened, may be easily done at this step.
- Uterines are clamped, cut and ligated.
- Cornual clamps may be applied in case the adnexa are to be spared, after clamping, cutting and being held long.
- In case adnexa is to be removed, then begin with the routine round ligament, to reduce the bulk of tubo-ovarian pedicle and access the infundibulopelvic ligament.
- Seth's ovarian clamps are used to go beyond the ovaries. A poor cousin is usually the Kocher's at this stage.
- After a good review to rule out any bleeding from pedicles, vaginal closure is done.
- The vaginal angles are sutured, on both sides and one or two sutures are taken in between the two angles in the midline may be taken keeping opening for drainage.
- Vagina packed with betadine soaked roller gauze.

## MODIFICATIONS

- In cases where there is fear of vault prolapse; simultaneous sacrospinous fixation may be done.
- Lateral vaginal mucosa should be taken with the uterosacrals.

- In case of long cervix, cut may be taken just below the bladder reflection.
- Cystocele may be repaired before mucosa closure.
- Excision of excessive posterior peritoneum during peritoneal closure cares for the enterocele.
- In cases of previous cesarean section. Adhesions are usually at the isthmus. So, sharp dissection should be done.

## POSTOPERATIVE

- Ambulation out of bed after 12 hours.
- Pack removal after 12 hours.
- Fluids after 4–6 hours followed by a soft diet at night.
- Remove catheter after 24 hours.
- Antibiotics for 5–7 days.
- Discharge after 48–72 hours.

### TIPS

- Careful evaluation of uterine size and mobility.
- Challenging to-do size over 12 weeks and requires experience.
- Transverse breadth of uterus important while deciding the case.
- Associated adnexal pathology may decide in favor of TLH or at least diagnostic laparoscopy.
- Use of long narrow single bladed Sim's speculum for anterior retraction and broad long single bladed Sim's speculum for posterior retraction especially for removal of nondescent bulky uterus. Due to groove of Sim's speculum anteriorly, the needle movement becomes very easy.
- No need to open the anterior pouch initially. Only confirm that the bladder is pushed up. After uterines, peritoneum will get opened up automatically.
- Closure of visceral peritoneum is usually not advocated.
- Continuous traction on cervix on contralateral side before applying clamp is very improtant.

Chapter

38

# Newer Concepts of Anterior and Posterior Vaginal Prolapse Repair

*Ajay Rane*

## PELVIC ORGAN SUPPORTS

The pelvic organs are supported by pelvic floor muscles; such as levator ani and iliococcygeus, connective tissues such as cardinal (Mackenrodt's), uterosacral, pubourethral, pubocervical and puborectal ligaments, and a horizontal vaginal axis. These can all be disrupted by birth trauma. The vaginal axis is nearly horizontal when the woman is standing. Hence any intra-abdominal downward force will oppose the vagina on the pelvic floor muscles preventing descent. This is aided by fascial and ligamentous support around the vagina (Fig. 38.1).

This support is divided into three levels:

**Level 1:** Includes uterosacral and cardinal ligaments supporting the upper vagina.

**Level 2:** Includes levator ani muscles via fascial attachments to the arcus tendineus ("white line") supporting the middle vagina.

**Level 3:** Includes the pubourethral and pubocervical ligaments supporting the lower vagina and posteriorly—the perineal body.

Damage at different levels of vaginal support thus leads to different types of prolapse:

**Level 1:** Vault and uterovaginal prolapse.

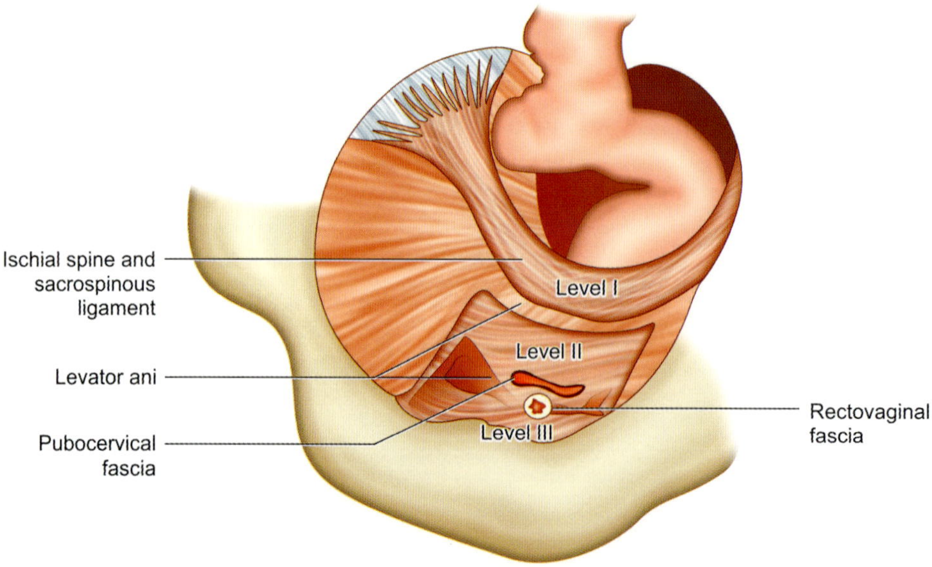


**Fig. 38.1:** Levels of fascial and ligamentous support (Reproduced from DeLancey JOL. 1992)

**Level 2:** Cystocele and rectocele.

**Level 3:** Urethrocele and perineal body hypermobility. Therefore, treatment should aim to correct the specific anatomical defects in order to optimize outcome.

## DIAGNOSIS

Prolapse is often asymptomatic and an incidental finding, and clinical examination may not necessarily correlate with symptoms. A comprehensive pelvic floor assessment should include a detailed history taking and POP physical examination that documents the maximum protrusion. There are validated pelvic organ prolapse questionnaires that may be used to assess patients' symptoms, bladder, bowel and sexual functions pre- and postoperatively. There are specific questionnaires to address each of these functions separately.

In women with established POP, a standardized, validated system should be used. The traditional assessment tool is called Baden Walker Classification described in 1968. In this classification:

**level 1:** Is described as prolapse extending half way to the hymen

**level 2:** Extending to the hymen, and

**level 3:** Extending outside the hymen. This classification is simple and easy to follow but the drawback is that it is subjective. The POP-Q assessment was first described in 1996 (Fig. 38.2) and is more complex but objective, site specific, quantifiable and reproducible. This system is approved by International Continence Society and followed universally. There is still a 30 percent chance of under diagnosing prolapse in the clinic set up.

## POP-Q SYSTEM

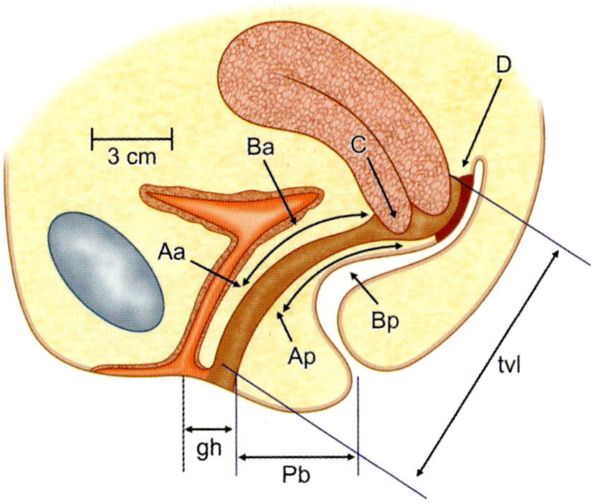


**Fig. 38.2:** POP-Q system

## INVESTIGATIONS

Evaluation for research purposes is often different from evaluation of clinical care. While most of the clinical care worldwide is done by physical examination alone, additional tools are useful in complex patients and for research purposes. Some of these modalities are urodynamics and imaging.

## URODYNAMICS

Urodynamic stress incontinence (USI) is diagnosed in 70–75 percent of these patients. Occult urodynamic stress incontinence (OUSI) is diagnosed in about 50 percent of the patients with genital prolapse not reporting stress incontinence before surgery. Performing urodynamic investigation in patients undergoing prolapse surgery may be valuable if diagnosing USI or OUSI results in the selection of the optimal treatment strategy. In women with severe prolapse ring pessary, reduction of prolapse during urodynamics is useful to determine symptomatic and occult conditions.

## IMAGING

Defecography or evacuation proctography is probably the most important imaging technique used in the assessment of POP. It is a study of voluntary bowel evacuation, and therefore, yields both anatomic and functional information. Traditionally defecography has mainly been used in the study of anorectal dysfunction as evacuation proctography. The equipment required includes a thick barium paste, a radiolucent toilet, and video equipment. Images are taken at rest, during straining effort, and during and after evacuation. Rectocoele is seen as an anterior rectal bulge and postevacuation barium trapping which may help to explain any evacuation dysfunction. It may suggest diagnosis of anismus as the main contributor to a patient's bowel dysfunction rather than rectocoele. The former is treated with biofeedback rather than surgery. An enterocoele is noted as a herniation of the small bowel into the cul-de-sac, into the vagina, rectovaginal space, or both.

## ULTRASOUND

Over the recent years, there has been an interest in MRI and ultrasound of the pelvic floor using 3D and quite a few papers have now been published. Using transperineal ultrasound, it is also possible to visualize the pelvic floor muscles in a dynamic fashion. CT scan also plays a role where there is any suspicion of associated pelvic pathology.

## SURGICAL MANAGEMENT

There is no specific indication or standardization for treatment of POP. For the purpose of this chapter, we have restricted to mesh-based pelvic reconstructive surgery. Since the introduction of the mesh over the last decade, there has been a steady increase in the types of mesh and different techniques associated with them. In this chapter, we discuss the transobturator mesh repair (Perigee) for anterior vaginal prolapse and transobturator sling (Monarc) and posterior defect specific repair.

## TRANSOBTURATOR MESH (PERIGEE)

### Instruments

- Perigee graft (large-pore polypropylene or a biologic porcine) has a tail that can be cut to fit the length of the patient's vagina and 4 arms that are attached to the pelvic sidewall.
- Needles used for anterior wall repair.

### Procedure

1. Patient is placed in modified lithotomy position.
2. Local anesthetic can be injected into the anterior vaginal wall
3. A midline skin incision is made and the bladder is dissected from the vaginal wall up to the bladder neck.
4. The entry points for superior needles are marked at the lateral edge of the pubic ramus at the level of the clitoris just below the insertion of adductor longus tendon.
5. The inferior needle entry points are also at the medial edge of the pubic ramus but at its inferior most point of the obturator foramen. The superior needles are identified by the pink color and the inferior needles are grey in color and sides are marked using arrows.
6. The right superior needle is the first one to be inserted with the needle tip perpendicular to skin and handle positioned at 45°.
7. The needle is advanced through the obturator muscle and membrane with gentle pressure and the needle tip should be palpated as it moves around the pubic ramus.
8. The needle is then guided through the vaginal incision until the needle tip is through the incision.
9. Before attaching the mesh, the mesh should be oriented so that the tail end is positioned down towards the table.
10. The mesh is then attached to the needle tip and pulled through along with the sheath.
11. The same is repeated on the other side.
12. The right inferior needle is then passed with the needle perpendicular to the skin and the handle parallel to the vertical axis of the patient.
13. The needle is then advanced through the obturator muscle and membrane.
14. The needle handle is rotated upwards constantly palpating the tip of the needle until the handle is horizontal. The needle is then brought out in the vagina. Check should be made to detect fornicial puncture.
15. The mesh is then attached to the needle tip and the mesh is pulled through.
16. A cystourethroscopy should be performed at this stage to ensure no mesh through the bladder or urethra.
17. The mesh should be positioned to lie flat.
18. Excess mesh should be trimmed.
19. Skin closed with absorbable sutures.

### Posterior Defect Specific Repair

1. Patient positioning is done.
2. Local anesthetic is given to the skin.
3. A midline incision is made on the posterior vaginal wall.
4. Rectum dissected off the vaginal wall.
5. The rectovaginal septum is identified at the lower end of the posterior vaginal wall.
6. The septum is then attached to the iliococcygeus muscle on the lateral vaginal wall bilaterally using 2-0 PDS.
7. A per rectal examination is performed to ensure no suture material is through the rectum.
8. Skin is closed with absorbable sutures.

## TRANSOBTURATOR SLING (MONARC)

1. Patient positioned in open lithotomy position.
2. Empty the bladder.
3. Recommend local anesthetic injection into the anterior vaginal wall at the level of the midurethra.
4. A 2 cm incision is made on the skin extending from about 1 cm from the external urethral meatus.
5. Para urethral tunnels should be created.
6. The Monarc needles are blue in color and sides can be identified by the direction of the arrow.
7. The right needle is usually placed first with the handle at 45° and passed through gently around the pubic ramus.
8. The tip of the needle should be felt through the vaginal incision and be guided through the incision.
9. Ensure the fornices are clear and the sling is attached after orientation.
10. The same is repeated on the other side too.
11. Recommend check cystourethroscopy for beginners.
12. The sling should be placed relatively loose so as to avoid any voiding problems in postoperatively.
13. Skin closed with absorbable sutures.

### Postoperative Care

- Ensure adequate analgesia
- Postoperative antibiotics for 5 days
- Ensure spontaneous voiding with a trial of voiding prior to discharge
- Vaginal estrogen may be prescribed postoperatively.

#### *Tips in the Management of Pelvic Prolapse*

- *Anatomy*
  - Surgeons should be familiar with the pelvic anatomy
  - Bony landmarks: Ischial spine, adductor longus tendon and ischial tuberosity
- *Patient positioning*
  - Flexion of the hip by 45° decreases the incidence of perioperative neuropathy
  - Avoid hyperflexion to prevent hip pain

- *To minimize mesh exposure*
  - Preoperative (more than 2 fold decrease in mesh extrusion) and postoperative estrogen cream
  - Full thickness vaginal dissection
  - Minimal vaginal skin excision
- *Minimize dyspareunia*
  - Place the mesh tension-free
  - Ensure that mesh lies flat and not bunched up
  - Release any bands of tissue under tension
- *Combined procedures*
  - If performing Perigee and Monarc at the same time, leave the upper arms of the plastic sheaths of Perigee in situ and perform Monarc. Remove the sheaths of both Perigee and Monarc at the end
- *Mesh exposure management*
  - Vaginal estrogen
  - Trimming in the clinic
  - Excise only the exposed mesh
  - Tension-free suturing of the vaginal skin
- *Preventing complications*
  - Preoperative evaluation
  - Antibiotic prophylaxis
  - Compression devices and/or clexane
  - Patient positioning
- *Postoperative care*
  - Early ambulation
  - Pain control
  - Trial of voiding
  - Postoperative antibiotics/estrogen
- *Avoid adductor* longus tendon to minimize groin pain
- If in doubt, take it out! (this applies to needles of monarc or perigee)
- Ensure objective and subjective follow-up for up to three years.

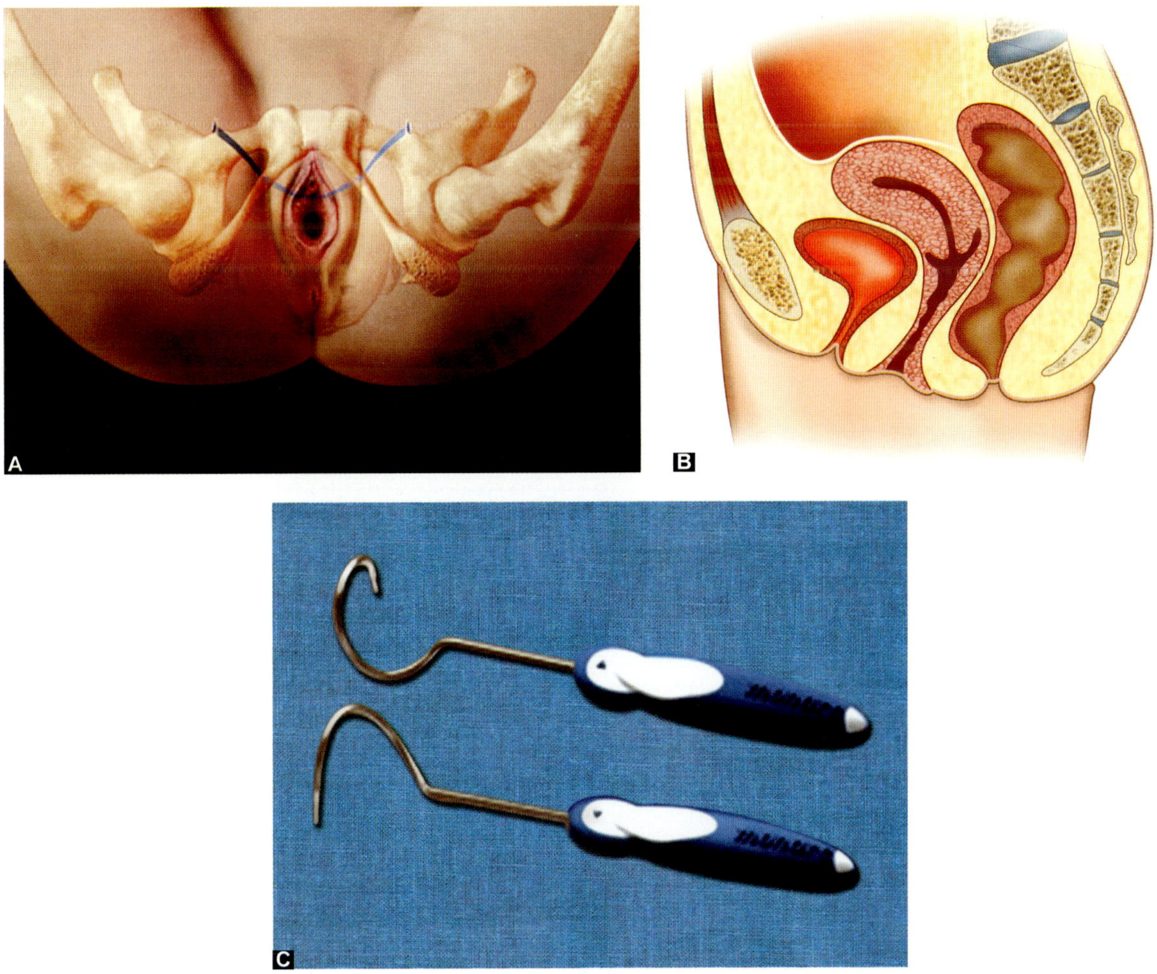

**Figs 38.3A to C:** Monarc

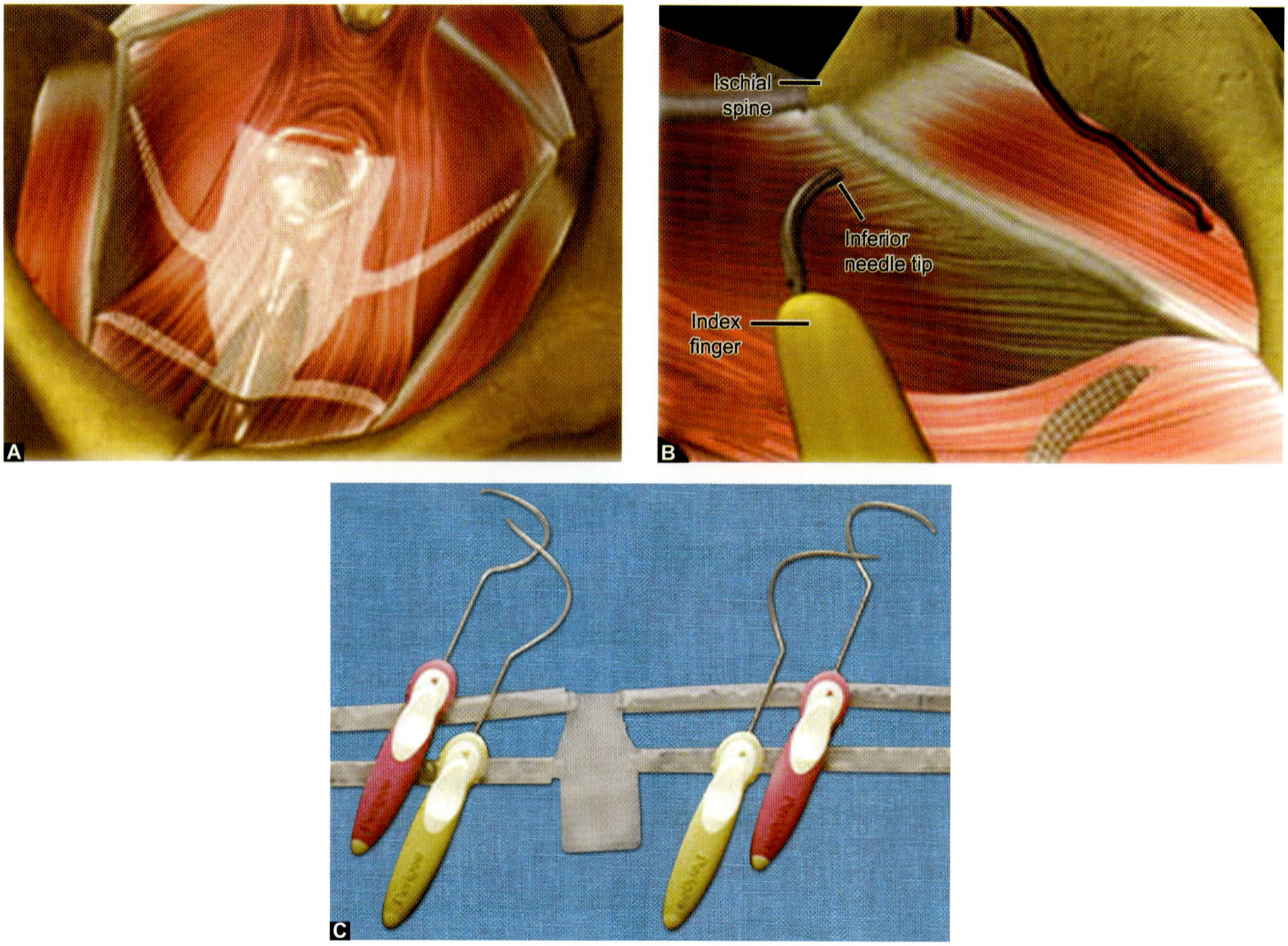


**Figs 38.4A to C:** Perigee

Chapter

39

# Apical and Posterior Vaginal Wall Repair

*Andri Nieuwoudt*

## INTRODUCTION

The sequence in which the surgery is done can have an influence on the outcome. In the author's experience the following sequence give the best results:

First do the apical repair, then the posterior wall and lastly the anterior wall.

In repairing the anterior wall, the securing of the pericervical ring is done first, before side wall dissection and side-specific repair is done.

## APICAL AND POSTERIOR VAGINAL WALL REPAIR

The extraperitoneal native tissue repair recreates the posterior cervical ring (apical repair) and re-attaches the severed rectovaginal septum to the posterior cervical ring and uterosacral/cardinal ligament complex. Bilateral uterosacral cervicopexy (BUSCer) describes the apical repair and Bilateral uterosacral colpopexy (BUSCol) describes the posterior wall repair.

### Bilateral Uterosacral Colpopexy (BUSCol) and Bilateral Uterosacral Cervicopexy (BUSCer)

Pathology to be repaired will include:

1. **High transverse defect** (HTD) of the rectovaginal fascia/septum *(Posterior Cervical Ring Defect)*

#### *Vaginal Topographic Mapping*

- Decreased/absent rugae on posterior wall pericervically
- Cervix can point anteriorly if anterior pericervical ring (PCR) is still intact
- If anterior pericervical ring (PCR) is also defective due to an anterior HTD, the cervix will be centrally placed at the vaginal apex with no ant/post fornixes.

2. Defective uterosacral (USL)—cardinal ligament (CL) complex

#### *VTMap*

- Increased distance between cervical external os and lateral fornix dimple.
- Bilateral: Cervix placed centrally.
- If unilateral, the cervix will point away from the defective area.

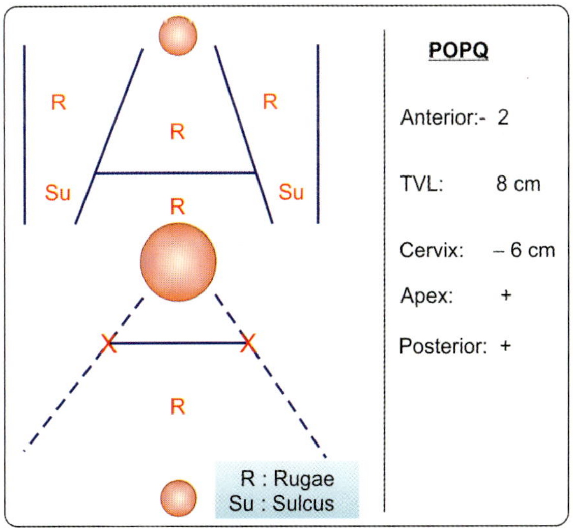


**Fig. 39.1**

- There is no need to differentiate between a "rectocele and "enterocele": The defective compartment—posterior or apical, is what needs to de addressed. If this is done, the sagging posterior wall ("rectocele") will be corrected, the perineum will be supported and the gap between the two severed USL ("enterocele") will be closed.
- The stabilization of the apical compartment is an essential part of defect correction of the posterior compartment as well as for the anterior compartment.

- The uterosacral ligament is never avulsed from the pericervical ring, it is more stretching of the medial third of that ligament. The USL can always be found at or near the attachment on the posterior aspect of the cervix.
- Defect correction of the apical segment will involve two steps:
  - If the connection between the CL and the USL is broken, this need to be corrected
  - Followed by re-establishing the connection between USCL complex and the cervix: This involves plicating the USL towards its posterior attachment area on the cervix. This will support the posterior cervical ring and the cervix in its normal position between the ischial spines.
- By plicating the medial portion of the USL, the gap between the two is closed—as with a McCall—resulting in closure of the "enterocele".
- After the BUSCol procedure—see below a roll of dissolvable xenograft is sutured onto the pericervical ring, running from USL to USL on both sides hugging the cervix—this can be strengthened by a piece of mesh-1/2 cm wide that is sutured to both USL and centrally to the cervix augmenting the postcervical ring.

## Opening the Posterior/Apical Vaginal Surgical Field

1. Starting at the introitus, the posterior vaginal wall is split longitudinally; ending just above the torn edges of the rectovaginal septum, this is being judged to be were the rugae stopped; *see* vaginal topographic mapping.

   Care is taken not to enter the rectovaginal space - if this is inadvertently entered, it is closed with interrupted Vicryl 000 sutures.

   The upper and lower end of the skin incision is supported with 2 hooks on each end attached to a Lone Star or TLC vaginal retractor frame.
2. The vaginal skin is split from the underlying condensation of collagen tissue that constitutes the rectovaginal fascia.

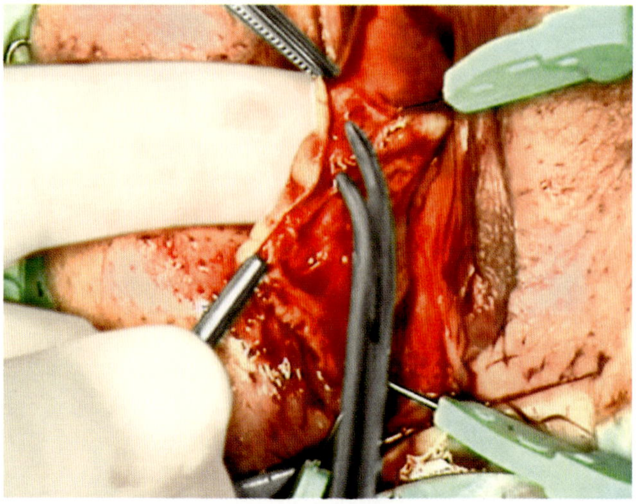

**Fig. 39.2:** Dissection is done with a fine scissors with the index finger of the surgeon supporting the vaginal skin

With the help of a Lone Star or TLC retractor facilitating stretching/counterstretching the dissection is taken laterally until the venous plexus of the rectum is reached on both sides. Two Lone Star hooks are placed, one on each side.

- After the initial skin cut is made, the upper end and lower ends are stabilized with 4 hooks that are anchored to the Lone star frame.
- If one do a transverse incision on the posterior vaginal wall-compare with anterior wall dissections—the closure of the skin can result in shortening of the vaginal canal.
- Transverse incisions can be done, but then two incisions will be needed: one 2 cm below the cervix and one on the perineum.
- Dissection will then involve tunnelling under the vaginal skin from proximal to distal incision—the Zimmermann-Yagi scissors (Marina Medical Instruments) is essential for this. This will enable the retracted rectovaginal septum to be pulled upwards with the BUSCol procedure, without compromising vaginal length.
- In the elderly acoital patient in whom vaginal length is no issue, only a transverse incision 2 cm below the cervix can be done, from here the dissection is taken downwards over the edge of the septum and upwards to the cervix—compare anterior wall dissection. In these cases, one need to trim vaginal skin at the end of the procedure.
- The rationale for transverse incisions is to decrease postoperative scarring of the vaginal cavity. The skin must be closed with interrupted sutures and not continual, as one will do with vertical vaginal wall incision closure.

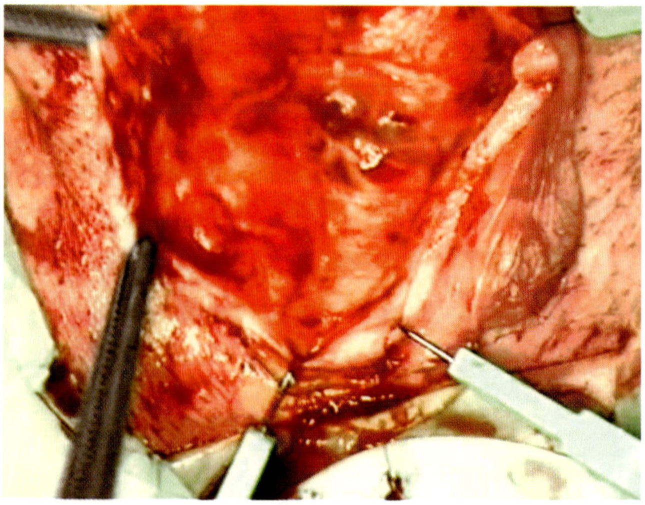

**Fig. 39.3**

3. At the distal end of the vaginal skin incision, the dissection is taken over the fascial edge—here only a peritoneal cover lines the vaginal skin, blunt dissection is usually sufficient. This dissection is taken up to the posterior pericervical ring, it usually is not necessary to split the overlying vaginal skin.

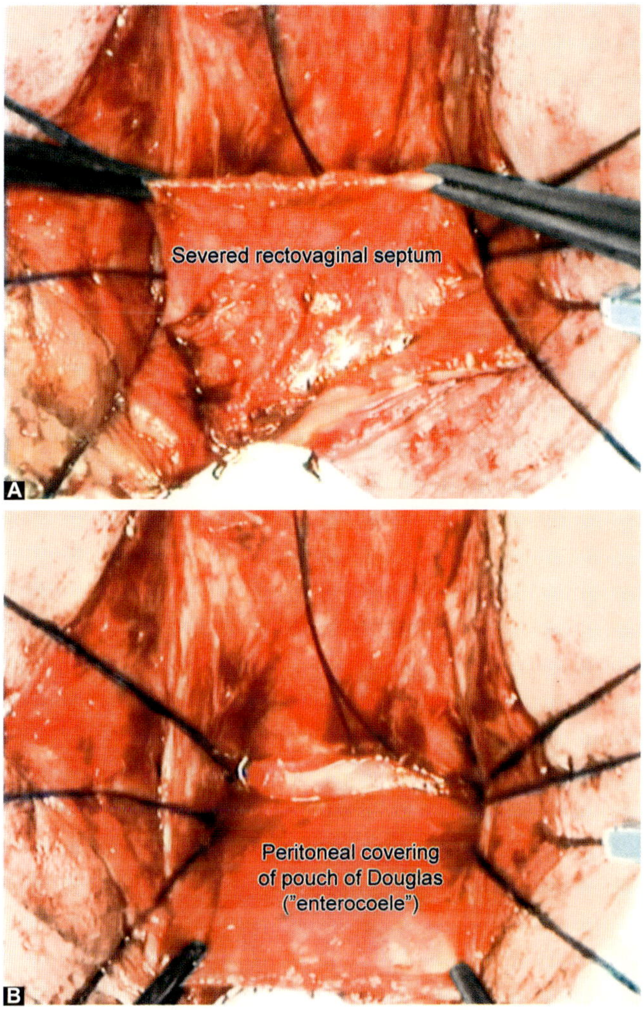


**Figs 39.4A and B:** Defective Posterior Cervical ring (HTD) to be repaired

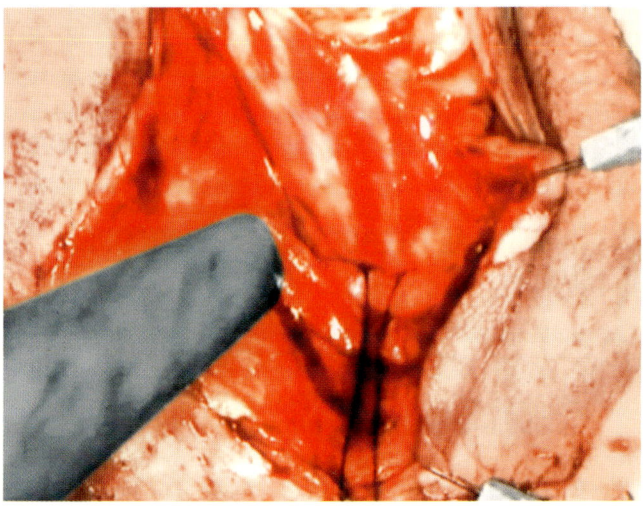

**Fig. 39.5:** Central cervical anchor suture in place

4. A Maxon 0 suture (Monofilament Polyglyconate Synthetic Absorbable Suture) using a HGU-46 needle (serial number: 6455-61) is used for a central cervical anchor. Care is taken not topierce the vaginal skin in the posterior fornix. This anchor is used to put traction on the pericervical ring, uterosacral ligaments (USL) and the cardinal ligaments (CL) during the procedures that are to follow. A small-toothed Kocher is put on the end of this surure, the needle is kept on the suture material.

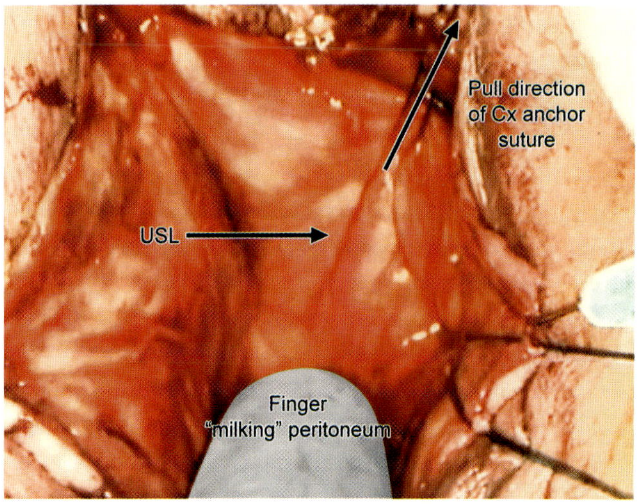


**Fig. 39.6:**

5. By pulling the central cervical anchor suture to one side, strain is put on the contralateral USL, it can be palpated at its origin on the posterior aspect of the cervix. Starting centrally on the left side at the pericervical ring where the US ligaments originate on the posterior aspect of the cervix, a clamp (preferably a curved Zeppelin) is put very superficially onto this stretched portion of the US ligament.

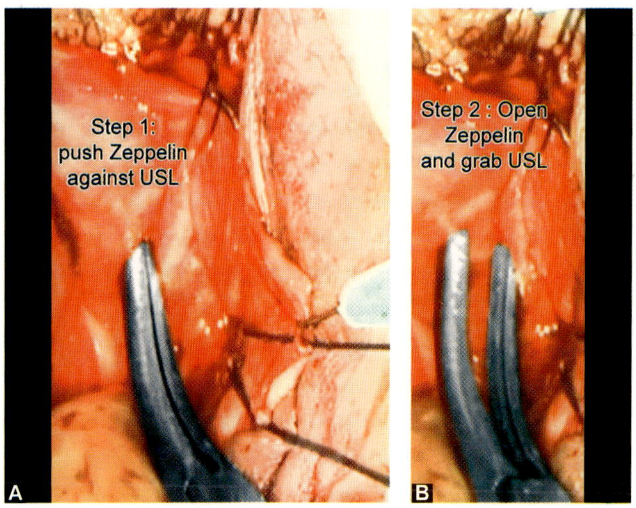


**Figs 39.7A and B:** The closer one stays to the cervix, the lesser the risk for ureter injury

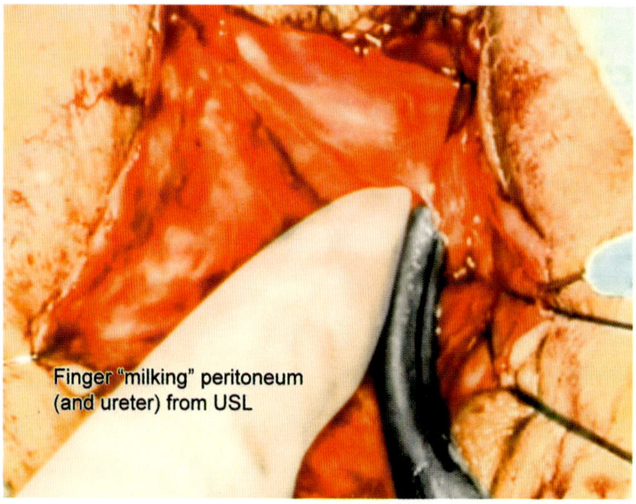


**Fig. 39.8:** Finger "milking" peritoneum (and ureter) from USL

6. Traction to the contralateral side by this clamp makes digitally palpation of the stretched ligament possible.
7. The index and middle finger of the surgeon is put on both sides of this ligament and by pushing medio-lateral along the palpable ligament, the peritoneum (and ureter) is pushed laterally. A second Zeppelin is applied.

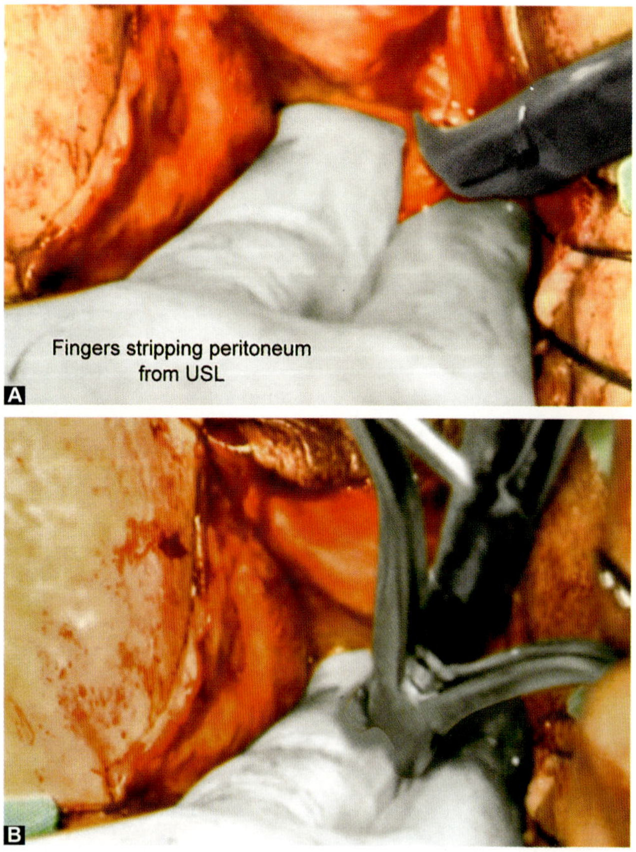


**Figs 39.9A and B:** Fingers stripping peritoneum from USL

8. The first clamp can be released and re-applied deeper to the second clamp on the ligament: "walking" up the ligament with these two clamps until a solid feel to the ligament is found. While doing this, the surgeons' finger is kept in place pushing the peritoneum (and ureter) laterally.
9. This is continued as high as possible. The further these clamps move away from the cervix, lesser is the risk of injuring the ureter, and the stronger is the ligament as it nears its attachment on the lateral aspects of the sacrum. The ligament broadens as it moves away from the cervix and spread out before it attaches to the side of the sacrum. The part of the ligament involved in the procedure is its inferior third: the peritoneal surface where one will find the ureter is thus not involved.

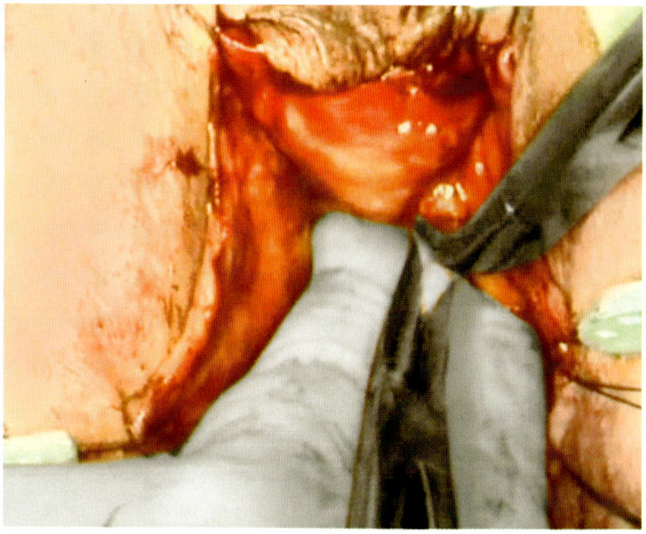

**Fig. 39.10**

10. Two clamps will now be on the USL—one superficial and one deep.

## I. BILATERAL UTEROSACRAL CERVICOPEXY (BUSCer)

The uterosacral/cardinal ligament complex is anchored to the cervix with delayed absorption and permanent sutures—this can be augmented with a synthetic mesh strip and/or xenograft. This will position the cervix in its' normal midpelvic cavity position at the interspinous level. The BUSCer procedure also closes the gap between the uterosacral ligaments reducing the "enterocele".

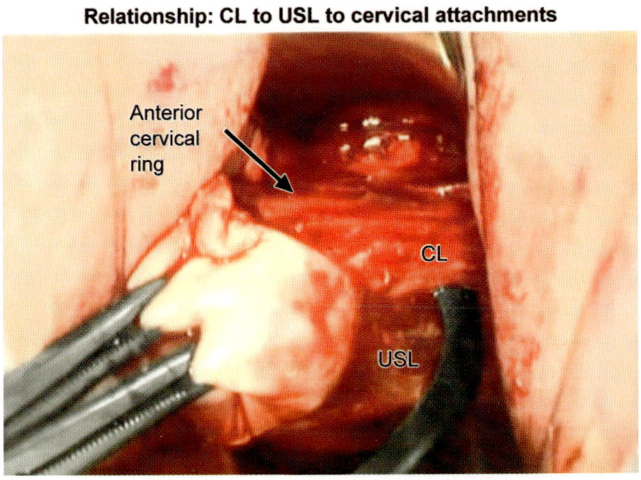


**Fig. 39.11:** Normal anatomy: Relationship of uterosacral ligament (USL) and cardinal ligament (CL) to each other and pericervical ring. With the BUSCer procedure and the HTD repair of the anterior vaginal wall, this normal anatomy is recreated

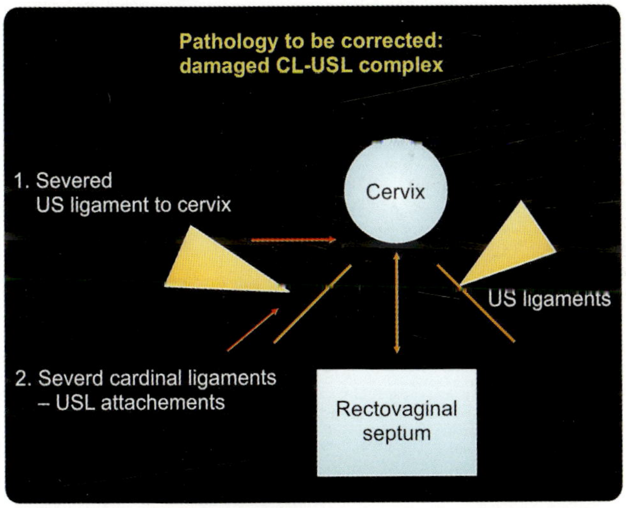


**Fig. 39.12:** BUSCer

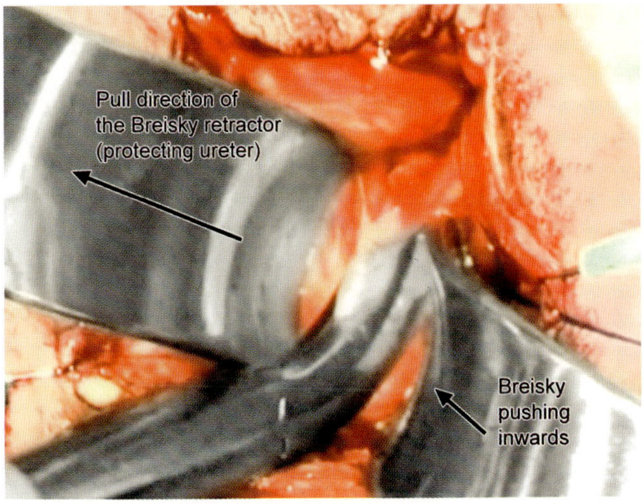


**Fig. 39.13:** Two Breisky-Navratil Vaginal Retractors can be useful to improve visualization

1. A deep uterosacral suture is placed: Maxon 0 (serial: 6455-61) is used for all sutures. The suture is placed from lateral to medial through the USL deep to the Zeppelin and pulled through. It is marked with a Mosquito clamp for identification purposes. This suture will be utilized when the BUSCol is done.

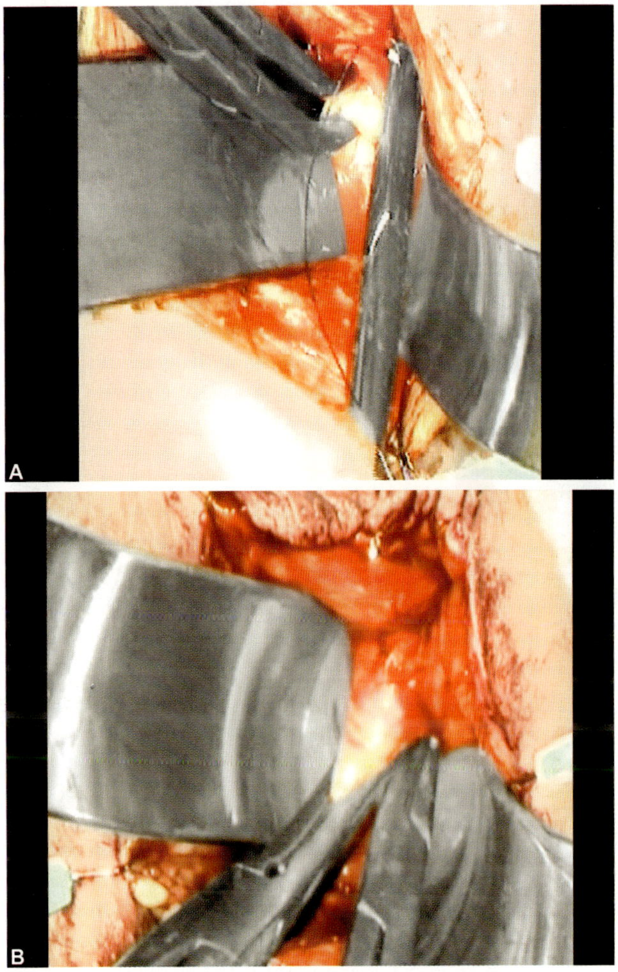

**Fig. 39.14A and B:** Placing the deep USL suture (Maxon 0)

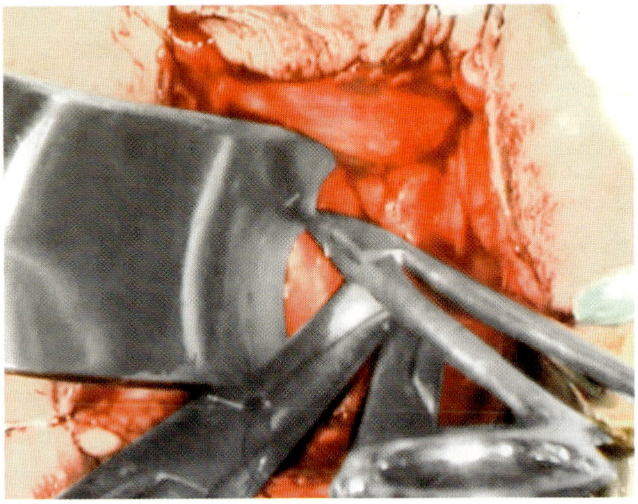

**Fig. 39.15:** A second needle holder is utilized in support of suturing

2. In marked decent of the cervix and apex, 1 or 2 Prolene sutures are placed—Prolene 2-0 on a UR-6 needle (VC 5673). This is done on the left side by turning the needle around in the needle holder ("back hand") and starting from medial to lateral (inside-out) in the deep and coming back superficially from lateral to medial (outside-in). The needle is kept on the suture. The deep Zeppelin clamp on the US ligament can be removed after the first is in place. The second Prolene suture is placed likewise. The same procedure is done on the right side, also from medial to lateral (inside-out) and back from lateral to medial (outside-in).

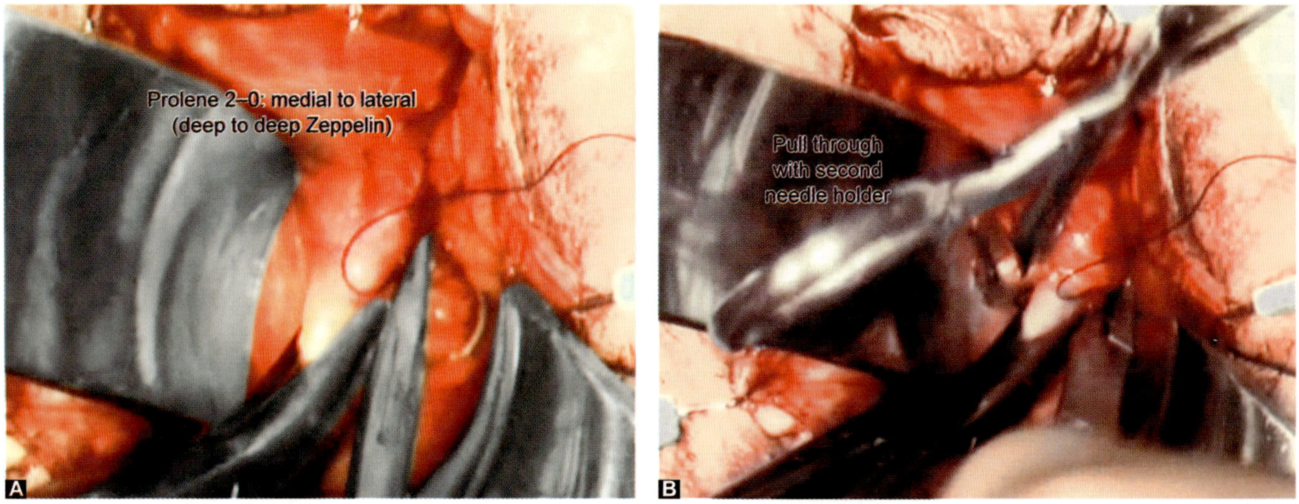


**Figs 39.16A and B:** Inside-out placing on right USL

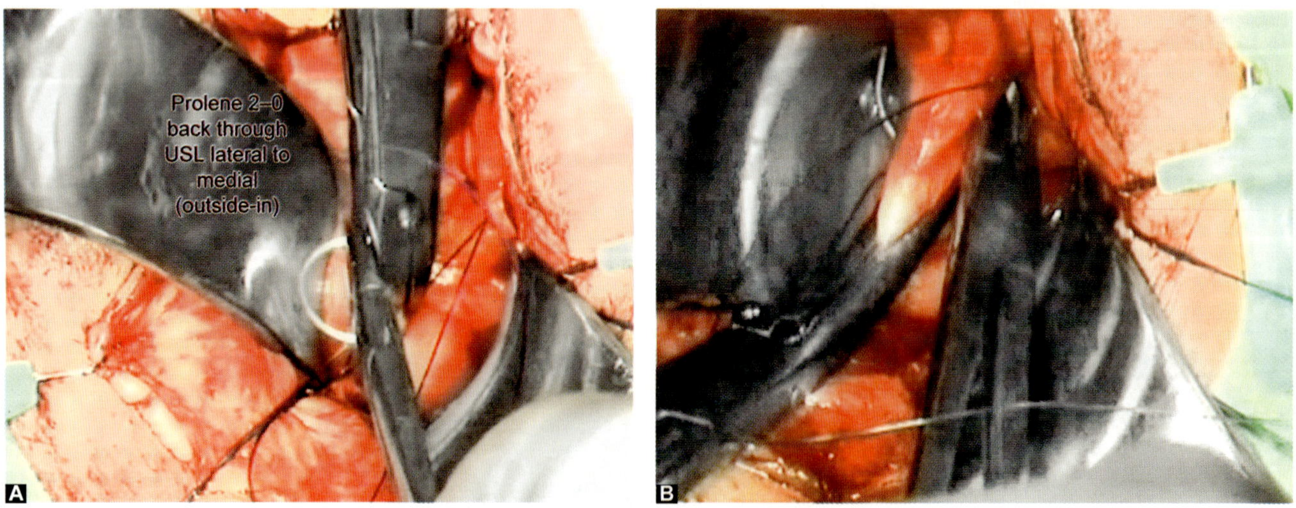


**Figs 39.17A and B:** Outside-in placing

3. ***The superficial uterosacral suture:***
   With the superficial USL clamp still in position, a Maxon 0 suture is place from medial to lateral (inside-out) and then back (outside-in). This suture is marked with a Rochester-Pean.

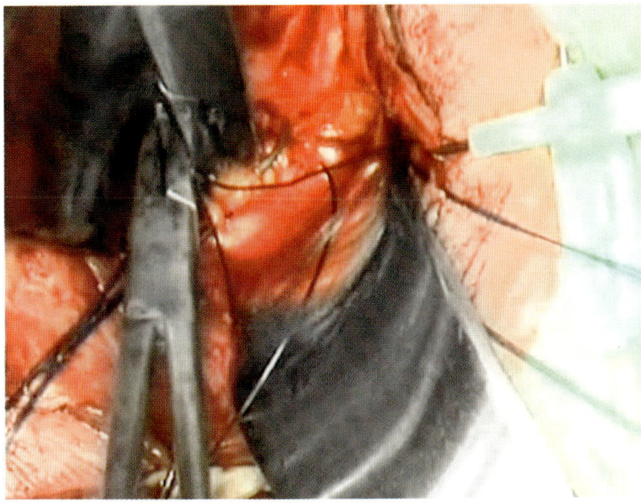

**Fig. 39.18:** Maxon 0: outside-in back through USL

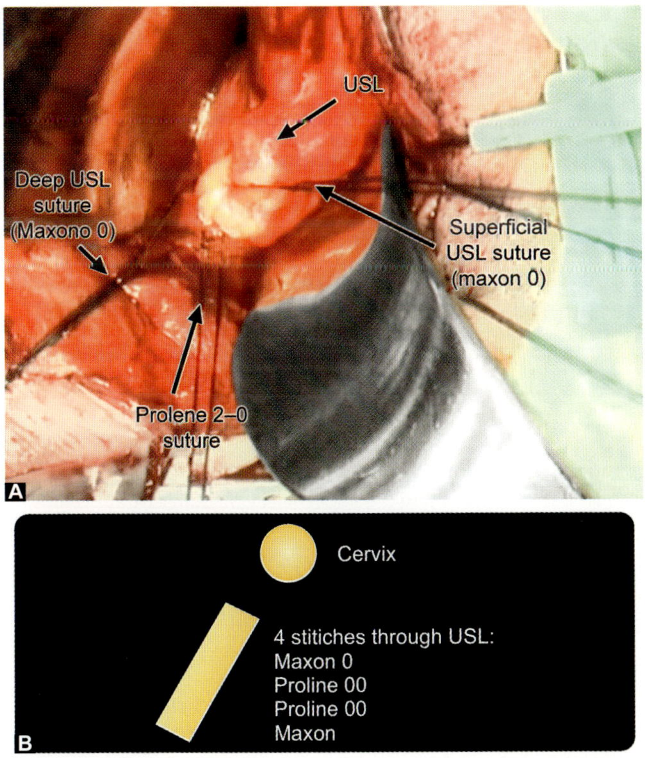


**Figs 39.19A and B:** *Note* that both the strands of both the superficial Maxon and the Prolene sutures are medial to the ligament. If a second Prolene is deemed necessary it will be placed between these two

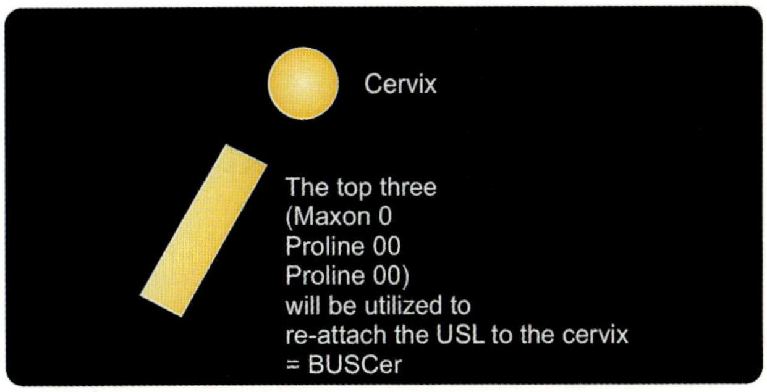


**Fig. 39.20:** Here 2 Prolene sutures are placed- this is only in patients where poor tissue quality is expected e.g. procidentia. One is usually sufficient in younger patients

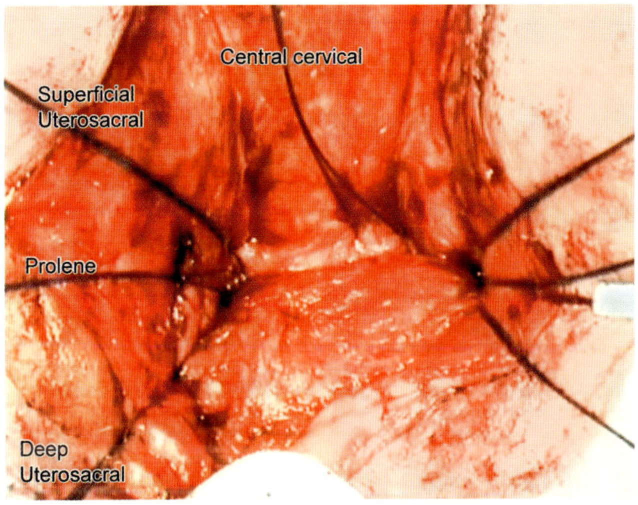


**Fig. 39.21:** Sutures to be utilized for BUSCer: Superficial uterosacral (Maxon 0) and the Prolene sutures: In this case only one Prolene 00 was placed on both sides

4. If the CL-US ligament complex is severed, this can be tested by pulling on the externally placed Vicryl suture and see if the two clamps on the USL move—the CL and USL must be reconnected: the deep Prolene suture or the deep USL Maxon suture is used to go laterally and take a bite into the vaginal skin where the external Vicryl suture is placed. Care is taken not to pierce the skin, if Prolene is used, or go too deep laterally into the CL, this is ureter country!

   Above procedures (placing of the Zeppelin clamps on the USL and placing of the different sutures) are done on the patients' left side first and then on the right side.

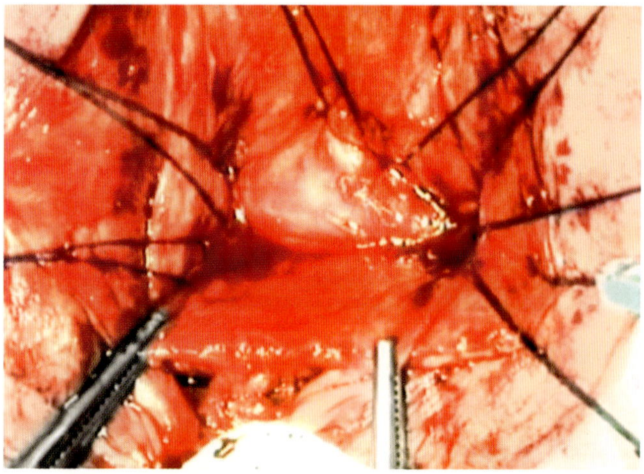

**Fig. 39.22:** Superficial USL sutures before placement into cervical stroma

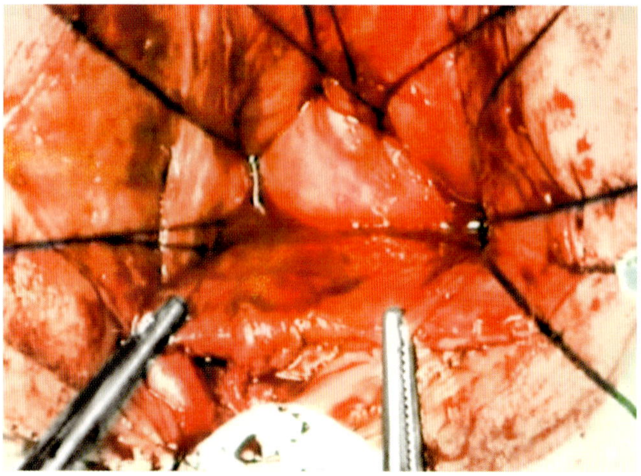

**Fig. 39.23:** Superficeal USL sutures after placement into cervical stroma

5. The two or three sutures (Maxon and Prolene) on the superficial aspect of the USL must now be attached to the posterior surface of the cervix: starting with the Maxon 0 on both sides, followed by the Prolene sutures. The needle is taken deep into the cervical stroma in the midline just below the central cervical sutures' attachment.

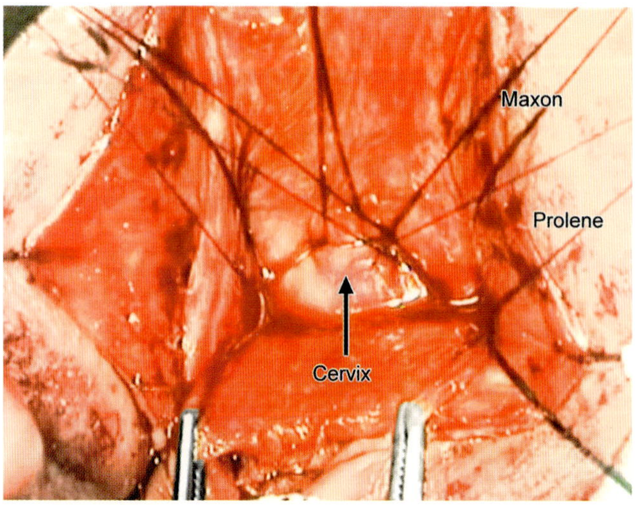


**Fig. 39.24:** Before tying the Maxon and Prolene sutures

6. This procedure is repeated on both sides without tying the sutures; these are only tied after all sutures are place on both sides, starting with the two superficial Maxon sutures (the two deep Maxon sutures are not utilized during the BUSCer procedure). This will plicate the proximal part of the US ligaments, anchoring the cervix and thus stabilizing the vaginal apex. Both the strands of the Prolene are cut as they are tied.

Rationale of the usage of suture materials: The Maxon sutures will keep the USL plicated to the cervix for 3 months to allow for strengthening of the attachments by normal wound healing to occur. The Prolene is to keep it approximated for a more enduring effect. With surgical auditing, it was found that if only Maxon is used, the attachment comes down after 3 months. But with the introduction of the Prolene, the desired effect was more lasting: initially 2 Prolene sutures were placed on each USL, but the same effect was found when one on each USL was placed. The thicker Maxon allows for more initial strain to be placed on the Cervix hugging it to the USL. The nonabsorbable Prolenes' knots will be hidden behind the rectovaginal septum as it is pulled upwards with the BUSCol procedure to be followed.

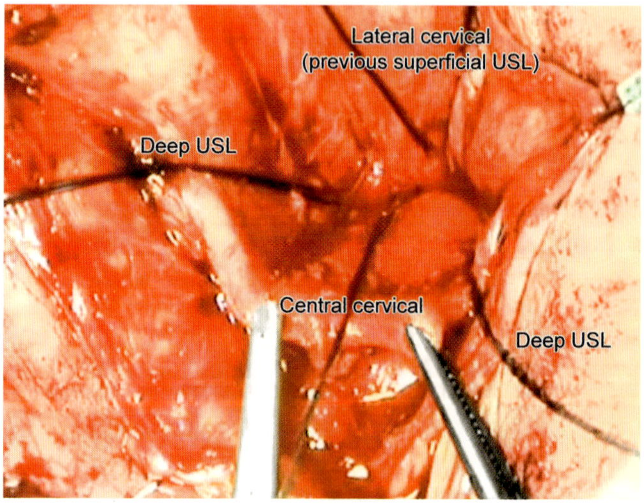


**Fig. 39.25:** After tying the superficial USL Maxon and Prolene sutures (BUSCer procedure)

5 Maxon sutures (with needles) will be present: 2 deep USL and 3 from the Cervix, these will be utilized for the BUSCol procedure.

Before the sutures are tied all the hooks from the Lonestar frame must be released to allow mobility of the vaginal skin. The plication of the two USL to the midline closes the pouch of Douglas and obliterates the central peritoneal sac—referred by some to as an "enterocele"—compare this to a McCall procedure.

This extraperitoneal procedure can take an externally placed cervix, e.g. with procedentia- 5 to 8 cm inside the vaginal canal, placing it in its correct anatomical position midway between the two ischial spines in the midpelvis. In these cases, it would be advised to use two Prolene sutures per USL.

7. In the very old or if there is marked decent of the cervix it is essential to build a strong posterior pericervical ring by augmenting the USL-Cervix attachments. This is done with a 1/4 cm by 4 cm piece of polyvinylidenfluoride (PVDF) (DynaMesh). It is centrally anchored by taking the strands of the 3 cervical Maxon sutures through the mesh and anchoring it laterally by doing the same with the deep USL placed Maxon. By not tying these, the mesh is tension-free placed running from one USL to the other with a central anchor on the cervix.

   The purpose of this piece of mesh is to stimulate adhesion formation on the posterior cervical ring, strengthening the attachment of the plicated USL
8. The mesh will be covered by the rectovaginal septum with the BUSCol procedure to be described next.

## II. BILATERAL UTEROSACRAL COLPOPEXY (BUSCOL)

Pathology to be repaired will include:

High transverse defect (HTD) of the recto-vaginal septum-pericervical ring attachment (defective posterior PCR).

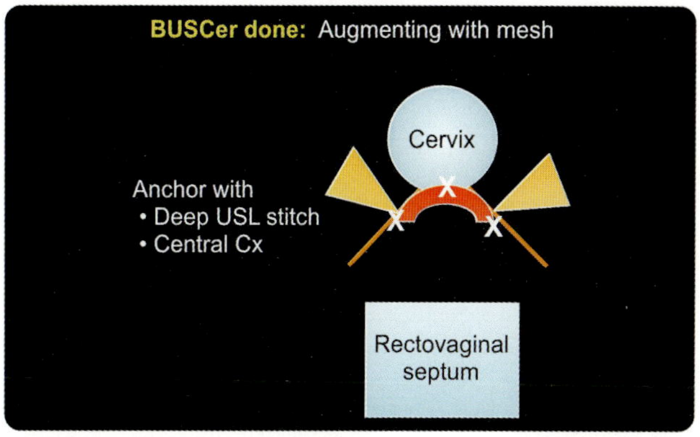


**Fig. 39.26**

Vaginal topographic (VTMap): Loss of rugae in the posterior vaginal fornix.

Once the apical segment is stabilized by the BUSCer procedure, the gap between the pericervical ring and the severed edge of the rectovaginal septum is closed by pulling this septum up and attaching it to the posterior aspect of the cervix and the two USL on both sides: this will stabilize the posterior vaginal wall

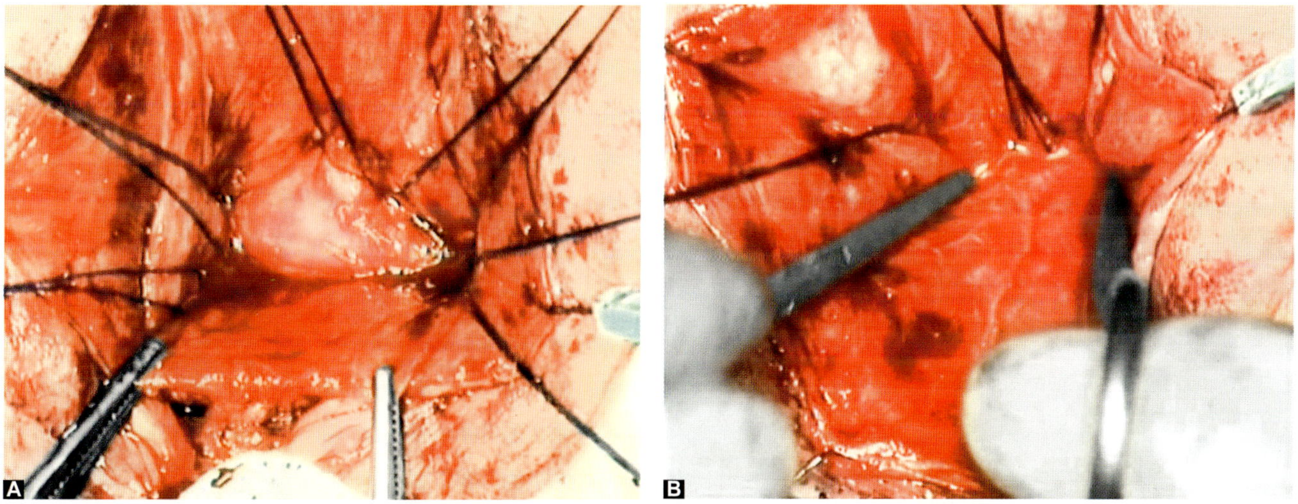


**Figs 39.27A and B:** The rectovaginal septum/fascia that was freed from the vaginal skin is resutured to the cervix centrally, and to the US ligaments bilaterally with 5 Maxon 0 sutures: The 3 cervical sutures and the two deep USL placed during the BUSCer procedure. The fascial plate that will be pulled up to the cervix with these sutures will bury the Prolene knots and the mesh, if that was placed

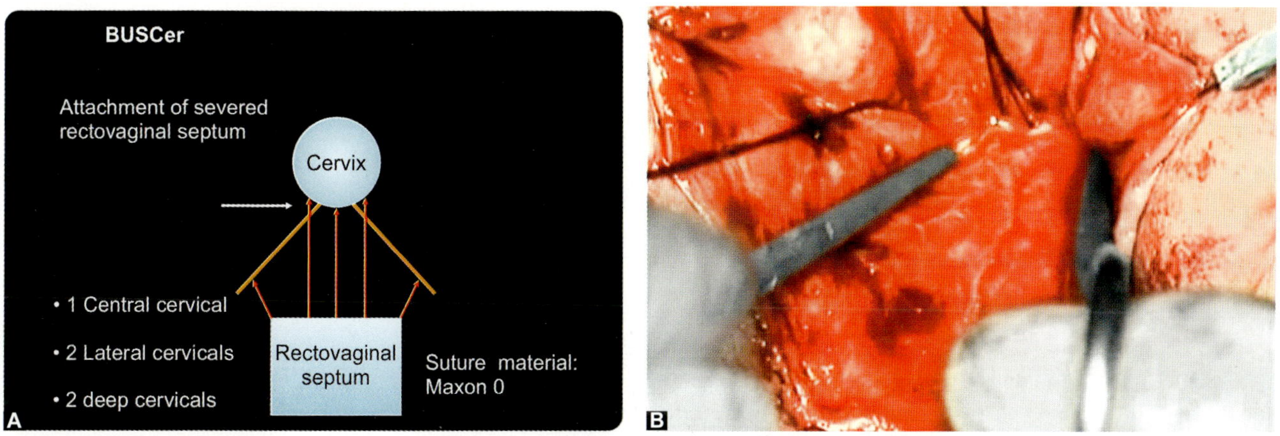


**Figs 39.28A and B**

1. The central cervical stitch (both strands) is brought through the septum centrally—the knot will be on the septum when tied.

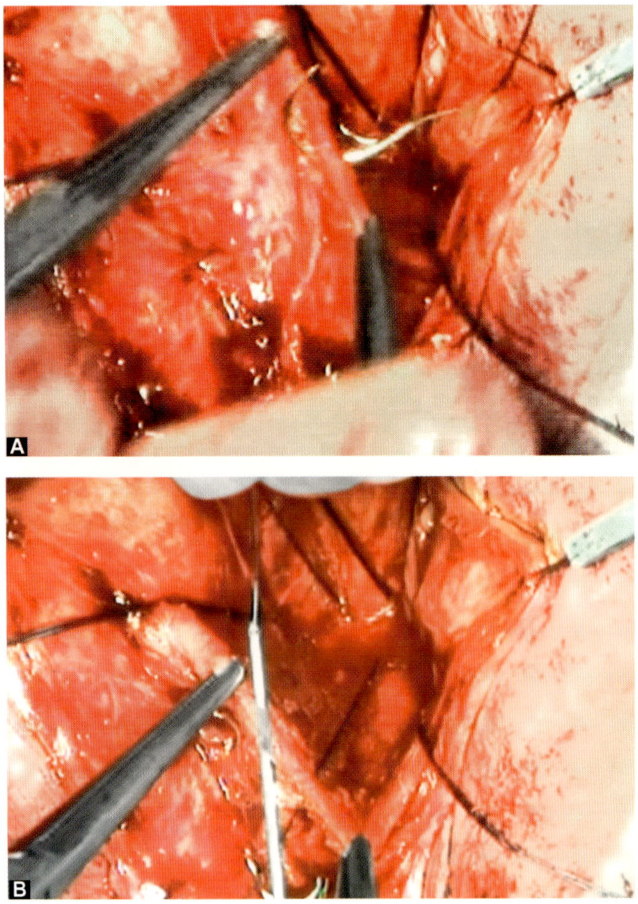

Figs 39.29A and B

2. The two lateral cervical stitches are placed in a similar manner.

The "superficial" USL sutures that anchored the USL to the posterior aspect of the cervix during the BUSCer procedure are the " lateral " cervical stitches.

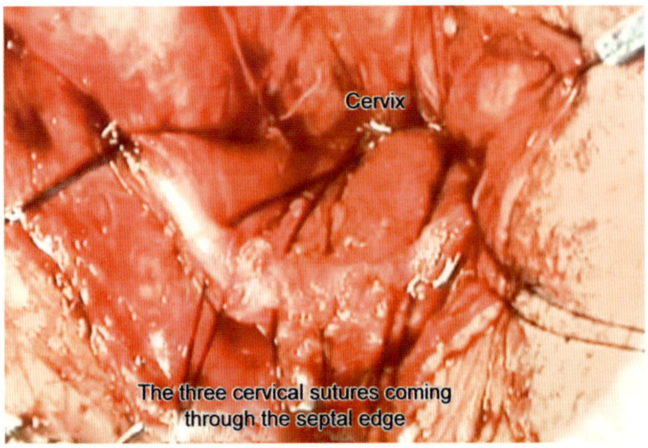


**Fig. 39.30:** These two lateral stitches not only help anchoring the rectovaginal septum onto the cervix, but also bury the Prolene sutures to counter their tendency to perforate through the overlying vaginal skin

3. The deep US stitch (only one strand) is pulled laterally on each side through the septum at the vaginal skin attachment

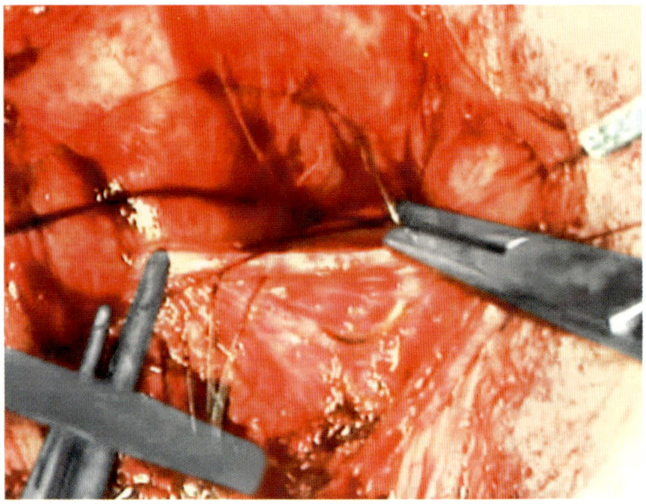

**Fig. 39.31:** These are extremely important for they will give length to the posterior vaginal wall. They are tied last

4. All 5 stitches are tied with the effect that the septum, plus the prolapsed posterior compartment is pulled upwards, supporting the rectum and the perineum.

Before tying of these all tension provided by the Lone Star hooks must be released.

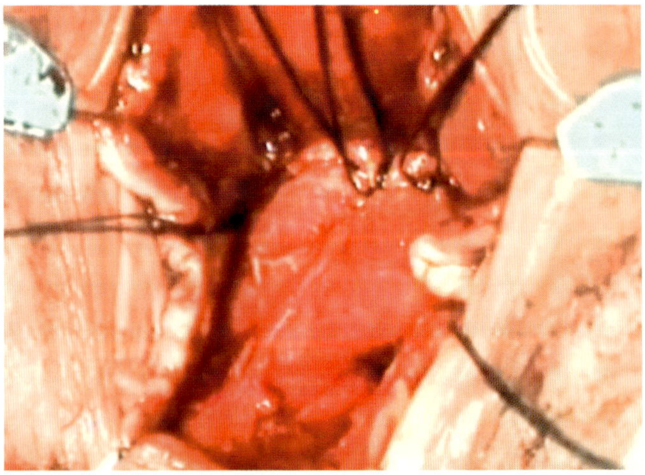

**Fig. 39.32:** The end result: Rectovaginal septum is pulled up and attached to the cervix and USL

## Augmenting the Posterior Cervical Ring with Xenograft

To strengthen and splint the suture lines, a roll of an absorbable xenograft (e.g. Biodesign, Cook Medical) can be sutured onto the posterior pericervical ring, running from USL to USL and hugging the cervix. The 5 previously used Maxon sutures can be used to achieve this. This is a temporary splint that will be in place for at least 3–6 months, before it is absorbed. It is advised in especially the older patient and those with depleted fascial tissue.

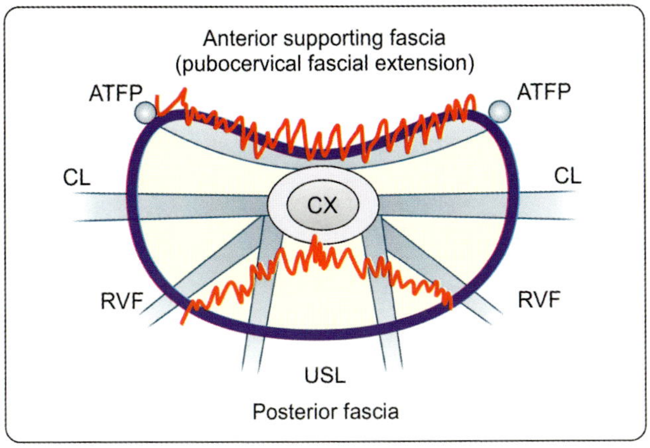


**Fig. 39.33:** Modified from Petros

- The use of an absorbable xenograft (non-crosslinked) has a primary role to act as a temporary splint for the suture lines against intra-abdominal pressure changes.
- Certain xenografts (e.g. Biodesign Cook Medical) also have an anti-inflammatory action and thus, decrease adhesion formation and can act as a matrix for the in growth of blood vessels, harvesting thus collagen from the surrounding cells via mast cell in growth.
- This and the temporary nature of the graft make it superior and safer, than permanently placed meshes and grafts.

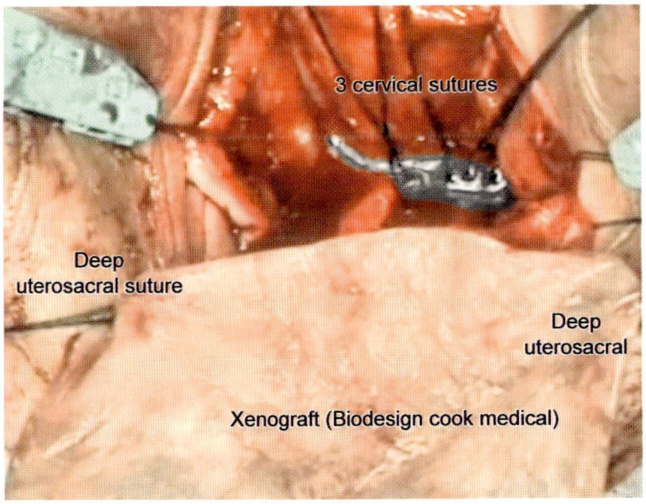


**Fig. 39.34**

1. A sheet of 10 × 7 cm Biodesign (Cook Medical) is laid over the surgical field. The two deep uterosacral sutures are placed through the top edges and re-catch the graft on both sides a quarter way down and at the halfway mark.
2. The needle ends of the three central cervical sutures are taken through the graft at its central point halfway down. All three sutures are thus split, three to the top and three to the bottom: the central ones will have Kochers on and the lateral ones Peans. The needles can be cut from the sutures.

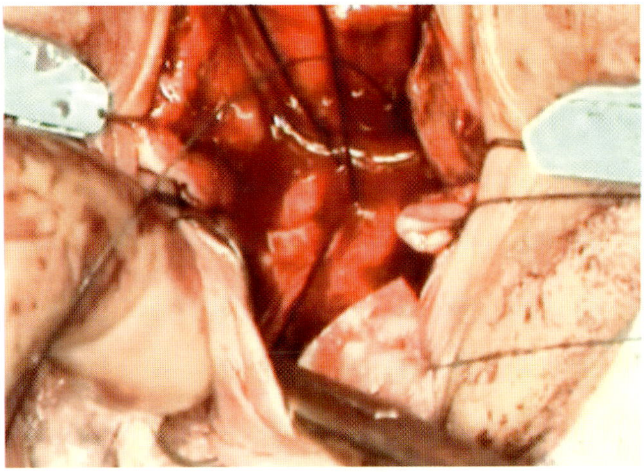

**Fig. 39.35**

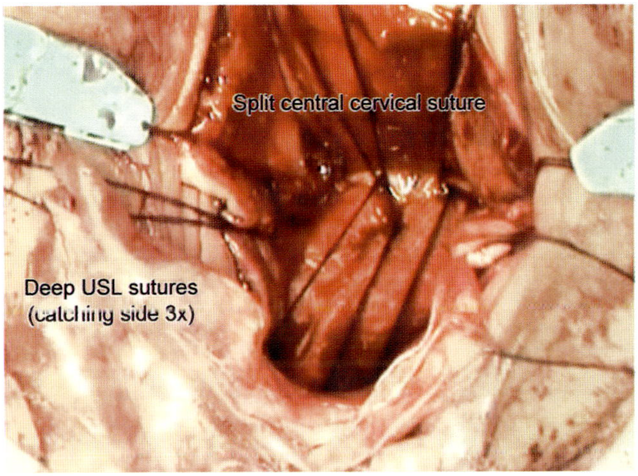


**Fig. 39.36**

3. All sutures are tied: First the two on the deep uterosacral ligaments, anchoring the folded graft onto the USL, and then the three central sutures, anchoring the graft firmly onto the cervix supporting the underlying suture line.

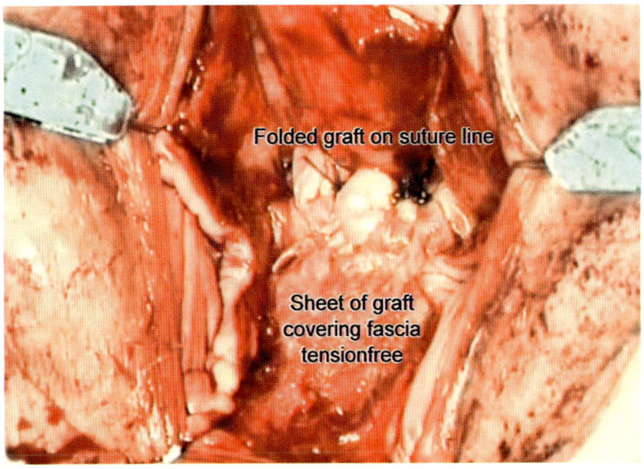


**Fig. 39.37**

The vaginal skin is closed with interrupted Vicryl 000

Chapter 40

# Transvaginal Tape Obturator (TVTO) for Stress Urinary Incontinence

*Prakash Trivedi, Sunita R Tandulwadkar*

## PREOPERATIVE EVALUATION

- Confirmation of diagnosis on table with full bladder. Bonney's and Marshall Marchetti test may help to give prognostic value of surgery.
- Urine routine, culture and sensitivity.
- Urodynamic studies.

## PREOPERATIVE PREPARATION

- It is preferred to do the procedure in immediate post-menstrual period.
- Insert a urethral catheter with aseptic precautions to keep the bladder empty.
- Anesthesia—can be carried out under local/regional/general.

## IMPORTANT EQUIPMENT

- TVT obturator device
- TVT helical passers
- TVT atraumatic winged guide
(All come together in disposable packet).

## PROCEDURE

1. Position of the patient: Dorsal lithotomy with hyperflexed hips over the abdomen and buttocks should be positioned flushed with the edge of the table. This position is very important as it gives better access to obturator membrane.
2. Marking of the exit point: An imaginary horizontal line is drawn at the level of the urethral meatus and second line drawn parallel and 2 cm above the first line. Locate the exit point on the 2nd line 2 cm lateral to the folds of thighs. 5 mm incision may be made at each exit point at this stage or may be later.
3. Midline vaginal incision of 1 cm is made on the middle 1/3rd of the urethra (1 cm proximal to the external urethral meatus).
4. With the help of pointed curved scissors, sharp dissection is done by using a 'push spread technique' through a path (should be approximately 5–7 mm in diameter and no deeper than 5 cm) which is as follows:
   i. First piercing the superior surface of perineal membrane and traveling underway from dorsal nerve of clitoris.
   ii. Pathway continues through para-urethral connective tissue (path of lateral dissection should be oriented at a 45° angle toward the medial edge of the obturator foramen) toward inferior pubic ramus and origin of pubococcygeous and pubo-rectalis muscle.
   iii. This continues below arcus tendinous, levator ani, obturator internus muscle through connective tissue and fat of the anterior recess of ischio-anal fossa, laterally along the inferior pubic ramus (Dissection beyond 5 cm may allow unintended entry into the retropubic space).
   iv. When the junction between the body of pubic bone and inferior pubic ramus is reached, loss of resistance is felt when obturator membrane is perforated.
   v. Path continues through obturator externus muscle, adductor magnus and brevis and the upper margin of gracilis muscle followed by fascia lata, subcutaneous tissue and skin at the exit point (which was marked previously).
   vi. Insert the TVT winged guide into the dissected tract (after removing from the pack with aseptic precautions). If difficulty is encountered, reconfirm the direction of the tract with scissors.
   vii. Insert the TVT helical passer into the dissected tract following the channel of TVT winged guide.

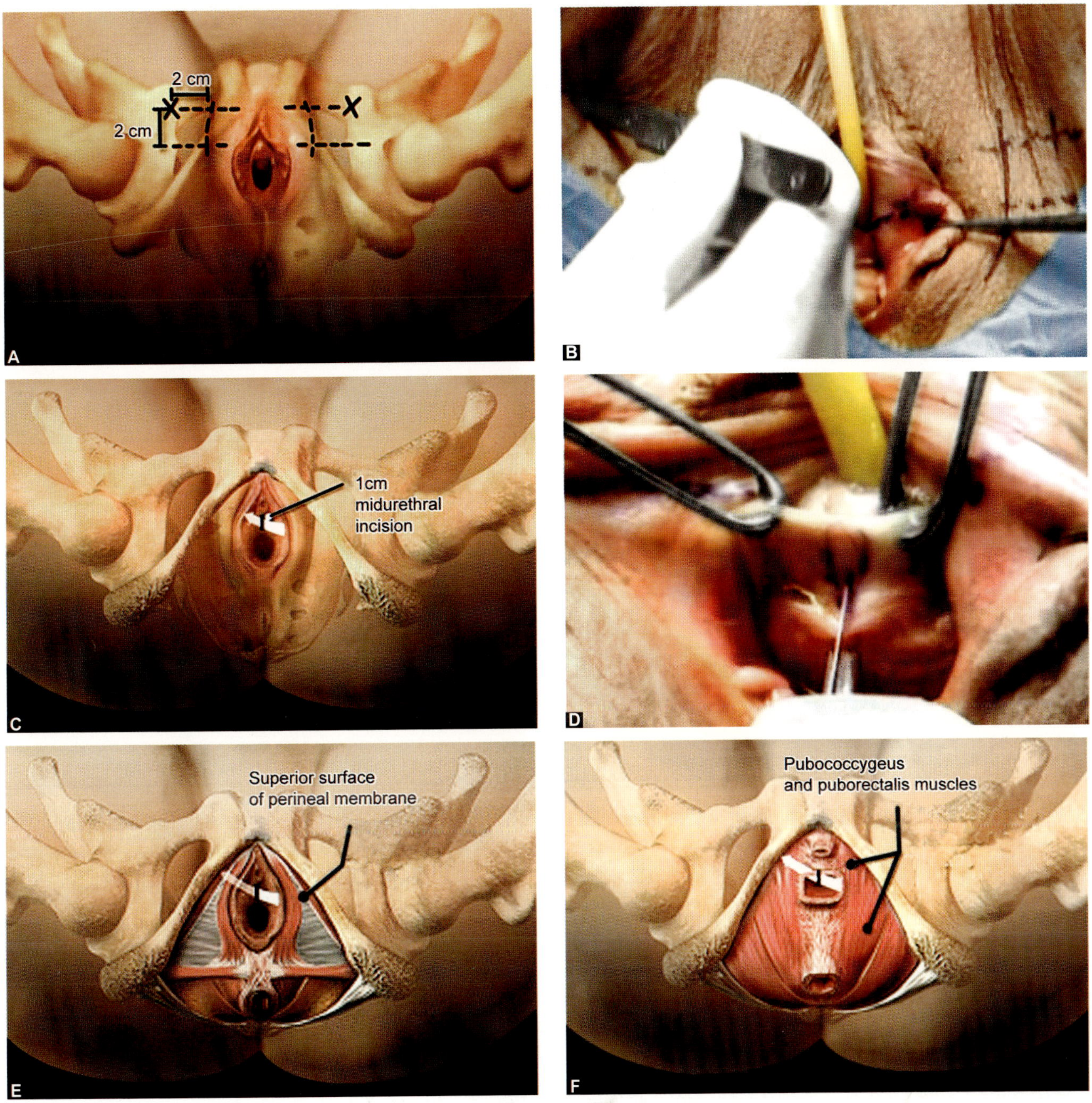


**Figs 40.1A to F**

Push the device inward, traversing and slightly passing the obturator membrane.

viii. Once in the above position, TVT winged guide is removed and the handle of the helical passer is moved toward the midline, until the handle is vertical to the floor.

ix. The point of the helical passer should exit near the previously determined exit points. When the tip of the plastic tube appears at the skin opening, grasp the pointed tip of the plastic tube with a clamp while stabilizing the tube near urethra with thumb, remove the helical passer by a reverse rotation of the handle.

x. Pull the plastic tube completely through the skin until the tape appears.

xi. Repeat the above technique on the other side, ensuring that the tape lies flat under the urethra.

xii. When both tubes have been extracted, through the skin incision, cut the plastic tubes from the tape and plastic sheath. Cough test can be performed at this stage which allows adjustment of the tape so that only a few drops of urine are lost during the cough.

xiii. Remove the plastic sheath that covers the tapes.

xiv. Close the vaginal and skin incision.

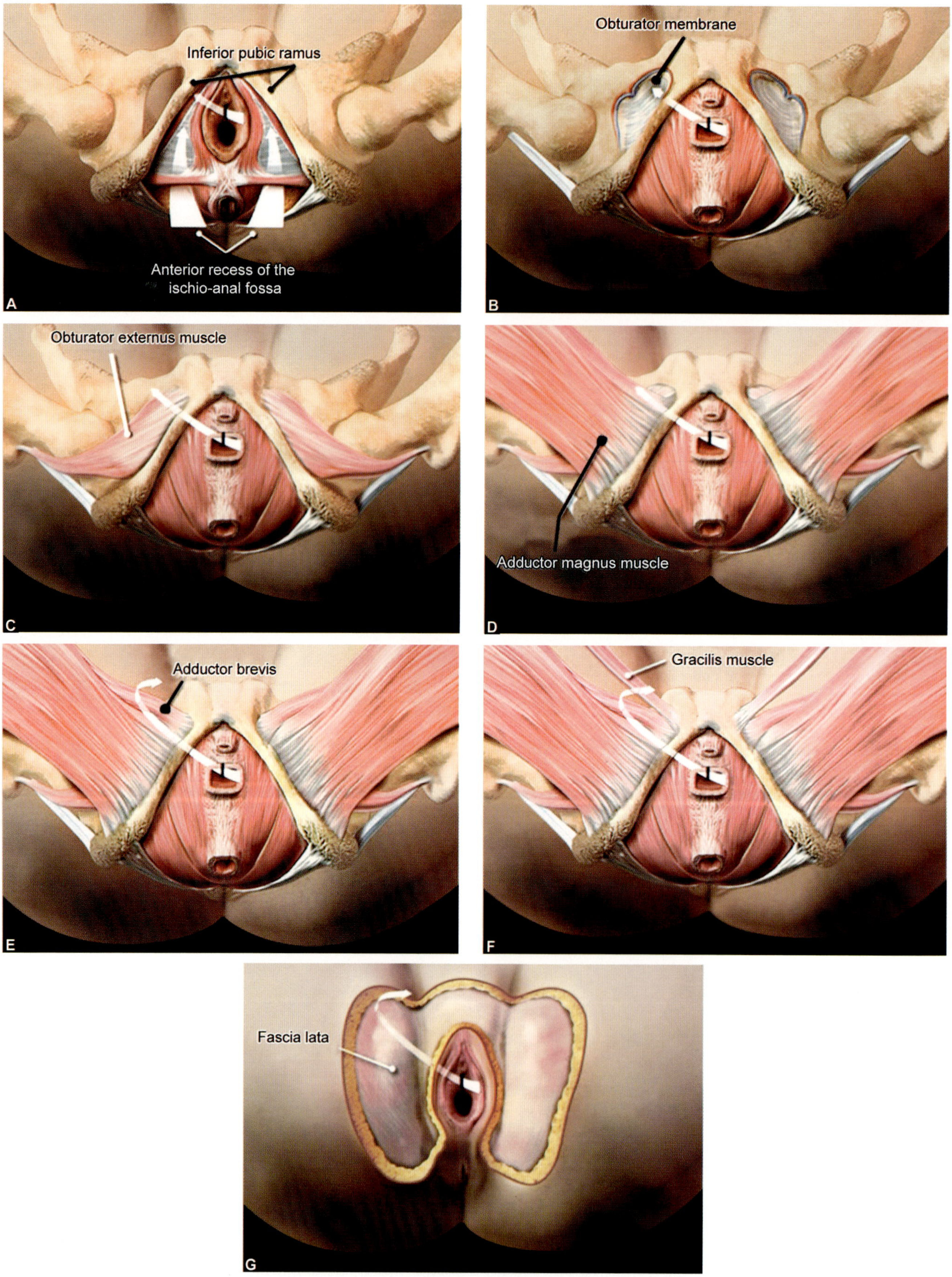


**Figs 40.2A to G**

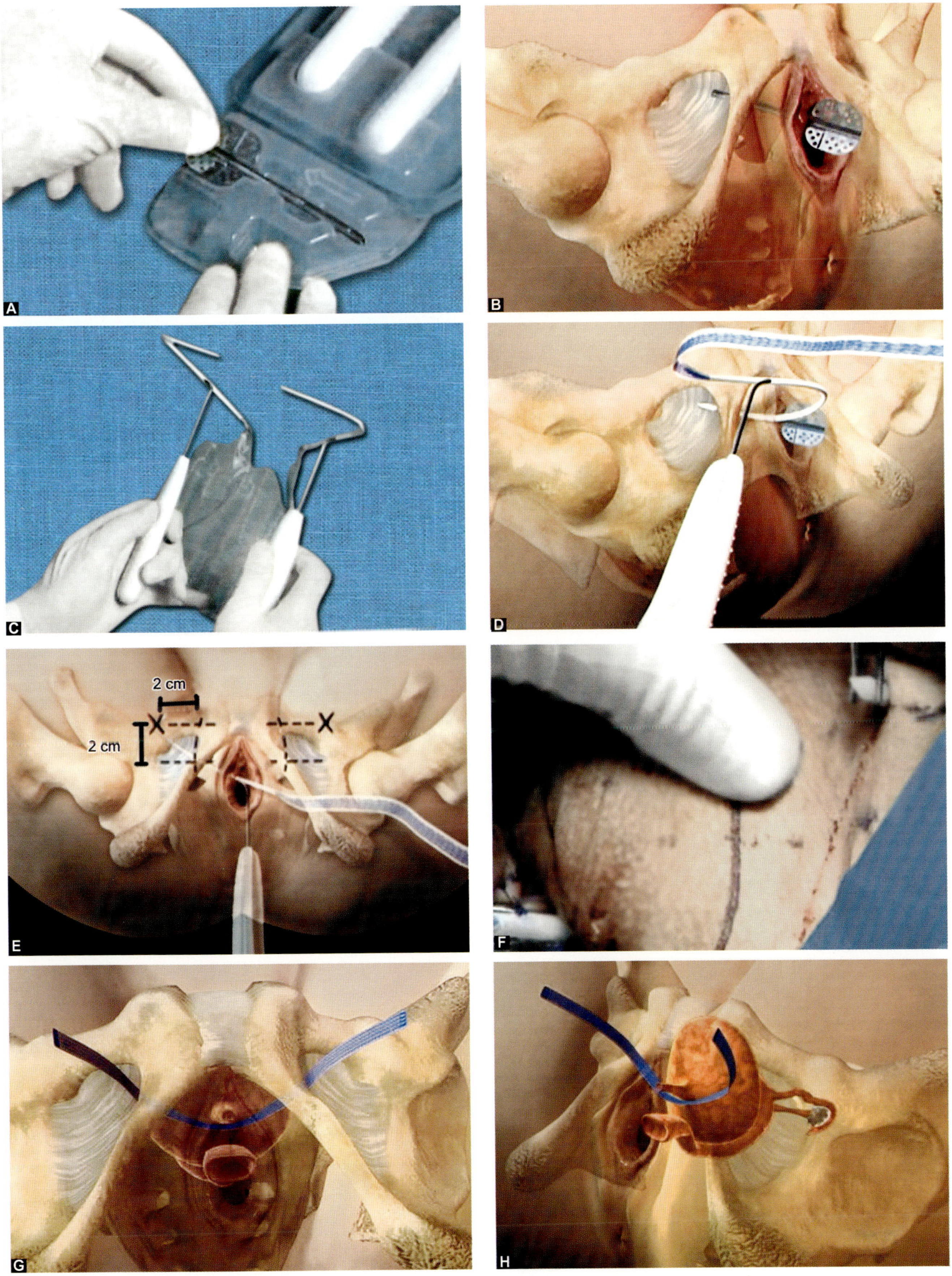


**Figs 40.3A to H**

*Contd...*

*Contd...*

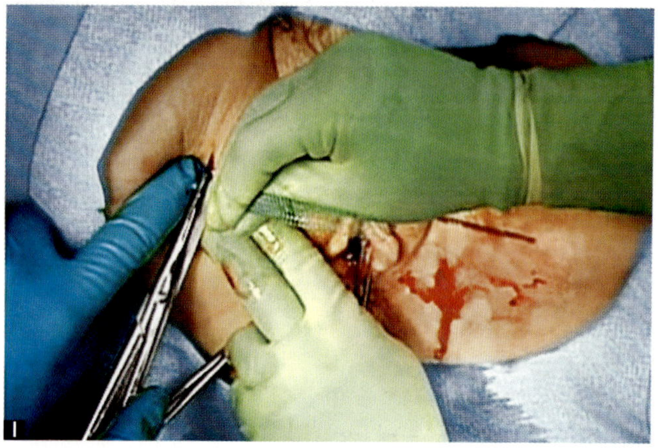

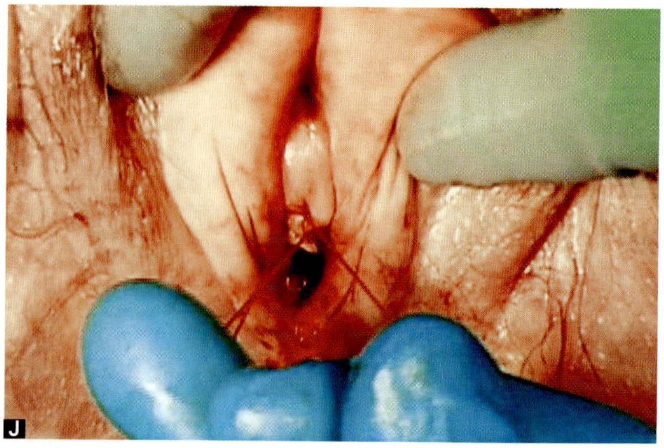

Figs 40.3I and J

## TIPS

- Dissection beyond 5 cm should be avoided as it will give unintended entry into space of Retzius.
- The open site of winged guide should always be facing the surgeon so that bendable tab can be bent to increase the length of the guide (originally 6 cm) to 7 cm, if needed.
- Device insertion to be completed on one side before beginning the dissection on the other side.
- Ensure correct orientation of the helical passers and tape by identifying logo and thumb indent on the plastic handle, which should be facing surgeon. The helical passer in the surgeon's left handle must be used on the patient's right side.
- Never allow the handle of the helical passer to be oriented horizontal to the floor.
- Position of the tape should be lose without tension and flat under the midurethra.
- Blunt instrument like a scissor/forceps can be placed between the urethra and the tape during removal of plastic sheath to avoid tension over the sheath. Overcorrection (i.e. too much tension) may cause temporary or permanent lower urinary tract obstruction.
- Cystoscopy can be performed at the discretion of the surgeon.

# Transobturator Tape

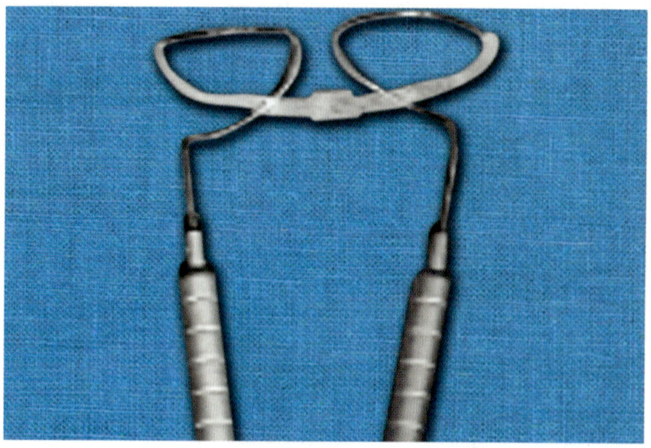

**Fig. 40.4:** Tr-O tape and needle

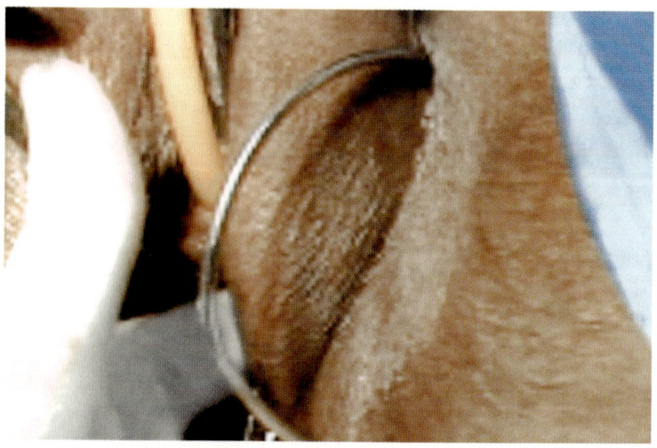

**Fig. 40.5:** Left needle insertion at the upper and medial most area of obturation parameter

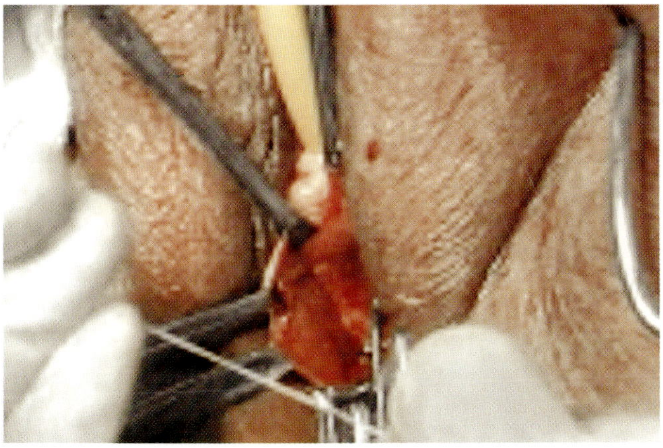

**Fig. 40.6:** Needle seen coming out below the midurethra

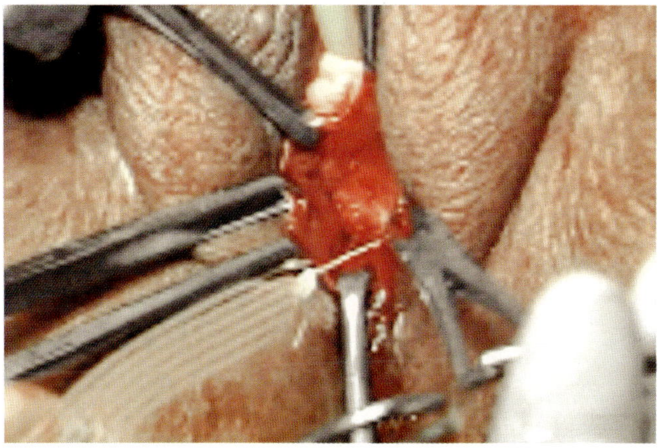

**Fig. 40.7:** Loading of Tr-O tape on the TrOt needle's eye

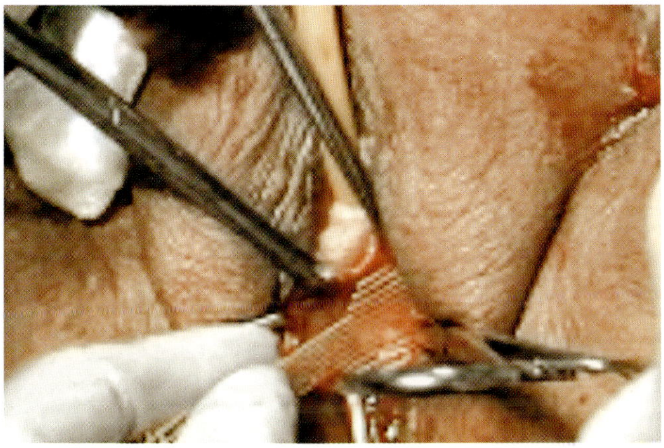

**Fig. 40.8:** Withdrawing the TrOT needle by pulling the TrOT sling

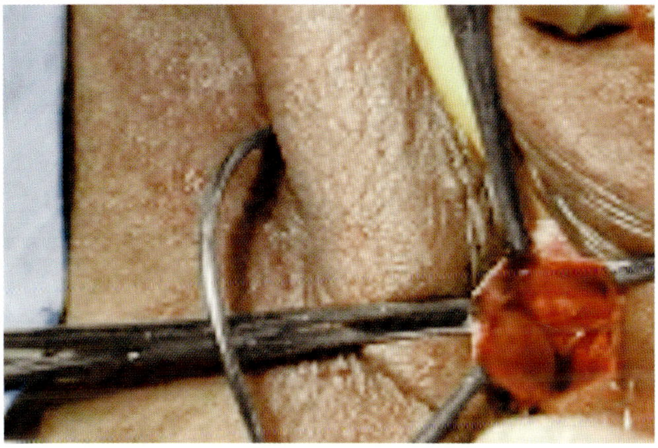

**Fig. 40.9:** Right TrOT needle insertion

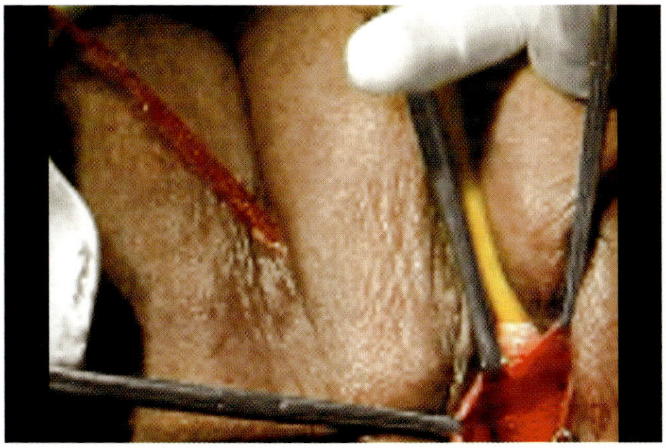

**Fig. 40.10:** TrOT seen pulled out of the obturator foramen with tension free suburethral placement

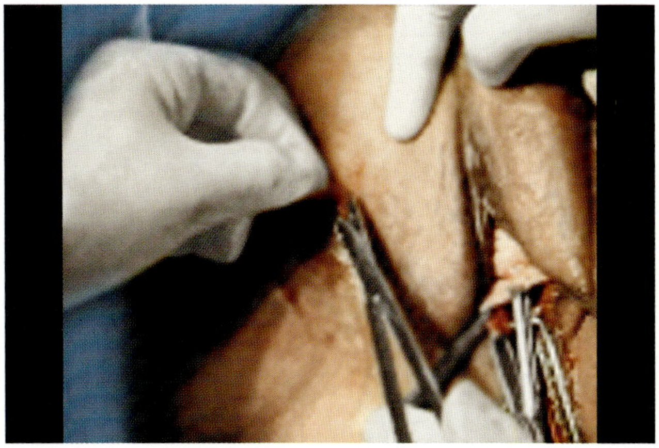

**Fig. 40.11:** Cutting the extra tape at skin level

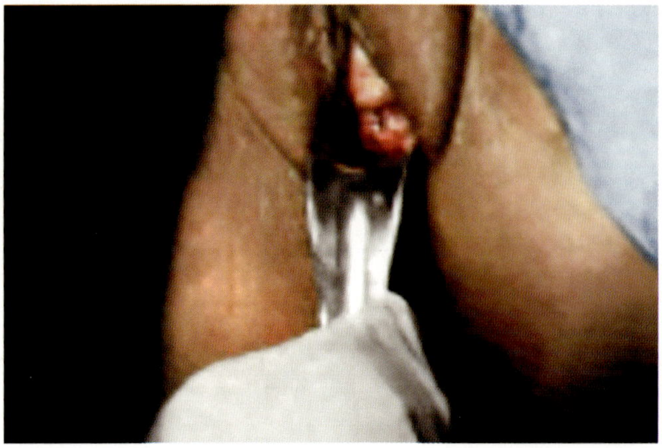

Fig. 40.12: Final view after vaginal incision closure

# T-SUIT

## Dynamic Sling Action of T-SUIT on Muscle Contraction

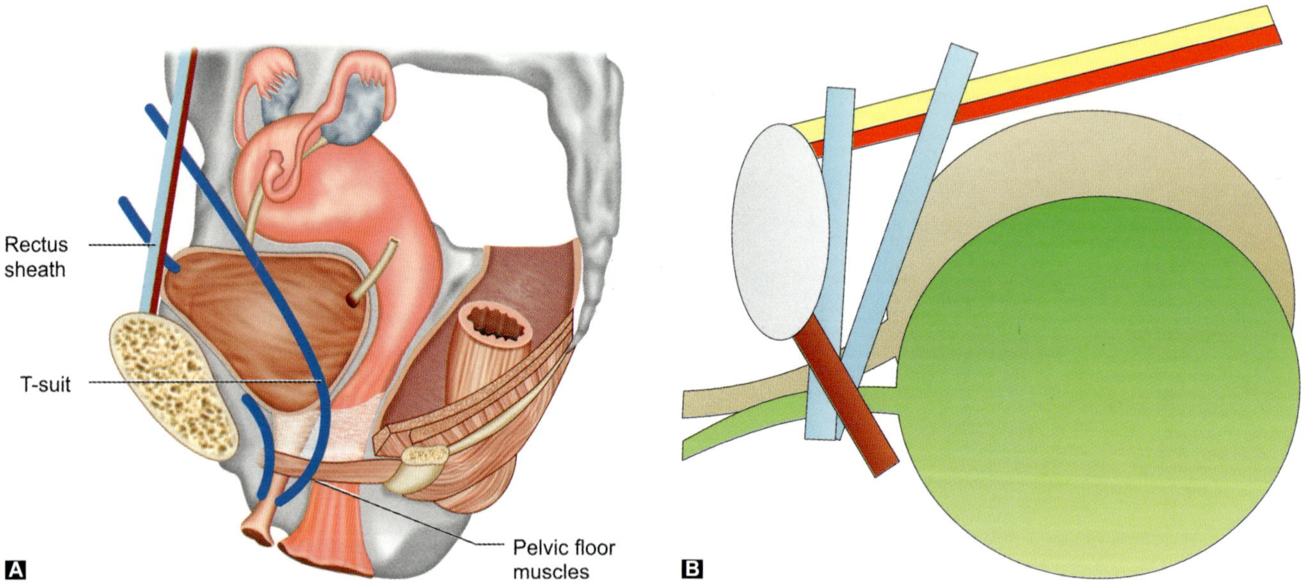


Figs 40.14A and B: Narrowing of tape at pelvic floor and rectus

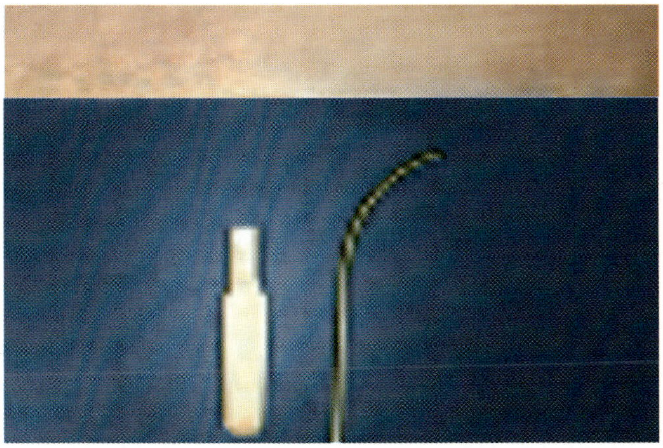

**Fig. 40.14:** T-SUIT handle, needle and tape

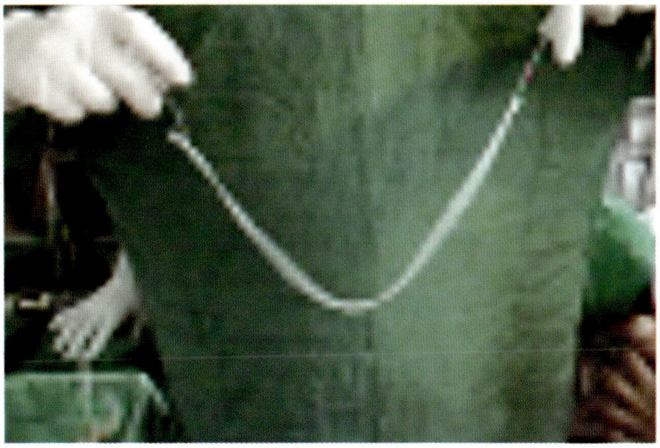

**Fig. 40.15:** T-SUIT tape

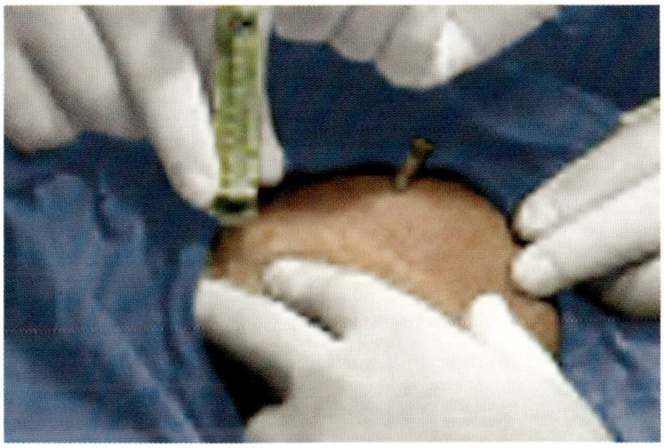

**Fig. 40.16:** Suprapubic infiltration of 10–15 ml 2% lignocaine with adrenaline 3 cm lateral to the midline

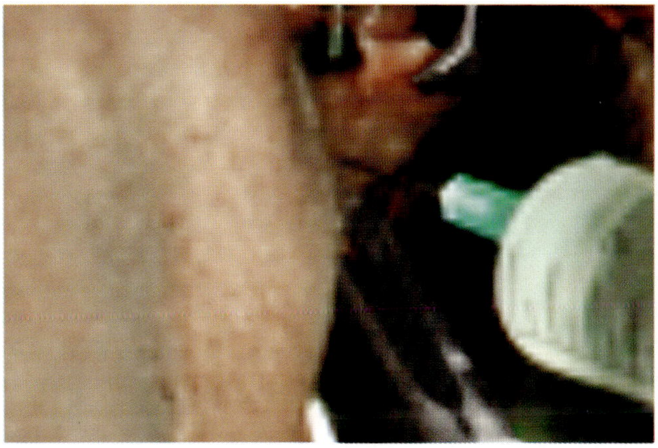

**Fig. 40.17:** Anterior vaginal wall infiltration and then 1.5 cm vertical vaginal incision is made 1.5 cm from the external urethral meatus

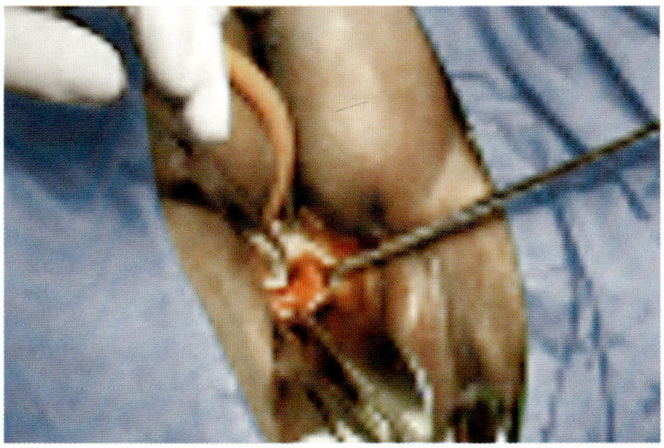

**Fig. 40.18:** Para urethral dissection

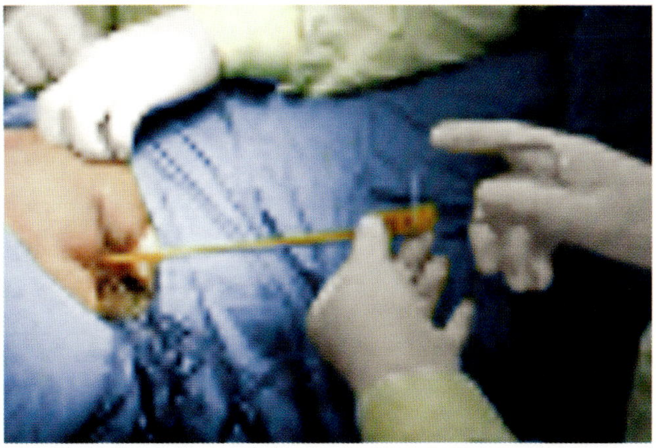

**Fig. 40.19:** Insertion of metal guide and pushing bladder neck

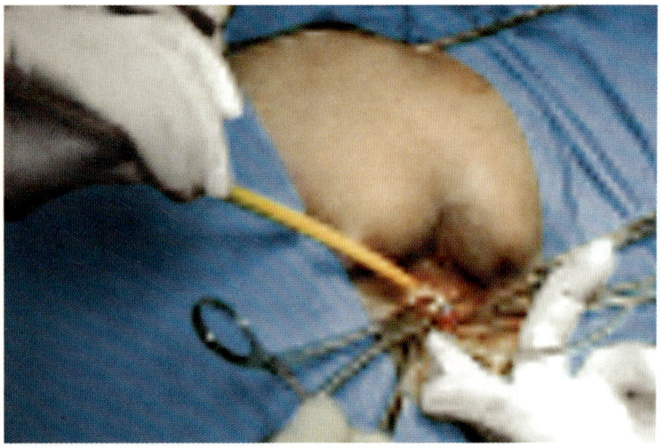

**Fig. 40.20:** Insertion of left and right T-SUIT needles

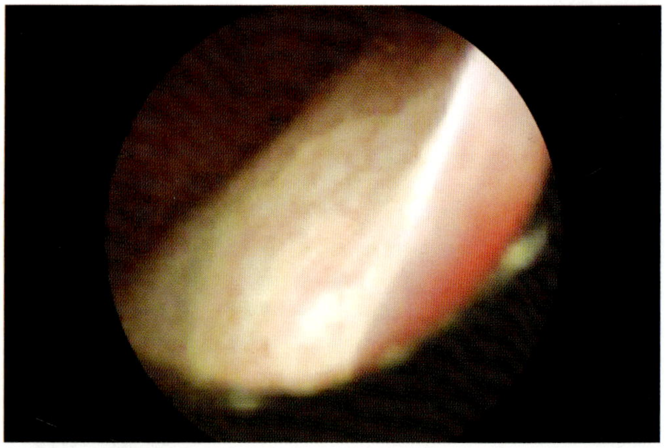

**Fig. 40.21:** 70° hysteroscopy/cystoscopy to confirm correct placement of needles

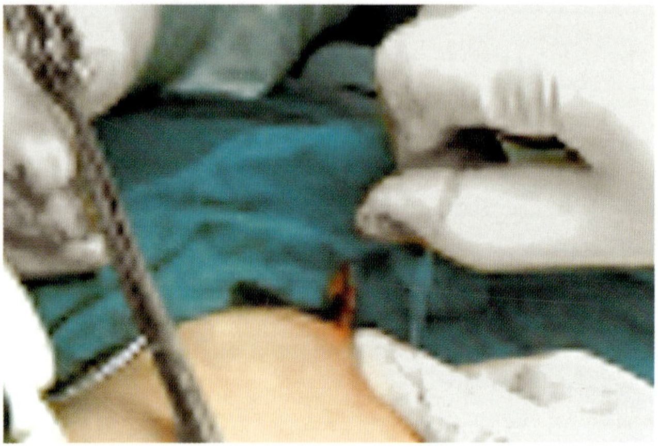

**Fig. 40.22:** Pulling of left tape

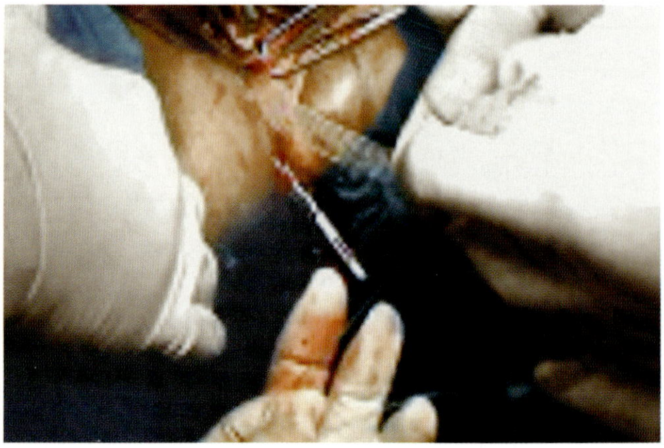

**Fig. 40.23:** Loading of the sutures of T-SUIT

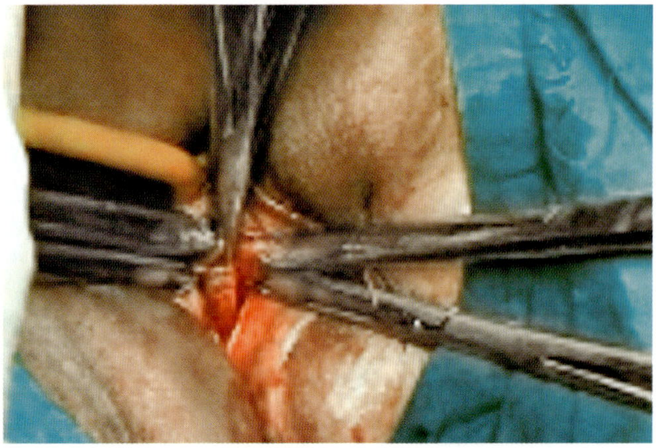

**Fig. 40.24:** Tension free positioning of T-SUIT with long artery forceps

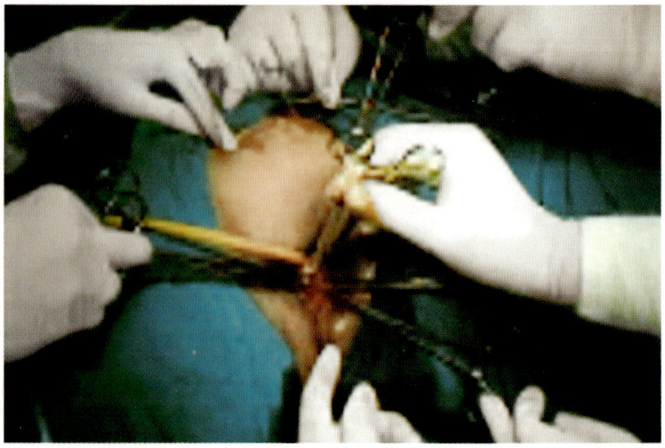

**Fig. 40.25:** Both tapes pulled abdominally

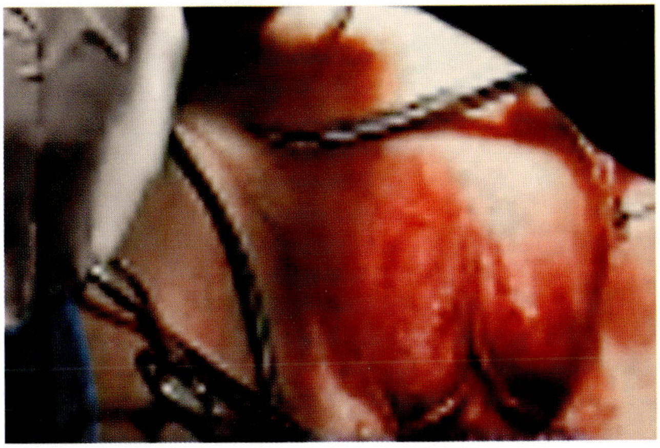

Fig. 40.26: Cutting of the tape close to skin

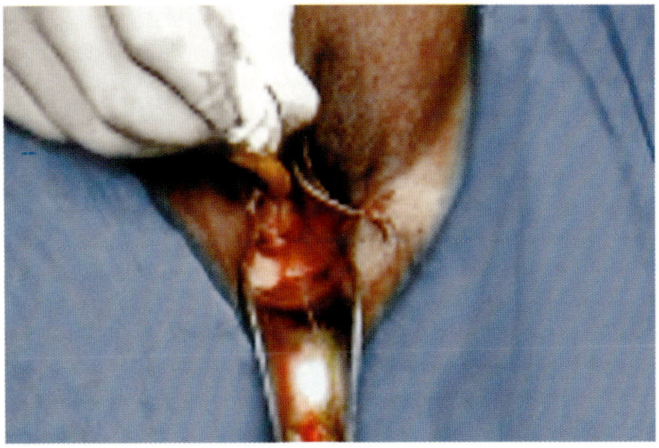

Fig. 40.27: Closure of vagina

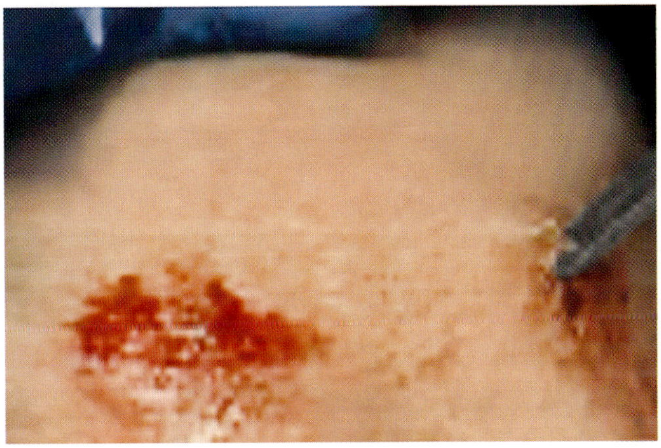

Fig. 40.28: Sites of tapes after cutting

## TVT ABBREVO™

The TVT Abbrevo™ continence system is a tension-free suburethral sling system devised for women with stress urinary incontinence.

The mesh transverses the obturator internus, obturator membrane, and obturator externus muscles. It supports the midurethra by acting as a buttress under it and allows the mobile bladder neck to descend and rotate with increased abdominal pressure, compressing the urethra under the sling.

### Instruments and Materials

- Gynecare TVT Abbrevo™ set comprising of two helical sheaths with helical passers; winged guide with insertion zone and a 12 cm polypropylene mesh with a placement loop at its center.
- Allis forceps, artery forceps.
- Scalpel.
- Skin marker.
- Scale.
- Weighted speculum.
- Metzenbaum scissors.

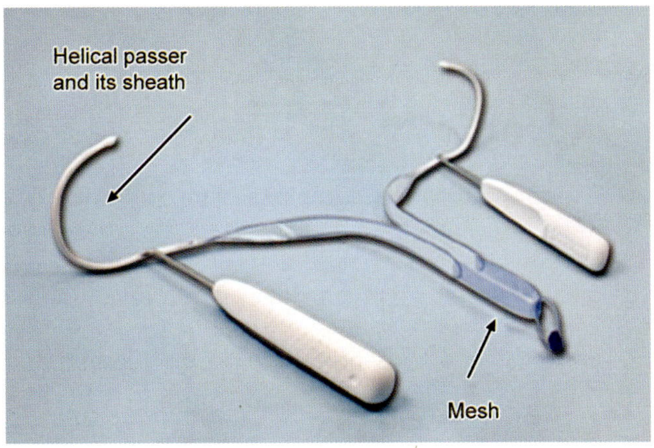


Fig. 40.29: TVT Abbrevo™ system

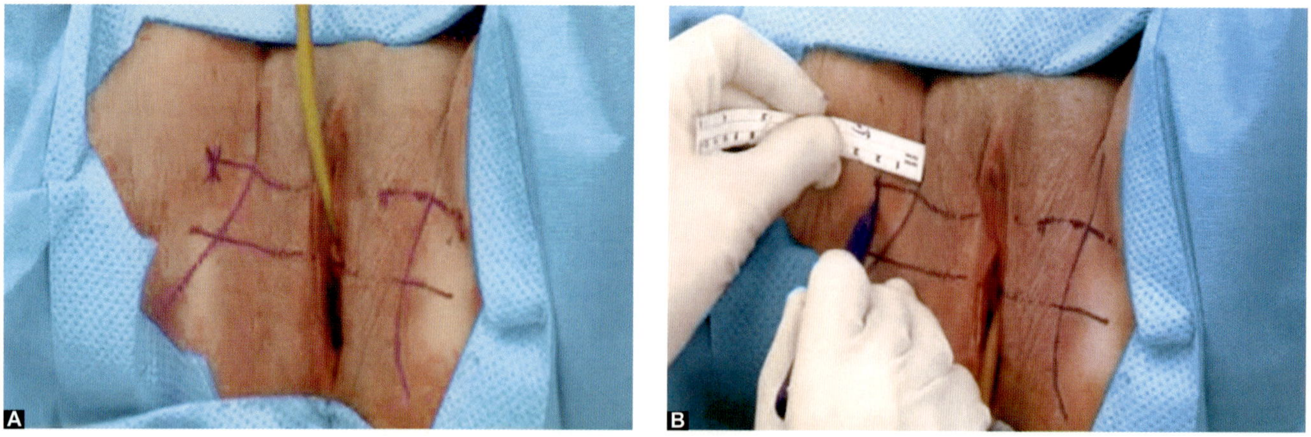

**Figs 40.30A and B:** Marking of skin lines and reference points: First line at level of external urethral meatus and second line 2 cm above and parallel to first. Reference points on second line, 2 cm lateral to thigh fold.

## Preoperative Evaluation

- Confirmation of diagnosis on table with full bladder. Bonney's and Marshall-Marchetti test may help to give prognostic value of surgery.
- Urine routine, culture and sensitivity.
- Urodynamic studies.

## Preoperative preparation

- It is preferred to do the procedure in immediate postmenstrual period.
- Insert a urethral catheter with aseptic precautions to keep the bladder empty.
- Anesthesia—can be carried out under local/regional/ general.

## Procedure

1. Tracing a horizontal line at the level of the urethral meatus. Then trace a second line 2 cm parallel and above to the first line.
2. Mark reference points on the second line 2 cm lateral to the thigh folds. (Incision is NOT to be made at this point during the procedure)
3. Posterior vaginal wall is retracted with speculum
4. Anterior vaginal wall held with Allis forceps for traction and vertical incision of about 1.5 cm is taken on the vagina 1 cm proximal to external urethral meatus.
5. Apply Allis forceps on both lips of the incision and with the help of curved scissors, dissect a tunnel in a direction towards the descending pubic ramus on either side.
6. Dissection is continued up to the ischio-pubic ramus into the obturator internus muscle, but taking care not to perforate the obturator membrane.
7. The winged guide is inserted along the dissection tract, avoiding perforation of the obturator membrane, and the insertion zone (3–4 cm) marked on the guide should remain visible.
8. The helical passer is then passed along the winged guide, following its curvature and is allowed to perforate the obturator membrane, but not beyond it.
9. Once the membrane has been perforated, the helical passer is rotated in a manner that its handle lies vertical in the midline.
10. Now proceed to rotate the helical passer towards the skin, staying close to the pubic ramus, until the skin is pierced.
11. Once the helical passer appears through the skin piercing, its sheath is grasped and held firmly. The urethral end of the sheath is stabilized and the helical passer and gently pulled out from within the sheath.
12. The sheath is then pulled through the skin incision so that the mesh is pulled through the tunnel on that side. Ensure that there is no twisting of the mesh during this step.
13. The similar steps are repeated on the other side and the placement loop of the mesh is brought to lie in the center (placement loop should be brought at the center). The mesh should lie in contact with the urethra.
14. The mesh sheath enclosing the two positioning lines is cut medial to the helical sheath on both sides and then is grasped with an artery forceps (without holding the positioning lines).
15. To adjust and tighten the mesh, place a scissor or a no. 8 Hegar dilator under the centre and then pull on either side for adjustment. (Cough test can be performed at this stage, which allows adjustment of the tape so that only a few drops of urine are lost during coughing.)

16. Once the adjustment has been made, the plastic sheaths are removed from both sides, without pulling the positioning lines.
17. The TVT Abbrevo™ system has a placement loop at the center of the mesh, which helps in adjustment of the mesh (loosening or tightening) as per surgeon's requirement.
18. Pulling both positioning lines on either side can do final minor adjustments for mesh placement. Once the final positioning has been done, pulling one end of the positioning line on both side will enable its removal.
19. The placement loop is then cut with scissors and the vaginal incision closed with no 1 Vicryl continuous interlocking sutures.

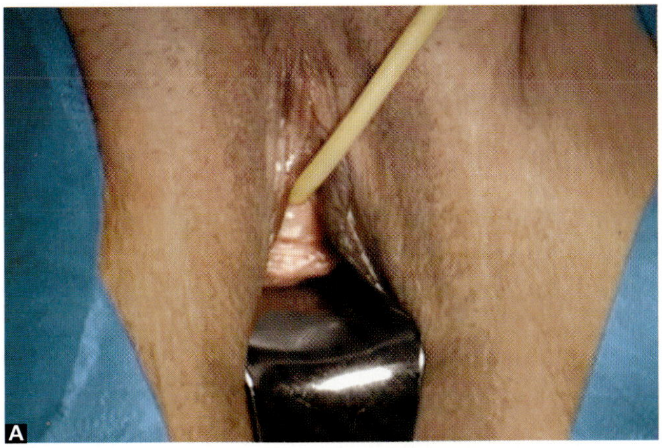


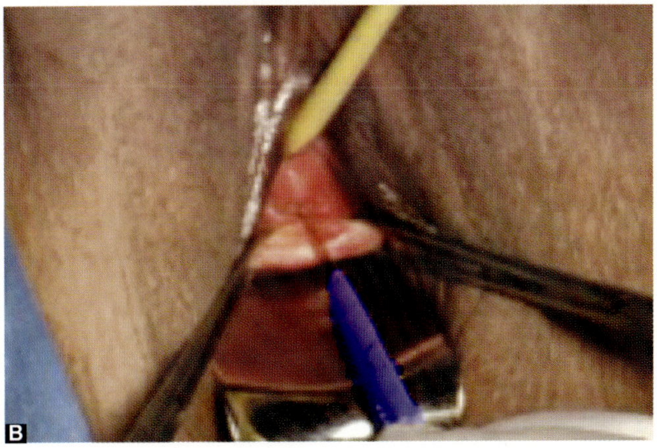


**Fig. 40.31A and B:** Posterior vaginal wall retracted and an incision made on the anterior vaginal wall, 1 cm proximal to the external urethral meatus. Traction is applied with Allis forceps

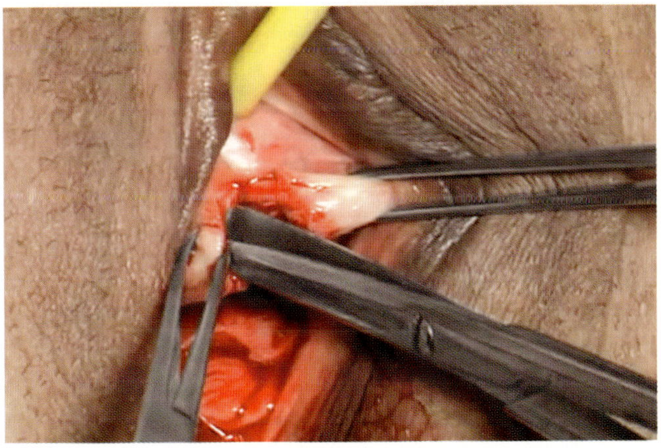

**Fig. 40.32:** Tunnel is dissected in a direction towards the descending pubic ramus on either side with a curved scissor, taking care not to perforate the obturator membrane

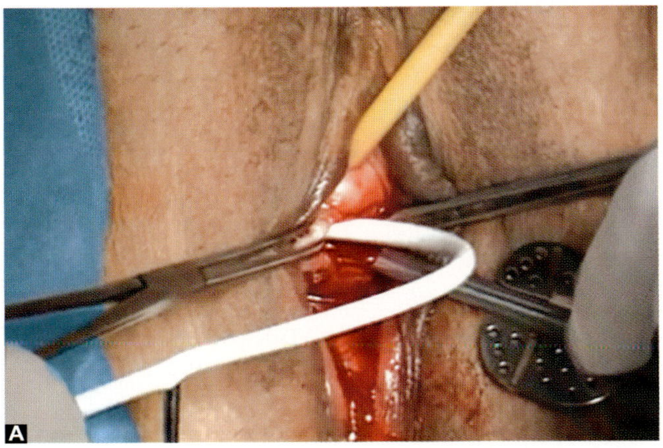


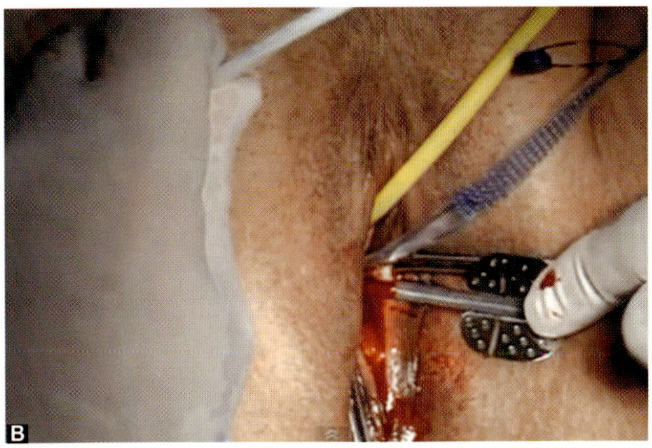


**Figs 40.33A and B:** Winged guide is inserted along the tunnel without perforating obturator membrane. The helical passer with sheath is passed over the guide and obturator membrane is pierced with it. The passer is removed from the sheath after rotating it in the midline

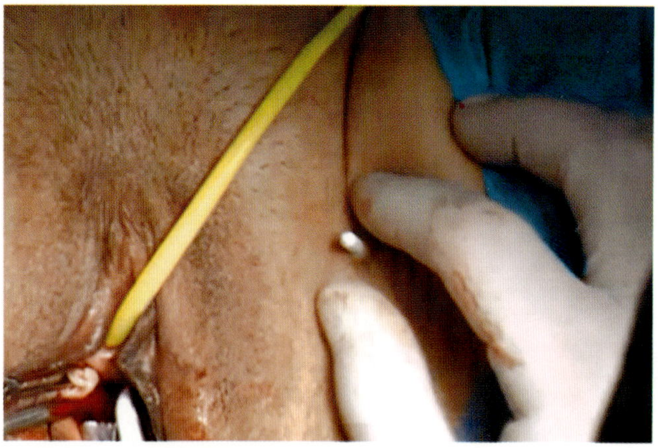

**Fig. 40.34:** Similar procedure is repeated on the other side

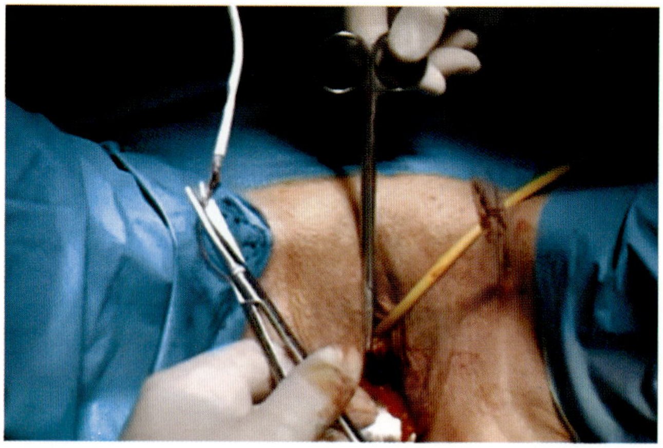

**Fig. 40.35:** Mesh centralized by pulling the positioning lines on either side

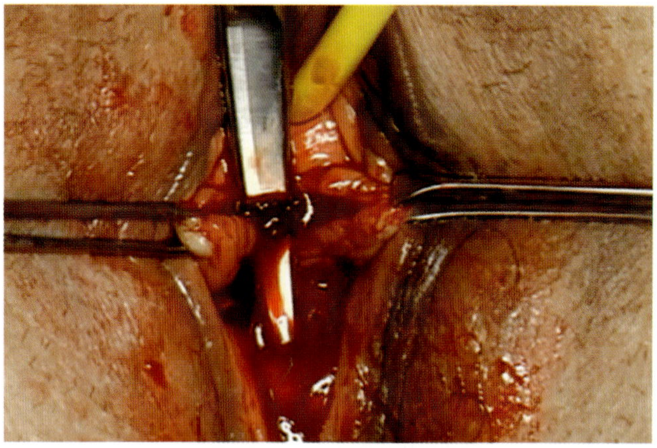

**Fig. 40.36:** Mesh is then appropriately tightened keeping Metzenbaum scissors as a guide

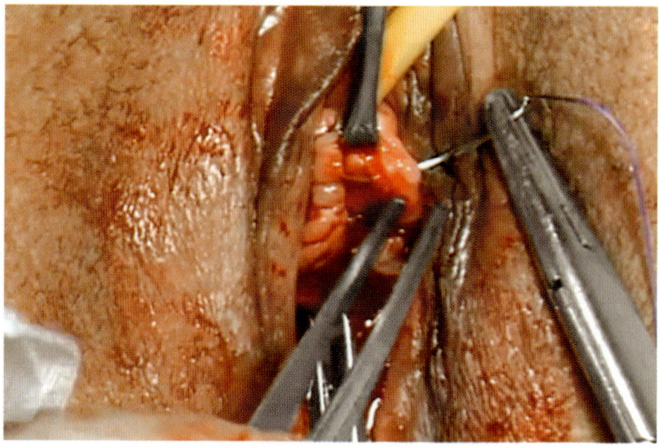

**Fig. 40.37:** Vaginal incision closed using interlocking continuous no.1 Vicryl sutures

Section

5

# Unusual Cases

Chapter

41

# Uterus Didelphys with Abnormally Placed Ovaries

*Sunita R Tandulwadkar*

A 30-year-old female with primary infertility came to Ruby Hall IVF/Endoscopy Center for evaluation.

TVS revealed uterus didelphys and inability to visualize the ovaries. Transabdominal USG revealed huge multicystic ovaries of approximately 10 × 15 cm each in lumbar region (as she had taken 3 cycles of clomiphene citrate outside). Findings were confirmed on MRI.

Patient was evaluated laparohysteroscopically—Uterus didelphys confirmed. Both the ovaries were found in paracolic gutters and were multicystic (cysts ranging from 4-6 cm). Cysts were punctured. Ovaries could not be mobilized or transfixed in the pelvic region due to extremely short infundibulopelvic ligaments.

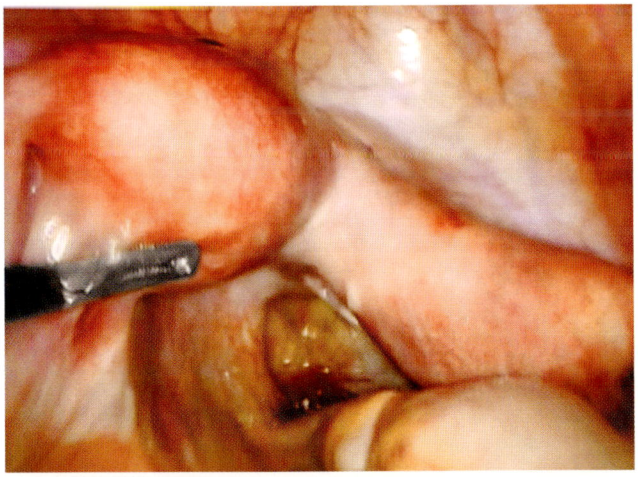

**Fig. 41.1:** Didelphic uterus with absent ovaries in pelvis

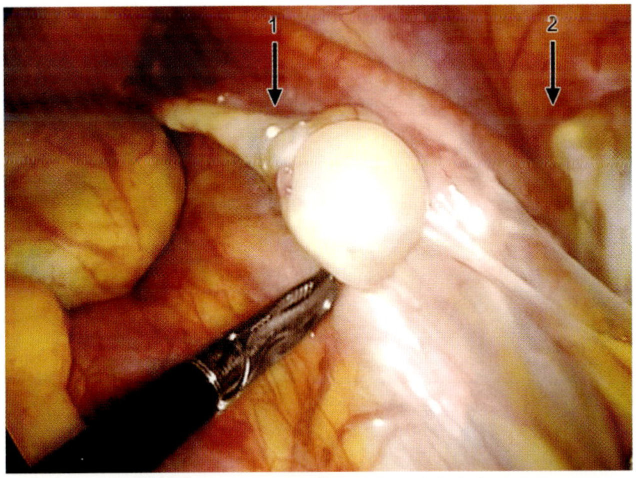



**Fig. 41.2:** 1 → small cyst at pelvic brim
2 → remaining right ovary in the lumbar region

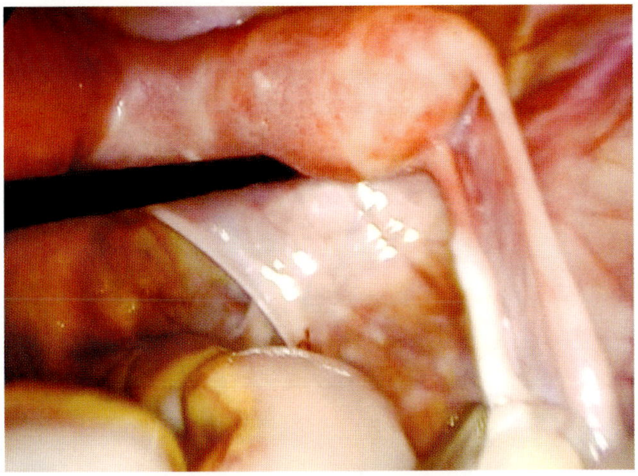

**Fig. 41.3:** Lengthened right ovarian ligament

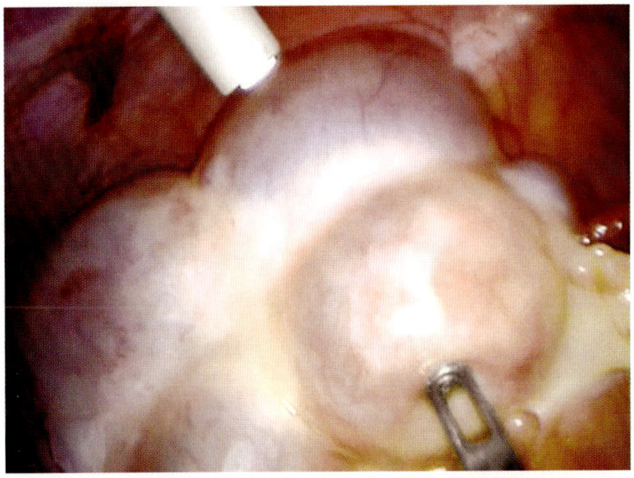

**Fig. 41.4:** Panaromic view of left ovary

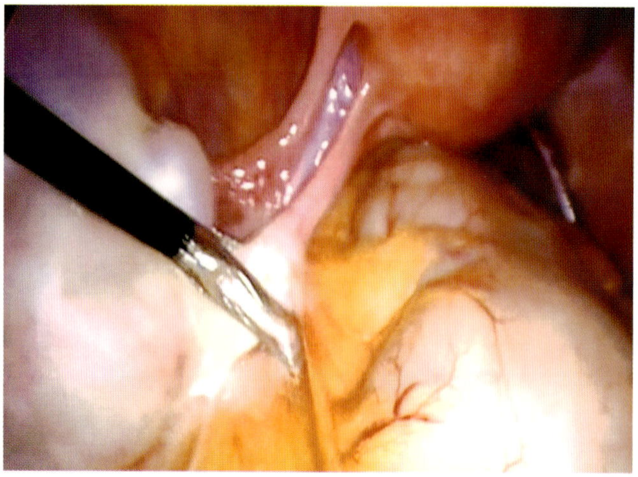

**Fig. 41.5:** Left ovary in left paracolic gutter

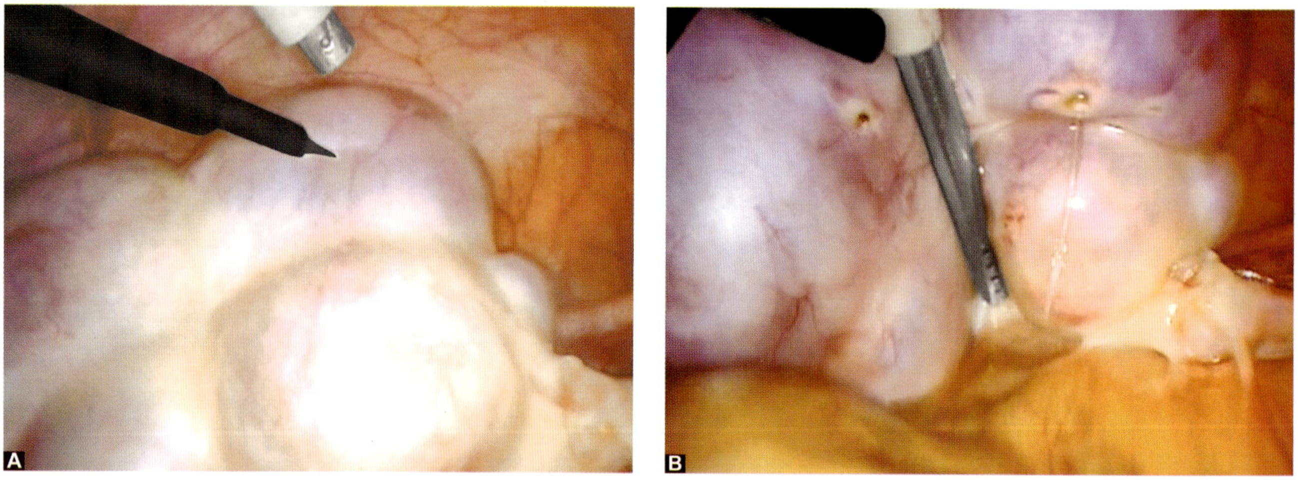

**Figs 41.6A and B:** Drilling of cysts

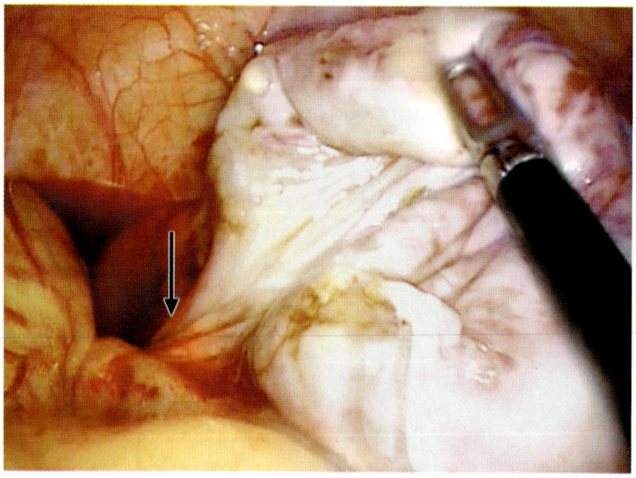

**Fig. 41.7:** Short infundibulopelvic ligament

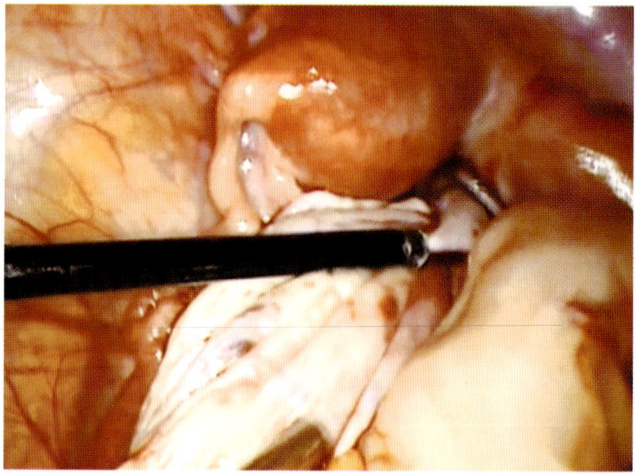

**Fig. 41.8:** Collapsed left ovary

Chapter

42

# Case of Chronic Twisted Adnexa

*Sunita R Tandulwadkar*

A 30-year-old female had torsion of right adnexa. Patient refused surgical intervention and was managed with painkillers and serial USG and color Doppler studies. Over a period of time, the hydrosalpinx resolved and the ovary came back to normal size. But throughout, she had dragging pain in the lower abdomen. After 4 months, patient gave consent for laparoscopic evaluation.

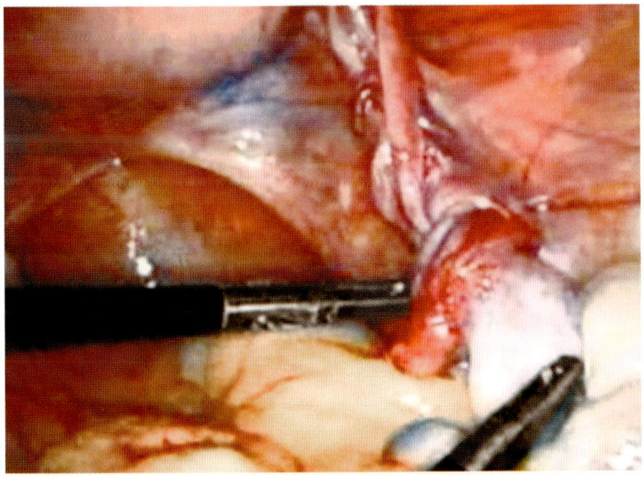

**Fig. 42.1:** Twisted right adnexa

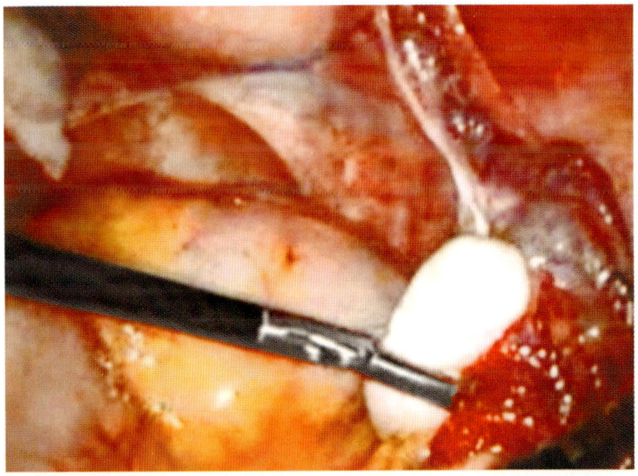

**Fig. 42.2:** Detorsion done. Note the lengthening of the right ovarian ligament

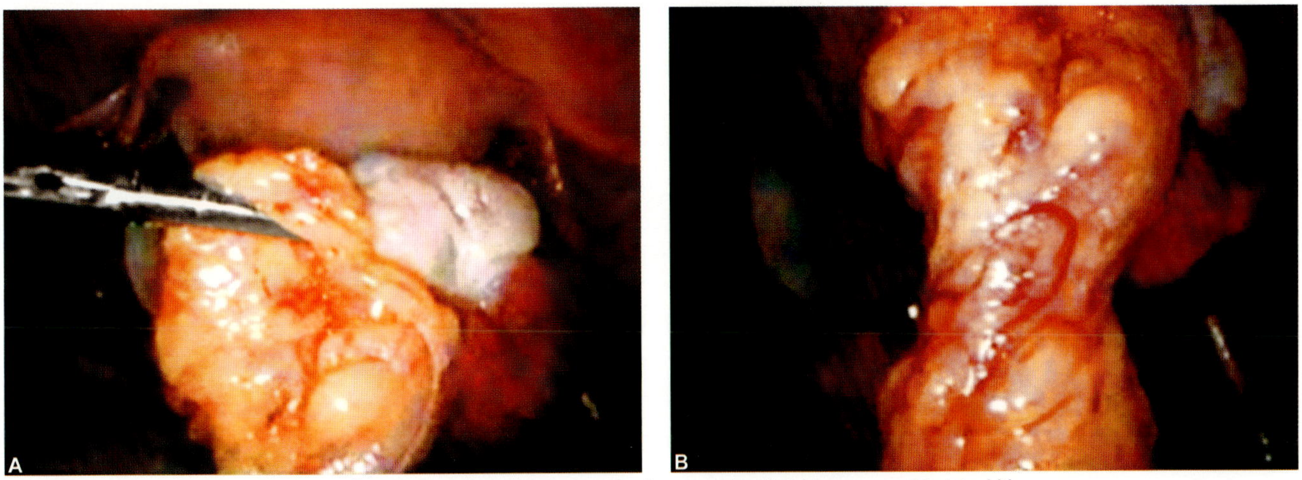

**Figs 42.3A and B:** Omentum adherent to the lower pole of right ovary and twisted like a rope.

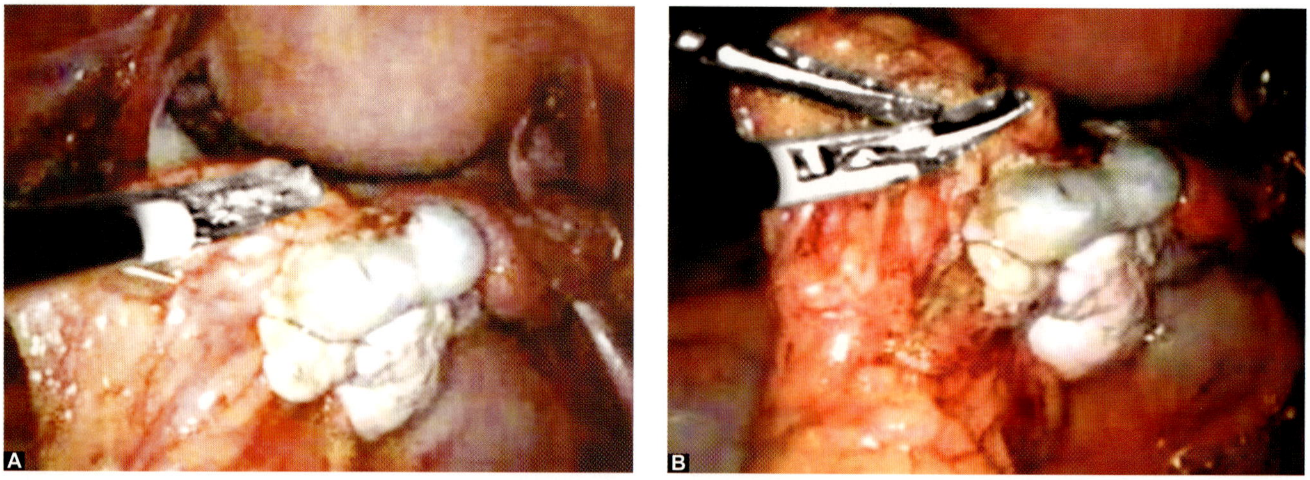

**Figs 42.4A and B:** Omentum released from the lower pole of the ovary, keeping small portion adherent to it, to be utilized later for anchoring it back to its ligament

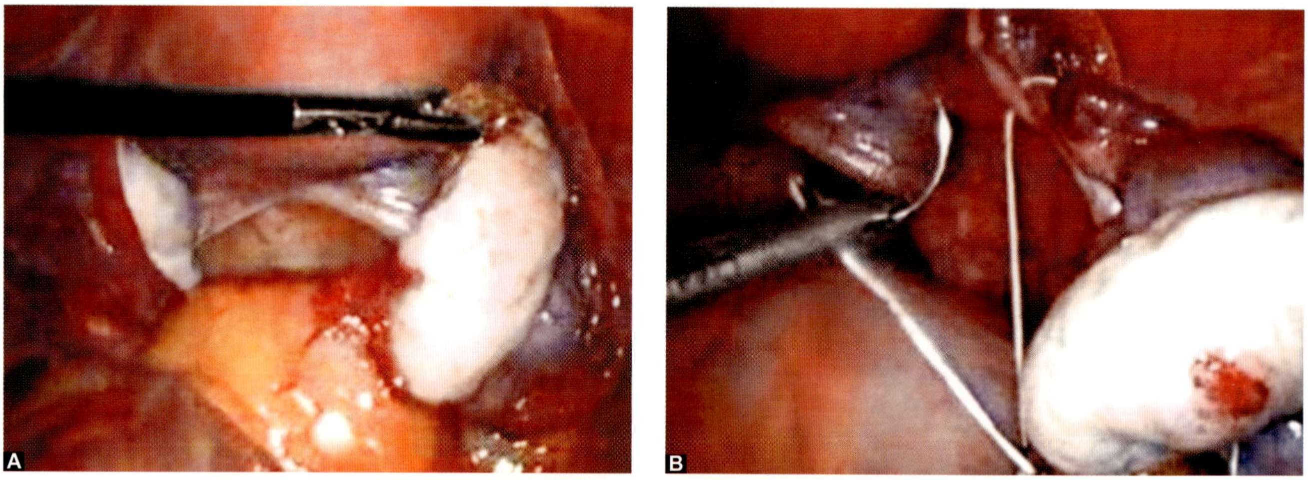

**Figs 42.5A and B:** Ovary taken back in pelvis and sutured with nonabsorbable suture material—Gortex

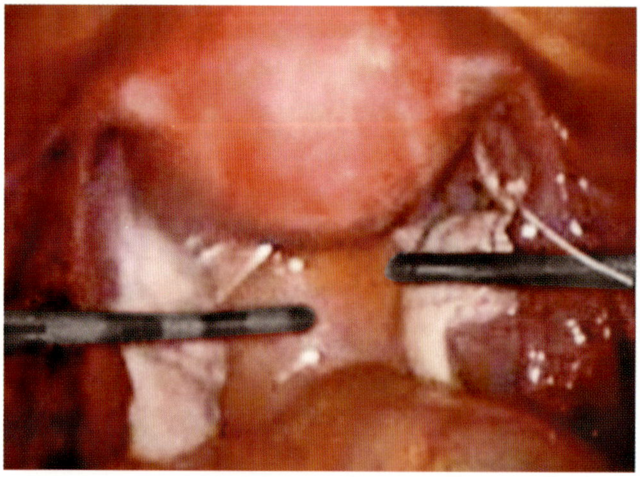

**Fig. 42.6:** End result

Chapter

43

# 27-Year-old Female with Bad Obstetric History with Unicornuate Uterus

*Sunita R Tandulwadkar, Pooja Lodha*

A 27-year-old female has a bad obstetric history with recurrent abortions/preterm deliveries between 12 and 24 weeks, last 2 abortions at 24 weeks inspite of cervical encirclage. She was diagnosed to have unicornuate uterus. The only alternative for her was to increase the intrauterine capacity.

So we decided to perform metroplasty on her so as to convert tubular cavity into triangular one.

Patient was put on Tab Premarin 1.250 mg, 6 weeks + Duphaston 20 mg for latter 4 weeks.

Second look hysteroscopy was performed after 6 weeks to see the outcome of surgery.

It showed very good cavity with increasead intrauterine capacity.

Patient conceived after 4 months and could continue pregnancy till 35 weeks.

We have performed 7 cases like this and quite satisfied with the results.

This surgery is not recommended for infertility.

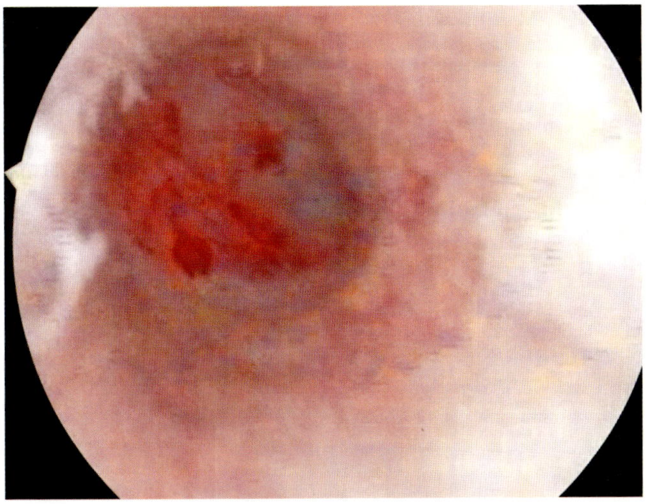

**Fig. 43.1:** Unicornuate uterus

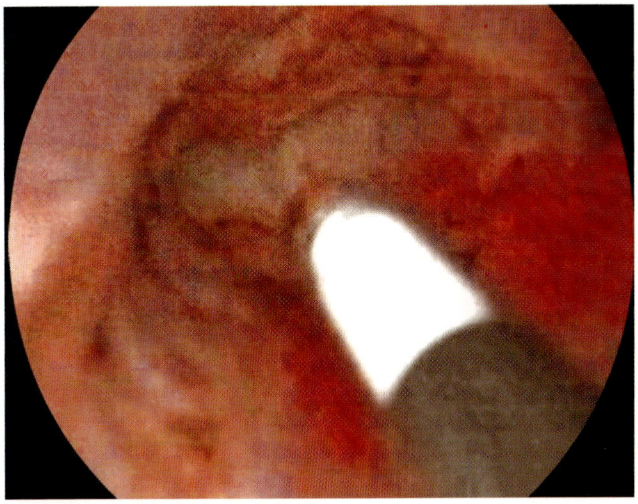

**Fig. 43.2:** Metroplasty done with versa point so as to increase intrauterine capacity

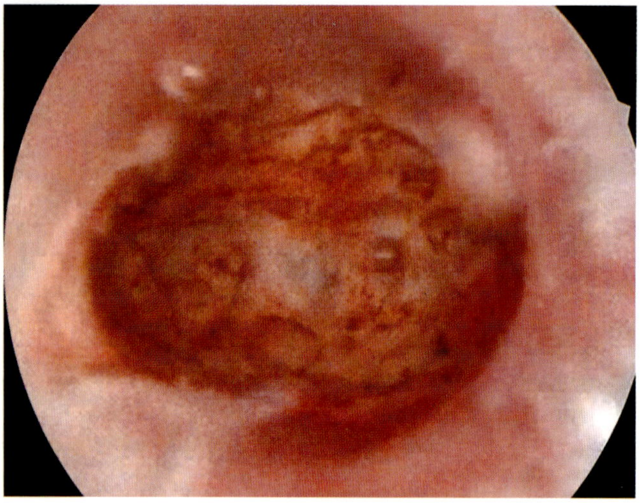

**Fig. 43.3:** Good cavity formed as an end result

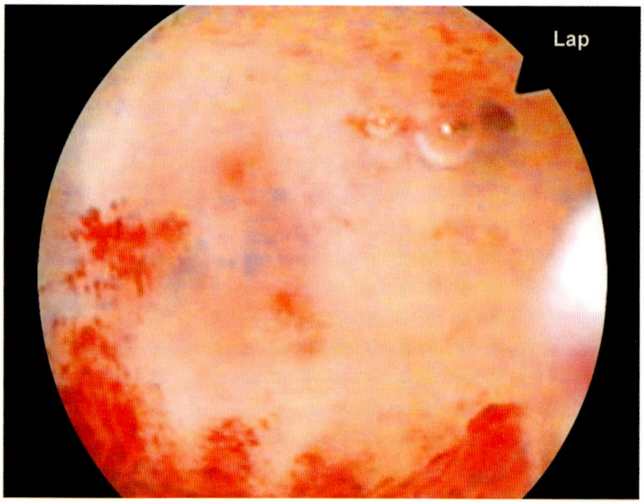


**Fig. 43.4:** Second look hysteroscopy done after 6 weeks

Chapter

# 44

# Case of Ovarian Fibroma

*Prakash Trivedi, Sunita R Tandulwadkar*

A patient schedule for open myomectomy and laparoscopy done in view of age and future fertility. A large solid ovarian mass of 12.3 cm was identified and the other ovary was normal. Oophorectomy was done with 5 mm vessel sealing device. Specimen removed by electronic morcellator and histopath revealed ovarian fibroma. Postoperative period uneventful.

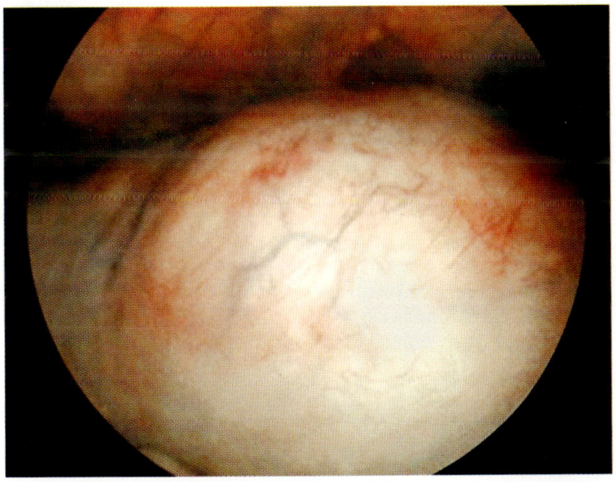

**Fig. 44.1:** Large pelvic mass

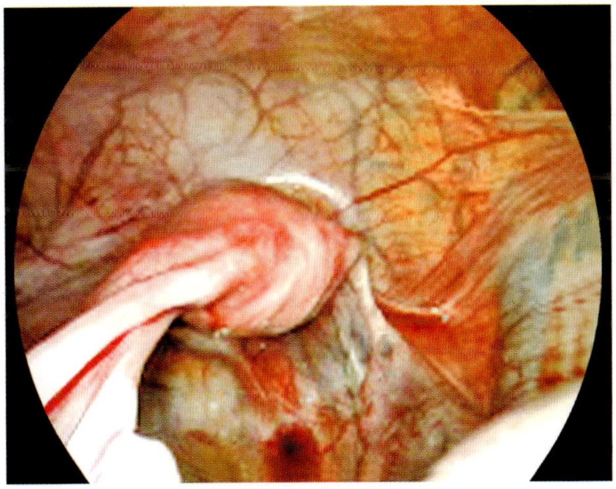

**Fig. 44.2:** Small uterus seen

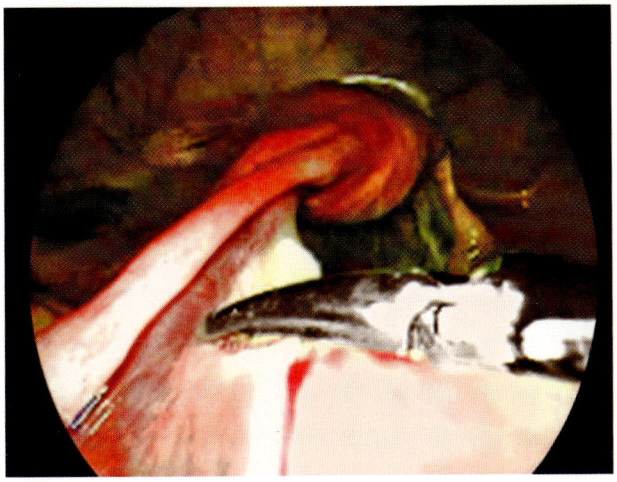

**Fig. 44.3:** Base of left ovarian mass

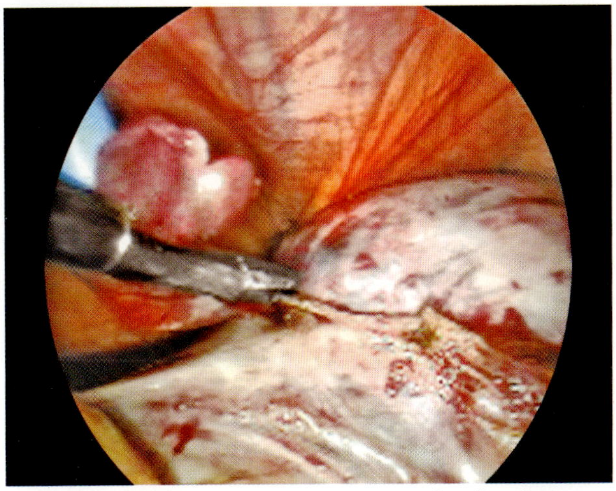

**Fig. 44.4:** Mass separated by 5 mm vessel sealing device

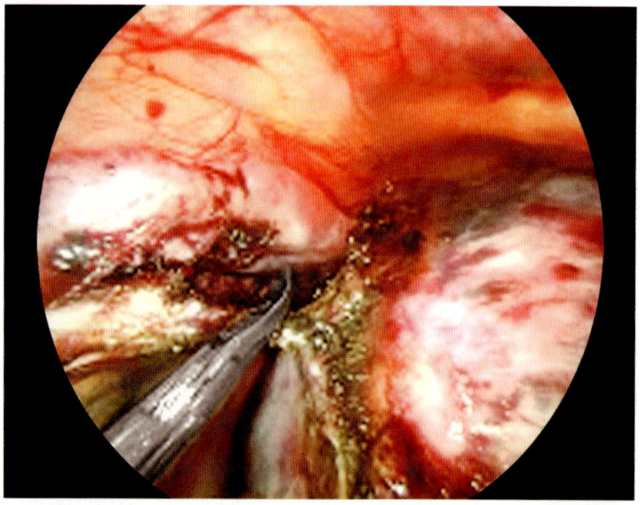

**Fig. 44.5:** Mass separated by 5 mm vessel sealing device

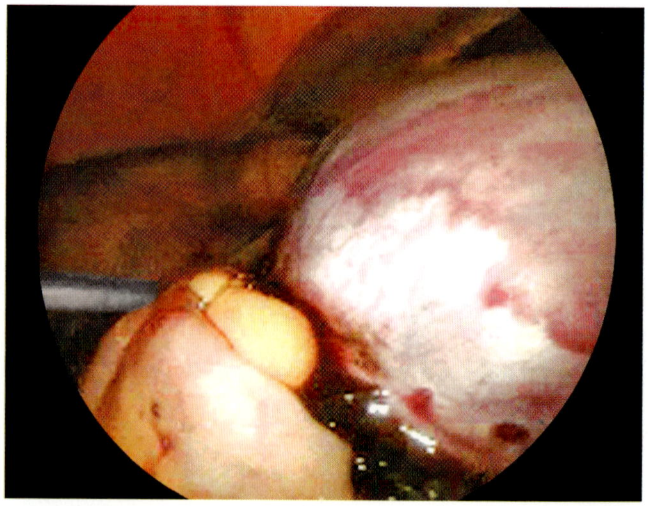

**Fig. 44.6:** Ovarian mass detached

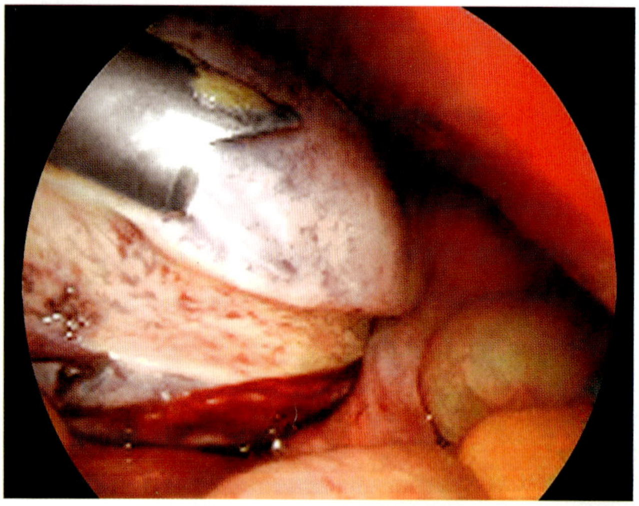

**Fig. 44.7:** Morcellation of ovarian mass

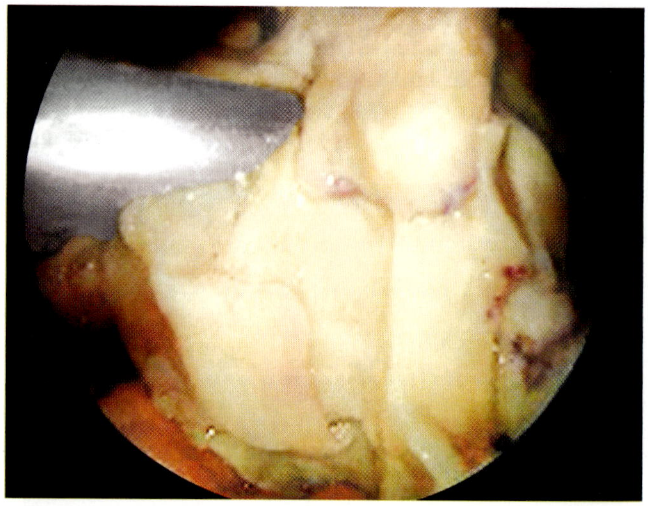

**Fig. 44.8:** Last part of morcellation

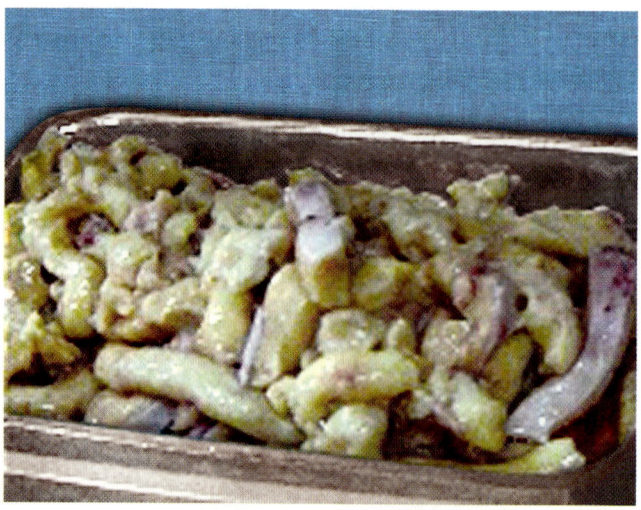

**Fig. 44.9:** Morcellated pieces of ovarian mass

# Laparoscopic Excision of an Ovarian Fibroma in a 16-year-old girl

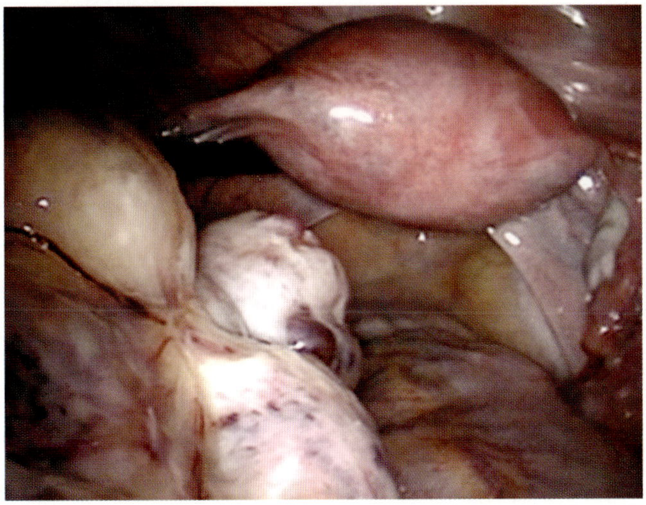

**Fig. 44.10:** Examination of pelvic cavity

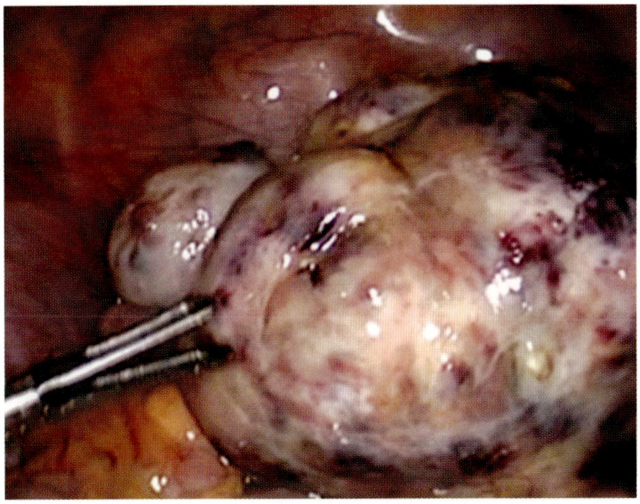

**Fig. 44.11:** Large ovarian fibroma of left ovary

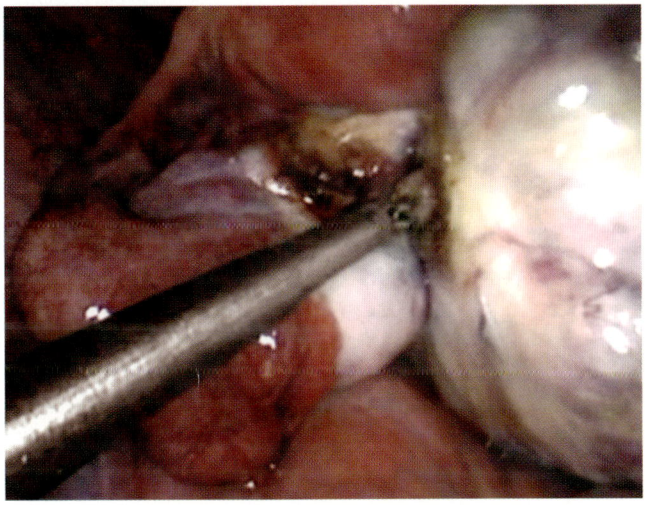

**Fig. 44.12:** Excision of mass from ovary taking care not to cauterize the ovarian blood supply

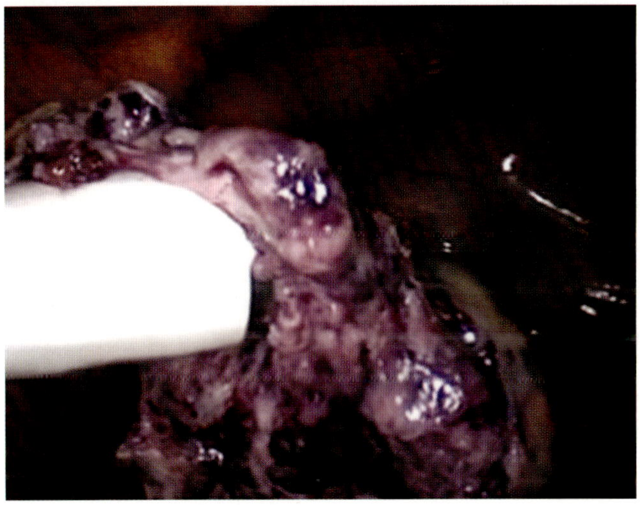

**Fig. 44.13:** Morcellation in progress

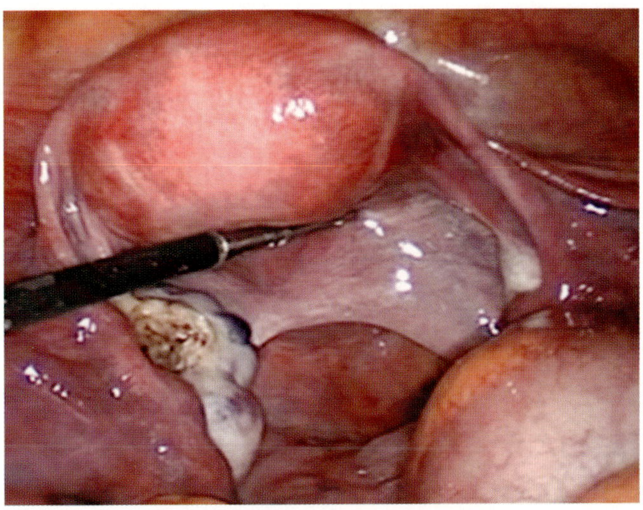

**Fig. 44.14:** End result: Clean cavity

Chapter

45

# Laparoscopy for Benign Uterine, Tubal and Ovarian Pathologies in Adolescent Age Group

*Sunita R Tandulwadkar, Nirzari Mangeshikar*

Laparoscopy has now been widely accepted as the most minimally invasive technique to treat a multitude of pelvic pathologies. It is a safe, less invasive and a feasible method to treat benign uterine, tubal and ovarian pathologies even in the adolescent age group.

In this young set of patients aged 10 to 19 years, laparoscopy is still feasible and does offer many advantages such as:

- Good hemostasis due to sealing of blood vessels prior to cutting the pathological tissue.
- Minimal handling of unaffected surrounding tissues and organs.
- Magnified view by laparoscopic camera, enabling the surgeon to have precise dissection planes so as to preserve normal tissue, keeping in mind the future fertility of these young patients.
- Less post-operative discomfort, which allows early ambulation and thus adhesion prevention.
- Less importantly, it offers more cosmetic scars.

## PRE-OPERATIVE PREPARATIONS

- A good imaging study to know the exact extent and location of the pathology.
- Good bowel preparation.
- Written informed consent should be taken regarding the possibility of uterine manipulation, as most of these are young, unmarried girls.

## INTRA-OPERATIVE CONSIDERATIONS

- Basic surgical principle remains the same.
- Entry should be made with a Veress needle, as patients in this age group tend to have lean body mass.
- Uterine manipulation should be preferably avoided.
- Try to use 3 mm instruments whenever possible.
- Minimal handling of the normal tissues and organs to avoid edema and inflammation.
- Thorough irrigation and lavage of the pelvic cavity to clean any debris and blood clots which can act as a focus of infection and then future adhesions.

## POST-OPERATIVE CONSIDERATIONS

- Early ambulation to prevent any adhesion formation over raw areas.

Following are a series of cases of various benign uterine, tubal and ovarian pathologies in adolescent girls that were treated laparoscopically.

Note that uterine manipulation was not done during any of the procedures.

## Laparoscopic Excision of a Symptomatic Adenomyoma of Uterus in an 18-year-old Girl

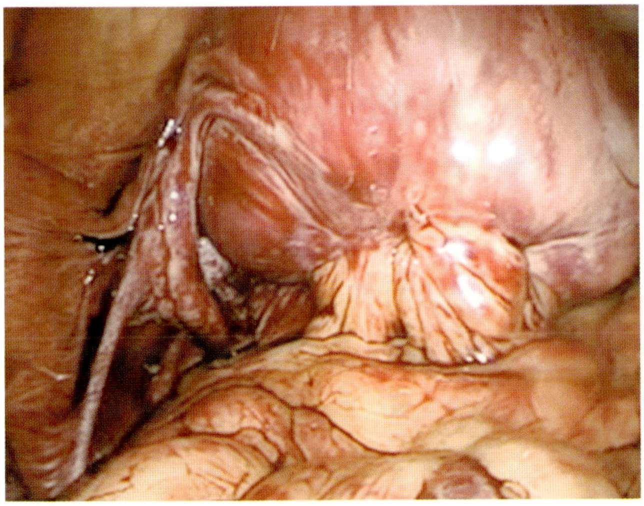

**Fig. 45.1:** Extensive bowel adhesions to posterior uterine wall released

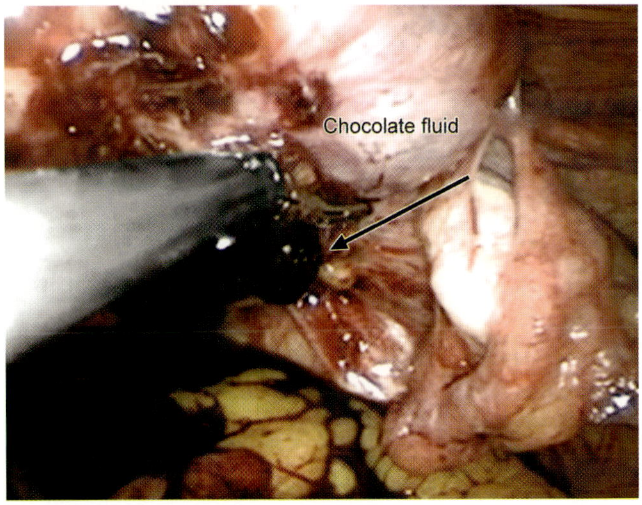


**Fig. 45.2:** Horizontal incision taken over adenomyoma; chocolate fluid drained

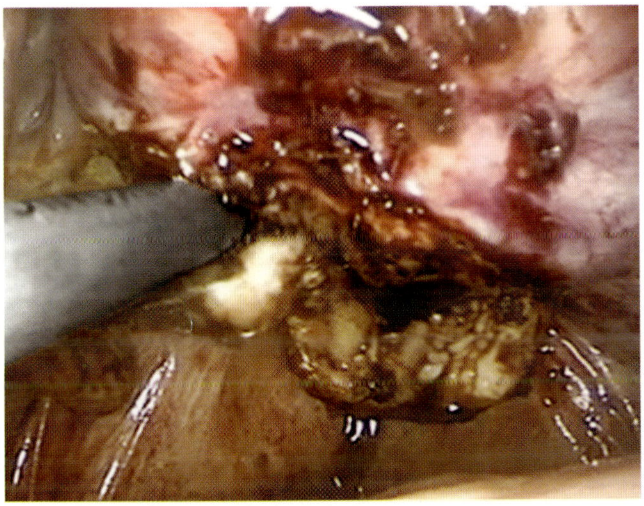

**Fig. 45.3:** Excision of adenomyoma in progress

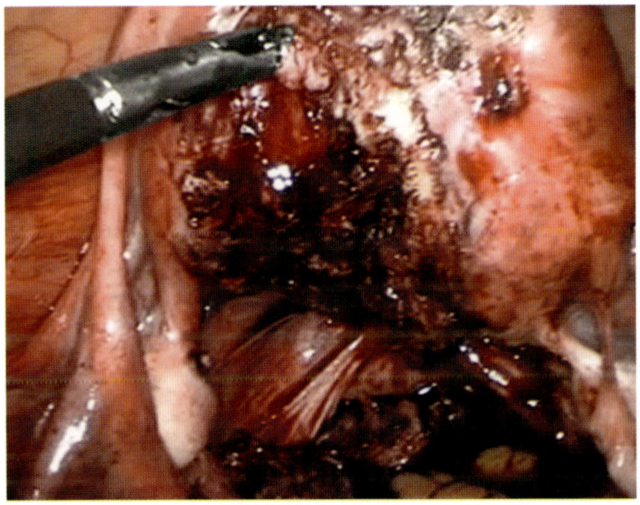

**Fig. 45.4:** Bed of the adenomyoma

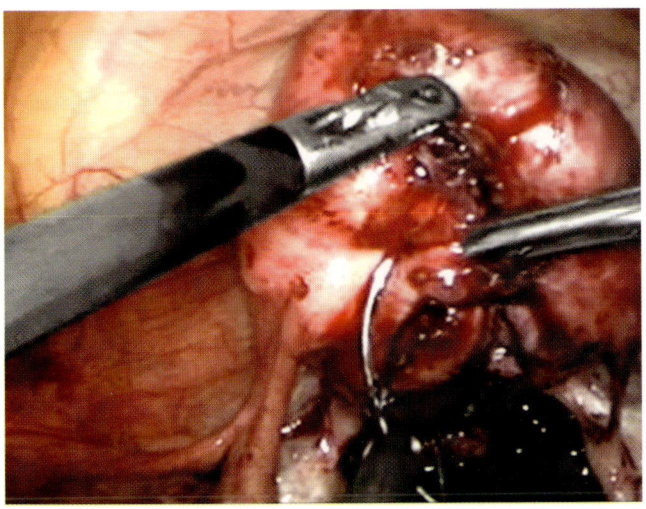

**Fig. 45.5:** Morcellation of specimen

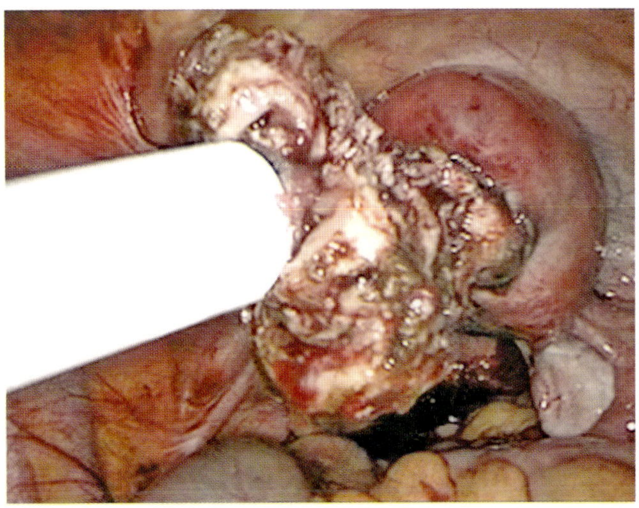

**Fig. 45.6:** Suturing done vertically

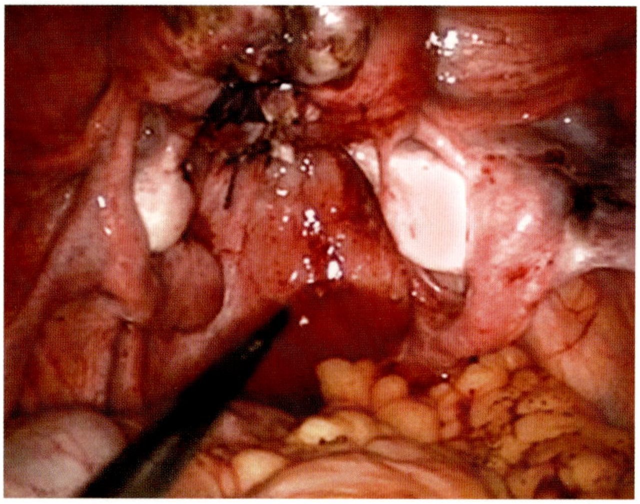

**Fig. 45.7:** Thorough irrigation and lavage given

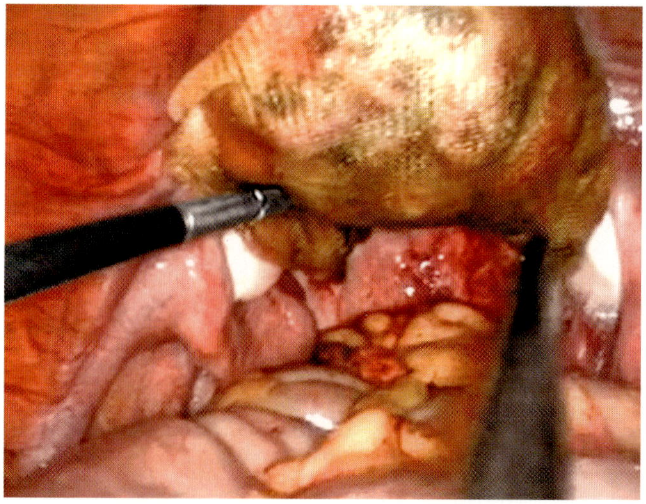

**Fig. 45.8:** Adhesion barrier placed to prevent future bowel adhesions. End result: Clean cavity

## Laparoscopic Excision of a Large Uterine Myoma in a 17-year-old Girl

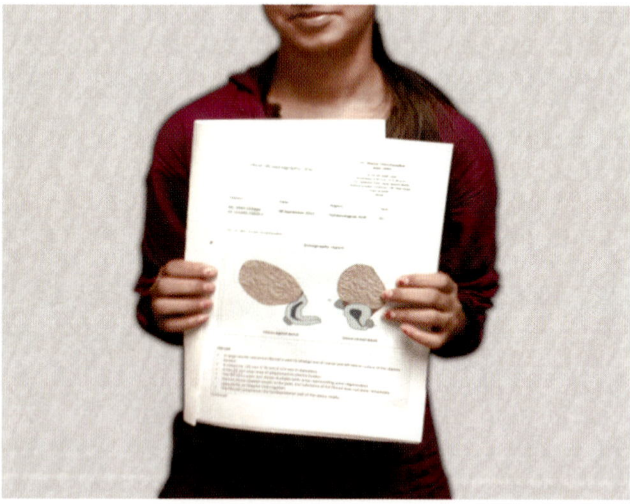

**Fig. 45.9:** Patient with sonography

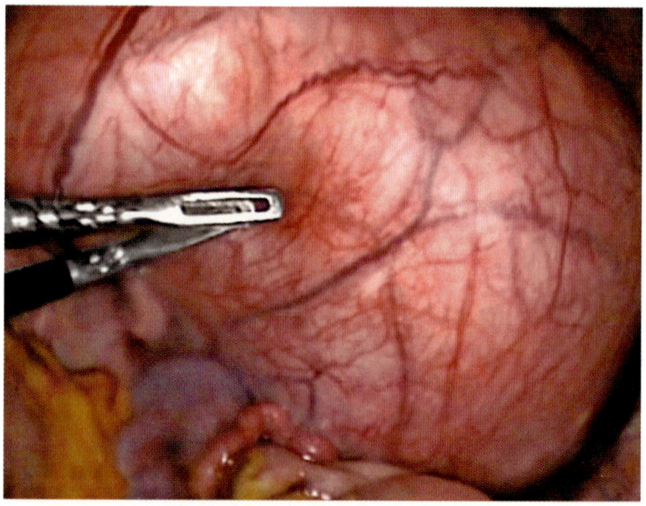

**Fig. 45.10:** Examination of myoma

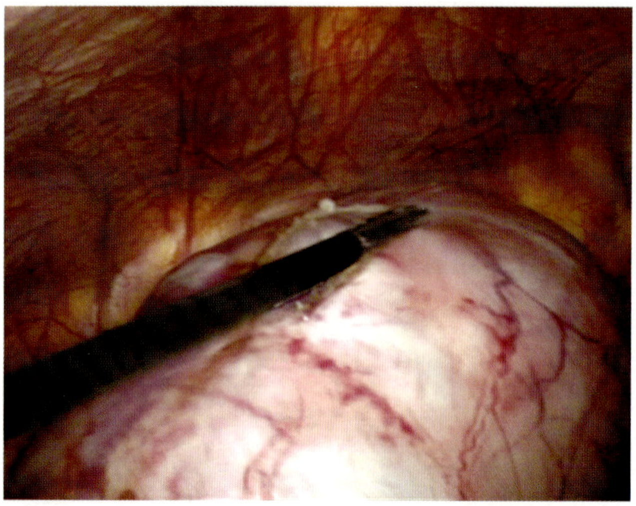

**Fig. 45.11:** Incision over myoma with enseal

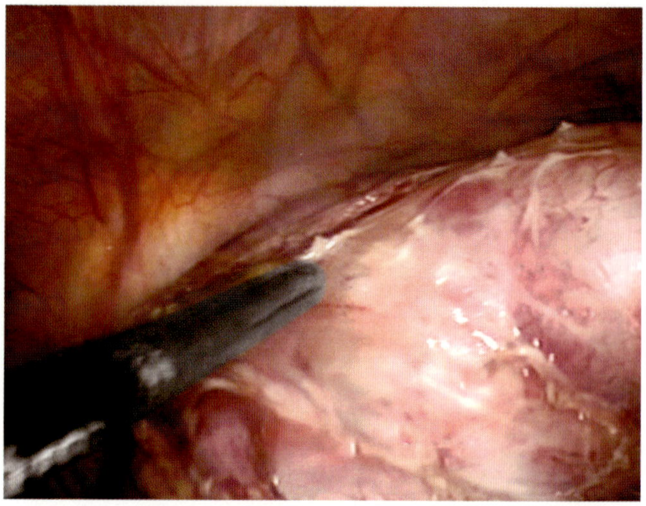

**Fig. 45.12:** Enucleation in progress

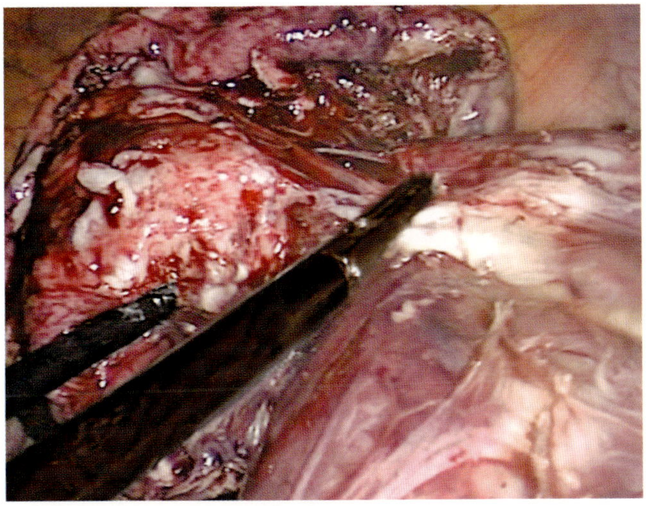

**Fig. 45.13:** Excision of base

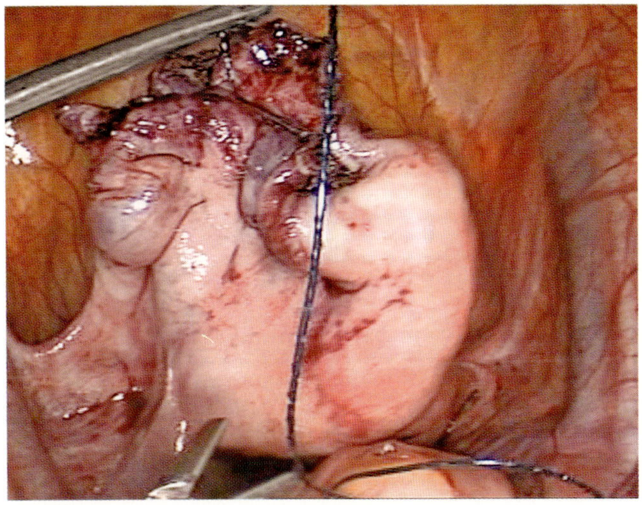

**Fig. 45.14:** Suturing the uterus

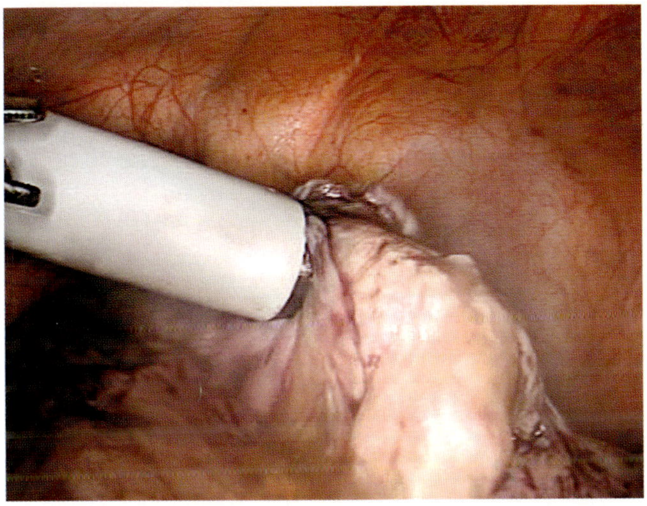

**Fig. 45.15:** Morcellation in progress

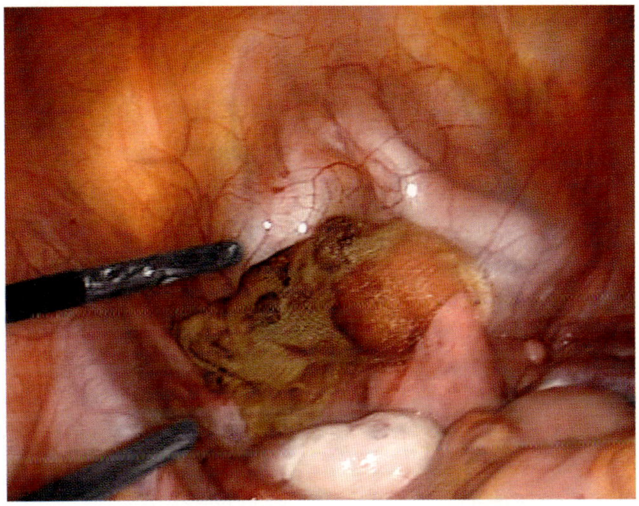

**Fig. 45.16:** End result: Clean cavity

## Laparoscopic Excision of a Non-communicating Functional Rudimentary Horn of Uterus in a 16-year-old Girl

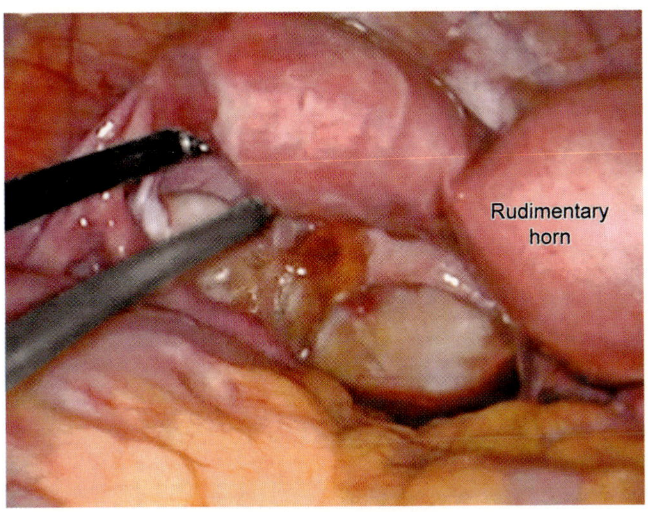


**Fig. 45.17:** Examination

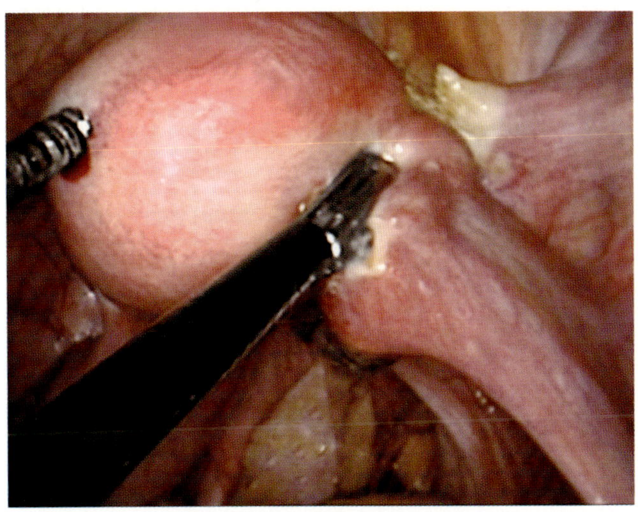

**Fig. 45.18:** Excision of medial side

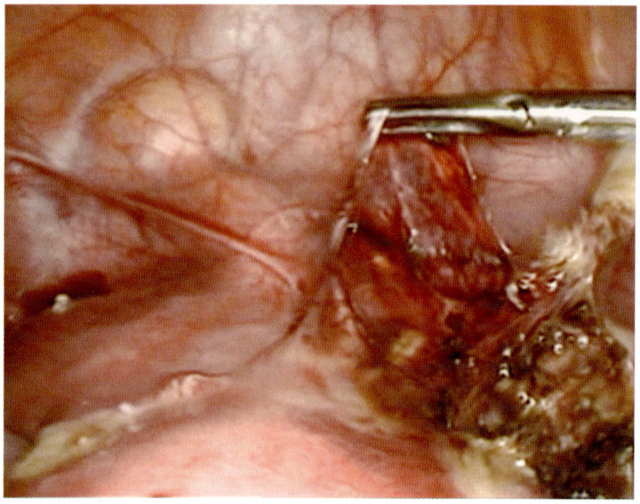

Fig. 45.19: Bladder dissection

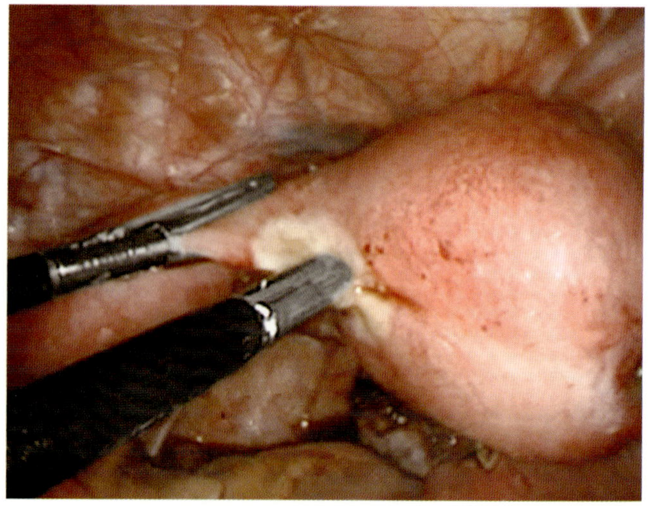

Fig. 45.20: Excision of lateral side

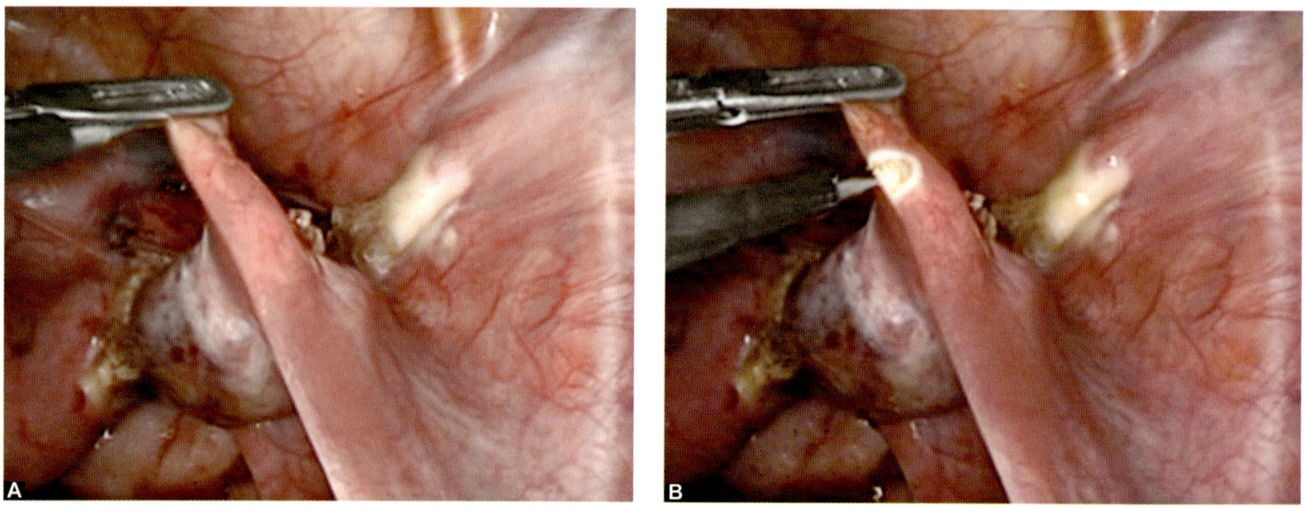

Figs 45.21A and B: Salpingectomy done with monopolar needle to avoid any compromise to the ovarian blood supply

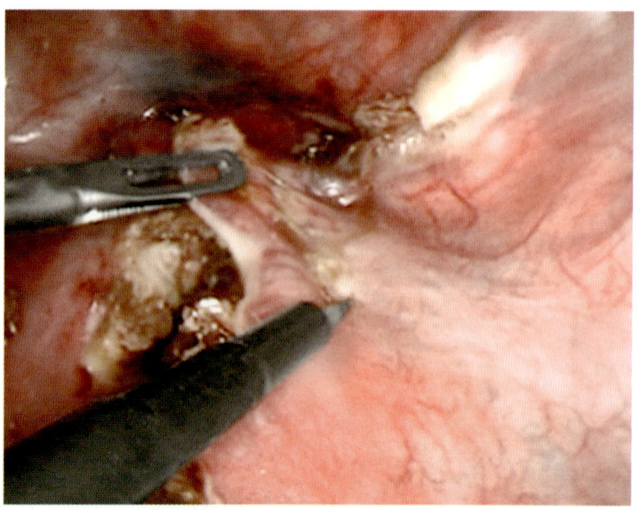

Fig. 45.22: Salpingectomy in progress

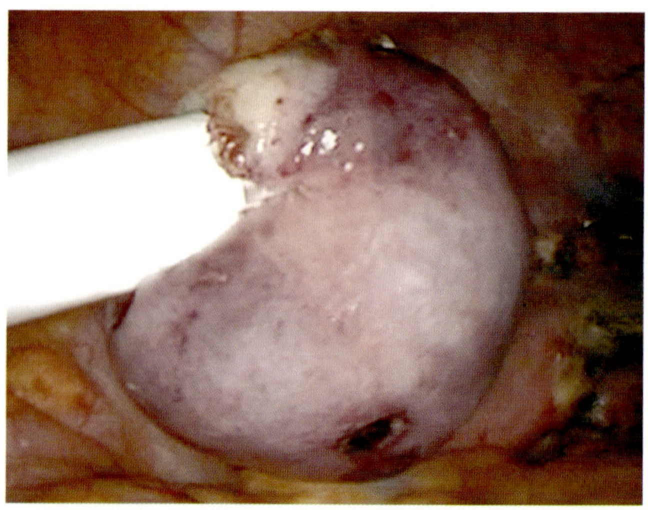

Fig. 45.23: Morcellation

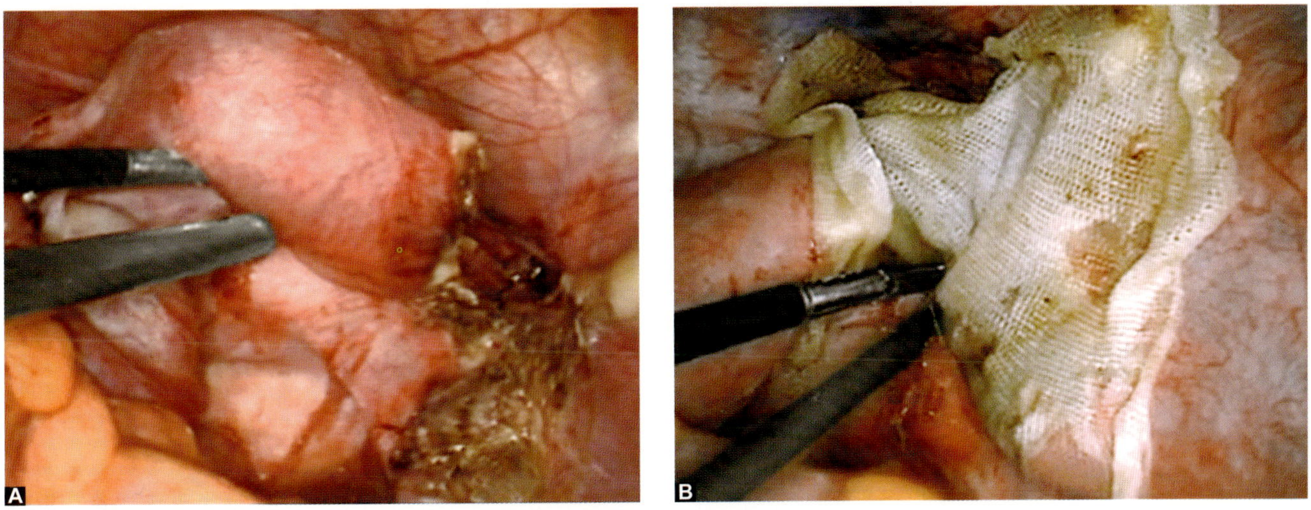

**Figs 45.24A and B:** End result

## Laparoscopic Management of Twisted Hydrosalpinx in a 17-year-old Girl

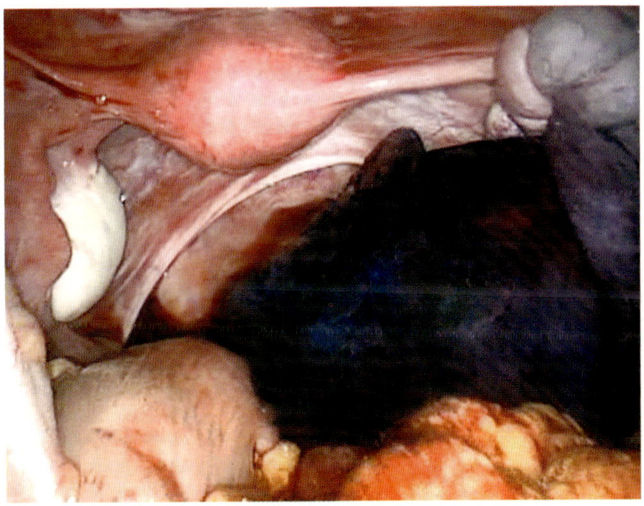

**Fig. 45.25:** Twisted hydrosalpinx in young girl, which probably became a hematosalpinx after torsion

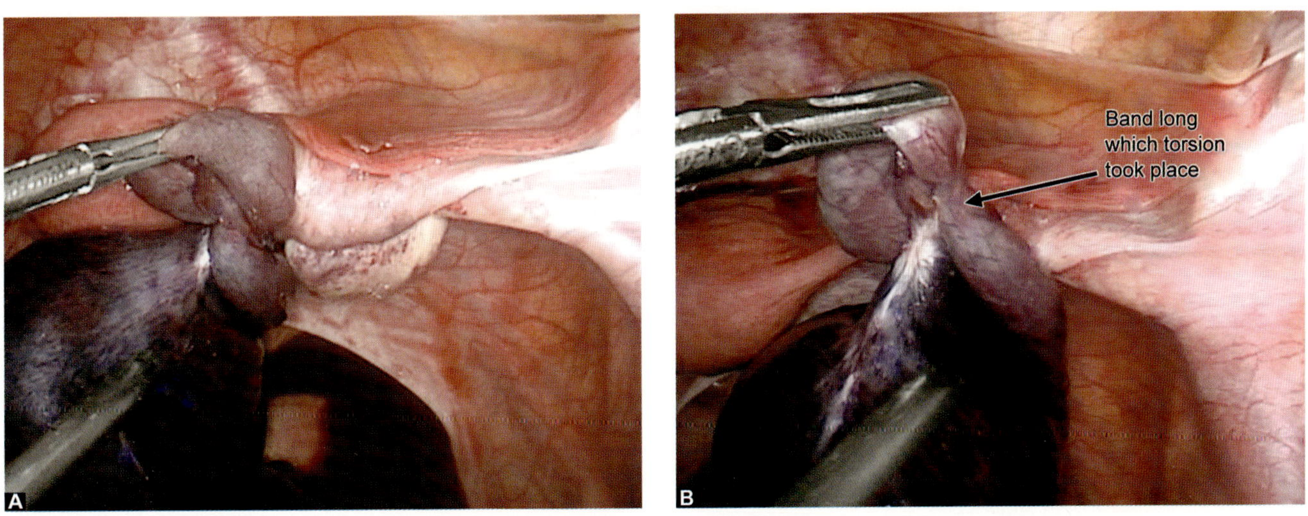


**Figs 45.26A and B:** De-torsion done and salpingectomy performed. Specimen retrieved with EndoBag

## Laparoscopic Excision of A Large Endometrioma In An 18-year-old Girl

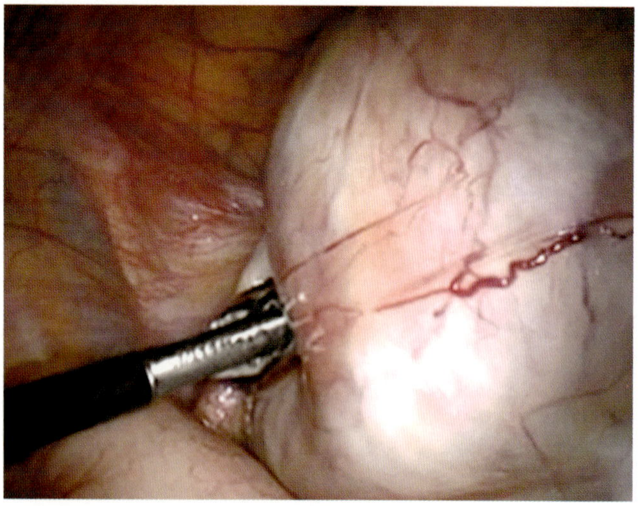

Fig. 45.27: Examination

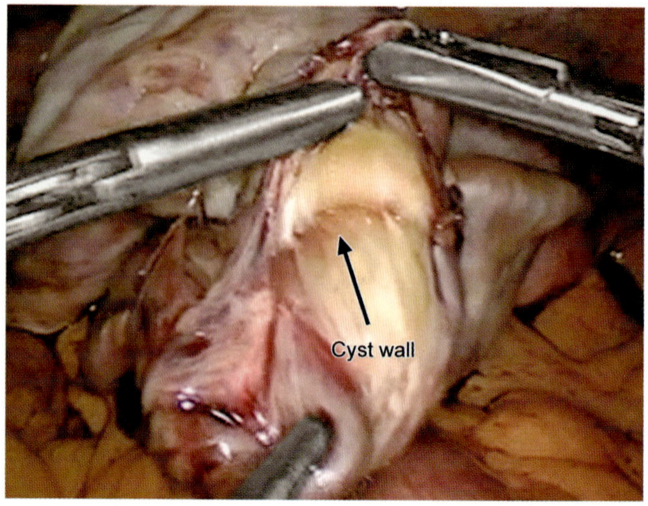


Fig. 45.28: CVT wall excised from normal ovary

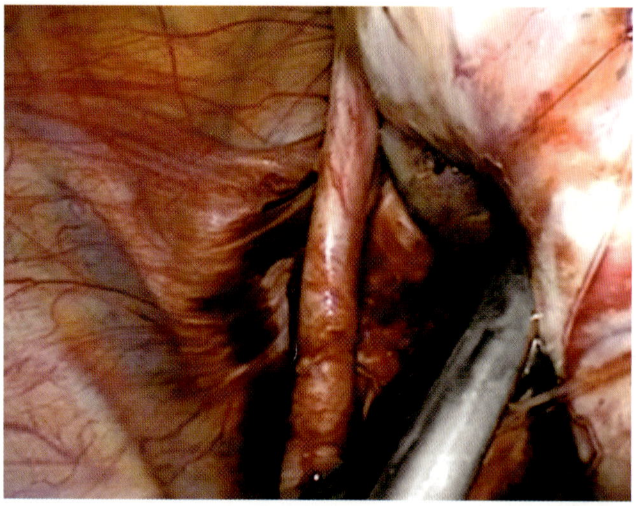

Fig. 45.29

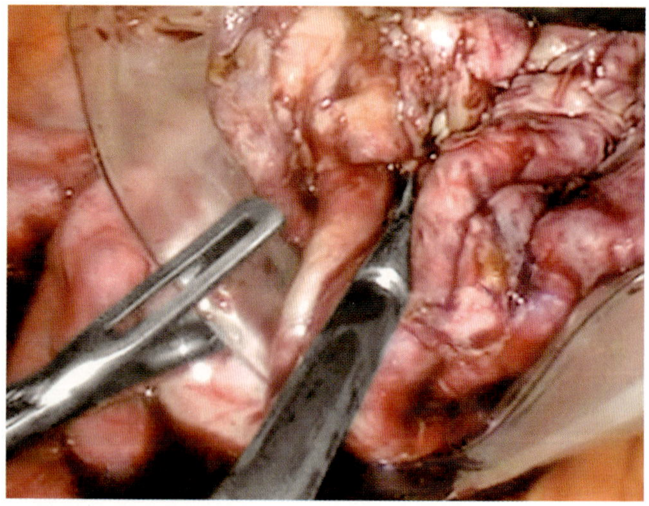

Fig. 45.30: CVT wall remove in endobage

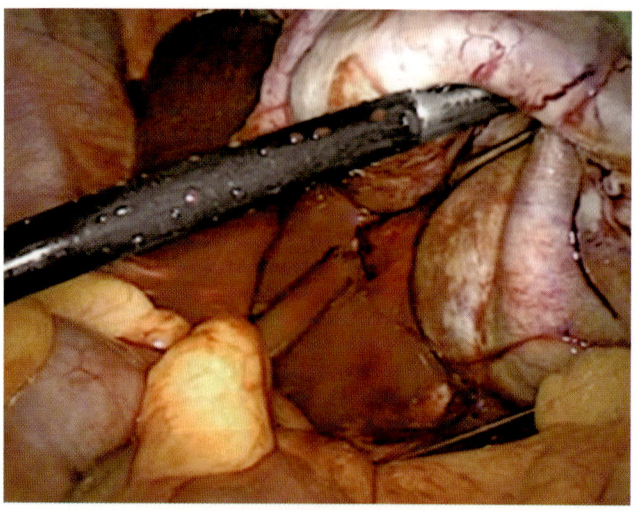

Fig. 45.31: 'Chocolate' Fluid drained

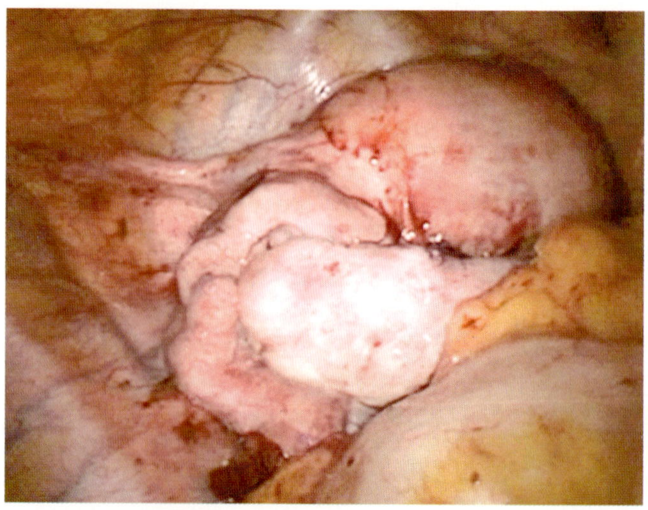

Fig. 45.32: End result: Clean cavity

## Laparoscopic Excision of a Large Ovarian Cyst in a 17-year-old Girl

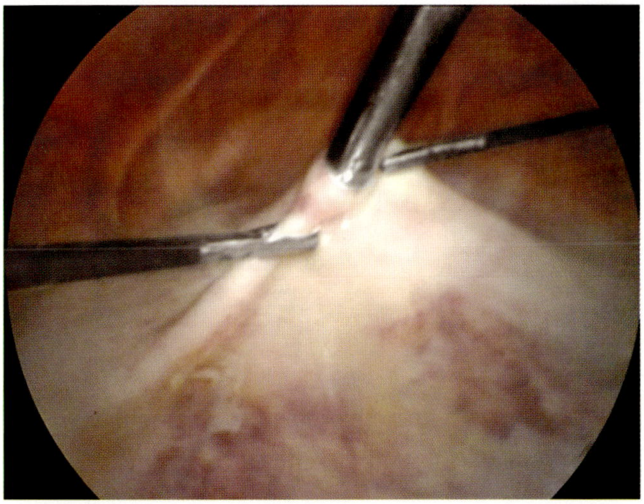

**Fig. 45.33:** Large ovarian cyst occupying whole pelvic cavity; fluid drained

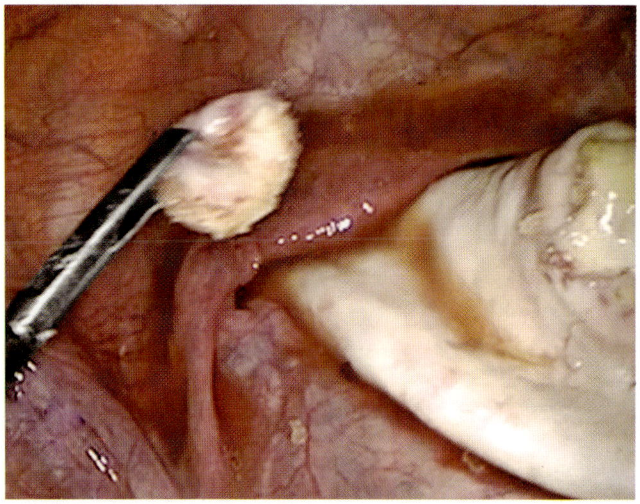

**Fig. 45.34:** Piece of cyst wall sent for frozen section: Benign nature

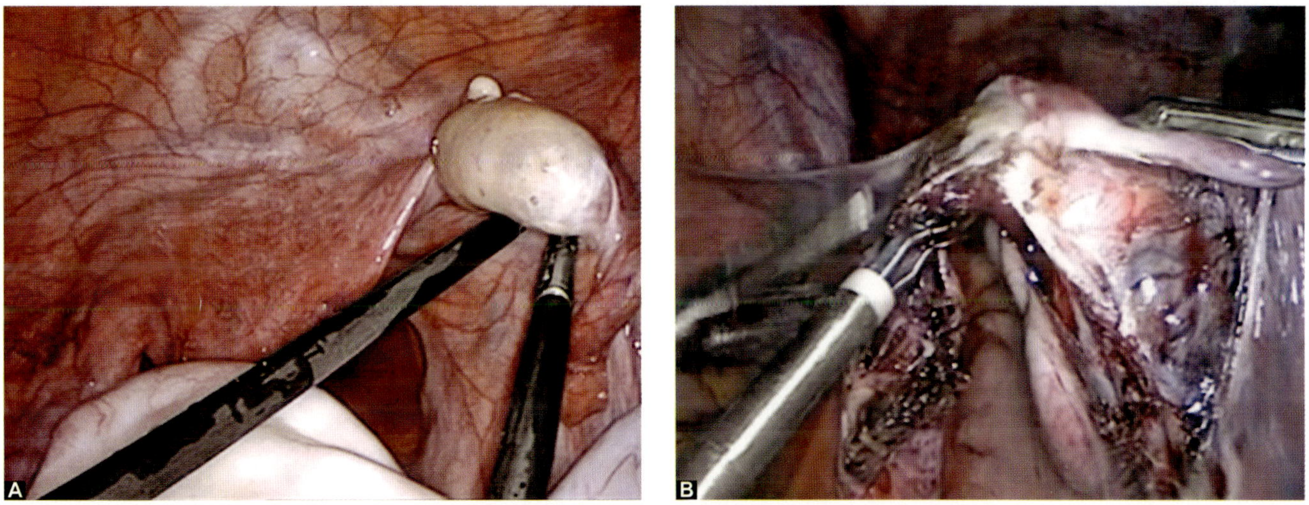

**Figs 45.35A and B:** Contralateral ovary normal

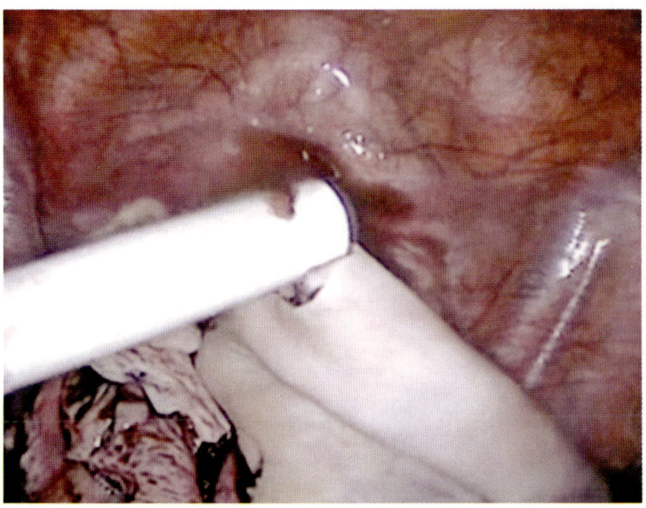

**Fig. 45.36:** Morcellation of cyst wall

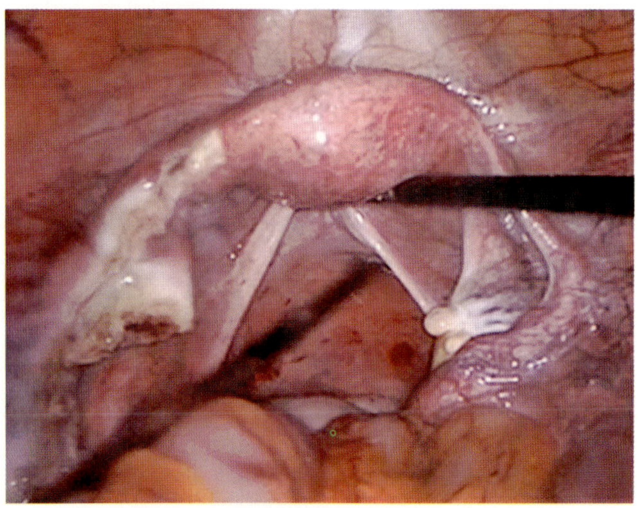

**Fig. 45.37:** End result

# Laparoscopic Excision of an Ovarian Fibroma in a 16-year-old Girl

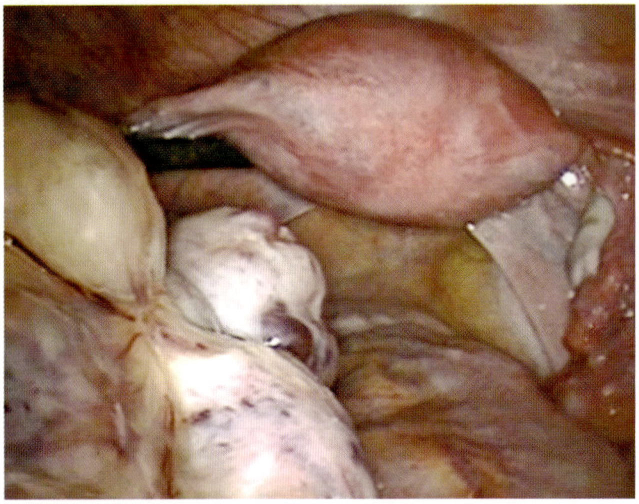

**Fig. 45.38:** Examination of pelvic cavity

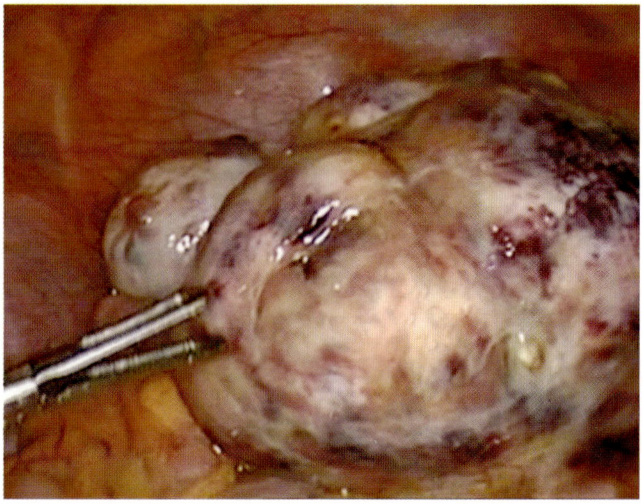

**Fig. 45.39:** Large ovarian fibroma of left ovary

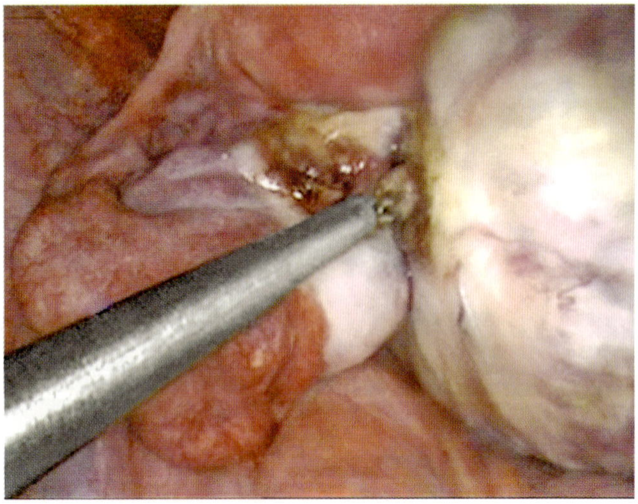

**Fig. 45.40:** Excision of mass from ovary taking care not be cauterize the ovarian blood supply

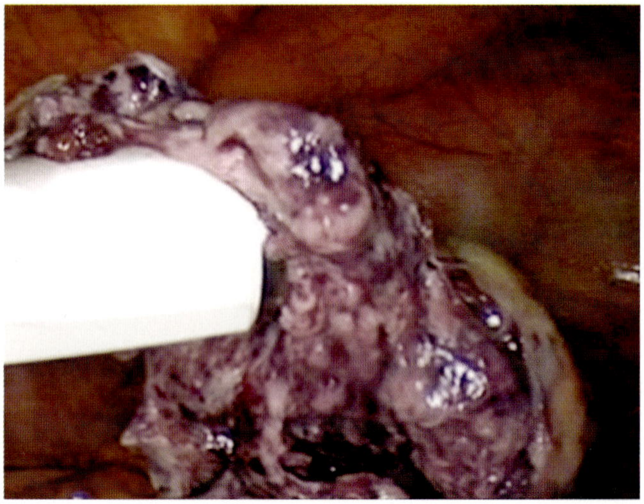

**Fig. 45.41:** Morcellation in progress

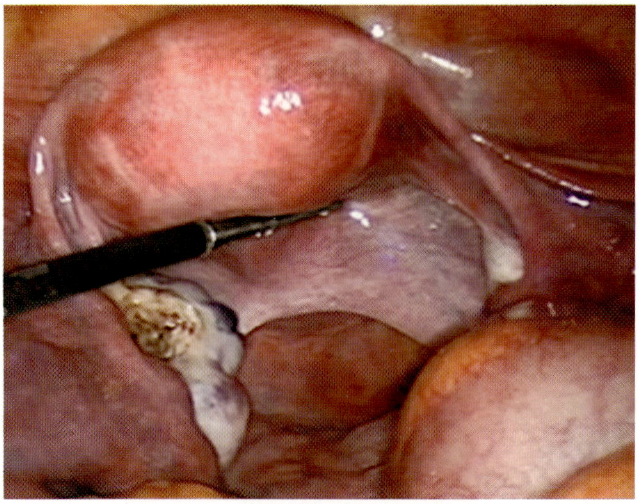

**Fig. 45.42:** End result: Clean cavity

## Laparoscopic Excision of a Retention Cyst of the Ovary in a 15-year-old Girl

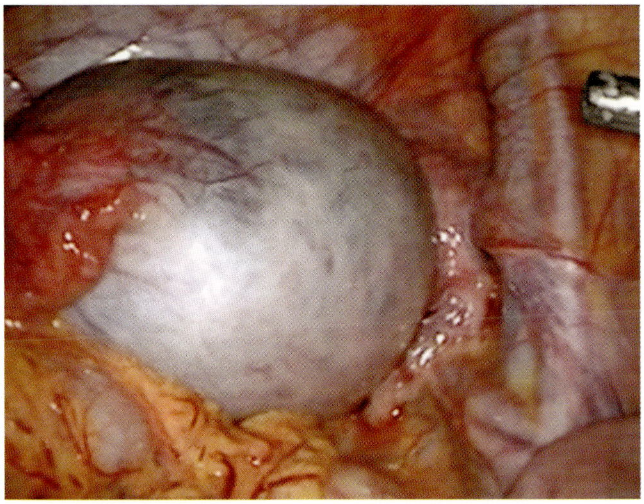

**Fig. 45.42:** Large retention cyst of the left ovary

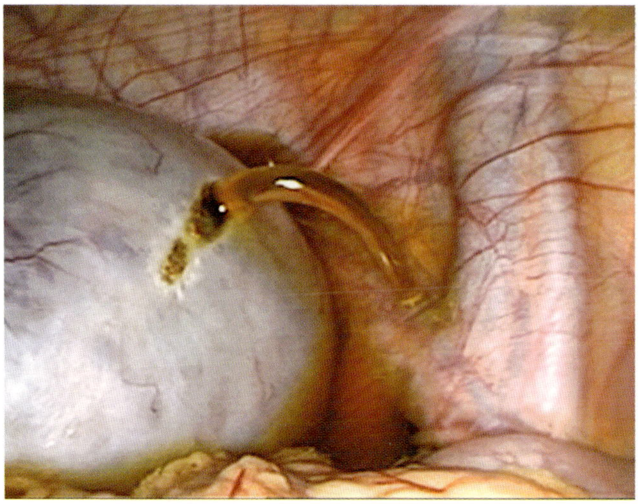

**Fig. 45.44:** Cyst punctured and follicular fluid drained

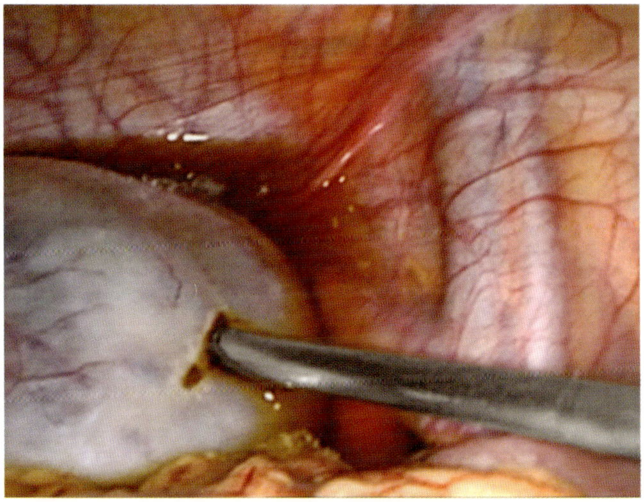

**Fig. 45.45:** Cyst drained with suction

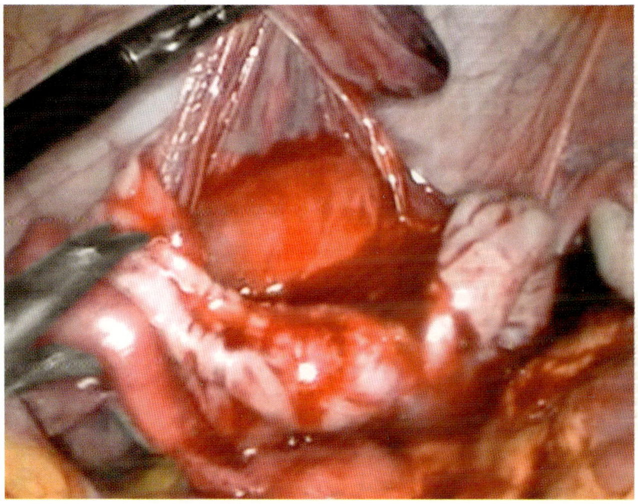

**Fig. 45.46:** Excision of cyst wall

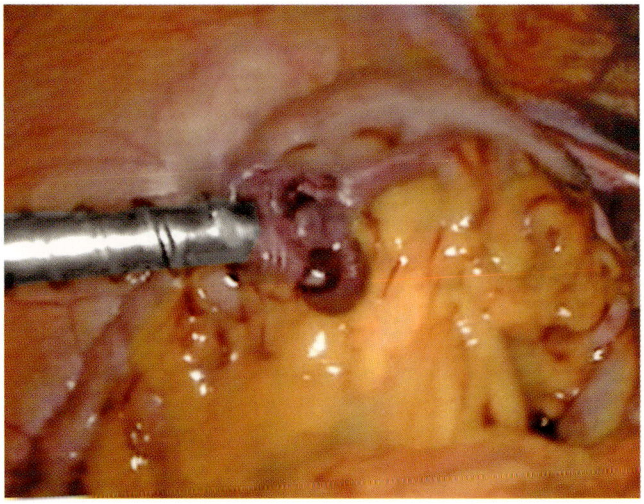

**Fig. 45.47:** Specimen removed through 5 mm port

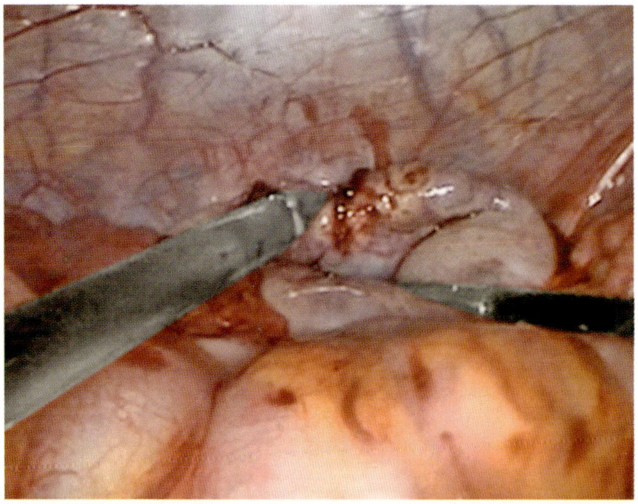

**Fig. 45.48:** Compression of the normal tissue to achieve hemostasis

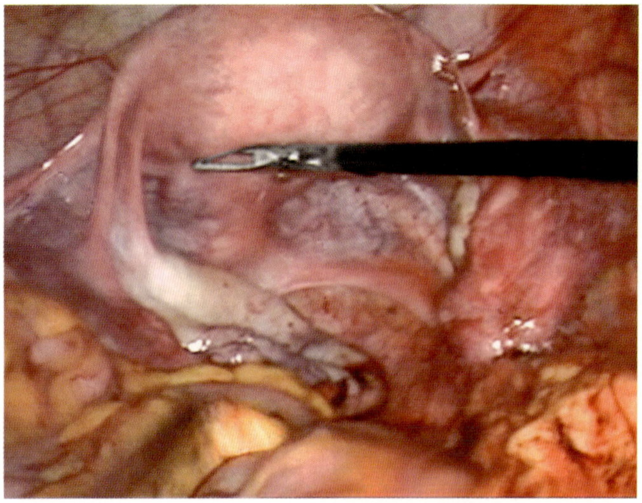

Fig. 45.49: End Result: Clean cavity

## Laparoscopic Excision of a Benign Ovarian Cyst with Papillary Projections in a 12-year-old Girl

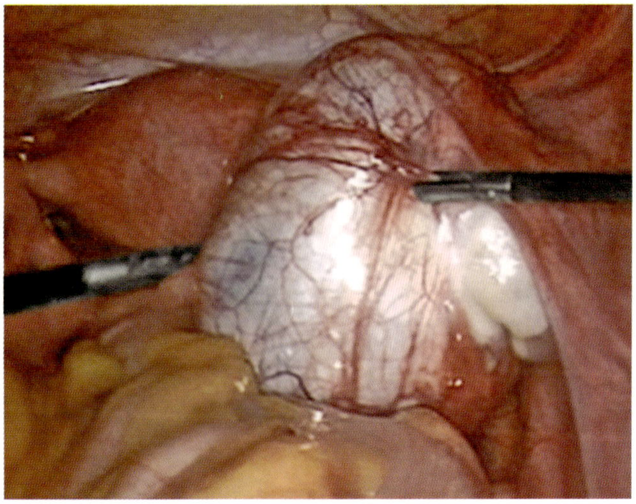

Fig. 45.50: Large cyst of the right ovary

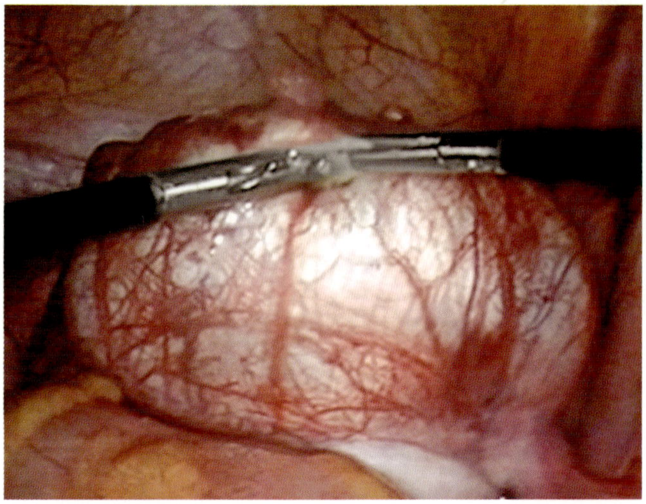

Fig. 45.51: Incision made over cyst and fluid drained out

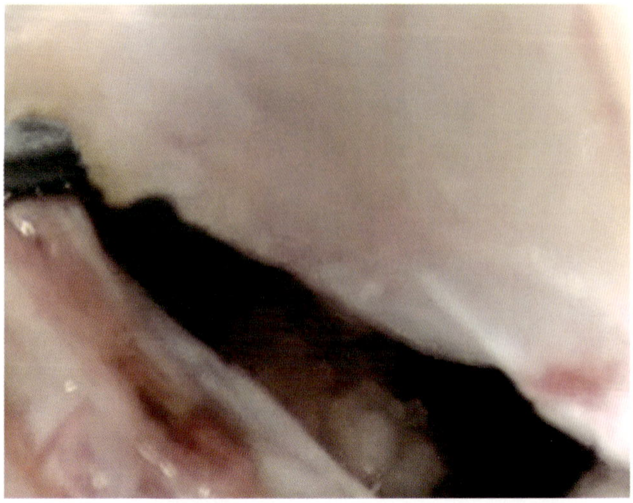

Fig. 45.52: Cystoscopy showed a papillary growth in the cyst

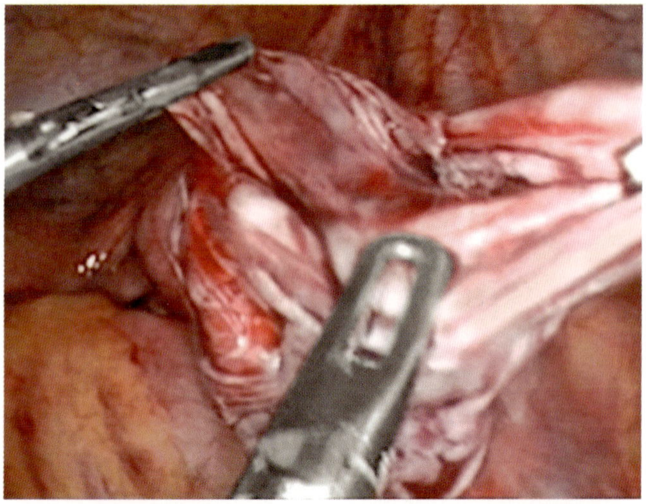

Fig. 45.53: Cyst wall excised. Frozen section sent: Benign pathology

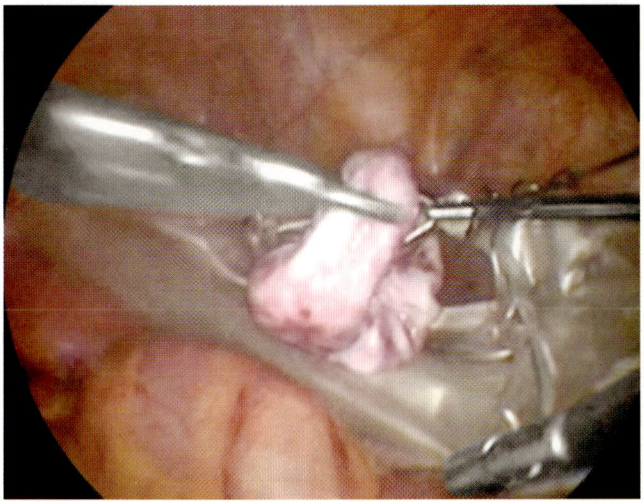

**Fig. 45.54:** Cyst wall removed in Endobag

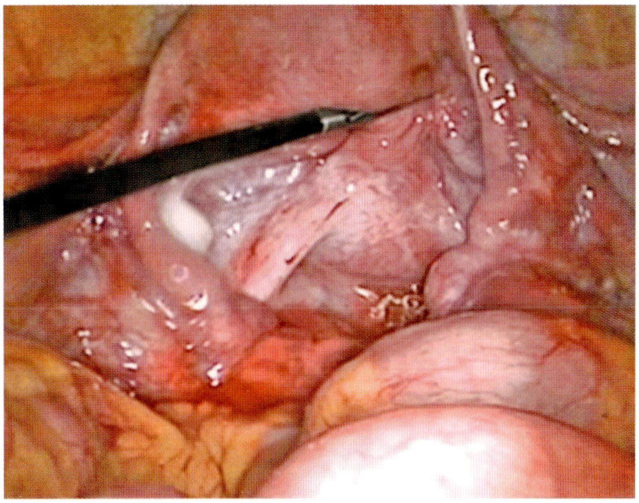

**Fig. 45.55:** End result: Clean Cavity

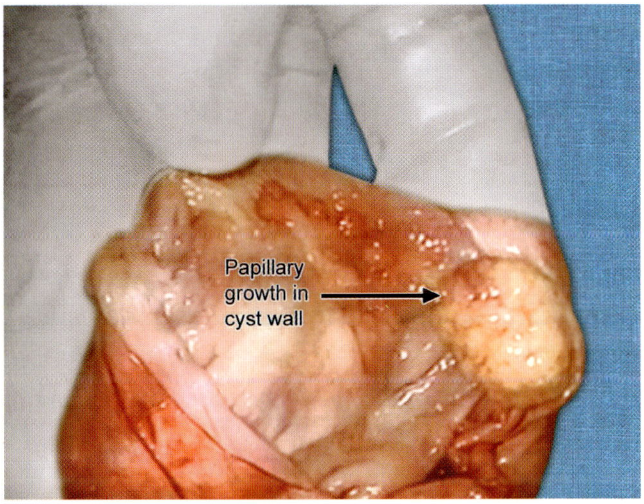


**Fig. 45.56:** Specimen seen after retrieval

Chapter

46

# Hysteroscopic Resection of a Large Type 0 Submucous Myoma

*Sunita R Tandulwadkar, Nirzari Mangeshikar*

A 25-year-old unmarried girl from Iraq came with sonography report of a large 8 × 8 cm type 0 submucous myoma.

When large type 0 submucous myoma is there, one can perform hysteroscopy in multiple sitting or one can go ahead and perform it by laparoscopy.

Considering her marital status, decision of performing hysteroscopy was taken. Though preoperative consent of multiple sittings should be taken, because of availability of bipolar energy source (and hence normal saline as a distention media) one can still try and perform in one sitting.

Pre-operative GnRH therapy may help.

Avoiding laparoscopy helps in decreasing the morbidity during her future pregnancies as large incision over the uterus entering the cavity is needed to remove such myoma.

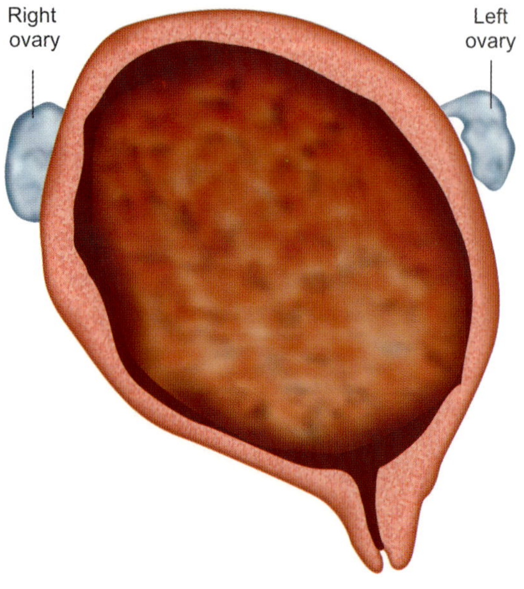


**Fig. 46.1:** Preoperative sonographic image of the myoma: Type 0 myoma

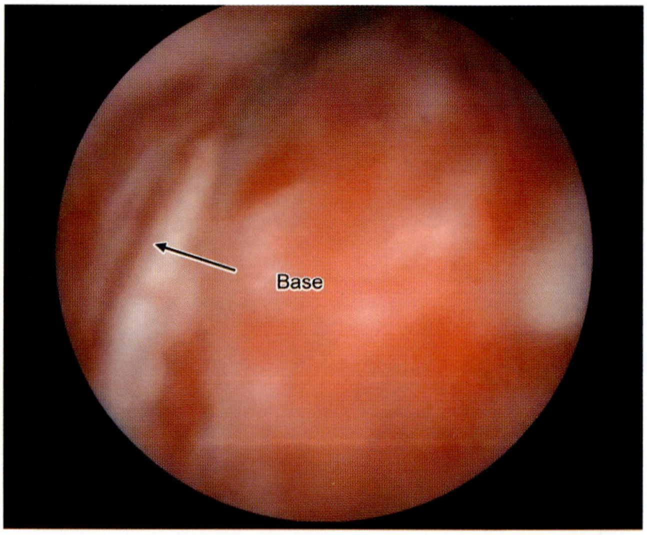


**Fig. 46.2:** Large type 0 submucous myoma with base on the right lateral wall

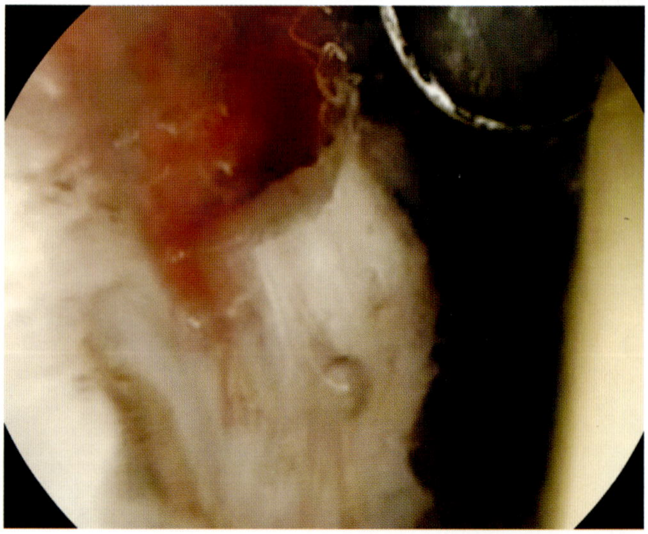

**Fig. 46.3:** Resection of the myoma done using bipolar resectoscope

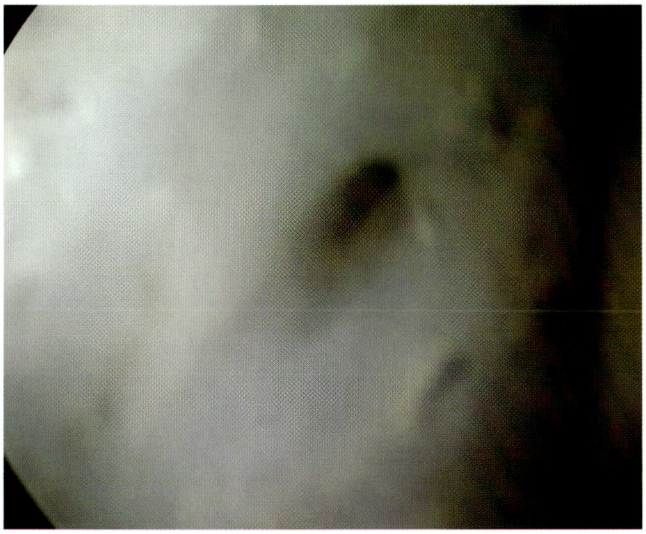

**Fig. 46.4:** Open vessel channels may be encountered

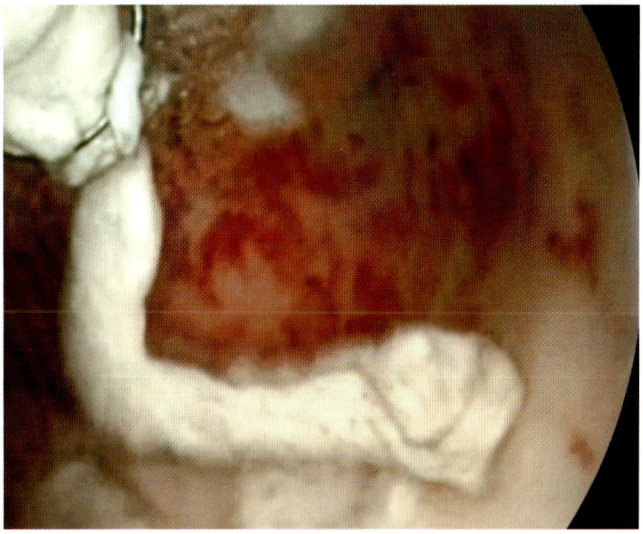

**Fig. 46.5:** End result: Entire myoma removed in one sitting

## TIPS

- In case of large type 0 myomas, one can perform a mini-hysteroscopy initially to discern the extent and identify the base of the myoma.
- Due to large size, there will be overcrowding of the resected pieces; this can be overcome by continuing the resection without wasting time in removal of those pieces. With the flow of fluid, pieces will automatically move laterally maintaining good surgical speed and avoiding blood in the cavity.
- One may encounter large open vessel channels, owing to increased vascularity of the myoma. Again speedy surgery will reduce the risk of complications related to irrigation fluid entering vascular channels, as will as potential hemorrhage.
- One can think of giving preoperative GnRH analogues, which can shrink the myoma and make it less vascular. This may also allow one to complete the surgery in one go.

Chapter

# 47

# Anti-NMDA Receptor Antibody Encephalitis—A Rare Condition Associated with Ovarian Teratoma

*Sunita R Tandulwadkar, Devika Chopra*

## INTRODUCTION

A 19-year-old unmarried female came with complaints of hyperthermia (100°F), severe headache, anxiety, and agitation, loss of consciousness, seizures, hypoventilation and prominent autonomic instability. The patient was intubated, catheterized, sedated and admitted in intensive care. A spinal tap was performed for examination of cerebrospinal fluid (CSF), as meningitis/ encephalitis was suspected. Apart from routine investigations, studies for autoimmune and infectious etiology, electroencephalogram (EEG), ultrasound and Computerized tomography (CT) scan were ordered. The initial differential diagnoses varied between Whipples' disease to viral meningitis.

CSF examination revealed mild pleocytosis, normal glucose values (72 mg/dL) and a raised protein concentration (55 mg/dL). No organisms were found on gram stain or negative staining. The CT scan revealed a well-defined, right adnexal lesion (0.9 × 1.4 cm) with fat and calcification. The right ovary was not separately seen, making the diagnosis most likely to be an ovarian teratoma. The uterus, left ovary and remaining pelvic organs were normal.

The medical management included administration of intravenous antibiotics (Imipenem, 500 mg IV 6 hourly), intravenous anti-epileptics (phenytoin sodium, loading dose: 15 mg/kg = 750 mg, maintenance dose: 6 mg/kg = 300 mg twice daily), immunoglobulins (IVIG 2 gm/kg = 100 g IV) and steroids (cortisone 100 mg intramuscular daily). The patient was posted for laparoscopic salpingo-oophorectomy for removal of the ovarian teratoma.

## INVESTIGATIONS

Routine laboratory tests, toxicology screening, studies for autoimmune and infectious etiologies, lumbar puncture, electroencephalogram, whole-body CT scan and abdominal ultrasound were performed.

## DIAGNOSIS

Paraneoplastic encephalitis associated with immature teratoma of the ovary and N-methyl- D-aspartate receptor (NMDAR) antibodies.

### Laparoscopic Right Salpingo-oophorectomy

After obtaining anesthesia fitness and a valid informed consent from the family members, the patient was posted for a laparoscopic right salpingo-oophorectomy.

- The procedure was performed under general anesthesia.
- The patient was placed in modified lithotomy position and pneumoperitoneum was created using Veress needle.
- A primary 10 mm port (infraumbilical) was taken after adequate pneumoperitoneum. Three accessory 5 mm ports were made.
- Since the patient was unmarried, no vaginal manipulation was performed.
- The right ovary showed a 2 cm mass, which was excised along with the right Fallopian tube using Harmonic scalpel and bipolar cautery.
- An Endobag was inserted via the 10 mm port and the mass was placed inside.
- The mass was removed piecemeal while still in Endobag via the 10 mm port.
- The pieces were then sent for histopathology.
- Ports were closed using 3-0 monocryl subcuticular stitches.

## HISTOPATHOLOGY

The histopathology revealed a benign cystic teratoma.

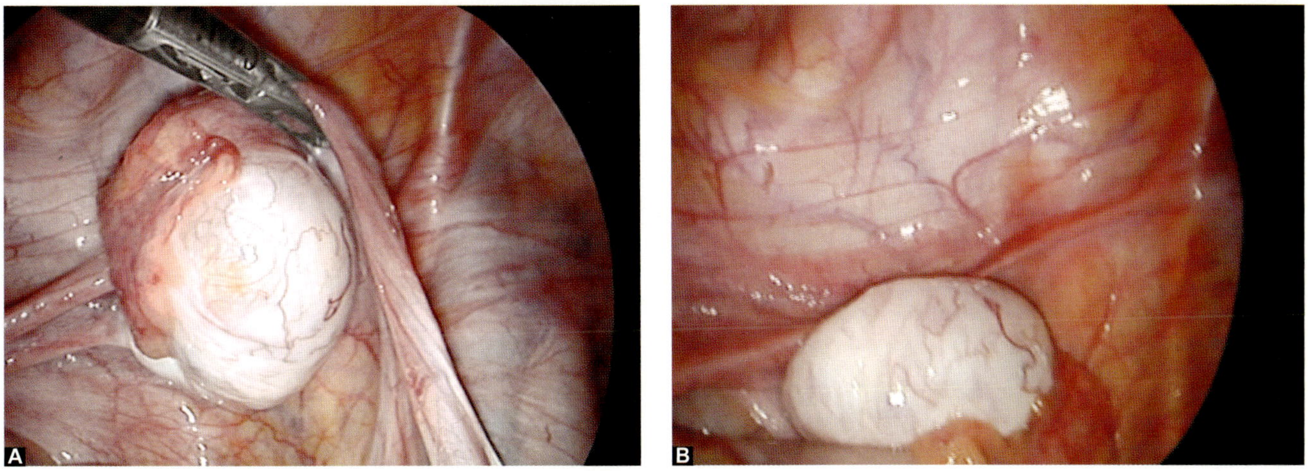

**Figs 47.1A and B:** Right ovary showing ovarian teratoma

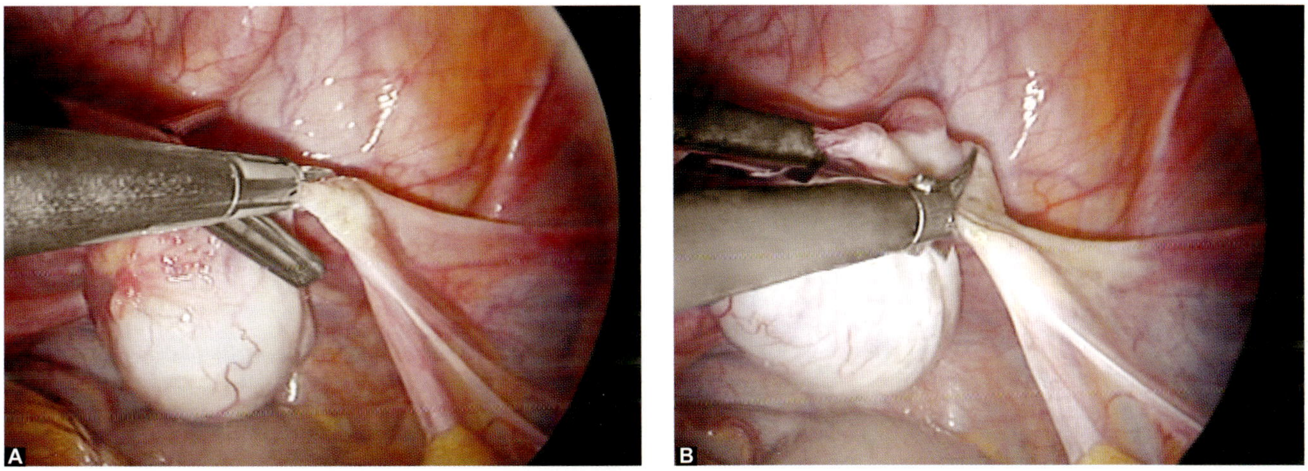

**Fig. 47.2A and B:** Right salpingo-oophorectomy with harmonic and bipolar

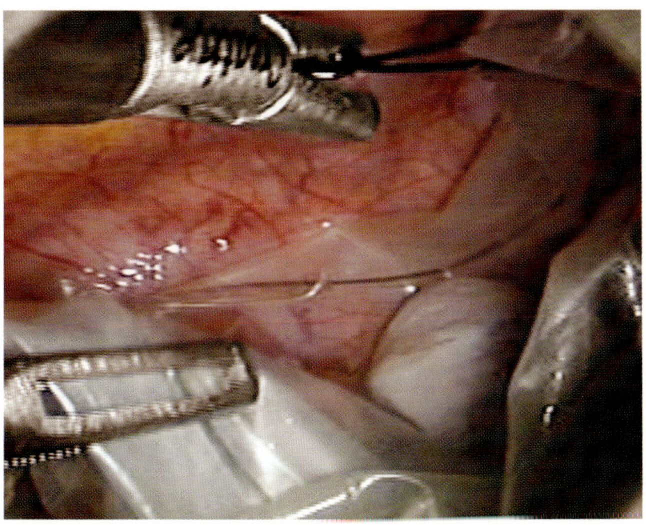

**Fig. 47.3:** Endobag was introduced via 10 mm port. Right ovarian teratoma was placed in the endobag and removed without spillage via the 10 mm port. The mass was sent for histological sections and examination

## PATIENT RECOVERY

The day following the right salpingo-oophorectomy, the patient regained consciousness and responded to verbal as well as tactile stimuli. The recovery was rapid and within a week, the patient was performing daily tasks. The patient was discharged 7 days post-op and was receiving weekly outpatient physiotherapy for treating remnant muscle rigidity.

NMDAR antibody encephalitis is a paraneoplastic syndrome, can be a potentially lethal disease, but prompt diagnosis and management may change the downhill prognosis of this condition. It should be suspected in young women with psychiatric symptoms, which proceed to autonomic instability, hypoventilation and dyskinesias. The CSF examination may be normal or show inflammatory changes. The associated tumor is a unilateral or bilateral ovarian teratoma (mature or immature). Preliminary data on this disease suggests that tumor resection, intensive care, immunotherapy along with physical therapy is the best treatment approach.

# Index

Page numbers followed by *t* refer to table and *f* refer to figure.


## A

Accessory fimbrial ostiae 202
Adenoma 45, 52*f*, 208, 208*f*
  coexisting pathologies 208
  diffuse adenomyosis 205, 213, 214
  endometrial polyps 44
  grade I 209
  grade II 209
  localized 213, 214
    adenomyoma 205
  on hysteroscopy 206
  on laparoscopy 206
  pitressin injected in 211*f*
  posterior wall 210*f*
  subendometrial 206
  transvaginal ultrasonography 205
Adenoma resection
  aim of 209
  technique of 209
    elliptical strip excision technique 209
    hood technique 209
    slice technique 209
Adnexectomy 165*f*, 166*f*
Allis forceps 135, 144, 224, 285
Ancillary trocar 121
Anti-NMDA receptor antibody encephalitis 314
  diagnosis 314
  histopathology 314
  investigations 314
Argon beam coagulator 15
Argon gases 15
Ashermann's syndrome 23
Assistant trocar 243
Atypical hyperplasia 51*f*

## B

Benign
  adnexal mass, excision of 163
  cystic teratomas 168
  endometrial polyp 40*f*
  lesions 44, 45
  ovarian mass 160
  polyps 40*f*
Bilatreral uterosacral
  cervicopexy (BUSCER) 265, 268, 269*f*
  colpopexy (BUSCOL) 265, 273
Bimanual palpation 66
Bipolar
  coagulation forceps 118
  diathermy 184, 185*f*
  forceps 120*t*, 135, 171, 176, 180, 193, 224
  modality 12*t*
  needles 68
Bladder peritoneum 98*f*, 101*f*
Bonney's and marshall-marchetti test 286
Boyle's apparatus 3, 5*f*
Braided suture 115
Broad ligament 78*f*, 89, 92*f*, 96*f*, 97*f*, 113, 144
Brosen's classification 184
Bupivacaine hydrochloride 155
Burch colposuspension 220, 223*f*
Buscol procedure 266

## C

Calibre veins 252
Capacitive coupling 14
Carcinoma 50
Carcinoma endometrium 41*f*
Cardinal ligaments (CL) 121, 132*f*, 260, 265, 266, 269
CCL vaginal extractor 143
Cervical canal
  extensive stenosis of 38*f*
  mild stenosis of 38*f*
  normal 38*f*
  palmate folds of 39*f*
Cervical ring 117*f*
  defect, posterior 265, 267*f*
Cervicovaginal junction 118
Chronic myeloid leukemia 85
Clermont-ferrand uterine manipulator 80, 127, 130
Clip applicator 8
C-loop technique 30, 31*f*
$CO_2$ insufflator 5
Cold knife
  enucleation 61*f*
  technique 57
Collin's knife 62, 68, 70
Colorectal integrity test 131, 134*f*
Colorectal nodule 132*f*
Colpotomy 130, 132*f*, 144
Corporal knot 102*f*
Curved scissors 120*t*
Cutting loop 99*f*
Cyst fluid 164*f*
Cystectomy 195*f*
Cystocele 261
Cystoscope 126

## D

Defecography 261
Defective uterosacral 265
Denonvilliers'fascia 138*f*
Diaphanoscopy 88
Didelphic uterus, with absent ovaries 291*f*
Direct coupling 14
Dysfunctional metrorrhagia 45

## E

Ectopic pregnancy
  ampullary 174*f*
  interstitial 174*f*
  isthmic 174*f*
  laparoscopic management of ovarian 175
Electric cutting loop 89
Electricity generator, monopolar 56
Electronic tissue morcellator 9
Electrosurgery forceps
  bipolar 12*f*
  monopolar 12*f*
Electrosurgery 11
  thermal effect 12
Electrosurgery machine 14*f*
Electrosurgical generator 6, 6*f*
  energy source 12
Electrosurgical injuries, prevention of 14
End tidal carbon dioxide 5
Endometrial
  adenocarcinoma 51*f*
  hyperplasia 41*f*, 45
  polyp 208
Endometrioma 196*f*
  laparoscopic management
    ablation of cyst wall 193
    cystectomy 194
    equipment 193
    port placement 193
    postoperative care 195
    preoperative
      evaluation 193
      preparation 193
  large laparoscopic excision of 197
  with extensive adhesions 196
Endometriosis 22, 208
  excision of 241
Endometriosis with frozen pelvis 126–134
  laprascopic hysterectomy
    equipment 126
    port placement 127*f*, 127
    postoperative management 133
    preoperative bowel preparation 126
    preoperative investigations 126
Endometritis 45, 48*f*
Endosalpingeal polyp 202, 203*f*
Endosalpinx 184, 200
  staining of 201*f*
Endoscopic camera 5
Endoscopic surgeries 20
  complications
    bowel injuries 21
    due to pneumoperitoneum 21
    during anesthesia 20
    during positioning of patient 20
    electrosurgical injuries 22
    morcellator related injuries 22
    postoperative 22
    preoperative 20
    trocar or veress needle injuries 21
    urinary tract injuries 21
  medicolegal issues 17
Endotip 7*f*
Enterocele 265, 268, 272

External os 43f
Extracorporeal knots 32, 108f
Extracorporeal sliding knots 32
  Ducanloop 32f
  Nicky's 32f
  Roeder 32f, 106f
  SMC knot 32f
  Tennessee slider 32f
  Weston 32f

## F

Falloposcopy 184
Falope ring excision 188f
Falope ring TL 184, 185f
Fiberoptic ureteric catheter 128f, 129f
Fibroid 208
  cervical 87
  development, role of genes in 85
  etiology of 84
  genotype 85
  large posterocervical 147
  phenotype 85
  recurrent 85
  small posterocervical 149
  viability 86
Figo staging 135
Figure of 8 suture 109f
Filshie's clip 184, 185f
Fimbriae 200f
Fimbrioplasty 180
Flimsy adhesions at cornu 39f
Flimsy adhesions in cavity 39f
Forceps 7
  bipolar 7, 9f
  claw 8f
  grasping 120t
  spoon 8f
  unipolar 9f
Fulcrum effect 184

## G

Genital tuberculosis 202, 203f
Genome wide scan, for fibroid genes 85
Gladiator rule 28, 30f
GnRH analogues 59, 133, 144, 195
Graspers 8f
Grounded electrosurgery systems 13
Gynecare TVT 285
Gyrus PK tissue management system 15

## H

Half-knot 27
Hamou micro hysteroflator 44
Hand instruments
  endoscopes 7
  trocars 7
  veress needle 6
Handlin's uterine manipulator 184, 184f
Harmonic scalpel 15, 15f, 80, 82f, 126, 130, 135, 194, 224
Hasson's technique of 25
Hasson's trocar 26f
Hematosalpinx 176, 178f
High transverse defect (HTD), of rectovaginal fascia 265
Hulkaclip 184
Hydromassage technique 60
Hydrosalpinx 176, 178f, 180f, 183, 293
Hyperplasia
  glandular cystic hyperplasia 48
  high-risk 48
    polypoid 50f
  low-risk 45, 50f
Hysterectomy 22
  intrafascial 130
  ovaries 86
  radical 241
  resection of fallopian tubes in 87
  supracervical 218, 219, 241
Hysterosalpingography 183
Hysterosalpinoscintigraphy 182f
Hysteroscopic cannulation technique 67
Hysteroscopic images, classification of 44
Hysteroscopic myomectomy 56
  preoperative
    evaluation 56
    preparation 56
    technique 56
Hysteroscopy
  diagnostic 37, 68
    trolley of 37f
  normal 45
  office
    preoperative
      evaluation 42
      preparation 42
    technique 42
    trolley of 42f
  pathologies diagnosed during 39
  preoperative prevention 23
  techniques 44

## I

Iliac artery ligation 134f
Iliococcygeus muscle 260
Infundibulo-pelvic ligament 76, 77f, 89, 113, 141f, 163f, 291
  short 292f
Insulation injury 14
Internal os 38f
Intracorporeal knots 28
Intracorporeal slip knot technique 212
Intraluminal adhesions 180
Intramyometrial cyst 206
Intrauterine adhesions 63f
  central 64
  flimsy 65
  hysteroscopic management of
    postoperative care 62
    preoperative evaluation 62
    preoperative preparation 62
    technique 62
Intrauterine manipulator 89, 90f, 98f
Isolated electrosurgical systems 14

## K

Kappa coefficient 53
Kevorkian curettes 44
Knot blocking sequence 28, 28f
KTP crystals 15

## L

Laparoscopes 8f
Laparoscopic cervical cerclage
  advantages 228
  disadvantages 228
  indications 228
  instruments 228
  preoperative evaluation 228
  preoperative preparation 228
  steps of 228
Laparoscopic excision
  of benign ovarian cyst 310
  of large ovarian cyst in 307
  of large uterine myoma 302
  of non-communicating functional rudimentary horn of uterus 303
  of ovarian fibroma 308
  of retention cyst of ovary 309
  of symptomatic adenomyoma 301
Laparoscopic hysterectomy 234
  equipment 75
  for previous cesarean sections
    adhesions and uterus ventrofixation 121
    bowel preparation 118
    equipment 118
    position of patient 118
    post hysterectomy inspection 125
    postoperative management 125
    preoperative evaluation 118
    preoperative preparation 118
    problems anticipated 125
    standard technique 118, 121f
  in endometriosis 126
  large uterus
    creating pneumoperitoneum 111
    optic used 112
    optical trocar placement 111
    secondary trocars 112
    uterine manipulator placement 111
  position of patient 75
  preoperative evaluation 75
  preoperative preparation 75
  steps of 76
  subtotal 84f, 84, 87
    ancillary trocars 88
    anticipated problems 91
    instruments 87
    optic trocar 88
    port placement 88
    postoperative management 91
    preoperative preparation 87
    prerequisites 87
    subtotal hysterectomy 89
  supracervical 120t
  technique 75
  ten steps 114–117
  total 84f, 84, 87
    anticipated problems 110
    basic set for 120t
    instruments 93
    postoperative inspection 104
    postoperative management 104
    preoperative preparation 91
    prerequisites 93
    steps for surgery 93
Twisted hydrosalpinx, laparoscopic management of 305
Laparoscopic myomectomy 146, 153
  closure of uterine flap 144
  definition 153
  extraction of myoma 144
  for intramural fibroids 153
    adhesion barriers 156
    advantages 153
    contraindications 153
    indications 153
    morcellation 155
    port placement 154
    postoperative management 156
    preoperative evaluation 154
    specific equipment 154
    surgical steps 154
    suturing 155
  for intramural myoma 158
  instruments 143
  modifications of techniques of 156
  preoperative evaluation 143
  preoperative preparations 143
  prerequisites 143
  procedure 143
  using single incisor 238
Laparoscopic needle holders 9f

Laparoscopic ovarian cystectomy 160
- preoperative preparation 135
- procedure 135
  - anterior u cut 135
  - dissection of pararectal space 138
  - dissection of rectovaginal space 137
  - lateralization of ureter 140
  - lymph node dissection 142, 142*f*
  - posterior u cut 135
- technique 135

Laparoscopic right salpingo-oophorectomy 314

Laparoscopic salpingectomy
- instruments 176
- preoperative evaluation 176
- preoperative preparation 176
- procedure 176
- using single incisor 238

Laparoscopic salpingoophorectomy, using single incisor 238

Laparoscopic sling surgery 224

Laparoscopic surgery
- single incision 231
  - equipment 231
  - port placement 232
  - postoperative management 238
  - preoperative evaluation 231
  - preoperative preparation 231
  - reconstruction of umbilicus 238
  - skin preparation 232
  - steps for 234
  - technique 231

Laparoscopic suturing 27
- extracorporeal 27
- intracorporeal 27

Laparoscopic tubotubal anastomosis
- absolute contraindications 183
- energy 183
- equipment 183
- indications 183
- intra-operative evaluation 184
- micro instrumentation 183
- needles 183
- preoperative evaluation 183
- selection of cases 184
- surgical technique 184
- sutures 183

Laparoscopy specimen retrieval bag 9

Laproscopic hysterectomy
- opening of vaginal vault 80
- post hysterectomy inspection 80
- postoperative management 80
- removal of large masses/leiomyoma 80

Lapsac bag 193

Large endometrioma, laparoscopic excision of 306

Laser 15
- advantages 15
- disadvantages 15
- precautions 15

Leg stirrups 6

Leiomyomatosis, hereditary 84

Levator ani muscle 220, 260

Ligasure system 16

Ligature sealer 115*f*

Lindere pair 116*f*

Llyod-davies position 126*f*

Lobular breast carcinoma, metastasis 50, 52*f*, 54*f*

Lone star aps retractor 253*f*

Long artery 224

## M

Mackenrodt's ligaments 139*f*, 140
- cauterization of 81*f*

Male
- factor infertility 183
- sterility 183

Malignant endometrial polyps 41*f*

Mangeshikar's
- manipulator 91, 111
- trocar 112*f*
- tube 104
- uterine manipulator 130

Manhes forceps 119

Maryland dissector 135

Maryland grasper 200*f*, 202

Maryland's forceps 180

Maxon sutures 272

Mayflower technique 134

Mccall procedure 272

Mersilene tape 228

Mesosalpinx 176, 188*f*

Metroplasty 295*f*

Metzenbaum scissors 285

Micro-salpingoscopy 200

Mini-hysteroscopy 313

Monopolar
- hook 120*t*, 147*f*, 149*f*
- modality 12*t*
- needles 8, 68
- spatula 8, 80
- diathermy 184

Motorized morcellator 143

Multiple fibroids 84, 144

Multiple polyps 40*f*

Myomas 44, 57, 144, 145*f*

Myomas resection, using bipolar resectoscope 312*f*

Myomas screw 8, 75, 135, 143, 147*f*, 231

Myomas
- above myoma 152*f*
- broad ligament myomectomy in 144
- fundal intramural globular 152*f*
- intramural 145, 146*f*
- morcellation of 158*f*
- multiple 152*f*
- recurrence rate of 156
- submucosal 45, 52*f*
- type 0 57, 57*f*, 59*f*, 313
  - hysteroscopic resection of 59
  - resection of 58
- type I 57, 57*f*
  - hysteroscopic resection of 60
- type II 57, 58*f*
  - hysteroscopic resection of 61
- vascular 152*f*

Myomatous uterus 103*f*

Myomectomy 23, 241
- incision for 145
- with vertical incision 151

## N

Nd:YAG laser 15

Needle holders 8, 120*t*

Non-traumatic graspers 135, 176, 180

## O

Obturator externus muscles 285

Obturator internus 285

Omega suture 116*f*, 117*f*

Omentum 293*f*

Oophorectomy 168

Open tubal re-canalization 192

Optical trocar 120*t*

Optimal manipulator 111

Ovarian cyst morcellation 165*f*

Ovarian cysthuge 166*f*
- removal of 167

Ovarian
- cystectomy 241
- dermoids 168*f*
- fibroma 297
- ligament 96*f*
- mass, morcellation of 298*f*
- teratoma 314

Ovary, carcinomas of 113

## P

Palmer point 24, 111, 112, 112*f*

Papillary renal cell carcinoma 84

Para-aortic lymph node dissection 241

Paracervical ring 116*f*

Parametrium 115*f*

Pathological tubes 187

PDS suture 102*f*

Pedunculated fibroid, myomectomy in 144

Pelvic floor, anatomy of 215

Pelvic mass 297*f*

Pelvic prolapse, management of 262

Pericervical ring, anterior 265

Perigee graft 262

Peritoneal suture 100*f*

Peritubal adhesions 183

Placental
- polyps 45
- remnants 45

Plasma kinetic cutting forceps 16

Pneumoperitoneum 24, 76, 88

Pneumoperitoneum pressure 21

Polycystic ovarian drilling 160

Pomeroy's method 184

Popliteal fossa, care of 20*f*

Pop-Q system 261

Port
- ancillary 24
- primary 24
- supraumbilical 24

Pouch of douglas 137

Presacral neurectomy 241

Prolene mesh 224

Prolene sutures 271, 271*f*

Proximal tubal block, hysteroscopic cannulation for 66

Pseudohyperplasia 45

Pubocervical fascia 80, 82*f*

Pubocervical ligament 76, 260

Puborectal ligaments 260

Pubourethral ligaments 260

Pulse oximeter monitoring 3

Pulse oxymeter 5

Purse string 89

Pyosalpinx 176

## R

Rectal probe 126, 193

Rectocele 261, 265

Renal cell carcinoma syndrome 84

Resectoscope loop 57

Retrograde dye pusher 202

Retrograde dye tester 199*f*

Retropubic colposuspension 241

Right corneal block 40*f*

Right uterine artery 79*f*

Robotic surgery
- advantages 247
- disadvantages of 247
- equipment used 243
- instruments for
  - hysterectomy 244
  - myomectomy 247
  - sacrocolpopexy 247
- preparation for surgery 241
- robotic components 241
- selection of cases 241
- technique 243

Robotic trocars 243

Rotocut morcellator 102*f*

Round ligaments 76, 77*f*, 92*f*, 96*f*, 127

Rumi/hulka's uterine manipulator 193
Ruptured ectopic 173
  instruments 172
  procedure 172

## S

Sacrocolpopexy 241
Sacro-uterine ligaments 104, 105*f*, 106*f*, 107*f*, 113
Salpingectomy 172, 173*f*, 177*f*, 192, 304*f*
  for ectopic 177*f*
  indications 172
  procedure 172
Salpingo-oophorectomy 129*f*
Salpingoscopy 180, 184, 187, 198, 200
  grade 1 184, 185*f*, 198
  grade 2 184, 186*f*, 200*f*, 200
  grade 3 184, 186*f*, 200*f*, 200
  grade 4 184, 186*f*, 201*f*, 202*f*
  grade 5 184, 186*f*, 201*f*, 202*f*
  instruments 198
  procedure of 198
Salpingostomy 171, 192
  incision 171
Sarcomatous fibroid 143
Scissors 7, 8*f*, 193
Septum
  complete resection of 69
  hysteroscopic resection of 68
  partial broad 70*f*
    base resection of 70
Sim's speculum 259
Simple ovarian cystectomy 162
Sims curettes 44
Slipknot 27
Sonography 176
Square knot 27
Sterilization, with sialistic bands 179*f*
Storz cutting loop 99*f*
Submucosal fibroid, classification of 56
Suction irrigation cannula 8, 9*f*, 171
Suction irrigation system 6, 176, 180, 224
Suction-irrigator probe 118
Suprapubic trocars 118
Surgical knot 27
Synechiae
  connective tissue 45
  endometrial 45, 48*f*
  multiple 53
  myofibrous 45, 48*f*

## T

Tenaculum 120*t*
  forceps 143
Ternamian endotip cannula 121
Tooth grasper 176
Transobturator
  mesh 262
  sling 262
  tape 280, 280*f*
Transvaginal tape obturator
  for stress urinary incontinence 276
    equipment 276
    preoperative evaluation 276
    preoperative preparation 276
    procedure 276
Trendelenburg position 88, 195
Trocars 7*f*
  primary 143
  secondary 143
T-suit 282, 284*f*
  handle 283*f*
  needles 283*f*, 284*f*
  tape 283*f*
Tubal block
  mid 183
  proximal 192*f*
Tubal
  diverticulum 202, 204*f*
  edema 202, 204*f*
  infertility 183
  orifice 38*f*
  reanastomosis 241
Tubectomy 183
Tuberculous salpingitis 177*f*
Tubotubal anastomosis
  ampullo-ampullary 187
  isthmo-ampullary 187
  isthmo-isthmic 187
  tubo-cornual 187
Tumor markers 162*f*
  alpha fetoprotein 160
  beta hCG 160
  Ca125 160
  CEA 160
TVT ABBREVO system 285, 285*f*
  instruments 285
  preoperative evaluation 286
  preoperative preparation 286
  procedure 286
TVT atraumatic winged guide 276
TVT helical passers 276
TVT obturator device 276
Twisted adnexa, chronic 293
Twisted adnexa, right 293*f*
Ultrasound dissector 15
  principle 15

## U

Unicornuate uterus 39*f*, 295, 295*f*
Unipolar diathermy needle 143
Unruptured ectopic
  instruments 171
  preoperative evaluation 171
  preoperative preparation 171
Ureteric stents 126
Ureteric tunnel dissection 131, 132*f*
Urethrocele 261
Urodynamic stress incontinence (USI) 261
USL maxonsuture 271
USL sutures 269*f*, 274
Uterine adhesions 208
Uterine artery 78, 89, 113
  ligation 79*f*
Uterine ligation 83*f*
Uterine malformations 45
Uterine malignancy 143
Uterine manipulator 81*f*, 118, 120*t*, 127, 154, 231
  clermont-ferrand 9*f*
  essential requirements 120*t*
  self-designed manipulator 9*f*
Uterine pedicles 98*f*
Uterine prolapse
  diagnosis 261
  laparoscopic prolapse repair 215
    instruments 215
    key steps of procedure 216
    port placements 216, 216*f*, 217*f*
    postoperative management 223
    preoperative evaluation 215
    preoperative preparation 215
  laparoscopic sacro-spinous fixation for 224
    instruments 224
    preoperative evaluation 224
    preoperative preparation 224
    procedure 224
  types of 260
Uterine septa 45
Uterine septum 39*f*
Uterocervical prolapse, 3rd degree 225*f*
Uterosacral ligament 80, 82*f*, 101*f*, 260, 266, 269
Uterosacral ligament suspension 241
Uterosacral suture, superficial 271
Uterosacral/cardinal ligament complex 265, 271
Uterosacral angle 80
Uterovaginal prolapse 260
Uterovesical fold 76, 78*f*, 137*f*
Uterus didelphys 45

## V

Vaginal cerclage 228
Vaginal hysterectomy
  nondescent
    anesthesia 258
    modifications 258
    position 258
    postoperative 259
    preoperative evaluation 258
    preoperative preparation 258
    technique 258
Vaginal probe 126, 193
Vaginal prolapse repair 260
Vaginal reconstruction surgery 252
Vaginal surgery 251
Vaginal topographic mapping 265
Vaginal wall repair
  apical 265
  posterior 265
Vaginoscopy 42
Vapor pulse coagulation (VPC) 15, 16
Vasopressin 128*f*, 143
Veress needle 7*f*, 121
Vesicouterine fold 118
Vesicouterine ligament 89
Vessel sealing device 78
Vessel sealing system 126
Vtmap 265

## W

Washing-suction device 120*t*
Weighted speculum 285
Xenograft 274

## X

Xenon bulbs 5

## X

Z technique 88
Zeppelin clamps 270, 271